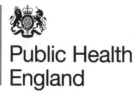

Public Health
England

McCance and Widdowson's

The Composition of Foods

Seventh summary edition

Compiled by

Institute of Food Research
and
Public Health England

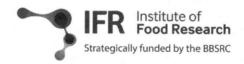

IFR Institute of
Food Research
Strategically funded by the BBSRC

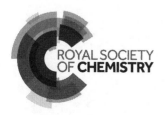

ROYAL SOCIETY
OF CHEMISTRY

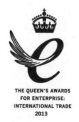

THE QUEEN'S AWARDS
FOR ENTERPRISE:
INTERNATIONAL TRADE
2013

CONTENTS

Dedicated to

Professor R A McCance (1898-1993)

And

Dr E M Widdowson (1906-2000)

FOREWORD TO THE 7th EDITION

I welcome the publication of the 7th summary edition of *The Composition of Foods*. This series has been the key reference tool for the nutritional composition of foods in the UK since the first edition was published in 1940. Data in these tables have a wide range of applications including food labelling, menu design and weight management tools and are invaluable to the health professionals, researchers and students that rely on their accuracy and extensive coverage.

I am proud that Public Health England is associated with the publication of this latest edition, working with a consortium led by the Institute of Food Research (IFR) and including the Royal Society of Chemistry and other interested bodies.

This new edition is dedicated, like its predecessor, to the memory of Professor McCance and Dr Widdowson whose pioneering work led to the establishment of the first UK food composition tables and laid the foundations for public health nutrition as a modern scientific discipline in this country. To summarise the history of these tables we can do no better than include their own foreword to the 5th edition of *The Composition of Foods* published in 1991. As they themselves say, a publication like this represents the work of many people, and I thank everyone involved in producing this edition for their efforts.

Professor Kevin Fenton
Director of Health and Wellbeing
Public Health England

FOREWORD TO THE 5TH EDITION

By R. A. McCance and E. M. Widdowson

In 1926 I (R. A. McC) was a medical student at King's College Hospital, London. Dr R. D. Lawrence, himself a diabetic, was in charge of the diabetic patients, and he was writing a book 'The Diabetic Life'. He wanted to include some values for the carbohydrate content of fruits and vegetables, which were then an important part of diabetic diets, but there were problems with this. First the values that were being used were derived from Atwater and Bryant's tables published in America in 1906, and these were nearly all obtained 'by difference', that is, water, fat, nitrogen and ash were determined, nitrogen was multiplied by 6.25 to obtain protein, the percentages of these were added together and the sum subtracted from 100 to give the percentage of carbohydrate. Carbohydrate calculated in this way contained not only sugar and starch which were important to the diabetic, but also the 'unavailable carbohydrate' or dietary fibre. Another problem in using the American tables was that most of the analyses had been made on raw materials, whereas people eat most of their vegetables cooked and their composition is altered by cooking. So a grant of £30 a year was obtained from the Medical Research Council for me to analyse raw and cooked fruits and vegetables for total 'available carbohydrate', that is sugars plus starch, which was the value needed for calculating diabetic diets. I analysed 109 different plant materials, each on six separate occasions, in the time I had to spare from my medical studies and the results were published in 1929 as a Medical Research Council Special Report No. 35 'The Carbohydrate Content of Foods' by R. A. McCance and R. D. Lawrence.

When Professor Cathcart, Professor of Physiology at Glasgow University, read the report he suggested that the work should be extended, and that protein and fat should be determined in meat and fish. The Medical Research Council agreed to provide a grant to cover the salaries of a chemist, H. L. Shipp and a technician, Alec Haynes, and a study of meat and fish began. Sixty-two varieties of fish were analysed, all except oysters cooked, 26 different cuts of meats, 9 varieties of poultry and game and 9 different kinds of 'offal', all cooked in standard ways. Besides total nitrogen, purine N, amino-N and extractive-N were determined and the analyses included fat, carbohydrate when present and minerals Na, K, Ca, Mg, Fe, P and Cl. We also investigated the losses of various constituents when meat and fish were cooked in various ways. Shrinkage caused most of the losses from meat, but not from fish. All the results were published in 1933 as a second Medical Research Council Special Report No. 187 'The Chemistry of Flesh Foods and their Losses on Cooking' by R A McCance and H. L. Shipp.

At the end of this study H. L. Shipp left and was replaced by L. R. B. Shackleton, and it was at this point that I (E. M. W.) joined the team. We four started again on fruits, vegetables and nuts. The analyses included 56 varieties of fruit, 9 of nuts, 28 of raw vegetables and 44 of vegetables after cooking. We analysed them for water, total nitrogen, glucose, fructose, sucrose and starch and for 'unavailable carbohydrate'. The same minerals were determined as in the meat and fish. Losses of sugars, nitrogen and minerals from vegetables while being boiled were also investigated. These results made a third Medical Research Council Special Report, No. 213, published in 1936 'The Nutritive Value of Fruits, Vegetables and Nuts' by R. A. McCance, E. M. Widdowson and L. R. B. Shackleton. The stock of all these reports was destroyed in a fire resulting from an air raid on London during World War II and they have been out of print ever since.

In 1938 we moved to Cambridge. L. R. B. Shackleton left but Alec Haynes came with us. We finished the analyses we had begun in London on cereals, dairy products, beverages and preserves and we put the results of all our analytical work together to make the first edition of 'The Chemical Composition of Foods' by R. A. McCance and E. M. Widdowson. This was published in 1940 as the fourth Medical Research Council Special Report No. 235. The working notebooks containing the details of all the analyses have been deposited with the Wellcome Institute for the History of Medicine.

Since one of the uses of the tables was likely to be the calculation of the composition of diets, and diets generally include cooked dishes we gave some information about their composition. Most of the recipes were taken from standard cookery books, and 90 are to be found in that first edition.

A second edition appeared in 1946, which included values for wartime foods, Household milk, dried eggs and National wheatmeal flour and bread made from it. Values for the composition of about 20 'economical' dishes were included.

In the 1950s we began to work on a third edition. By then many new foods had become available, and those introduced in wartime had disappeared from the market. Alec Haynes had left, and Dr. D. A. T. Southgate joined us. He, with the help of a technician, Janet Adams, was responsible for analysing more than 100 new foods for the same constituents as we had previously done.

By the 1950s methods for the determinations of vitamins had improved, and many foods had been analysed for one or more of them. We decided to depart from our original principle of including only the results of our own analyses in the tables, and to use values taken from the literature. Dr. W. I. M. Holman, who knew a great deal about the determination of vitamins in foods, undertook the task of reading every paper he could find on the vitamin content of foods published in the past 15 or 20 years. This involved abstracting well over 1000 papers. He selected those reporting results which he believed to be reliable, and then he left us and his abstracts to take up a post in South Africa. Miss I. M. Barrett joined us, and she constructed the tables of the vitamin content of foods from the information Dr. Holman had collected together.

Values for the amino-acid content of the main protein-containing foods, cereals, meat, fish, eggs, milk and its products, and of some nuts and vegetables were also included in the third edition. These were partly taken from the literature and partly from analyses made by Dr. B. P. Hughes who was working with us at the time. The third edition was published in 1960, with a change of title to 'The Composition of Foods'. As time had gone on some cookery experts had been rather critical of our original recipes, so the whole of the section on the composition of cooked dishes was revised with the help of members of the cookery department of King's College of Household and Social Science.

Up to the third edition we had the ultimate responsibility for the tables. I (R. A. McC) retired in 1966 and it became clear that a decision had to be made about the future of 'The Composition of Foods'. Tables such as these must be revised from time to time or they become obsolete and therefore useless. In the late sixties I (E. M. W) raised the matter at a meeting of the Interdepartmental Committee on Food Composition. It was unanimously agreed that the tables must not be allowed to die. The Interdepartmental Committee on Food Composition accepted responsibility for the revision of the tables, and appointed a Steering Panel under the chairmanship of Dr. D. A. T. Southgate to advise those responsible for the revision, leading to the fourth edition. In the event meats were completely reanalysed. The conformation of farm animals had altered and methods of butchering had changed since the 1930s when the original samples were collected. Cereals, milk and milk products were also extensively revised, but most other foods were not reanalysed, and about a third of the values in the fourth edition, published in 1978, were our original figures, obtained by what are regarded nowadays as very primitive methods 40 years before. Those methods were no less accurate than the modern automated ones, but they took a much longer time.

Since 1978 several supplements to the tables have been published covering the composition of different groups of foodstuffs as these have been revised, and tables showing the composition of foods used by immigrants in the United Kingdom were made available. Now a fifth summary edition of 'The Composition of Foods' has been prepared. This represents the work of many people including those who were responsible for making the analyses as we had done half a century ago. We are happy that we are still part of it.

July 1991

ACKNOWLEDGEMENTS

The compilers and editors would like to thank the numerous experts who have helped during the preparation of this book.

Some values in this book are based on the detailed supplements to previous editions of *The Composition of Foods*. The editors of this summary edition are therefore indebted to all the experts who have contributed towards the series of books. In particular, we would like to acknowledge the huge contribution and efforts made by the late Professor David Southgate in developing and updating the UK series of food tables from 1955 until his death in 2008.

Most of the new analyses were carried out by a consortium led by the Institute of Food Research and including British Nutrition Foundation (BNF), Laboratory of the Government Chemist (LGC), Eurofins Laboratories and supported by Susan Church, an independent nutritionist. The project formed part of Public Health England's (and previously the Department of Health's) rolling programme of nutrient analysis, which provides up-to-date and reliable information on the nutrient content of foods and supports the National Diet and Nutrition Survey (NDNS). The BNF team, led by Prof Judy Buttriss, with key contributions from Bridget Benelam and Dr Emma Williams, contributed significantly to stakeholder engagements, dissemination and survey designs. We also gratefully acknowledge the contributions of Margaret Walker and analysts from Eurofins Laboratories, and Selvarani Elahi, Madhumita Mittra, Dionisis Theodosis and analysts from LGC.

Many current and former professional and support staff at PHE, the Department of Health and the Food Standards Agency have been involved in the work leading to the production of this book, from design of the analytical projects on which most of the data are based, through data collation and checking, to the final compilation. In particular we would like to thank Natasha Powell, Mark Bush, Mary Day, Dr Rachel Allen, Alette Addison, David Townsend, and Victoria Targett. In addition, Jackie Hughes, Wendy Nimmo, Dawn Wright, Aliceon Blair and Yvonne Clements, of IFR, all assisted with various aspects of the projects associated with this publication.

We wish to especially acknowledge numerous manufacturers, retailers and other organisations for information on the range and composition of their products. In particular, we would like to thank Amanda Cryer and Dr Juliet Gray from the British Egg Industry Council, who provided additional funding and facilitated sampling for the 2011 survey of eggs, and Seafish UK and the Shellfish Association of Great Britain, who advised on the 2010/11 survey of fish and fish products. The design of the 2011/12 survey of fruit and vegetables was aided by individual trade associations who provided information on products consumed in the UK. The Federation of Bakers provided information on salt content in bread and morning goods.

An Expert User Group (EUG) provided valuable opinions and advice on survey design, sources of data and foods to be included. The EUG included representatives from key stakeholders and users including food manufacturers, retailers, academia and public health nutrition, and consisted of: Susan Church (chair), Prof Ashley Adamson (University of Newcastle), Marjorie Dixon (Great Ormond Street Hospital for Children), Wendy Duncan (Unilever), Helen Farnsworth (Bidvest 3663), Emily Fitt (formerly MRC Human Nutrition Research), Tanya Footman (Unilever), Bridie Holland (West Essex PCT), Dr Orla Kennedy (University of Reading), Dr Santosh Khokhar (University of Leeds), Dr Joanne Lunn (Waitrose), Charlotte Radcliffe (McDonalds), Prof Siân Robinson (University of Southampton), Jo Sweetman (formerly Premier Foods) and Dr Ailsa Welch (University of East Anglia). We are also grateful for the contributions from Joanne Holden (United States Department of Agriculture) and Jayne Ireland (Danish Food Information), who acted as international expert advisors to the project Steering Group.

We also acknowledge the contribution from members of the European Food Information Resource (EuroFIR), who have made their national data available for comparison and who have contributed to the development of standards for the production and management of food composition data. The Food Databanks National Capability at the IFR has received funding from the British Biotechnology and Biological Sciences Research Council, which has supported the production of this publication.

INTRODUCTION

1.1 Background

"A knowledge of the chemical composition of foods is the first essential in the dietary treatment of disease or in any quantitative study of human nutrition" (McCance & Widdowson, 1940)[1].

1.1.1 This seventh summary edition of the UK food composition tables extends and updates a series which began with the vision of R A McCance and E M Widdowson in the 1930s, under the auspices of the Medical Research Council. From 1978, the publications were the responsibility of the Ministry of Agriculture, Fisheries and Food (MAFF). Responsibility for maintenance of the tables and the associated programme of nutrient analysis transferred to the Food Standards Agency (FSA) in 2000. In 2010, management of the work moved to the Department of Health as part of the transfer of responsibility for nutrition policy in England. From April 2013, responsibility transferred to the Department of Health's executive agency, Public Health England (PHE). The data for this seventh summary edition were compiled, under contract, by a consortium led by the Institute of Food Research (IFR) and including the British Nutrition Foundation (BNF), Royal Society of Chemistry (RSC), Laboratory of the Government Chemist (LGC) and Eurofins Laboratories. The work is also supported by BBSRC's Food Databanks National Capability (FDNC), based at IFR.

1.1.2 This edition is intended to be a convenient single volume of the most recent nutrient values for a range of commonly consumed foods in the UK. Since the publication of the sixth edition in 2002, 12 analytical surveys have been undertaken. This edition includes the majority of the new data from these surveys. In addition to new analytical values, all foods have been reviewed to check that the values are representative of foods currently consumed. Many processed foods have been reformulated to reduce the content of salt, sugar and fat in line with government public health initiatives and, where necessary, values have been updated with industry data to reflect those changes in composition.

1.1.3 The most comprehensive version of the UK National Nutrient Databank is freely available as the Composition of Foods Integrated Dataset (CoFID), which comprises the most recent values for the energy and nutrient content for a more extensive number of foods than covered in this summary edition. CoFID brings together all the data from the Composition of Foods series of publications in a single electronic file with a single entry for each food. In addition to the nutrients presented in the main tables within this book, the CoFID includes information, where available, on fatty acid fractions, vitamin fractions, phytosterols and organic acids. Further, in CoFID, values have been recalculated in the format required for nutrition labelling. The Dataset, which was first published in 2008, has been updated as part of the process of producing this new summary book, and a new version will be released after publication of this edition.

1.2 Sources of data and methods of evaluation

1.2.1 It is essential that food composition data are regularly updated for a number of reasons. Since the sixth summary edition was published, many new fresh, ambient, frozen and processed foods have become familiar items in our shops, and values for these have been included where possible. In addition, the nutritional value of some raw foods, many processed foods and composite dishes have changed. This can happen when there are new varieties or new sources of supply for the raw materials. New farming practices can affect the nutritional value of both plant and animal products. New manufacturing practices, including changes in the type and amounts of ingredients and changes in fortification practice can affect the content of processed foods. Many foods have been reformulated in line with government public health initiatives, including reductions in the amount of fat, *trans* fatty acids, saturated fat, sugar and salt added. Methods of preparation and cooking in the home have also changed and can affect the nutrient content of foods consumed.

1.2.2 To ensure that the UK food composition data could continue to have as wide a coverage, and be as up to date as possible, MAFF decided in the early 1980s to set up a rolling programme of food analysis, the responsibility for which now lies with PHE. The analytical survey reports from 2002 onwards and some earlier reports are available in electronic form from http://www.ifr.ac.uk/fooddatabanks/. These reports comprise raw laboratory data and have not been evaluated to the same extent as data incorporated into the *Composition of Foods*.

1.2.3 Many of the values included in these Tables have been taken from the sixth summary edition and detailed supplements, themselves mainly derived from the government's series of analytical surveys. However, this edition includes new and previously unpublished analytical data for over 400 key foods, particularly cereals and cereal products, eggs, fish, vegetables, fruit, and a range of processed foods. Further details are given in the introduction to each food group. The main data source for each food is provided, where known, in the 'main data reference' column and refers to the *References* section (Section 4.6) which lists the reports from which new data were taken. In addition, foods for which new or updated data are included can be identified through the new food code in the *Food index* (Section 4.7). Where updated values have not been included, the previous values were reviewed and judged to be valid.

1.2.4 Where new analytical data were not available, and previous values were judged not to be valid, values have been taken from a number of sources including manufacturers' data, scientific literature, food composition datasets from other countries and calculations based on previous values and/or ingredients. In particular, the values for sodium, sugars, saturated and *trans* fat content of many processed foods have been updated, to reflect the reductions achieved by food manufacturers since the sixth summary edition was published in 2002 (FSA, 2002)[18]. Fortified products have also been reviewed against label data and values updated where necessary to reflect current practices for the range and amounts of nutrients added. All recipes have been recalculated, using the most recent available data for ingredients, and ingredients used have also been updated where appropriate.

1.2.5 Where the values in the Tables were derived by direct analysis of the foods, care was taken when designing sampling protocols to ensure that the foods analysed were representative of those consumed by the UK population. For most foods a number of samples were purchased at different shops, supermarkets or other retail outlets, and, where appropriate, foodservice outlets or catering suppliers. Samples analysed were composite samples, consisting of equal quantities of each sub-sample purchased. When the composite sample was made up from a number of different brands of food, the proportion of the individual brands purchased was related to their relative shares of the retail market. Full details of samples are available in the reports given as main data references. If the food required preparation prior to analysis, techniques such as washing, soaking, cooking, etc. were as similar as possible to normal domestic practices. Cooking methods were based on manufacturer's recommendations for pre-packaged foods and methods for non pre-packed foods were based on review of 'usual' consumer preparation. Details of preparation procedures are available in the reports given as main data references.

1.2.6 A summary of the analytical techniques used for this edition is given in Section 4.1.

1.2.7 Where data from literature sources were included, preference was given to reports where the food was similar to that in the UK, where the publication gave full details of the sample, method of preparation and analysis, and where the results were presented in a detailed and acceptable form. EuroFIR (European Food Information Resource) datasets and tools (www.eurofir.org) were used to help evaluate existing or new data values, and to calculate values for foods where suitable analytical or literature data were not available.

1.2.8 Where processed foods with brand names are included, they are restricted to leading brands with an established composition. No inference should be drawn from the inclusion of data for a particular brand.

1.2.9 The final selection of values published here is dependent on the judgement of the compilers and their interpretation of the available data. Due to the large natural variability of foods, it is unlikely that a particular item will have precisely the same composition as given in these tables. This is particularly true for unprocessed foods such as cereals, dairy products, eggs, meat, fish, fruit and vegetables.

1.2.10 Users are advised to consult other sources of data (e.g. product labels, manufacturers' data, published analytical reports) where appropriate, depending on their particular needs or interests, for the food item under consideration. It should be noted that manufacturers can and do change or reformulate their products and this will influence nutrient content. This is particularly relevant for foods where nutrients are added for fortification purposes, or for technological purposes, such as antioxidants or colouring agents. Information on processed foods, including fortification levels and reformulations, is often available from manufacturers' websites and from retailers.

1.3 Arrangement of the Tables

1.3.1 This book is composed of three parts, the Introduction, the Tables and a number of Additional Tables and Appendices.

1.3.2 Foods have been arranged in groups with common characteristics. Each food group is preceded by text covering points of specific relevance to the foods in that group. Generally the order within the groups is similar to that in previous editions and supplements.

The arrangement of the food groups in the Tables are as follows:

Cereals and cereal products
Milk and milk products
Eggs and egg dishes
Fats and oils
Meat and meat products
Fish and fish products
Vegetables
Herbs and spices
Fruits
Nuts and seeds
Sugars, preserves and snacks
Beverages
Alcoholic beverages
Soups, sauces and miscellaneous foods

1.3.3 The values are presented over four pages of information for each food with footnotes providing additional information where necessary.

The **first page** gives the food number, name and description along with the main data reference and the major constituents (water, nitrogen, protein, fat, carbohydrate and energy).

Food number
For ease of reference, each food has been assigned a consecutive publication number for the purposes of this edition only. In addition, each food has a unique food code number which is given in the index and allows cross-referencing to CoFID, the supplements or the fifth and sixth editions, where appropriate.

Food name
The food name has been chosen as that most recognisable and descriptive of the food referenced.

Description and main data sources
Information given under the description and main data sources describes the nature of the samples taken for analysis. Sources of values derived, either from the literature or by calculation, are also indicated under this heading.

Main data reference
The main data reference indicates the principal report or publication from which the majority of the data for the food code are taken. Values for individual nutrients within each code may be taken from different sources, calculated or estimated from other codes. For foods that do not have an analytical report or literature source that can be referred to as the main data reference, the food description should indicate how the data have been estimated (e.g. from manufacturer's data, calculated from related codes or calculated as a recipe). In some cases there is a main data reference referring to analytical data and the description indicates that industry data has also been used to update some nutrients, usually sodium, sugars, fats or added minerals and vitamins.

The **second page** gives starch, total and individual sugars (glucose, fructose, sucrose, maltose, lactose), dietary fibre (expressed as non-starch polysaccharide (NSP) and as total dietary fibre (AOAC)), fatty acid totals, and cholesterol.

The **third page** gives data for inorganic elements and the **fourth page** data for the vitamin composition of the foods.

1.3.4 **Additional tables** cover carotenoid fractions, vitamin E fractions and vitamin K.

1.3.5 Information contained in the **Appendices** includes a summary of analytical techniques, weight changes on the preparation of foods, cooked foods and dishes, the recipes, a table of alternative and taxonomic names for foods and references to the Tables and Introduction. This section provides useful supporting information for the data in the Tables.

In addition, the Appendices include edible conversion factors and information for the calculation of nutrient content for foods 'as purchased' or 'as served'. Many foods are purchased or served with inedible material and a factor is given which shows the proportion of the edible matter in the food. This refers to the edible material remaining after the inedible waste, e.g. the peel of a banana, bone attached to meat, has been trimmed away or discarded. For canned foods, such as vegetables, the factor refers to the edible contents after the liquid has been drained off.

1.3.6 A food index, with full coding list, is provided at the end of the appendices. This also includes cross-references from alternative food and taxonomic names to the food names used in the Tables.

1.4 **The definition and expression of nutrients**

1.4.1 *The expression of nutrient values*

For this summary edition, all foods are expressed per 100g edible portion, unless otherwise stated (alcoholic beverages expressed per 100ml). For foods that require an edible portion conversion factor, i.e. those that are generally purchased or served with waste, guidance and factors for calculating nutrient content 'as purchased' or 'as served' is given in Section 4.2.

Generally the values have been expressed to a constant number of decimal places for each nutrient with the number of significant digits in line with international recommendations (Greenfield & Southgate, 2003)[134]. Exceptions have been made where appropriate, either within groups of foods or for individual values. For example, the iron content of liquid milks has been expressed to 2 decimal places, because the amounts that can be consumed render this value significant.

1.4.2 *Water*

For most foods, water has been analysed using gravimetric methods. In some cases where protein, fat or carbohydrate have been updated based on industry data, the water value has been estimated by calculation (100 − (protein + fat + available carbohydrate + dietary fibre + ash)).

1.4.3 *Protein*

Protein has been calculated by multiplying the total nitrogen value by the factors shown in Table 1. For all foods not listed in Table 1, including foods containing more than one ingredient, a factor of 6.25 is used based on the assumption that proteins contain 16% nitrogen.

Table 1   *Factors for converting total grams of nitrogen in foods to protein*[a]

Cereals		Nuts	
Wheat		Peanuts, Brazil nuts	5.46
Wholemeal flour	5.83	Almonds	5.18
Flours, except wholemeal	5.70	All other nuts	5.30
Pasta	5.70		
Bran	6.31	Milk and milk products	6.38
Maize	6.25	Gelatin	5.55
Rice	5.95	All other foods	6.25
Barley, oats, rye	5.83		
Soya	5.71		

[a] Breese Jones (1941)[89]

The proportion of non-protein nitrogen is high in many foods, notably fish, fruits and vegetables. In most of these, however, this is amino acid in nature and therefore little error is involved in the use of a factor applied to the total nitrogen, although protein in the strictest sense is overestimated. For those foods which contain a measurable amount of non-protein nitrogen in the form of urea, purines and pyrimidines (e.g. mushrooms) the non-protein nitrogen has been subtracted before multiplication by the appropriate factor.

1.4.4 *Fat*

The fat in most foods is a mixture of triglycerides, phospholipids, sterols and related compounds. The values in the Tables refer to total fat and not just to triglycerides.

1.4.5 *Carbohydrates*

Total carbohydrate and its components, starch, total and individual sugars (glucose, fructose, sucrose, maltose, lactose) and oligosaccharides, but not fibre, are wherever possible expressed as their monosaccharide equivalent. The values for total carbohydrate in the Tables have generally been obtained from the sum of analysed values for these components of 'available carbohydrate', contrasting with figures for carbohydrate 'by difference', which are sometimes used in other food tables or on the labels of processed foods. Such figures are obtained by subtracting the measured weights of the other proximates from the total weight and many include the contribution from any dietary fibre present, as well as errors from the other analyses.

Available carbohydrate is the sum of total sugars (glucose, fructose, galactose, sucrose, maltose and lactose), oligosaccharides and complex carbohydrates (dextrins, starch and glycogen). It should be noted, however, that values for galactose are not reported in this summary edition.

Carbohydrates are classified based on chemistry but that does not allow a simple translation into nutritional effects since each class of carbohydrate has overlapping physiological properties and effects on health (Cummings & Stephen, 2007)[95].

Carbohydrate values expressed as monosaccharide equivalents can exceed 100g per 100g of food because on hydrolysis 100g of a disaccharide, such as sucrose, gives 105g monosaccharide (glucose and fructose). 100g of a polysaccharide such as starch gives 110g of the corresponding monosaccharide (glucose). Thus white sugar appears to contain 105g carbohydrate (expressed as monosaccharide) per 100g sugar. For conversion between carbohydrate weights and monosaccharide equivalents, the values shown in Table 2 should be used.

Any known or measured contribution from oligosaccharides and/or maltodextrins has been included in the total carbohydrate value but not in the columns for starch or total sugars. In most foods oligosaccharides are present in relatively low quantities. In vegetables and some processed foods where glucose syrups and maltodextrins are added, oligosaccharides will make a significant contribution to carbohydrate content. Because of this, the sum of starch and total sugars will be less than the total carbohydrate for these foods, and where this occurs, the values have been marked in the Tables with footnotes.

Oligosaccharides that occur naturally in foods include raffinose, stachyose, verbascose, inulin and fructo-oligosaccharides. These oligosaccharides are not α-1,4 or α-1,6 glucans and are not susceptible to digestion by pancreatic or brush border enzymes. Maltodextrins are mostly derived from starch and are widely used as sweeteners, fat substitutes and texture modifiers and are absorbed like other α-glucans (Cummings & Stephen, 2007)[95]. Where oligosaccharides are present in foods, they are not always measured separately and may be included in the starch, sugar or fibre fractions, depending on the nature of the oligosaccharide and on the analytical methods used.

Table 2 *Conversion of carbohydrate weights to monosaccharide equivalents*

Carbohydrate	Equivalents after hydrolysis g/100g	Conversion to monosaccharide equivalents
Monosaccharides e.g. glucose, fructose and galactose	100	no conversion necessary
Disaccharides e.g. sucrose, lactose and maltose	105	x 1.05
Oligosaccharides e.g.		
raffinose (trisaccharide)	107	x 1.07
stachyose (tetrasaccharide)	108	x 1.08
verbascose (pentasaccharide)	109	x 1.09
Polysaccharides e.g. starch	110	x 1.10

Non-milk extrinsic sugars (NMES) were defined by the Committee on Medical Aspects of Food Policy (COMA) as sugars contributing to the development of dental caries. The UK Dietary Reference Value for sugar intake (Department of Health, 1991)[98] is based on NMES. For the purpose of estimating intakes in national dietary surveys, NMES are taken as the sugars in fruit juices, honey and sugars (excluding lactose) added to foods as a sweetener, plus 50% of the naturally occurring sugar in canned, dried and stewed fruit. NMES values have not been included in the tables because it is not analytically possible to distinguish between intrinsic and extrinsic sugars. Instead values are estimated based on available information about the sources of sugars in processed foods, but there is no definitive method for this.

1.4.6 *Dietary fibre*

Different methods give different estimates of the total fibre content of food, and recent editions of the *Composition of Foods* have presented values for total non-starch polysaccharides (NSP) (Englyst *et al.*, 1994)[105] on which the UK Dietary Reference Value for fibre (Department of Health, 1991)[98] is based. For this edition, values are also given for total dietary fibre (AOAC, 2011)[78] either analysed or estimated from label information. AOAC determinations include resistant starch and lignin in the estimation of total fibre, rather than only the non-starch polysaccharides (Westenbrink *et al.*, 2013)[171]. For nutritional labelling purposes, it is recommended that fibre values obtained by AOAC methodology are used (Food Standards Agency, 2000)[126].

1.4.7 Alcohol

The values for alcohol in alcoholic beverages are given as g/100ml. Pure ethyl alcohol has a specific gravity of 0.79 and dividing the values by 0.79 converts them to alcohol by volume (i.e. ml/100ml). The specific gravities of the alcoholic beverages are given in the introduction to the Alcoholic Beverages section of the Tables so that calculations can be made if the beverages are measured by weight. The alcohol contents of a range of strengths 'by volume' are also given in that section.

1.4.8 Energy value - kcal and kJ

The metabolisable energy values of all foods are given in both kilocalories (kcal) and kilojoules (kJ). These energy values have been calculated from the amounts of protein, fat, carbohydrate and alcohol in the foods using the energy conversion factors shown in Table 3.

Table 3 *Metabolisable energy conversion factors used in these Tables[a,b]*

	kcal/g	kJ/g
Protein	4	17
Fat	9	37
Available carbohydrate expressed as monosaccharide	3.75	16
Alcohol	7	29

[a] Royal Society (1972)[162]
[b] See Section 1.9 for the conversion factors that should be used in food labelling

These factors permit the calculation of the metabolisable energy of a typical UK mixed diet with a level of accuracy which compares well with values obtained in human subjects using calorimetry (Southgate and Durnin, 1970)[167].

It has been suggested that the contribution of fibre (measured using the AOAC method) to energy should be taken into account using a factor of 2 kcal/g or 8 kJ/g (FAO, 2003)[122]. This has been incorporated into food labelling regulations (see Section 1.9), together with factors for organic acids and sugar alcohols. No contribution from fibre or sugar alcohols is included in the values for energy content presented in the main Tables. However, the CoFID update will also include energy values that have been recalculated to include the contribution from fibre.

The energy value of foods in kilojoules can also be calculated from the kilocalorie value using the conversion factor 4.184 kJ/kcal. Whilst it is more accurate to apply the kilojoule factors in Table 3 to protein, fat, carbohydrate and alcohol, a direct kcal/kJ conversion produces differences of little nutritional significance (1-2 per cent).

1.4.9 *Fatty acids*

For this edition, only total saturated (including branched chain), monounsaturated (*cis* + *trans*), and polyunsaturated (*cis* + *trans*) and total *trans* unsaturated fatty acids are given. In this edition *trans* fatty acids appear under total *trans* fats and are also included in total monounsaturated and total polyunsaturated fatty acids. For food labelling purposes *trans* fats are not included in the values for monounsaturated and polyunsaturated fats. More detailed information on individual fatty acids is available in the CoFID.

The fat in most foods contains non fatty acid material such as phospholipids and sterols. To allow the calculation of the total fatty acids in a given weight of food, the conversion factors shown in Table 4 were applied.

A worked example is shown below (TFA = total fatty acids)

	Total fat in Mackerel, grilled	= 22.4g/100g
	Conversion factor (for fatty fish)	= 0.900
	Total fatty acids = 22.4 x 0.900	= **20.2**g/100g

Saturates	at 25.3g/100g	TFA x 20.2 ÷ 100	= 5.1g/100g food
Monounsaturates	at 41.3g/100g	TFA x 20.2 ÷ 100	= 8.3g/100g food
Polyunsaturates	at 26.6g/100g	TFA x 20.2 ÷ 100	= 5.4g/100g food
Unidentified[a]	at 6.8g/100g	TFA x 20.2 ÷ 100	= 1.4g/100g food

[a] Unidentified fatty acids are fatty acid isomers that are not identified by gas chromatography with quantification by reference to standard calibration mixtures of fatty acids.

Table 4   *Conversion factors to give total fatty acids in fat*[a]

Wheat, barley and rye[b]		Beef lean[d]	0.916
whole grain	0.720	Beef fat[d]	0.953
flour	0.670	Lamb, take as beef	
bran	0.820	Pork lean[e]	0.910
		Pork fat[e]	0.953
Oats, whole[b]	0.940	Poultry	0.945
Rice, milled[b]	0.850	Heart[e]	0.789
Milk and milk products	0.945	Kidney[e]	0.747
Eggs[c]	0.830	Liver[e]	0.741
		Fish, fatty[f]	0.900
		white[f]	0.700
Fats and oils		Vegetables and fruit	0.800
all except coconut oil	0.956	Avocado pears	0.956
coconut oil	0.942	Nuts	0.956

[a] Paul & Southgate (1977)[156]   [b] Weihrauch *et al.* (1976)[170]   [c] Posati *et al.* (1975)[160]
[d] Anderson *et al.* (1975)[75]   [e] Anderson (1976)[76]   [f] Exler *et al.* (1975)[120]

1.4.10 *Cholesterol*

Cholesterol values are included for all foods in this publication and are expressed as mg/100g food. To convert to mmol cholesterol, divide the values by 386.6.

1.4.11 *Inorganic constituents*

Details of the inorganic constituents covered in the Tables are given in Table 5. Further information on variability can be found in Section 1.5 and on bioavailability in Section 1.6.

Table 5 *Inorganic constituents*

Atomic symbol	Name	Units	Atomic weight[a]
Na	Sodium[b]	mg/100g	23
K	Potassium	mg/100g	39
Ca	Calcium	mg/100g	40
Mg	Magnesium	mg/100g	24
P	Phosphorus[c]	mg/100g	31
Fe	Iron	mg/100g	56
Cu	Copper	mg/100g	64
Zn	Zinc	mg/100g	65
Cl	Chloride	mg/100g	35
Mn	Manganese	mg/100g	55
Se	Selenium	µg/100g	79
I	Iodine	µg/100g	127

[a] To convert the weight of a mineral to mmol or µmol divide by the atomic weight
[b] To convert mg Na to mg salt equivalent (NaCl) multiply by 2.5
[c] To convert mg P to mg PO_4 multiply by 3.06

1.4.12 *Vitamins*

Details of vitamins covered in the Tables are given in Table 6.

Vitamin A: retinol and carotene

The two main components of the vitamin are given separately in the Tables.

Retinol is found in many animal products, the main forms being all-*trans* retinol and 13-*cis* retinol. The latter has about 75% of the activity of the former (Sivell *et al.,* 1984)[165]. Eggs and fish roe also contain retinaldehyde which has 90% of the activity of all-*trans* retinol. Retinol is expressed in the Tables as the weight of all-*trans* retinol equivalent, i.e. the sum of all-*trans* retinol plus contributions from 13-*cis* retinol and retinaldehyde after correction to account for their relative activities.

All-*trans* retinol equiv = all-*trans* retinol + (0.75 x 13-*cis* retinol) + (0.90 x retinaldehyde)

Where the retinol profile was incomplete, because values for 13-*cis* retinol and/or retinaldehyde were not available, it has been assumed that only all-*trans* retinol is present, leading to a possible underestimate in some cases.

Table 6 *Vitamins*

Vitamin	Units	International Units (IU)[a]
Vitamin A		
Retinol	µg/100g	0.3µg
Carotene (β-carotene equivalents)	µg/100g	0.6µg
Vitamin D	µg/100g	0.025µg
Cholecalciferol, ergocalciferol		
Vitamin E	mg/100g	0.67mg
α-Tocopherol equivalents		
Vitamin K$_1$ (phylloquinone)	µg/100g	
(additional table only)		
Thiamin	mg/100g	
Riboflavin	mg/100g	
Niacin		
Total preformed niacin	mg/100g	
Tryptophan (mg) divided by 60	mg/100g	
Vitamin B$_6$	mg/100g	
Total of all forms (pyridoxine, pyridoxal, pyridoxamine, and relevant phosphorylated forms)		
Vitamin B$_{12}$	µg/100g	
Folate	µg/100g	
Total folate		
Pantothenate	mg/100g	
Biotin	µg/100g	
Vitamin C	mg/100g	
Total ascorbic and dehydroascorbic acids		

[a] Amount equivalent to one International Unit

Approximately 600 carotenoids are found in plant products and milks but few have vitamin A activity (Olson, 1989)[155]. Of these, the most important is β-carotene. The other main forms with vitamin A activity are α-carotene and α- and β-cryptoxanthins, which have approximately half the activity of β-carotene. Carotene is expressed in the Tables in the form of β-carotene equivalents, that is the sum of the β-carotene and half the amounts of α-carotene and α- and β-cryptoxanthins present.

β-carotene equivalents = β-carotene + (α-carotene x 0.5) + (α and β-cryptoxanthins x 0.5)

Where the carotenoid profile was incomplete, because only values for β-carotene were available, it has been assumed that only β-carotene is present. This may result in an underestimate of β-carotene equivalents, but as α-carotene and cryptoxanthin are usually present in low levels in foods without complete carotenoid profiles, it is likely that any error is small. Analysis of individual carotenoids is difficult because of several factors, including extraction from the food matrix and instability, and can lead to inconsistencies in data (Rodriguez-Amaya, 2001)[161].

Retinol equivalents

In the UK the requirement for vitamin A is expressed as retinol equivalents (Department of Health, 1991)[98]. This measure of the overall potency of vitamin A relates to the lower biological efficiency of carotenoids compared with retinol. The absorption and utilisation of carotenes vary, for example with the amount of fat in the diet and β-carotene concentration (Thurnham, 2007)[168], and there has been much debate about use of retinol equivalents (Scott & Rodriquez-Amaya, 2000)[163]. However, the generally accepted relationship is still that 6μg β-carotene or 12μg of all other active carotenoids are equivalent to 1μg retinol (Department of Health, 1991; Castenmiller & West, 1998)[98,92], so that:

$$\text{Vitamin A potency as } \mu\text{g retinol equivalents} = \mu\text{g retinol} + \frac{\mu\text{g } \beta\text{-carotene equivalents}}{6}$$

In 2001, the U.S. Institute of Medicine recommended a new unit, the retinol activity equivalent (RAE) where each μg RAE corresponds to 1 μg retinol, 12 μg of dietary β-carotene, or 24 μg of α-carotene and β-cryptoxanthin (Institute of Medicine, 2001)[136].

The relationship between the different units used to express vitamin A is shown in Table 7.

Vitamin D

Few foods contain vitamin D from intrinsic sources. All those which contain vitamin D naturally are products of animal origin and contain D_3 (cholecalciferol) derived, as in humans, from the action of sunlight on the animal's skin or from its own food. Vitamin D_2 (ergocalciferol) made commercially has the same potency as D_3 in man. Both vitamin D_2 and vitamin D_3 are used to fortify a number of foods.

Meat can contain vitamin D_3 (cholecalciferol) derived from the action of sunlight or, for pigs and poultry, from the feed. Vitamin D_3 in meat may also be present in the form of the more active 25-hydroxy vitamin D_3. For meat, meat products, and poultry, therefore, the total vitamin D activity has been taken as the sum of vitamin D_3 (cholecalciferol) and five times 25-hydroxy vitamin D_3 (25-hydroxy cholecalciferol), where data are available. There is, however, some debate about the factor that should be used for 25-hydroxy vitamin D_3 when estimating total vitamin D activity (Jakobsen, 2007)[140].

Table 7   *Relationship and conversion between the units used to express retinol and carotene*

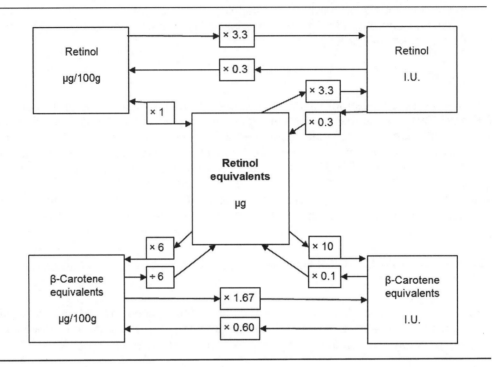

Vitamin E

The vitamin E in food is present as various tocopherols and tocotrienols, each having a different level of vitamin E activity. In most animal products the α-form is the only significant form present, but in plant products, especially seeds and their oils, γ-tocopherol and other forms are present in significant amounts. The values for vitamin E are expressed as α-tocopherol equivalents, using the factors shown in Table 8.

Table 8   *Conversion factors for vitamin E activity[a]*

α-tocopherol	x	1.00
β-tocopherol	x	0.40
γ-tocopherol	x	0.10
δ-tocopherol	x	0.01
α-tocotrienol	x	0.30
β-tocotrienol	x	0.05
γ-tocotrienol	x	0.01

[a] McLaughlin and Weihrauch (1979)[149]

Thiamin

The majority of values for thiamin are expressed as thiamin chloride hydrochloride using either the direct thiochrome method, HPLC with fluorimetric detection or microbiological assay (see Section 4.1).

Niacin

The values are the sum of nicotinic acid and nicotinamide, which are collectively known as niacin.

Tryptophan

Tryptophan is converted in the body to nicotinic acid with varying efficiency. On average, 60mg tryptophan is equivalent to 1mg niacin, so the tryptophan content of the protein in each food has been shown after division by 60. This may be added to the amount of niacin to give the niacin equivalent for the food.

Vitamin B$_6$

Vitamin B$_6$ occurs in foods as pyridoxine, pyridoxal, pyridoxamine and their relevant phosphorylated forms. A proportion of the vitamin B$_6$ present in plant-based foods is biologically unavailable because it is present as pyridoxine glycosides that are not hydrolysed by intestinal enzymes. These glycosides may therefore be absorbed, but are not used by the body and are excreted unchanged in the urine (Gregory *et al.*, 1991)[133]. However, the active form in human blood and tissues is pyridoxal phosphate. Pyridoxine is expressed in the Tables as pyridoxine hydrochloride by microbiological assay, or the sum of the individual forms by HPLC, and expressed as the sum of total pyridoxine hydrochloride, pyridoxal hydrochloride and pyridoxamine dihydrochloride (see Section 4.1). The HPLC values for vitamin B$_6$ do not always agree closely with total B$_6$ values obtained by microbiological assay. This can be due to the different extraction procedures employed for the methods, and the varying response of the organism to the different forms of the vitamin in the microbiological assay (Ollilainen *et al.*, 2001)[154]. Where an acid hydrolysis step is used with a microbiological assay, pyridoxine glycosides may be converted to pyridoxine (Gregory, 1988)[132].

Folate

For folates, the value refers to total folates measured by microbiological assay after deconjugation of the polyglutamyl forms. Folic acid (PteGlu) is the predominant form used for fortification purposes. Other major folates present in food are 5-methyltetrahydrofolates (5-CH$_3$H$_4$PteGlu$_n$; mainly plant- and dairy-based foods), 5- and 10-formyltetrahydrofolates (5- and 10-CHOH$_4$PteGlu$_n$; mainly animal-based foods) and tetrahydrofolates (H$_4$PteGlu$_n$). Some HPLC-derived values are available for 5-methyltetrahydrofolate (Laboratory of the Government Chemist, 1996)[52], but the values for other folates are much less reliable. Other sources of folate data, e.g. composition datasets from other countries, scientific publications or manufacturer's data may present data using different terminology or methods and may not be directly comparable (Bouckaert *et al.*, 2011)[87].

Pantothenate

The majority of values for total pantothenate are expressed as calcium D-pantothenate.

Vitamin C

Values include both ascorbic and dehydroascorbic acids, as both forms are biologically active. In fresh foods, the reduced form is the major one present but the amount of the dehydro-form increases during cooking and processing. Total ascorbate (ascorbic acid + dehydroascorbic acids) has been determined using either the fluorimetric procedure and/or HPLC with UV or fluorescence detection (see Section 4.1).

1.4.13 Missing, trace and zero values for nutrients

Missing values in the tables are denoted by 'N'. N is used when there is considered to be a significant amount of the nutrient in the food but there is no reliable information on the amount present. This may be because the food has not been analysed for the nutrient (such as micronutrients in processed foods that are relatively new on the market or a new unprocessed food that has not been analysed for the full range of nutrients) or because the levels vary so much that it is not possible to give a typical value. This may occur if some brands are fortified with the nutrient but others are not. The compilers of this edition have tried to minimise the use of N values as much as possible.

Zero values are used when there is no known source of the nutrient in the food (e.g. vitamin B_{12} in non-animal products) or as a result of analysis. Trace values are used when a small amount of the nutrient has been found on analysis (below the lowest reportable level) or when the food is thought to contain an insignificant amount of the nutrient.

1.5   The variability of nutrients in foods

1.5.1   Although values in these Tables have been derived from analyses of composite samples, representative of each food available, it is important to appreciate that the composition of any individual sample may differ considerably from this. There are two main reasons for the variability, apart from the apparent differences caused by analytical variations.

1.5.2   *Natural variation*

All natural products vary in composition. Two samples from the same animal or plant may well be different, but the composition of meat, milk and eggs are also affected by season, feeding regime and age of the animal. Different varieties of the same plant may differ in composition, and their nutritional value will also vary with the country of origin, growing conditions and subsequent storage (Greenfield & Southgate, 2003)[134]. In general, those nutrients that are closely associated with structure and metabolic function show rather less variation than those which accumulate in particular locations of the plant or animal, or those which are unstable. For instance, nitrogen and phosphorus tend to show less variation than vitamin A, iron or vitamin C.

A major influence on the nutrient concentration in foods is the water content, and this is particularly important in plant foods where water is the main constituent. As the duration and conditions of food storage affect the water content of foods, they also impact on the nutrient content per 100g. Many individual nutrients will also be affected by storage conditions with the greatest effect being on the more labile vitamins such as vitamin C, vitamin E and folate (Greenfield & Southgate, 2003)[134]. Thus, if the storage conditions of a food item differ from those for the samples analysed for the Tables, the nutrient values may differ from those given.

The level of fat in food can vary greatly and result in large variations in the nutrient content of each 100g of the food. It will also influence energy and the level of fat-soluble vitamins. An example of how fat and moisture content vary (in minced meat) is given in Table 9.

Table 9 *Fat and moisture content of minced meats*

	No. samples	Moisture % mean (range)	Fat % mean (range)
Beef mince, raw[a]	10	64.0 (57.3-70.0)	16.6 (7.8-26.5)
Beef mince, extra lean, raw[a]	10	69.6 (63.8-72.6)	8.3 (3.9-16.9)
Lamb mince, raw[b]	10	66.8 (58.1-71.6)	13.5 (8.1-22.8)
Pork, mince, raw[c]	10	70.6 (64.3-73.2)	9.3 (5.4-19.5)

[a] Laboratory of the Government Chemist (1992-1993)[36]
[b] Laboratory of the Government Chemist (1993-1994)[42]
[c] Laboratory of the Government Chemist (1992-1993)[37]

1.5.3 *Extrinsic differences*

Further differences in composition can be introduced by food manufacturers, caterers, and in the home. For example, manufacturers may change both their recipes and their fortification practices, and dishes prepared in the home or by caterers may vary widely in the amounts and types of ingredient used, and thus differ in nutritional value from those included here.

Examples of some external influences on nutrient contents are shown below:

Sodium	The level found in many foods will depend upon the amount of salt and other sodium-containing compounds used in cooking or added by manufacturers, and can therefore be very variable. The sodium content of processed foods has been revised extensively in this edition, using information from analysis, manufacturers and food labels, reflecting a general reformulation of products to lower salt content in line with government health recommendations. Vegetables analysed for the food tables were cooked in distilled water without salt. Recipes used to calculate values do not contain added salt (see Section 4.4). The Table values are adequate for planning low-sodium diets.
Potassium	The potassium content of boiled vegetables is dependent on the amount of water, length of cooking time and the state of preparation of the vegetable. The user should refer to the description and main data sources for the foods in the Tables to ensure sample foods are comparable.
Calcium	Most vegetables in the Tables were cooked in distilled water. Foods cooked in and prepared with tap water, which contains variable amounts of calcium, may not have the same levels as in these Tables. The concentration of calcium in baking powder is high and variations in the quantity used will affect the calcium content of some cereal products.
Iron	Food can become contaminated with iron from knives, pans, soil particles and processing machinery. This has the greatest effect on the iron content of ground foods such as spices.
Chloride	Chloride variation will be similar to that of sodium.
Iodine	Iodine levels in milk and dairy products are affected by the levels in animal feedstuffs, and to a lesser degree by the iodine levels in the solutions used for teat dips, sanitizers and the lactation promoter iodinated casein (Phillips et al., 1988; Bath et al., 2011)[158,79]. Average iodine levels in UK cows' milk have not changed substantially since the late 1990s but are higher than in the 1980s.
Selenium	The selenium content of soil has a large effect on the foods harvested from it. The levels of selenium in UK soils are low and analysed values reflect this. Data from literature sources have been taken from those countries with similar soil profiles to the UK.
β-Carotene	β-Carotene is sometimes used as a food colouring additive (E160a). In certain processed foods, such as orange squash, samples may contain added β-carotene.
Vitamin C	Vitamin C is added to a number of foods for fortification or antioxidant purposes (E300, L-ascorbic acid), and so may be present in unexpectedly high levels in some foods, including some meat products and soft drinks.

1.6 Bioavailability of nutrients

The term bioavailability (biological availability) is used to describe the proportion of a nutrient in food that is utilised for normal body function (Fairweather-Tait, 1998)[121]. There are many factors, both dietary and physiological, that influence nutrient bioavailability, and because these interactions are so variable, it is not possible to provide an accurate measure of bioavailability in these Tables.

Dietary-related factors include:

- The physical form of the nutrient within the food structure, and the ease with which the nutrient can be released from that structure.

- The chemical form of the nutrient in a food and its solubility in the lumen.

- The presence of enhancers of absorption (e.g. ascorbic acid for iron, some organic acids, sugars, amino acids, bulk lipid for fat-soluble vitamins and specific fatty acids).

- The presence of inhibitors (primarily of inorganic absorption, e.g. phosphates (especially phytate), polyphenols including tannins, oxalate and carbohydrate (especially dietary fibre)).

Physiological factors include the composition and volume of gastric and intestinal secretions, and a number of host-related variables, many of which are essential parts of the body's homeostatic regulatory mechanism (e.g. nutritional status, development state, mucosal cell regulation and gut microflora (Fairweather-Tait, 1998)[121].

Allowance has been made for reduced biological activities of different forms of three of the vitamins given in the Tables: 13-cis-retinol and retinaldehyde (vitamin A), carotenes other than β-carotene, and tocopherols and tocotrienols other than α-tocopherol (vitamin E), as described in Section 1.4. Other nutrients in the tables, which are absorbed and utilised with varying degrees of efficiency, include iron, calcium, magnesium, zinc, copper, manganese, selenium, folate, niacin and vitamin B_6. No allowance is made in the Tables for the potential lower availability of these nutrients, and the values quoted represent the actual content in foods.

1.7 Calculation of nutrient intakes

1.7.1 *Calculation*

The values in this edition form part of the more extensive electronic dataset, CoFID (see Section 1.1.3). In addition, there are numerous commercial nutrition analysis packages available that facilitate the manipulation of CoFID and other food composition data to, for example, analyse food diaries, calculate the nutrient content of recipes, or produce values for nutrition labelling.

There are several steps involved in the calculation of nutrient intake from the Tables. The first is to choose the item in the Tables which corresponds most closely with the food consumed. The index includes many alternative names and it should be noted that a food may be found in a different food group from the one in which it is expected.

If the food consumed is not in this edition or CoFID, then it is necessary to choose a suitable alternative by consideration of the food type, general characteristics and likely nutrient profile. The results, however, are likely to be less accurate. Alternatively, users might wish to seek other sources of data (e.g. manufacturers, composition data from other countries).

Once the food has been chosen, calculation of nutrient intake is achieved by multiplying the nutrient figure quoted in the Tables by the weight of the food consumed (nutrients are expressed either per 100g of the edible portion of the food, or per 100ml for alcoholic beverages), e.g. if 80g food has been consumed, the nutrient should be multiplied by 0.8, and if 120g consumed, it should be multiplied by 1.2. The results from these calculations are then summed to give the total intake.

1.7.2 Recipes

If the sample of food consumed is a cooked dish prepared with a different recipe from any of those in this book, the nutrients for the new recipe can be calculated using the methods given in Section 4.3.

1.7.3 Portion sizes

If the weight of food consumed has not been recorded or if an estimate is required, publications such as FSA (2002)[127], and Wrieden and Barton (2006)[175] may be used to provide information on typical portion sizes consumed or equivalent weights for household measures. In fieldwork, representations such as pictures (Nelson et al., 2002; Foster et al., 2011)[153,128], models or household measures may also be used to obtain estimates of portion size.

1.8   Potential pitfalls when using the data

"There are two schools of thought about food tables. One tends to regard the figures in them as having the accuracy of atomic weight determinations; the other dismisses them as valueless on the ground that a foodstuff may be so modified by the soil, the season, or its rate of growth that no figure can be a reliable guide to its composition. The truth, of course, lies somewhere between these two points of view." (Widdowson & McCance, 1943)[173].

1.8.1 Those who are unfamiliar with the uses of these tables should note the following points which can reflect on the accuracy of the information obtained from them. Further details are available in Greenfield & Southgate (2003)[134] and Church (2009)[94].

1.8.2 Missing nutrient values (see Section 1.4.13) in food composition databases should not be treated as zero values during calculations, otherwise an underestimation of nutrient intake will result. However, the major sources of any nutrient are likely to have been analysed and included in these Tables.

1.8.3 Errors will arise if foods are classified incorrectly and it is important to ensure that sufficient detail about each food is available to allow the best match to be selected. Factors that should be considered include:

- Are there different versions of a food? For example, the type of milk (whole, semi-skimmed, 1% fat, skimmed) will affect the content of fat, fatty acids, energy and fat-soluble vitamins.

- Is the food raw or cooked, and, if cooked, which cooking method was used?

- Is the food known by alternative names or are there local variations in the food name? For example, in Scotland, swede is sometimes referred to as turnip.

- Which part of the food was consumed? For example, a chicken breast could be consumed with or without the skin.

1.8.4 Users should consider whether the values presented in these tables are appropriate for the intended use. In particular, users are advised to check the labels of processed foods for any changes in formulation or fortification and for nutrients that may have been added as antioxidants or colorants.

1.8.5 When comparing the nutrient values in these Tables with those of other countries or literature reports, nutrient definitions (e.g. whether carbohydrate is total or available), the expression of units and conversion factors used in calculations may vary.

1.8.6 When using the Tables to estimate nutrient intake, users should also consider how the accuracy of these estimates is affected by limitations in dietary assessment methods used to collect food consumption data, including the measurement and recording of the quantities of foods consumed and the duration of the recording period and misreporting of food consumption (Gibson, 2005; DAPA toolkit (http://dapa-toolkit.mrc.ac.uk/))[130,99].

1.9 Food labelling

1.9.1 Nutrition information is increasingly being provided on food labels and from 2016 will be mandatory on the majority of pre-packed foods. Values from these food composition tables may be used for this purpose, but only if certain conditions are met. Values that meet the criteria below are included in CoFID, where possible.

1.9.2 *Regulations applying until (and including) 12 December 2014*

The rules governing nutrition labelling are contained in Directive 90/496/EEC[106] on Nutrition Labelling for Foodstuffs, as amended by Commission Directives 2003/120/EC[107] and 2008/100/EC[108]. In Great Britain, these rules are implemented by the Food Labelling Regulations 1996 (as amended). Northern Ireland has similar, but separate, legislation. These rules are in place to ensure consistency and accuracy of labelling, and to prevent misleading claims. At the time of publication (2014), nutrition labelling is not compulsory unless a nutrition and/or health claim is made, or vitamins and/or minerals have been added to the foodstuff.

1.9.3 *Regulations applying from 13 December 2014*

New food information regulations (the EU Food Information for Consumers Regulation (EU FIC) No. 1169/2011)[119], which bring EU rules on general and nutrition labelling together into a single regulation (replacing the previous food labelling regulations after a transition period), came into force in November 2011. ,Under the new regulations (available at:
http://ec.europa.eu/food/food/labellingnutrition/nutritionlabel/index_en.htm), 'back of pack' nutrition labelling will become mandatory for the majority of pre-packed foods from 13 December 2016.

If a nutrition declaration is provided prior to 13 December 2016 on a voluntary basis, or is required because a nutrition and/or health claim has been made or vitamins and/or minerals have been added to the foodstuff, it must comply with EU FIC from 13 December 2014.

The mandatory declaration will comprise:

- energy (kJ, kcal)
- fat
- saturates
- carbohydrate
- sugars
- protein
- salt

Salt is calculated as total sodium content multiplied by 2.5. Supplementary information on other nutrients listed in the Regulation can be provided on a voluntary basis. The additional listed nutrients are: monounsaturates; polyunsaturates; polyols; starch; fibre; and specified minerals and vitamins, present in significant amounts (as defined in the Regulation). If a claim is made for any of these nutrients, or if minerals and/or vitamins are added to a food, then the amount of the respective nutrient(s) must be declared in addition to the mandatory declaration outlined above.

Declared values for nutrients should be average values derived using one or more of the following methods:

- manufacturer's analysis of food;
- a calculation from the known or actual average values of the ingredients used in the preparation of the food; or
- a calculation from generally established and accepted data.

Generally established and accepted data for the UK include values published in this edition and/or CoFID, if the product or its ingredients are similar to those described. Nevertheless, it is important to note the following differences:

- Protein should be given as total nitrogen x 6.25 for every food, whereas more specific factors have been used in this edition;
- Carbohydrate is to be declared as the weight of the carbohydrates themselves and not their monosaccharide equivalents.

The following factors may be used to convert monosaccharide equivalents from this edition to actual weights:

Total carbohydrate	Divide by 1.05 (unless it is known to be mainly starch or mainly oligosaccharide)
Starch	Divide by 1.10
Sucrose and lactose	Divide by 1.05
Glucose, etc.	As given

Different factors are to be used to calculate energy values. These are shown in Table 10.

Table 10   *Energy conversion factors to be used in food labelling*

	kcal/g	kJ/g
Carbohydrate (except polyols), expressed as weight	4	17
Polyols	2.4	10
Protein	4	17
Fat	9	37
Salatrims	6	25
Alcohol (ethanol)	7	29
Organic acid	3	13
Fibre	2	8
Erythritol	0	0

1.9.4   *'Front of pack' nutrition labelling*

EU FIC allows elements of the mandatory nutrition declaration which are of importance to public health to be repeated on the 'front of pack' in one of the following formats:

- Energy value alone; or
- Energy value plus amounts of fat, saturates, sugars and salt

Guidance on providing 'front of pack' labelling in line with the UK Governments' 2013 Recommendation can be found at: www.gov.uk/government/publications/front-of-pack-nutrition-labelling-guidance.

1.9.5   *Tolerances for nutrient values declared on a label*

It is widely recognised that it is not possible for foods to always contain the exact quantity of nutrients declared on the label, owing to natural variation, and variations during food production and storage. However, in order to avoid consumers being misled, it is important that the deviation from declared values should be minimal. EU guidance has therefore been produced on tolerances, i.e. the acceptable differences between the nutrient values declared on a label and those established in the course of official controls by enforcement authorities. The tolerances, which vary by nutrient, by the amount present and take account of the uncertainty of measurement, can be found at: http://ec.europa.eu/food/food/labellingnutrition/nutritionlabel/index_en.htm.

The
Tables

SYMBOLS AND ABBREVIATIONS USED IN THE TABLES

Symbols

0	None of the nutrient is present
Tr	Trace amounts of the nutrient are present
N	The nutrient is present in significant quantities but there is no reliable information on the amount

Abbreviations

g	grams
mg	milligrams
ml	mililitres
µg	micrograms
kcal	kilocalories
kJ	kilojoules
Gluc	Glucose
Fruct	Fructose
Sucr	Sucrose
Malt	Maltose
Lact	Lactose
NSP	Non-starch polysaccharides
AOAC	Association of Official Analytical Chemists
Satd	Saturated
Monounsatd	Monounsaturated
Polyunsatd	Polyunsaturated
Na	Sodium
K	Potassium
Ca	Calcium
Mg	Magnesium
P	Phosphorus
Fe	Iron
Cu	Copper
Zn	Zinc
Cl	Chloride
Mn	Manganese
Se	Selenium
I	Iodine
Trypt	Tryptophan

Cereals and cereal products

Section 2.1

Cereals and cereal products

A substantial proportion of the data in this section is new, taken from analytical surveys of flours and grains (including rice)[68], pasta[66], breakfast cereals[67], and biscuits, buns, cakes and pastries[70] undertaken since 2002. There are also analytical data for several new foods, including couscous[68], polenta[68], wild rice[68], American style cookies[70], chocolate covered caramel shortcake[70], and filo pastry[70]. In addition, data from manufacturers has been used to update bread and other processed cereal-based foods to reflect reductions made in salt, sugar, and/or fat content. Manufacturers' data has also been used to validate data from the 2004 breakfast cereals survey[67] and updated to reflect reformulation and changes in fortification practice. Where breakfast cereal fortification differs between brands, values reflect the brand leader(s) and footnotes provide clarification or more detail. Data for sandwiches has been calculated based on ingredients typically included in retail sandwiches.

Values for wheat flours and their products were restricted to those from the UK because flours are required to be fortified by law (The Bread and Flour Regulations, 1998)[88]. UK flour must contain at least 1.65mg iron, 0.24mg thiamin and 1.60mg niacin per 100g and so these nutrients are added to all white flours and most brown flours in the UK. Calcium carbonate must also be added to all flours except wholemeal and certain self-raising flours at a rate equivalent to 94-156mg calcium per 100g flour.

Sources of variation pertinent to cereals and cereal products include soil type and fertiliser use (which particularly affects inorganics) and the practice of allowing for losses, during handling and storage, of nutrients added as fortificants (overages). In addition, the range and levels of added nutrients do change with time (e.g. for breakfast cereals) and also vary by brand. Users requiring details of possible recent changes in fortification practices and brand-specific information should contact manufacturers directly.

Losses of labile vitamins assigned on recipe calculation were estimated using figures in Section 4.3. Changes in weight on toasting bread and boiling rice and pastas are shown in Section 4.3. Taxonomic names for foods included in this part of the Tables can be found in Section 4.5.

Composition of food per 100g edible portion

No.	Food	Description and main data sources	Main data reference	Water g	Total nitrogen g	Protein g	Fat g	Carbohydrate g	Energy value kcal	Energy value kJ
Flours, grains and starches										
1	**Bran**, wheat	Analytical data, 2003	68	10.4	2.35	14.8	5.5	20.6	186	785
2	**Cornflour**[a]	Analytical data, 2003; and MW4, 1978	68, 4	12.5	0.09	0.6	0.7	92.0	354	1508
3	**Couscous**, plain, raw	Wheat. Analytical data, 2003	68	9.9	2.10	12.0	2.1	79.2	364	1549
4	plain, cooked	Wheat. Calculated from raw		53.8	1.26	7.2	1.0	37.5	178	759
5	**Flour, chapati**, brown	Analytical data, 2003	68	11.2	1.81	10.3	1.9	73.0	332	1413
6	**Flour, rye**	Analytical data, 2003	68	10.7	1.25	7.3	1.6	73.5	319	1359
7	**Flour, soya**	Analytical data, 2003	68	5.9	6.02	34.3	22.4	18.7	409	1711
8	**Flour, wheat**, brown	81% extraction. Analytical data, 2003	68	11.6	2.15	12.2	2.0	72.5	339	1441
9	white, bread/strong	Analytical data, 2003	68	11.7	1.98	11.3	1.2	79.2	353	1504
10	white, plain, soft	Analytical data, 2003	68	11.6	1.60	9.1	1.4	80.9	352	1501
11	white, self raising	Analytical data, 2003	68	11.3	1.55	8.9	1.5	79.6	348	1480
12	wholemeal	Analytical data, 2003	68	11.1	1.98	11.6	2.0	69.9	327	1390
13	**Polenta**, hydrated, raw	Corn based. Analytical data, 2003	68	77.1	0.30	1.9	0.4	15.2[b]	68	290
14	**Quinoa**, raw	Seeds from a species of goosefoot. Literature sources, FAN Supplement, 1992	11	11.5	2.21	13.8	5.0	55.7[c]	309	1311
15	**Wheatgerm**	Analytical data, 2003	68	9.1	4.69	27.3	8.4	44.7	352	1490
Rice										
16	**Rice, brown, wholegrain**, raw	Analytical data, 2003	68	11.9	1.30	7.7	1.5	77.0	333	1418
17	boiled in unsalted water	Analytical data, 2003	68	67.0	0.60	3.6	0.9	29.2	132	562

[a] Content of custard powder, not instant, as for cornflour

[b] Oligosaccharides may be present, but levels are unknown

[c] Includes oligosaccharides

Cereals and cereal products

Composition of food per 100g edible portion

No.	Food	Starch	Total sugars	Individual sugars					Dietary fibre		Fatty acids				Cholesterol
				Gluc	Fruct	Sucr	Malt	Lact	NSP	AOAC	Satd	Mono-unsatd	Poly-unsatd	Trans	
		g	g	g	g	g	g	g	g	g	g	g	g	g	mg

Flours, grains and starches

No.	Food	Starch	Total sugars	Gluc	Fruct	Sucr	Malt	Lact	NSP	AOAC	Satd	Mono-unsatd	Poly-unsatd	Trans	Cholesterol
1	**Bran**, wheat	18.3	2.3	Tr	Tr	2.3	Tr	0	33.0	41.3	0.9	0.7	2.9	Tr	0
2	**Cornflour**[a]	92.0	Tr	Tr	0	Tr	0	0	0.1	N	0.1	0.1	0.3	0	0
3	**Couscous**, plain, raw	76.9	2.3	Tr	Tr	0.8	1.4	0	3.6	3.7	0.3	0.3	0.8	Tr	0
4	plain, cooked	36.5	1.0	Tr	Tr	0.2	0.8	0	1.9	2.2	0.2	0.2	0.5	Tr	0
5	**Flour, chapati**, brown	71.9	1.1	Tr	Tr	0.9	0.2	0	7.3	7.9	0.3	0.2	0.8	Tr	0
6	**Flour, rye**	72.0	1.5	Tr	Tr	1.2	0.2	0	11.8	14.1	0.2	0.2	0.7	Tr	0
7	**Flour, soya**	12.3	6.4	Tr	Tr	6.4	Tr	0	12.9	18.0	2.7	3.8	11.4	Tr	Tr
8	**Flour, wheat**, brown	71.5	1.0	Tr	Tr	0.9	0.1	0	6.9	7.7	0.3	0.2	0.8	Tr	0
9	white, bread/strong	78.7	0.5	Tr	Tr	0.4	Tr	0	3.1	3.3	0.3	0.2	0.3	Tr	0
10	white, plain, soft	80.3	0.6	Tr	Tr	0.5	0.1	0	3.4	4.0	0.4	0.2	0.2	Tr	0
11	white, self raising	79.0	0.6	Tr	Tr	0.5	0.1	0	3.1	4.0	0.4	0.2	0.4	Tr	0
12	wholemeal	68.5	1.4	Tr	Tr	1.0	0.3	0	8.8	10.1	0.3	0.2	0.9	Tr	0
13	**Polenta**, hydrated, raw	15.2	Tr	Tr	Tr	Tr	0	0	0.6	1.7	0.1	0.1	0.2	Tr	0
14	**Quinoa**, raw	47.6	6.1[b]	2.7	0.6	2.8	0	0	N	7.0	0.5	1.4	2.1	Tr	0
15	**Wheatgerm**	28.7	16.0	0.7	0.5	14.8	0	0	11.6	13.9	1.1	0.8	4.1	Tr	Tr

Rice

No.	Food	Starch	Total sugars	Gluc	Fruct	Sucr	Malt	Lact	NSP	AOAC	Satd	Mono-unsatd	Poly-unsatd	Trans	Cholesterol
16	**Rice, brown, wholegrain**, raw	76.3	0.7	Tr	Tr	0.7	0	0	1.8	3.0	0.3	0.5	0.5	Tr	Tr
17	boiled in unsalted water	29.0	0.1	Tr	Tr	0.1	0	0	0.9	1.5	0.2	0.3	0.3	Tr	Tr

[a] Content of custard powder, not instant, as for cornflour
[b] Not including oligosaccharides

Inorganic constituents per 100g edible portion

No.	Food	Na	K	Ca	Mg	P	Fe	Cu	Zn	Cl	Mn	Se	I
					mg							µg	
Flours, grains and starches													
1	**Bran**, wheat	3	1269	65	389	1078	8.6	1.04	5.6	95	5.9	14	Tr
2	**Cornflour**[a]	11	3	2	2	17	0.1	Tr	0.5	30	N	Tr	Tr
3	**Couscous**, plain, raw	4	287	28	59	238	2.0	0.36	1.8	93	1.1	5	Tr
4	plain, cooked	4	154	20	32	129	1.0	0.21	0.9	82	0.6	3	Tr
5	**Flour, chapati**, brown	14	280	54	110	377	4.6	0.75	3.0	126	2.1	32	Tr
6	**Flour, rye**	2	419	33	85	307	2.4	0.33	2.3	53	2.2	2	Tr
7	**Flour, soya**	1	1867	182	245	668	8.4	1.31	4.1	81	2.4	7	Tr
8	**Flour, wheat**, brown	2	295	28	72	256	2.4	0.32	2.2	82	2.3	6	Tr
9	white, bread/strong	2	166	134	26	128	1.9	0.15	0.8	98	0.7	9	Tr
10	white, plain, soft	2	175	96	23	114	1.9	0.15	0.7	143	0.7	3	Tr
11	white, self raising	342[b]	190	280[b]	25	463[b]	1.7	0.12	0.8	108	0.8	3	Tr
12	wholemeal	2	358	32	83	281	2.5	0.37	1.9	108	2.0	5	Tr
13	**Polenta**, hydrated, raw	541	27	6	7	20	0.1	Tr	0.1	813	Tr	Tr	N
14	**Quinoa**, raw	61	780	79	210	230	7.8	0.82	3.3	N	N	N	N
15	**Wheatgerm**	3	1045	45	240	1047	8.1	0.82	14.0	107	13.5	18	Tr
Rice													
16	**Rice, brown, wholegrain**, raw	Tr	243	11	116	323	1.1	0.22	1.8	56	2.5	10	Tr
17	boiled in unsalted water	4	62	17	48	125	0.5	0.08	0.7	35	0.9	4	Tr

[a] Inorganic content of custard powder, not instant, as for cornflour except for Na (320mg) and Cl (480mg)

[b] The amount present will depend on the nature and level of the raising agent used

Vitamins per 100g edible portion

No.	Food	Retinol µg	Carotene µg	Vitamin D µg	Vitamin E mg	Thiamin mg	Ribo-flavin mg	Niacin mg	Trypt 60 mg	Vitamin B$_6$ mg	Vitamin B$_{12}$ µg	Folate µg	Panto-thenate mg	Biotin µg	Vitamin C mg

Flours, grains and starches

No.	Food	Retinol	Carotene	Vit D	Vit E	Thiamin	Riboflavin	Niacin	Trypt 60	Vit B$_6$	Vit B$_{12}$	Folate	Pantothenate	Biotin	Vit C
1	**Bran**, wheat	0	0	0	1.02	0.93	0.33	26.1	5.9	1.15	0	76	2.5	32	0
2	**Cornflour**[a]	0	0	0	Tr	0.02	Tr	Tr	0.1	Tr	0	2	Tr	Tr	0
3	**Couscous**, plain, raw	0	0	0	0.13	0.28	0.06	2.6	2.7	0.15	0	28	0.6	3	0
4	plain, cooked	0	0	0	0.06	0.13	Tr	2.1	1.2	0.08	0	13	0.4	2	0
5	**Flour, chapati**, brown	0	0	0	1.17	0.35	0.09	3.8	2.4	0.24	0	28	0.6	3	0
6	**Flour, rye**	0	0	0	0.64	0.35	0.12	0.9	1.8	0.36	0	60	0.7	7	0
7	**Flour, soya**	0	Tr	0	4.33	0.38	0.26	1.9	9.2	0.40	0	245	1.8	14	0
8	**Flour, wheat**, brown	0	0	0	0.90	0.39	0.10	3.7	2.6	0.41	0	44	0.7	4	0
9	white, bread/strong	0	0	0	0.43	0.30	0.03	1.8	2.3	0.15	0	16	0.3	1	0
10	white, plain, soft	0	0	0	0.59	0.28	0.05	1.7	2.0	0.18	0	16	0.4	2	0
11	white, self raising	0	0	0	0.63	0.28	0.05	1.7	2.0	0.18	0	18	0.4	2	0
12	wholemeal	0	0	0	0.69	0.36	0.10	5.0	2.9	0.50	0	27	1.0	7	0
13	**Polenta**, hydrated, raw	0	Tr	0	Tr	0.05	Tr	0.3	0.2	0.02	0	5	0.1	1	0
14	**Quinoa**, raw	0	N	0	N	0.20	0.40	2.9	1.9	N	0	N	N	N	0
15	**Wheatgerm**	0	0	0	16.20	1.80	0.63	6.7	6.0	2.58	0	277	2.6	23	0

Rice

| 16 | **Rice, brown, wholegrain**, raw | 0 | 0 | 0 | 0.37 | 0.30 | 0.06 | 4.3 | 2.2 | 0.19 | 0 | 22 | 0.7 | 4 | 0 |
| 17 | boiled in unsalted water | 0 | 0 | 0 | 0.14 | 0.11 | Tr | 2.0 | 1.2 | 0.04 | 0 | 7 | 0.2 | 1 | 0 |

[a] Vitamin content of custard powder, not instant, as for cornflour

Composition of food per 100g edible portion

No.	Food	Description and main data sources	Main data reference	Water g	Total nitrogen g	Protein g	Fat g	Carbo-hydrate g	Energy value kcal	kJ
	Rice continued									
18	**Rice, egg fried**, ready cooked, re-heated	Retail, not takeaway. Analytical data, 2003	68	59.9	0.66	3.9	5.3	28.1	169	712
19	**Rice, pilau**, plain, homemade	Recipe		69.9	0.41	2.5	3.7	24.3[a]	134	564
20	**Rice, ready cooked**, plain, re-heated	Analytical data, 2003	68	59.6	0.70	4.1	1.9	33.9	161	682
21	**Rice, savoury**, dried, cooked	Assorted meat and vegetable varieties. Cooked in water according to manufacturer's instructions. Analytical data, 2003; and industry data, 2013	68	59.0	0.62	3.7	1.4	34.0	155	659
22	**Rice, white**, basmati, raw	Analytical data, 2003	68	11.3	1.36	8.1	0.5	83.7	351	1495
23	basmati, boiled in unsalted water	Analytical data, 2003	68	69.5	0.47	2.8	0.7	26.5	117	498
24	basmati, easy cook, boiled in unsalted water	Analytical data, 2003	68	66.8	0.59	3.5	0.4	32.2	138	590
25	Italian Arborio risotto, raw	Analytical data, 2003	68	13.0	1.08	6.4	1.0	85.2	354	1509
26	Italian Arborio risotto, boiled in unsalted water	Calculated from raw		67.1	0.53	3.2	0.5	32.2	138	588
27	long grain, raw	Analytical data, 2003	68	11.3	1.12	6.7	1.0	85.1	355	1513
28	long grain, boiled in unsalted water	Analytical data, 2003	68	68.2	0.47	2.8	0.4	31.1	131	560
29	long grain, easy cook, boiled in unsalted water	Analytical data, 2003	68	67.0	0.51	3.0	0.4	34.7	146	621

[a] Includes oligosaccharides

Cereals and cereal products *continued*

No.	Food	Starch g	Total sugars g	Individual sugars					Dietary fibre		Fatty acids				Cholest-erol mg
				Gluc g	Fruct g	Sucr g	Malt g	Lact g	NSP g	AOAC g	Satd g	Mono-unsatd g	Poly-unsatd g	Trans g	

Rice continued

No.	Food	Starch	Total sugars	Gluc	Fruct	Sucr	Malt	Lact	NSP	AOAC	Satd	Mono-unsatd	Poly-unsatd	Trans	Cholesterol
18	**Rice, egg fried**, ready cooked, re-heated	28.1	Tr	Tr	Tr	Tr	0	Tr	1.2	2.8	0.7	2.6	1.8	Tr	53
19	**Rice, pilau**, plain, homemade	23.3	0.8[a]	0.3	0.2	0.3	0	Tr	0.3	0.6	0.5	0.8	2.3	Tr	0
20	**Rice, ready cooked**, plain, re-heated	33.9	Tr	Tr	Tr	Tr	0	0	Tr	1.1	0.3	0.4	0.9	Tr	0
21	**Rice, savoury**, dried, cooked	30.8	3.2	0.5	0.5	1.4	Tr	0.8	1.3	1.7	0.5	0.5	0.3	0.1	Tr
22	**Rice, white**, basmati, raw	83.6	0.1	Tr	Tr	0.1	0	0	0.9	1.1	0.1	0.1	0.2	Tr	0
23	basmati, boiled in unsalted water	26.5	Tr	Tr	Tr	Tr	0	0	0.6	0.6	0.2	0.1	0.3	Tr	0
24	basmati, easy cook, boiled in unsalted water	32.1	Tr	Tr	Tr	Tr	0	0	Tr	Tr	0.1	0.1	0.2	Tr	0
25	Italian Arborio risotto, raw	84.9	0.2	Tr	Tr	0.2	0	0	0.9	1.4	0.2	0.2	0.4	Tr	0
26	Italian Arborio risotto, boiled in unsalted water	32.1	Tr	Tr	Tr	Tr	0	0	Tr	Tr	0.1	0.1	0.2	Tr	0
27	long grain, raw	84.8	0.2	Tr	Tr	0.2	0	0	0.9	1.1	0.3	0.3	0.3	Tr	0
28	long grain, boiled in unsalted water	31.1	Tr	Tr	Tr	Tr	0	0	Tr	0.5	0.1	0.1	0.1	Tr	0
29	long grain, easy cook, boiled in unsalted water	34.7	Tr	Tr	Tr	Tr	0	0	Tr	0.7	0.1	0.1	0.1	Tr	0

[a] Not including oligosaccharides

Inorganic constituents per 100g edible portion

No.	Food	Na	K	Ca	Mg	P	Fe	Cu	Zn	Cl	Mn	Se	I
						mg						µg	
Rice continued													
18	**Rice, egg fried**, ready cooked, re-heated	409	88	28	12	77	0.4	0.09	0.5	531	0.3	7	3
19	**Rice, pilau**, plain, homemade	1	51	11	9	34	0.9	0.09	0.4	25	0.2	4	Tr
20	**Rice, ready cooked**, plain, re-heated	151	51	18	9	57	0.1	0.12	0.4	229	0.2	7	Tr
21	**Rice, savoury**, dried, cooked	290	154	28	18	92	0.5	0.14	0.6	420	0.4	6	3
22	**Rice, white**, basmati, raw	1	77	10	21	101	1.7	0.27	1.4	65	0.7	16	Tr
23	basmati, boiled in unsalted water	4	15	14	6	30	0.1	0.10	0.4	50	0.2	5	Tr
24	basmati, easy cook, boiled in unsalted water	4	16	18	6	38	0.1	0.11	0.3	54	0.1	7	Tr
25	Italian Arborio risotto, raw	1	86	5	30	125	0.2	0.20	1.4	46	0.7	5	Tr
26	Italian Arborio risotto, boiled in unsalted water	4	33	12	12	52	0.1	0.10	0.6	54	0.3	2	Tr
27	long grain, raw	1	87	16	25	117	0.3	0.18	1.4	46	1.1	13	Tr
28	long grain, boiled in unsalted water	11	12	9	5	28	Tr	0.07	0.4	84	0.3	5	Tr
29	long grain, easy cook, boiled in unsalted water	6	18	20	7	39	0.1	0.09	0.3	88	0.3	7	Tr

Cereals and cereal products *continued*

Vitamins per 100g edible portion

No.	Food	Retinol µg	Carotene µg	Vitamin D µg	Vitamin E mg	Thiamin mg	Ribo-flavin mg	Niacin mg	Trypt 60 mg	Vitamin B$_6$ mg	Vitamin B$_{12}$ µg	Folate µg	Panto-thenate mg	Biotin µg	Vitamin C mg
Rice continued															
18	**Rice, egg fried**, ready cooked, re-heated	Tr	24	Tr	2.08	0.11	0.06	1.7	0.9	0.08	Tr	8	0.5	2	Tr
19	**Rice, pilau**, plain, homemade	0	4	0	1.83	0.04	Tr	0.3	0.6	0.03	0	2	0.1	Tr	Tr
20	**Rice, ready cooked**, plain, re-heated	0	0	0	0.36	0.08	Tr	2.3	1.2	0.08	0	5	0.5	1	0
21	**Rice, savoury**, dried, cooked	Tr	159	Tr	0.45	0.20	0.09	2.5	1.1	0.12	Tr	22	0.5	2	1
22	**Rice, white**, basmati, raw	0	0	0	0.07	0.13	Tr	1.2	2.1	0.10	0	12	0.4	1	0
23	basmati, boiled in unsalted water	0	0	0	0.08	0.03	Tr	0.2	0.9	0.03	0	5	0.2	1	0
24	basmati, easy cook, boiled in unsalted water	0	0	0	0.01	0.06	Tr	1.0	0.8	0.06	0	8	0.2	1	0
25	Italian Arborio risotto, raw	0	0	0	0.03	0.09	Tr	1.6	2.0	0.11	0	13	0.3	1	0
26	Italian Arborio risotto, boiled in unsalted water	0	0	0	0.01	0.03	Tr	0.5	1.3	0.05	0	7	0.2	1	0
27	long grain, raw	0	0	0	0.03	0.12	Tr	1.4	1.9	0.12	0	14	0.4	2	0
28	long grain, boiled in unsalted water	0	0	0	0.01	Tr	Tr	0.3	0.9	0.03	0	4	0.1	Tr	0
29	long grain, easy cook, boiled in unsalted water	0	0	0	0.01	0.05	Tr	0.7	0.7	0.03	0	6	0.1	Tr	0

Cereals and cereal products *continued*

Composition of food per 100g edible portion

No.	Food	Description and main data sources	Main data reference	Water g	Total nitrogen g	Protein g	Fat g	Carbo-hydrate g	Energy value kcal	kJ
Rice continued										
30	**Rice, wild**, raw	Analytical data, 2003	68	8.3	2.06	12.2	1.1	75.8	343	1461
31	boiled in unsalted water	Analytical data, 2003	68	66.7	0.89	5.3	0.6	31.7	145	620
32	**Risotto**, plain, homemade	Recipe		56.2	0.55	3.3	4.7	35.6[a]	184	778
Pasta										
33	**Macaroni cheese**, homemade	Recipe		62.4	1.27	7.8	8.6	19.8	183	768
34	**Noodles, egg**, dried, raw	Fine, medium and thick. Analytical data, 2002	66	8.2	2.11	12.0	2.0	72.6	338	1440
35	medium, dried, boiled in unsalted water	Analytical data, 2002	66	57.0	1.02	5.8	1.0	35.7	166	707
36	**Noodles, rice**, fine, dried, boiled in unsalted water	Analytical data, 2002	66	73.2	0.33	1.9	0.2	21.3	89	381
37	**Pasta, egg**, fresh, raw	Including tagliatelle, penne, conchiglie, spaghetti and fusilli. Analytical data, 2002	66	27.1	1.86	10.6	2.9	57.0	282	1200
38	white, tagliatelle, fresh, boiled in unsalted water	Analytical data, 2002	66	64.0	1.01	5.8	1.6	30.6	152	647
39	fresh, filled with cheese only, boiled in unsalted water	Including tortelloni, tortellini and ravioli. Analytical data, 2002	66	52.0	1.64	10.5	6.7	30.2	216	910
40	fresh, filled with meat, boiled in unsalted water	Including tortellini and cappelletti and chicken, ham, beef bacon fillings. Analytical data, 2002	66	52.4	1.61	10.1	4.7	31.3	200	846

[a] Includes oligosaccharides

Cereals and cereal products continued

Composition of food per 100g edible portion

No.	Food	Starch	Total sugars	Individual sugars					Dietary fibre		Fatty acids				Cholesterol
				Gluc	Fruct	Sucr	Malt	Lact	NSP	AOAC	Satd	Mono-unsatd	Poly-unsatd	Trans	
		g	g	g	g	g	g	g	g	g	g	g	g	g	mg
Rice continued															
30	**Rice, wild,** raw	75.7	0.1	Tr	Tr	0.1	0	0	3.0	4.3	0.3	0.2	0.5	Tr	0
31	boiled in unsalted water	31.2	0.4	Tr	Tr	0.3	0	0	1.2	2.5	0.1	0.1	0.3	Tr	0
32	**Risotto,** plain, homemade	34.3	1.0[a]	0.3	0.3	0.4	0	0	0.5	0.9	0.7	1.0	2.7	Tr	Tr
Pasta															
33	**Macaroni cheese,** homemade	16.9	2.8	0	0	0.1	0.3	2.4	0.8	1.1	4.5	2.7	0.7	0.2	17
34	**Noodles, egg,** dried, raw	70.9	1.7	0.2	0.2	0.6	0.7	0	3.9	N	0.3	0.3	0.7	Tr	2
35	medium, dried, boiled in unsalted water	35.7	Tr	Tr	Tr	Tr	Tr	0	2.2	3.0	0.2	0.1	0.4	Tr	1
36	**Noodles, rice,** fine, dried, boiled in unsalted water	21.3	Tr	Tr	Tr	Tr	0	0	0.7	1.1	0.1	Tr	0.1	Tr	0
37	**Pasta, egg,** fresh, raw	54.9	2.1	0.3	0.4	Tr	1.4	0	3.4	3.3	0.7	0.9	0.8	Tr	15
38	white, tagliatelle, fresh, boiled in unsalted water	30.6	Tr	Tr	Tr	Tr	Tr	0	0.9	2.0	0.4	0.5	0.4	Tr	N
39	fresh, filled with cheese only, boiled in unsalted water	28.0	2.2	Tr	Tr	Tr	1.4	0.8	2.1	2.2	3.5	2.0	0.8	0.2	33
40	fresh, filled with meat, boiled in unsalted water	30.3	1.0	Tr	0.1	Tr	0.6	0.3	1.4	1.9	1.8	1.6	0.8	0.1	31

[a] Not including oligosaccharides

Inorganic constituents per 100g edible portion

No.	Food	mg										µg	
		Na	K	Ca	Mg	P	Fe	Cu	Zn	Cl	Mn	Se	I
Rice continued													
30	**Rice, wild**, raw	4	326	8	108	377	1.3	0.63	4.3	75	1.2	3	Tr
31	boiled in unsalted water	4	102	16	43	141	0.5	0.24	1.8	55	0.5	1	Tr
32	**Risotto**, plain, homemade	447	73	9	15	62	0.2	0.11	0.6	670	0.3	2	Tr
Pasta													
33	**Macaroni cheese**, homemade	149	140	172	19	157	0.4	0.07	1.0	250	0.2	6	21
34	**Noodles, egg**, dried, raw	500	378	73	49	187	2.7	0.20	1.3	710	1.1	16	6
35	medium, dried, boiled in unsalted water	141	75	43	25	89	1.1	Tr	0.6	186	0.5	10	Tr
36	**Noodles, rice**, fine, dried, boiled in unsalted water	4	3	22	3	19	0.1	Tr	0.4	65	0.1	1	3
37	**Pasta, egg**, fresh, raw	24	186	28	31	156	1.5	0.83	1.0	120	0.5	11	9
38	white, tagliatelle, fresh, boiled in unsalted water	9	40	29	16	76	0.6	Tr	0.5	65	0.3	5	8
39	fresh, filled with cheese only, boiled in unsalted water	242	99	124	21	147	0.7	Tr	0.9	406	0.3	11	18
40	fresh, filled with meat, boiled in unsalted water	298	115	69	20	124	0.9	0.10	0.9	445	0.3	9	8

Cereals and cereal products *continued*

Vitamins per 100g edible portion

No.	Food	Retinol µg	Carotene µg	Vitamin D µg	Vitamin E mg	Thiamin mg	Riboflavin mg	Niacin mg	Trypt 60 mg	Vitamin B6 mg	Vitamin B12 µg	Folate µg	Pantothenate mg	Biotin µg	Vitamin C mg
Rice continued															
30	**Rice, wild**, raw	0	0	0	0.24	0.25	0.27	4.4	3.6	0.15	0	65	0.7	2	0
31	boiled in unsalted water	0	0	0	0.10	0.13	0.08	2.2	1.9	0.04	0	24	0.2	1	0
32	**Risotto**, plain, homemade	0	2	0	2.01	0.04	Tr	0.4	0.9	0.04	Tr	3	0.8	Tr	0
Pasta															
33	**Macaroni cheese**, homemade	N	48	N	N	0.04	0.16	0.5	1.8	0.06	0.7	6	0.4	2	1
34	**Noodles, egg**, dried, raw	4	43	0.2	0.53	0.12	0.02	3.3	2.5	0.15	Tr	19	0.6	4	0
35	medium, dried, boiled in unsalted	Tr	Tr	0.1	0.35	Tr	Tr	0.6	1.4	0.01	Tr	6	0.3	1	0
36	**Noodles, rice**, fine, dried, boiled in unsalted water	0	0	0	0.09	Tr	Tr	0.1	0.8	0.01	0	3	Tr	Tr	0
37	**Pasta, egg**, fresh, raw	17	Tr	0.3	0.52	0.15	0.09	2.1	2.3	0.01	Tr	18	0.8	1	0
38	white, tagliatelle, fresh, boiled in unsalted water	8	Tr	0.1	0.26	0.08	0.04	0.7	1.1	0.01	Tr	6	0.4	2	0
39	fresh, filled with cheese only, boiled in unsalted water	77	21	0.3	0.91	0.07	0.10	0.8	2.1	0.02	Tr	10	0.5	2	0
40	fresh, filled with meat, boiled in unsalted water	22	11	0.3	0.62	0.58	0.09	1.4	2.0	0.12	Tr	24	0.5	2	Tr

Cereals and cereal products *continued*

41 to 52

			Composition of food per 100g edible portion						
		Main data		Total				Carbo-	Energy value
No.	Food	Description and main data sources	reference	Water	nitrogen	Protein	Fat	hydrate	kcal	kJ
				g	g	g	g	g		

Pasta continued

No.	Food	Description and main data sources	reference	Water g	Total nitrogen g	Protein g	Fat g	Carbohydrate g	kcal	kJ
41	**Pasta, ravioli**, meat filling, canned in tomato sauce	Analytical data, 2002; and industry data, 2013	66	78.4	0.41	2.3	1.4	14.8	77	328
42	**Pasta, spaghetti**, canned in tomato sauce	Analytical data, 2002; and industry data, 2013	66	80.5	0.37	2.1	0.3	16.2	72	306
43	**Pasta, white**, dried, raw	Including penne, fusilli, conchiglie, tagliatelle and spaghetti. Analytical data, 2002	66	8.7	1.98	11.3	1.6	75.6	343	1461
44	spaghetti, dried, boiled in unsalted water	Analytical data, 2002	66	64.9	0.78	4.4	0.6	31.5	141	601
45	twists/fusilli, dried, boiled in unsalted water	Analytical data, 2002	66	58.3	0.85	4.8	0.4	32.9	146	623
46	**Pasta, wholewheat, spaghetti**, dried, raw	Analytical data, 2002	66	9.5	2.15	12.6	2.5	68.3	329	1400
47	dried, boiled in unsalted water	Analytical data, 2002	66	63.7	0.90	5.2	1.1	27.5	134	569

Bread, rolls and morning goods

No.	Food	Description and main data sources	reference	Water g	Total nitrogen g	Protein g	Fat g	Carbohydrate g	kcal	kJ
48	**Bagels**, plain	Analytical data, 1993-1994; and industry data, 2013	50	32.1	1.60	10.0	1.8	57.8[a]	273	1161
49	**Bread, brown**, average	Analytical data, 1998; and industry data, 2013	61	41.2	1.40	7.9	2.0	42.1	207	882
50	**Bread, ciabatta**	Analytical data, 1998; and industry data, 2013	61	29.2	1.80	10.2	3.9	52.0	271	1150
51	**Bread, garlic and herb**	Retail, frozen and chilled. Analytical data, 2010	72	25.8	1.23	7.0	16.7	45.1	348	1459
52	**Bread, malt**, fruited	Analytical data, 1998	61	24.2	1.40	7.8	2.3	64.9	295	1256

[a] Includes oligosaccharides

Cereals and cereal products *continued*

Composition of food per 100g edible portion

No.	Food	Starch	Total sugars	Individual sugars					Dietary fibre		Fatty acids				Cholest-erol
				Gluc	Fruct	Sucr	Malt	Lact	NSP	AOAC	Satd	Mono-unsatd	Poly-unsatd	Trans	
		g	g	g	g	g	g	g	g	g	g	g	g	g	mg
Pasta continued															
41	**Pasta, ravioli**, meat filling, canned in tomato sauce	11.4	3.4	1.0	0.9	1.1	0.4	0	1.6	1.1	0.5	0.5	0.3	Tr	1
42	**Pasta, spaghetti**, canned in tomato sauce	10.7	5.5	1.3	1.4	2.4	0.4	0	1.3	0.9	0.1	Tr	0.1	Tr	0
43	**Pasta, white**, dried, raw	73.5	2.1	0.1	0.2	0.3	1.5	0	3.7	N	0.2	0.2	0.7	Tr	0
44	spaghetti, dried, boiled in unsalted water	30.5	1.0	Tr	0.1	Tr	0.9	0	1.5	1.7	0.1	0.1	0.3	Tr	0
45	twists/fusilli, dried, boiled in unsalted water	32.3	0.6	Tr	Tr	Tr	0.6	0	2.7	2.6	0.1	0.1	0.2	Tr	0
46	**Pasta, wholewheat, spaghetti**, dried, raw	64.4	3.9	0.4	0.4	0.5	2.6	0	8.1	11.7	0.4	0.3	1.1	Tr	0
47	dried, boiled in unsalted water	27.5	Tr	Tr	Tr	Tr	Tr	0	4.4	4.2	0.2	0.1	0.5	Tr	0
Bread, rolls and morning goods															
48	**Bagels**, plain	51.3	4.8[a]	0.8	1.0	Tr	3.0	0	2.4	3.0	N	N	N	N	0
49	**Bread, brown**, average	38.7	3.4	Tr	0.3	Tr	3.0	0	3.5	5.0	0.4	0.4	0.7	Tr	0
50	**Bread, ciabatta**	48.9	3.1	Tr	0.1	0.3	2.7	0	2.3	3.3	0.6	2.1	0.9	Tr	0
51	**Bread, garlic and herb**	42.2	2.9	0.1	0.2	Tr	2.5	Tr	0.8	2.7	8.6	5.4	1.6	0.3	31
52	**Bread, malt**, fruited	42.3	22.6	7.4	6.3	1.0	7.2	0.7	2.6	3.5	0.5	1.0	1.0	0.2	Tr

[a] Not including oligosaccharides

43

Cereals and cereal products *continued*

Inorganic constituents per 100g edible portion

No.	Food	Na	K	Ca	Mg	P	Fe	Cu	Zn	Cl	Mn	Se	I
		mg										µg	
Pasta continued													
41	**Pasta, ravioli**, meat filling, canned in tomato sauce	260	137	14	11	39	0.8	Tr	0.4	400	0.2	3	Tr
42	**Pasta, spaghetti**, canned in tomato sauce	190	122	13	9	27	0.6	Tr	0.2	300	0.1	2	Tr
43	**Pasta, white**, dried, raw	2	232	24	47	179	1.6	0.30	1.2	100	0.8	22	Tr
44	spaghetti, dried, boiled in unsalted water	3	41	27	21	66	0.6	Tr	0.5	55	0.3	8	Tr
45	twists/fusilli, dried, boiled in unsalted water	5	40	25	22	77	0.7	0.19	0.6	50	0.4	6	Tr
46	**Pasta, wholewheat, spaghetti**, dried, raw	3	426	39	103	333	3.3	0.54	2.8	118	2.5	15	Tr
47	dried, boiled in unsalted water	5	82	31	46	124	1.5	0.26	1.2	50	1.1	6	Tr
Bread, rolls and morning goods													
48	**Bagels**, plain	400	N	N	N	N	N	N	N	N	N	N	N
49	**Bread, brown**, average	400	216	186	45	157	2.2	0.17	1.3	710	1.1	4	6
50	**Bread, ciabatta**	350	152	121	22	100	1.4	0.09	0.7	540	0.6	19	10
51	**Bread, garlic and herb**	476	149	126	21	88	1.6	0.08	0.7	730	0.6	1	3
52	**Bread, malt**, fruited	246	234	104	37	125	1.7	0.14	0.7	408	0.7	10	27

Cereals and cereal products *continued*

Vitamins per 100g edible portion

No.	Food	Retinol	Carotene	Vitamin D	Vitamin E	Thiamin	Ribo-flavin	Niacin	Trypt 60	Vitamin B6	Vitamin B12	Folate	Panto-thenate	Biotin	Vitamin C
		µg	µg	µg	mg	mg	mg	mg	mg	mg	µg	µg	mg	µg	mg
Pasta continued															
41	**Pasta, ravioli**, meat filling, canned in tomato sauce	0	78	Tr	0.41	0.07	0.06	0.8	0.6	0.09	Tr	3	0.2	6	Tr
42	**Pasta, spaghetti**, canned in tomato sauce	0	88	0	0.29	0.09	0.01	0.9	0.3	0.06	Tr	4	0.2	1	Tr
43	**Pasta, white**, dried, raw	0	0	0	0.30	0.17	0.03	3.3	2.4	0.14	0	19	0.8	1	0
44	spaghetti, dried, boiled in unsalted water	0	0	0	0.11	0.08	0.01	0.9	0.8	0.01	0	8	0.2	1	0
45	twists/fusilli, dried, boiled in unsalted water	0	0	0	0.08	Tr	0.03	1.1	1.3	0.02	0	5	0.3	Tr	0
46	**Pasta, wholewheat, spaghetti**, dried, raw	0	0	0	0.60	0.33	0.06	5.6	3.2	0.31	0	29	0.8	4	0
47	dried, boiled in unsalted water	0	0	0	0.25	0.11	0.02	1.8	1.2	0.02	0	8	0.3	2	0
Bread, rolls and morning goods															
48	**Bagels**, plain	0	0	0	N	N	N	N	N	N	0	N	N	N	0
49	**Bread, brown**, average	0	0	0	0.01	0.22	0.07	2.8	2.1	0.17	0	45	0.5	3	0
50	**Bread, ciabatta**	0	0	0	0.47	0.24	0.06	2.0	2.2	0.07	0	21	0.4	1	0
51	**Bread, garlic and herb**	179	53	Tr	1.79	0.23	0.13	1.1	1.7	0.14	0.1	11	0.2	1	Tr
52	**Bread, malt**, fruited	Tr	Tr	Tr	0.18	0.24	0.32	2.4	1.9	0.11	0	34	N	N	Tr

Composition of food per 100g edible portion

No.	Food	Description and main data sources	Main data reference	Water g	Total nitrogen g	Protein g	Fat g	Carbo-hydrate g	Energy value kcal	kJ
	Bread, rolls and morning goods continued									
53	**Bread, malted wheat**	Sliced and unsliced, including granary products. Analytical data, 1998; and industry data, 2013	61	34.9	1.65	9.6	2.3	47.4	237	1005
54	**Bread, naan**	Retail, including garlic and coriander. Analytical data, 1998; and industry data, 2013	61	30.8	1.40	7.8	7.3	50.2	285	1206
55	peshwari	Takeaway and retail, with nuts and raisins. Analytical data, 2007	69	32.4	1.22	7.6	7.9	39.8	251	1058
56	**Bread, pitta**, white	Analytical data, 1998; and industry data, 2013	61	31.4	1.60	9.1	1.3	55.1	255	1084
57	**Bread, seeded**	Industry data, 2013; and calculated		33.0	1.74	9.9	7.4	43.8	270	1143
58	**Bread, wheatgerm**	Pre-packed and sliced. Analytical data, 1998; and industry data, 2013	61	39.7	1.90	11.1	3.1	39.5	220	935
59	**Bread, white**, Danish style	Including Nimble and Weight Watchers. Analytical data, 1998; and industry data, 2013	61	37.5	1.60	9.1	2.7	44.5	228	967
60	farmhouse or split tin	Analytical data, 1998; and industry data, 2013	61	36.8	1.60	9.0	2.0	49.9	241	1025
61	French stick	Baguette and flute, thick and thin. Analytical data, 1998; and industry data, 2013	61	29.0	1.60	9.0	1.9	56.1	263	1121
62	premium	Analytical data, 1998; and industry data, 2013	61	38.4	1.50	8.3	2.3	47.0	230	978
63	sliced	Analytical data, 1998; and industry data, 2013	61	38.6	1.40	7.9	1.6	46.1	219	931
64	sliced, toasted	Calculated using weight loss of 18%		25.1	1.71	9.7	2.0	56.2	267	1137

Composition of food per 100g edible portion

No.	Food	Starch	Total sugars	Individual sugars					Dietary fibre		Fatty acids				Cholesterol
				Gluc	Fruct	Sucr	Malt	Lact	NSP	AOAC	Satd	Mono-unsatd	Poly-unsatd	Trans	erol
		g	g	g	g	g	g	g	g	g	g	g	g	g	mg

Bread, rolls and morning goods continued

No.	Food	Starch	Total sugars	Gluc	Fruct	Sucr	Malt	Lact	NSP	AOAC	Satd	Mono-unsatd	Poly-unsatd	Trans	Cholesterol
53	**Bread, malted wheat**	44.5	2.9	0.1	0.3	Tr	2.5	0	3.3	5.3	0.6	0.6	0.8	Tr	0
54	**Bread, naan**	47.0	3.1	0.7	0.8	Tr	1.3	0.4	2.0	2.9	1.0	3.1	2.4	0.1	5
55	peshwari	38.2	1.6	Tr	Tr	1.6	Tr	Tr	3.0	5.6	3.1	2.6	1.7	Tr	41
56	**Bread, pitta**, white	52.2	3.0	0.5	0.5	Tr	2.0	0	2.4[a]	2.3[a]	0.2	0.1	0.5	Tr	0
57	**Bread, seeded**	40.0	3.8	N	N	N	N	0	N	6.2	1.0	N	N	Tr	0
58	**Bread, wheatgerm**	35.8	3.8	0.2	0.6	Tr	2.9	0	4.0	5.7	0.7	0.7	1.1	Tr	0
59	**Bread, white**, Danish style	41.6	3.0	0.1	0.2	Tr	2.7	0	2.4	3.1	0.5	0.5	0.9	Tr	0
60	farmhouse or split tin	47.0	2.9	Tr	0.2	Tr	2.7	0	2.1	2.9	0.5	0.4	0.6	0.1	0
61	French stick	53.3	2.8	Tr	0.2	Tr	2.7	0	2.4	3.3	0.3	0.3	0.7	Tr	0
62	premium	44.4	2.7	Tr	0.2	Tr	2.5	0	1.9	2.8	N	N	N	Tr	0
63	sliced	42.7	3.4	Tr	0.2	Tr	3.2	0	1.9	2.5	0.3	0.3	0.5	Tr	0
64	sliced, toasted	52.1	4.1	Tr	0.2	Tr	3.9	0	2.3	3.0	0.4	0.4	0.6	Tr	0

[a] Wholemeal pitta bread contains 5.2g NSP and 6.4g AOAC per 100g

47

Inorganic constituents per 100g edible portion

No.	Food	Na	K	Ca	Mg	P	Fe	Cu	Zn	Cl	Mn	Se	I
		mg										µg	

Bread, rolls and morning goods continued

No.	Food	Na	K	Ca	Mg	P	Fe	Cu	Zn	Cl	Mn	Se	I
53	**Bread, malted wheat**	400	191	209	39	138	1.9	0.18	1.1	580	0.8	6	8
54	**Bread, naan**	360	172	187	21	299	1.6	0.09	0.7	550	0.5	Tr	N
55	peshwari	390	197	226	28	310	1.4	0.17	0.7	601	0.5	Tr	N
56	**Bread, pitta**, white	400[a]	178	138[a]	22	99	1.9[a]	0.12	0.8[a]	640	0.5	2	N
57	**Bread, seeded**	360	226	150	80	180	2.3	0.47	1.5	554	0.8	13	N
58	**Bread, wheatgerm**	390	269	212	64	219	2.9	0.26	2.3	560	2.1	12	N
59	**Bread, white**, Danish style	400	110	130	21	93	1.7	0.14	0.6	710	0.4	11	N
60	farmhouse or split tin	400	135	172	19	89	1.3	0.12	0.8	550	0.5	5	4
61	French stick	400	152	121	22	100	1.4	0.09	0.7	630	0.6	5	10
62	premium	400	138	177	25	101	1.5	0.19	0.8	570	0.5	10	N
63	sliced	400	137	177	23	95	1.6	0.14	0.8	720	0.5	6	4
64	sliced, toasted	490	167	216	28	116	2.0	0.17	1.0	880	0.6	5	5

[a] Wholemeal pitta bread contains 400mg Na, 48mg Ca, 2.7mg Fe and 1.8mg Zn per 100g

Vitamins per 100g edible portion

No.	Food	Retinol µg	Carotene µg	Vitamin D µg	Vitamin E mg	Thiamin mg	Ribo-flavin mg	Niacin mg	Trypt 60 mg	Vitamin B₆ mg	Vitamin B₁₂ µg	Folate µg	Panto-thenate mg	Biotin µg	Vitamin C mg
	Bread, rolls and morning goods continued														
53	**Bread, malted wheat**	0	0	0	0.23	0.24	0.09	2.7	2.4	0.19	0	88	0.5	1	0
54	**Bread, naan**	5	11	0.1	0.64	0.27	0.05	3.0	1.8	N	Tr	15	N	N	Tr
55	peshwari	17	138	N	1.62	0.11	0.03	2.6	1.8	N	Tr	22	0.5	4	Tr
56	**Bread, pitta**, white	0	0	0	N	0.34	0.08	2.2	2.2	N	0	20	N	N	0
57	**Bread, seeded**	0	N	0	N	N	N	N	2.5	N	N	N	N	N	0
58	**Bread, wheatgerm**	0	0	0	0.48	0.34	0.11	3.6	2.5	0.09	0	38	0.5	2	0
59	**Bread, white**, Danish style	0	0	0	Tr	0.25	0.07	2.0	1.7	0.07	0	44	N	N	0
60	farmhouse or split tin	0	0	0	0.22	0.19	0.06	1.4	2.0	0.06	0	23	0.4	3	0
61	French stick	0	0	0	Tr	0.21	0.06	1.7	2.2	0.07	0	29	0.4	1	0
62	premium	0	0	0	0.17	0.23	0.07	1.5	2.1	0.07	0	23	0.5	1	0
63	sliced	0	0	0	Tr	0.24	0.08	1.6	2.0	0.08	0	25	0.4	1	0
64	sliced, toasted	0	0	0	Tr	0.25	0.10	2.0	2.4	0.10	0	30	0.5	1	0

Cereals and cereal products *continued*

Composition of food per 100g edible portion

No.	Food	Description and main data sources	Main data reference	Water g	Total nitrogen g	Protein g	Fat g	Carbo-hydrate g	Energy value kcal	Energy value kJ
Bread, rolls and morning goods continued										
65	**Bread, white**, 'with added fibre'	Including Hovis Best of Both, Kingsmill 50/50 and Warburtons Half & Half Toastie. Industry data, 2013; and calculated		39.2	1.50	8.7	2.2	45.1	224	951
66	'with added fibre', toasted	Calculated using weight loss of 16%		27.6	1.94	10.4	2.6	53.7	266	1132
67	**Bread, wholemeal**, average	Sliced and unsliced. Analytical data, 1998; and industry data, 2013	61	41.2	1.65	9.4	2.5	42.0	217	922
68	toasted	Calculated using weight loss of 14.6%		31.1	1.93	11.2	2.9	49.2	255	1084
69	**Bread rolls, brown**, soft	Analytical data, 1998; and industry data, 2013	61	36.4	1.70	9.9	3.2	44.8	236	1004
70	**Bread rolls, malted wheat**	Pre-packed and freshly baked, including granary products. Analytical data, 1998; and industry data, 2013	61	34.5	1.70	10.0	4.2	42.7	238	1009
71	**Bread rolls, white**, crusty	Analytical data, 1998; and industry data, 2013	61	29.7	1.60	9.2	2.2	54.9	262	1116
72	soft	Analytical data, 1998; and industry data, 2013	61	35.6	1.60	9.3	2.6	51.5	254	1078
73	**Bread rolls, wholemeal**	Analytical data, 1998; and industry data, 2013	61	37.2	1.80	10.4	3.3	46.1	244	1037
74	**Chapatis**, made with fat	Retail. MW4, 1978; and industry data, 2013	4	28.5	1.42	8.1	12.8	48.3	328	1383
75	**Croissants**	Analytical data, 1998; and industry data, 2013	61	24.8	1.50	8.3	19.7	43.3	373	1563
76	**Crumpets**, toasted	Analytical data, 1998; calculated using 16.5% weight loss; and industry data, 2013	61	40.3	1.20	6.9	1.0	45.4	207	881
77	**Currant buns**	Analytical data, 1998; and industry data, 2013	61	27.9	1.40	8.0	5.6	52.6	280	1185
78	toasted	Calculated using weight loss of 10%		19.9	1.56	8.9	6.2	58.4	311	1316
79	**Muffins, English style**, white	Analytical data, 1998	61	40.5	1.80	10.0	1.9	44.2	223	948

Composition of food per 100g edible portion

No.	Food	Starch g	Total sugars g	Individual sugars					Dietary fibre		Fatty acids				Cholest-erol mg
				Gluc g	Fruct g	Sucr g	Malt g	Lact g	NSP g	AOAC g	Satd g	Mono-unsatd g	Poly-unsatd g	Trans g	
	Bread, rolls and morning goods continued														
65	**Bread, white**, 'with added fibre'	41.6	3.5	0.1	0.3	Tr	3.0	0	3.5	4.8	0.4	0.6	0.9	Tr	0
66	'with added fibre', toasted	49.5	4.2	0.1	0.4	Tr	3.6	0	4.2	5.7	0.5	0.7	1.1	Tr	0
67	**Bread, wholemeal**, average	39.3	2.8	0.2	0.4	Tr	2.2	0	5.0	7.0	0.5	0.6	0.8	Tr	0
68	toasted	46.0	3.2	0.2	0.5	Tr	2.5	0	5.9	8.2	0.5	0.7	1.0	0.1	0
69	**Bread rolls, brown**, soft	42.0	2.8	0.5	0.4	Tr	2.0	0	3.8	4.3	1.1	1.0	1.0	Tr	0
70	**Bread rolls, malted wheat**	39.7	3.0	0.3	0.6	Tr	2.0	0	3.6	4.4	1.1	1.1	1.4	Tr	0
71	**Bread rolls, white**, crusty	52.1	2.7	Tr	0.2	Tr	2.6	0	2.4	2.9	0.5	0.5	0.7	Tr	0
72	soft	48.8	2.6	0.2	0.2	Tr	2.2	0	2.0	2.6	0.6	0.6	0.8	Tr	0
73	**Bread rolls, wholemeal**	43.5	2.6	0.5	0.5	Tr	1.7	0	4.4	5.5	0.8	0.9	0.7	Tr	0
74	**Chapatis**, made with fat	46.5	1.8	N	N	N	N	0	N	N	N	N	N	N	N
75	**Croissants**	38.0	5.3	1.2	2.0	Tr	1.9	0.2	1.6	3.1	9.8	5.9	1.8	0.8	52
76	**Crumpets**, toasted	42.3	3.1	1.1	0.3	Tr	1.7	0	2.0	3.1	0.1	0.1	0.5	Tr	0
77	**Currant buns**	36.6	16.0	8.2	7.0	Tr	0.9	Tr	2.2	2.9	1.9	2.0	1.2	Tr	2
78	toasted	40.7	17.8	9.1	7.8	Tr	1.0	Tr	2.4	3.2	2.1	2.2	1.3	Tr	2
79	**Muffins, English style**, white	40.8	3.4	0.5	0.8	Tr	2.1	Tr	1.9	2.6	0.4	0.5	0.6	Tr	0

Cereals and cereal products *continued*

Inorganic constituents per 100g edible portion

No.	Food	Na	K	Ca	Mg	P	Fe	Cu	Zn	Cl	Mn	Se	I
		mg										µg	

Bread, rolls and morning goods continued

No.	Food	Na	K	Ca	Mg	P	Fe	Cu	Zn	Cl	Mn	Se	I
65	**Bread, white, 'with added fibre'**	370	195	N	45	149	2.0	0.19	1.2	650	1.1	7	Tr
66	'with added fibre', toasted	440	232	N	54	177	2.4	0.23	1.4	770	1.3	8	Tr
67	**Bread, wholemeal, average**	400	253	106	66	202	2.4	0.23	1.6	660	1.8	7	N
68	toasted	470	296	124	77	237	2.8	0.27	1.9	770	2.1	11	N
69	**Bread rolls, brown**, soft	380	234	201	49	170	2.4	0.18	1.4	614	1.2	6	6
70	**Bread rolls, malted wheat**	370	191	209	39	138	1.9	0.18	1.1	520	0.8	4	8
71	**Bread rolls, white**, crusty	400	164	177	22	104	1.7	0.13	0.9	540	0.5	4	4
72	soft	400	145	184	23	99	1.5	0.13	0.9	660	0.5	6	4
73	**Bread rolls, wholemeal**	380	248	87	61	197	2.4	0.26	1.7	610	1.5	7	6
74	**Chapatis**, made with fat	300	160	66	41	130	2.3	0.20	1.1	580	1.4	4	N
75	**Croissants**	330	126	75	19	93	1.1	0.05	0.7	510	0.4	8	N
76	**Crumpets**, toasted	480	168	123	17	220	1.4	0.10	0.6	570	0.4	6	1
77	**Currant buns**	230	210	110	27	100	1.9	0.18	0.6	150	0.4	N	N
78	toasted	260	233	122	30	111	2.1	0.20	0.7	170	0.4	N	N
79	**Muffins, English style**, white	431	124	123	20	89	1.3	0.11	0.8	665	0.4	6	N

Bread, rolls and morning goods continued

No.	Food	Retinol µg	Carotene µg	Vitamin D µg	Vitamin E mg	Thiamin mg	Ribo-flavin mg	Niacin mg	Trypt 60 mg	Vitamin B6 mg	Vitamin B12 µg	Folate µg	Panto-thenate mg	Biotin µg	Vitamin C mg
65	**Bread, white**, 'with added fibre'	0	0	0	0.14	0.25	0.07	2.7	2.2	0.10	0	33	0.5	4	0
66	'with added fibre', toasted	0	0	0	0.17	0.25	0.07	3.1	2.6	0.09	0	20	0.5	4	0
67	**Bread, wholemeal**, average	0	0	0	0.28	0.25	0.05	3.8	2.3	0.11	0	40	0.6	6	0
68	toasted	0	0	0	0.33	0.25	0.06	4.5	2.7	0.13	0	46	0.7	7	0
69	**Bread rolls, brown**, soft	0	0	0	Tr	0.29	0.14	3.5	2.6	0.18	0	57	0.5	3	0
70	**Bread rolls, malted wheat**	0	0	0	0.23	0.24	0.09	2.7	2.4	0.19	0	78	0.5	1	0
71	**Bread rolls, white**, crusty	0	0	0	0.23	0.22	0.07	2.0	2.2	0.03	0	31	0.4	1	0
72	soft	0	0	0	0.20	0.20	0.06	1.8	2.0	0.03	0	27	0.4	1	0
73	**Bread rolls, wholemeal**	0	0	0	0.30	0.30	0.09	4.1	2.5	0.10	0	57	0.6	6	0
74	**Chapatis**, made with fat	N	0	N	N	0.26	0.04	1.7	1.7	0.20	0	15	0.2	2	0
75	**Croissants**	163	19	0.1	0.99	0.19	0.16	1.5	1.8	0.11	Tr	47	0.5	9	0
76	**Crumpets**, toasted	0	0	0	0.26	0.23	0.06	1.7	1.8	0.07	0	9	0.3	3	0
77	**Currant buns**	Tr	Tr	0	0.37	0.22	0.16	2.1	1.6	0.11	Tr	12	N	N	1
78	toasted	Tr	Tr	0	0.41	0.24	0.18	2.3	1.8	0.12	Tr	13	N	N	1
79	**Muffins, English style**, white	65	Tr	Tr	0.09	0.24	0.16	2.0	2.1	0.12	Tr	41	0.5	7	Tr

Cereals and cereal products *continued*

Composition of food per 100g edible portion

No.	Food	Description and main data sources	Main data reference	Water g	Total nitrogen g	Protein g	Fat g	Carbo-hydrate g	Energy value kcal	kJ
Bread, rolls and morning goods continued										
80	**Muffins, English style**, white, toasted	Calculated using weight loss of 12.6%		31.9	2.00	11.3	2.7	51.0	261	1108
81	**Puri**	Deep fried chapati, homemade and from cafes. Analytical data, 2007	69	25.0	1.15	7.2	22.3	36.5	366	1531
82	**Tortilla**, wheat, soft	Analytical data, 1998; and industry data, 2013	61	30.6	1.37	7.8	5.7	53.9	285	1206
Sandwiches										
83	**Sandwich, white bread**, bacon, lettuce and tomato	Recipe		51.5	1.39	8.2	11.9	24.1	230	965
84	cheddar cheese and pickle	Recipe		41.4	1.97	12.0	14.4	27.7	282	1184
85	chicken salad	Recipe		58.7	1.78	10.7	4.9	22.5	172	725
86	egg mayonnaise	Recipe		47.5	1.49	8.8	11.2	28.5	243	1020
87	ham salad	Recipe		58.5	1.38	8.2	4.1	25.0	163	690
88	tuna mayonnaise	Recipe		48.7	2.08	12.5	10.2	25.3	237	994
Breakfast cereals										
89	**Bran type cereal**, fortified	Including All-Bran and own brand. Analytical data, 2002; and industry data, 2013	67	4.0	1.97	12.4	3.4	49.7	267	1132
90	**Bran flakes**, fortified	Including Kellogg's and own brands. Analytical data, 2002; and industry data, 2013	67	4.0	1.65	9.6	2.2	73.3	333	1417

Cereals and cereal products *continued*

80 to 90

Composition of food per 100g edible portion

No.	Food	Starch g	Total sugars g	Individual sugars					Dietary fibre		Fatty acids				Cholesterol mg
				Gluc g	Fruct g	Sucr g	Malt g	Lact g	NSP g	AOAC g	Satd g	Mono-unsatd g	Poly-unsatd g	Trans g	
	Bread, rolls and morning goods continued														
80	**Muffins, English style**, white, toasted	47.3	3.8	0.5	0.8	Tr	2.4	Tr	2.2	3.0	0.4	0.5	0.7	Tr	0
81	**Puri**	35.3	1.2	Tr	Tr	0.5	0.6	0	4.0	3.5	2.7	7.3	10.9	Tr	30
82	**Tortilla**, wheat, soft	51.9	2.0	Tr	0.4	Tr	1.6	0	1.9	3.6	2.5	2.0	0.8	Tr	Tr
	Sandwiches														
83	**Sandwich, white bread**, bacon, lettuce and tomato	21.7	2.4	0.2	0.4	0.1	1.6	Tr	1.2[a]	1.5[b]	2.5	5.4	3.1	Tr	17
84	cheddar cheese and pickle	23.1	4.6	0.9	1.1	0.9	1.7	Tr	1.1[a]	1.5[b]	7.4	3.9	1.9	0.5	30
85	chicken salad	20.4	2.1	0.2	0.4	0	1.5	0	1.1[a]	1.4[b]	1.2	1.7	1.6	Tr	26
86	egg mayonnaise	26.2	2.2	0	0.1	0.1	2.0	0	1.2[a]	1.5[b]	1.9	5.0	3.2	Tr	103
87	ham salad	22.5	2.5	0.2	0.4	0.2	1.7	Tr	1.2[a]	1.6[b]	0.9	1.2	1.5	Tr	12
88	tuna mayonnaise	23.2	2.1	0	0.1	0.1	1.7	Tr	1.0[a]	1.4[b]	1.3	5.0	3.2	Tr	20
	Breakfast cereals														
89	**Bran type cereal**, fortified	29.7	20.0	0.7	0.7	17.5	1.1	0	23.0	24.6	0.5	0.5	1.8	Tr	Tr
90	**Bran flakes**, fortified	52.3	21.0	2.0	2.6	15.9	0.5	0	12.8	13.4	0.3	0.2	1.1	Tr	0

[a] Average NSP content of sandwiches made with wholemeal bread is 2.8g per 100g

[b] Average AOAC fibre content of sandwiches made with wholemeal bread is 3.9g per 100g

Inorganic constituents per 100g edible portion

No.	Food	Na	K	Ca	Mg	P	Fe	Cu	Zn	Cl	Mn	Se	I
						mg						µg	
Bread, rolls and morning goods continued													
80	**Muffins, English style**, white, toasted	493	142	141	23	102	1.5	0.13	0.9	760	0.5	7	N
81	**Puri**	279	180	109	39	153	2.5	0.22	1.1	430	1.4	4	Tr
82	**Tortilla**, wheat, soft	622	126	148	18	212	1.6	0.09	0.6	N	0.4	3	Tr
Sandwiches													
83	**Sandwich, white bread**, bacon, lettuce and tomato	477	177	95	17	84	1.0	0.09	0.7	795	0.3	5	4
84	cheddar cheese and pickle	591	107	321	22	206	1.0	0.08	1.7	883	0.3	5	11
85	chicken salad	235	196	91	20	105	1.0	0.10	0.8	414	0.3	7	4
86	egg mayonnaise	323	124	124	18	115	1.5	0.11	0.9	553	0.3	11	17
87	**ham salad**	405	190	98	19	126	1.0	0.11	0.8	639	0.3	6	4
88	tuna mayonnaise	350	151	100	21	108	1.4	0.10	0.7	617	0.3	26	7
Breakfast cereals													
89	**Bran type cereal**, fortified	360	757	329[a]	189	639	10.7[b]	0.82	5.1	550	5.8	7	3
90	**Bran flakes**, fortified	360	480	44	121	357	13.5	0.42	2.1	550	2.5	6	Tr

[a] Some products are not fortified with calcium and contain 34mg per 100g

[b] Value is average of fortified products (range 8.8mg to 14.0mg per 100g)

Vitamins per 100g edible portion

No.	Food	Retinol µg	Carotene µg	Vitamin D µg	Vitamin E mg	Thiamin mg	Ribo-flavin mg	Niacin mg	Trypt 60 mg	Vitamin B6 mg	Vitamin B12 µg	Folate µg	Panto-thenate mg	Biotin µg	Vitamin C mg
Bread, rolls and morning goods continued															
80	**Muffins, English style**, white, toasted	74	Tr	Tr	0.10	0.27	0.18	2.3	2.4	0.14	Tr	47	0.6	8	Tr
81	**Puri**	N	0	0	6.76	0.19	0.01	1.9	1.7	0.20	0	32	0.2	2	0
82	**Tortilla**, wheat, soft	0	0	0	N	0.27	0.01	1.4	1.5	0.07	0	8	0.1	1	0
Sandwiches															
83	**Sandwich, white bread**, bacon, lettuce and tomato	30	66	0.3	2.66	0.34	0.08	2.2	1.7	0.14	0.2	23	0.5	1	3
84	cheddar cheese and pickle	141	94	0.4	1.46	0.14	0.16	0.9	3.1	0.09	0.7	23	0.4	2	Tr
85	chicken salad	26	64	0.3	1.15	0.15	0.08	3.2	2.3	0.14	Tr	22	0.6	1	3
86	egg mayonnaise	66	21	1.1	3.10	0.17	0.18	1.0	2.2	0.08	0.6	24	0.6	5	Tr
87	ham salad	25	63	0.2	1.21	0.31	0.08	2.3	1.7	0.18	0.2	24	0.5	1	2
88	tuna mayonnaise	40	19	0.6	3.15	0.13	0.09	4.2	3.1	0.15	1.1	15	0.3	1	Tr
Breakfast cereals															
89	**Bran type cereal**, fortified	0	54	3.9[a]	N	1.00	1.20	13.4	3.1	1.30	1.7	200	N	N[b]	N[c]
90	**Bran flakes**, fortified	0	0	4.6[a]	8.30	1.10	1.40	15.6	2.4	1.40	2.3	367	N[d]	7	0

[a] Value relates to fortified products

[b] Products fortified with biotin contain 150µg per 100g

[c] Products fortified with vitamin C contain 58mg per 100g

[d] Products fortified with pantothenate contain between 6.0mg and 6.9mg per 100g

Composition of food per 100g edible portion

No.	Food	Description and main data sources	Main data reference	Water g	Total nitrogen g	Protein g	Fat g	Carbo-hydrate g	Energy value kcal	kJ
	Breakfast cereals continued									
91	**Cornflakes**, fortified	Including Kellogg's, other brands and own brands. Analytical data, 2002; and industry data, 2013	67	3.4	1.14	7.1	0.8	90.9	376	1605
92	unfortified	Organic. Analytical data, 2002; and industry data, 2013	67	3.4	1.14	7.1	0.8	91.4	378	1613
93	crunchy/honey nut coated, fortified	Including Crunchy Nut Corn Flakes and own brand. Analytical data, 2002; and industry data, 2013	67	2.9	0.85	5.3	4.2	86.6	384	1631
94	frosted, fortified	Including Frosties and own brand. Analytical data, 2002; and industry data, 2013	67	3.1	0.75	4.7	0.5	87.0	350	1490
95	**Crunchy clusters type cereal,** without nuts, unfortified	Including Jordans Country Crisp, Quaker Oat Granola and own brand. Analytical data, 2010	72	3.0	1.23	7.2	11.6	71.0[a]	399	1687
96	**Crunchy/crispy muesli type cereal,** with nuts, unfortified	Including Jordans Country Crisp, Kellogg's Crunchy Nut Clusters and own brand. Analytical data, 2010	72	3.3	1.45	8.4	20.5	61.9[a]	450	1892
97	**Fruit and fibre type cereal,** fortified	Including Kellogg's Fruit 'n Fibre and own brand. Analytical data, 2002; and industry data, 2013	67	5.7	1.38	8.0	5.8	70.3	348	1475
98	**Honey loops and hoops,** fortified	Including Honey Loops and own brands. Based on Honey Nut Cheerios and products containing nuts. Analytical data, 2002; and industry data, 2013	67	3.6	1.13	6.6	3.1	78.7[a]	349	1486
99	**Malted flake cereal,** fortified	Including Special K and own brand. Analytical data, 2002; and industry data, 2013	67	4.1	1.98	11.8	1.4	83.4	373	1587
100	**Malted wheat cereal,** fortified	Including Shreddies and own brand. Analytical data, 2002; and industry data, 2013	67	4.3	1.49	8.7	2.3	75.7[a]	339	1444

[a] Oligosaccharides may be present, but levels are unknown

Cereals and cereal products *continued*

Composition of food per 100g edible portion

No.	Food	Starch	Total sugars	Individual sugars					Dietary fibre		Fatty acids				Cholest-
				Gluc	Fruct	Sucr	Malt	Lact	NSP	AOAC	Satd	Mono-unsatd	Poly-unsatd	Trans	erol
		g	g	g	g	g	g	g	g	g	g	g	g	g	mg
Breakfast cereals continued															
91	**Cornflakes**, fortified	83.6	7.3	1.7	1.5	4.1	Tr	0	1.8	2.6	0.1	0.1	0.3	Tr	0
92	unfortified	88.4	3.0	0.7	0.6	1.7	Tr	0	1.8	2.6	0.1	0.1	0.3	Tr	0
93	crunchy/honey nut coated, fortified	49.2	37.4	2.7	1.6	33.1	Tr	0	1.2	3.8	0.7	2.3	1.0	Tr	0
94	frosted, fortified	48.7	38.3	1.1	1.0	36.2	Tr	0	N	2.0	0.1	0.1	0.2	Tr	0
95	**Crunchy clusters type cereal**, without nuts, unfortified	45.7	25.3	3.6	3.8	16.6	1.3	0	4.3	7.2	4.2	4.5	2.3	Tr	N
96	**Crunchy/crispy muesli type cereal**, with nuts, unfortified	38.7	23.1	1.4	1.6	20.2	Tr	0	4.4	7.9	4.6	10.6	4.2	Tr	N
97	**Fruit and fibre type cereal**, fortified	44.1	26.2	8.4	9.4	8.4	Tr	0	8.6	8.6	2.7	0.9	0.6	Tr	Tr
98	**Honey loops and hoops**, fortified	44.0	34.7	1.4	1.6	31.0	0.7	0	4.4	4.3	0.7	1.0	1.2	Tr	0
99	**Malted flake cereal**, fortified	66.2	17.2	0.3	0.5	14.9	0.5	1.0	2.7	3.0	0.3	0.2	0.6	Tr	Tr
100	**Malted wheat cereal**, fortified	55.4	20.3	0.3	0.4	18.9	0.7	0	8.3	8.6	0.3	0.5	0.8	Tr	Tr

Cereals and cereal products *continued*

Inorganic constituents per 100g edible portion

No.	Food	Na	K	Ca	Mg	P	Fe	Cu	Zn	Cl	Mn	Se	I
		mg										µg	
		Na	K	Ca	Mg	P	Fe	Cu	Zn	Cl	Mn	Se	I

Breakfast cereals continued

No.	Food	Na	K	Ca	Mg	P	Fe	Cu	Zn	Cl	Mn	Se	I
91	**Cornflakes**, fortified	450	88	3	12	46	11.8	Tr	0.2	690	0.1	9	Tr
92	unfortified	410	93	7	11	53	0.4	Tr	0.2	620	0.1	9	Tr
93	crunchy/honey nut coated, fortified	350	123	15	24	57	12.0	0.12	0.3	560	0.2	5	Tr
94	frosted, fortified	300	59	456[a]	9	33	12.0	Tr	0.1	470	0.1	5	9
95	**Crunchy clusters type cereal**, without nuts, unfortified	41	310	40	72	232	2.7	0.30	1.6	100	2.1	6	2
96	**Crunchy/crispy muesli type cereal**, with nuts, unfortified	138	290	46	83	245	N[b]	0.34	1.8	240	2.3	19	3
97	**Fruit and fibre type cereal**, fortified	350	444	47	71	209	10.9	0.40	1.3	490	1.7	4	2
98	**Honey loops and hoops**, fortified	280	219	265[c]	54	240	9.4	0.22	1.3	310	1.8	2	Tr
99	**Malted flake cereal**, fortified	380	216	66[d]	46	174	N[e]	0.16	1.6	600	1.4	8	14
100	**Malted wheat cereal**, fortified	250	348	36	70	229	10.6	0.28	1.5	400	1.7	4	3

[a] Value relates to fortified products, non-fortified products contain approximately 7mg per 100g

[b] Products fortified with Fe typically contain 5.3mg per 100g

[c] Value relates to fortified products

[d] Ca from dried skimmed milk powder, not from fortification. Where products are also fortified, Ca content is 315mg per 100g

[e] Products fortified with Fe contain between 11.6mg and 23.1mg per 100g

Vitamins per 100g edible portion

No.	Food	Retinol	Carotene	Vitamin D	Vitamin E	Thiamin	Ribo-flavin	Niacin	Trypt 60	Vitamin B6	Vitamin B12	Folate	Panto-thenate	Biotin	Vitamin C
		μg	μg	μg	mg	mg	mg	mg	mg	mg	μg	μg	mg	μg	mg
Breakfast cereals continued															
91	**Cornflakes**, fortified	0	125	4.7	0.14	1.10	1.40	15.8	0.6	1.50	1.9	N[a]	N[b]	2	0
92	unfortified	0	125	0	0.14	Tr	0.08	0.8	0.6	0.13	Tr	7	0.2	2	0
93	crunchy/honey nut coated, fortified	0	125	N[c]	0.44	1.10	1.40	15.5	0.6	1.50	2.0	396	N[c]	N	0
94	frosted, fortified	0	125	4.7	0.14	1.20	1.40	16.0	0.6	1.60	1.7	N[d]	N[d]	2	0
95	**Crunchy clusters type cereal**, without nuts, unfortified	0	Tr	0	1.38	1.02	1.06	4.0	2.8	0.17	0	90	0.3	9	Tr
96	**Crunchy/crispy muesli type cereal**, with nuts, unfortified	0	Tr	0	3.26	0.16	0.07	1.0	2.0	0.27	0	21	0.8	10	Tr
97	**Fruit and fibre type cereal**, fortified	0	Tr	N[e]	1.36	1.00	1.20	13.2	1.7	1.30	N[e]	210	N[e]	3	Tr
98	**Honey loops and hoops**, fortified	0	N	4.5[f]	N	1.00	1.20	14.0	N	1.20[f]	2.1[f]	170[f]	5.0[f]	N	67[f]
99	**Malted flake cereal**, fortified	0	0	8.3[g]	0.31	1.60	2.10	23.6	2.5	2.10	3.4	300	N[h]	2	134[i]
100	**Malted wheat cereal**, fortified	0	0	0.4	0.85	0.80	1.10	12.1	2.2	1.10	1.9	150	4.5	N	0

[a] Products fortified with folate contain between 166μg and 400μg per 100g

[b] Products fortified with pantothenate contain 6.0mg per 100g

[c] Fortified products contain 5.0μg vitamin D and 6.0mg pantothenate per 100g

[d] Fortified products contain between 166μg and 400μg folate and 6.0mg pantothenate per 100g

[e] Fortified products contain between 3.5μg and 5.0μg vitamin D;
0.9μg and 2.5μg vitamin B12 4.2mg and 6.0mg pantothenate per 100g

[f] Value relates to fortified products

[g] Value reflects brand leader. Fortification ranges from 5.0μg to 8.3μg per 100g

[h] Products fortified with pantothenate contain between 6.0mg and 9.9mg per 100g

[i] Value reflects brand leader. Fortification ranges from 80mg to 134mg per 100g

Cereals and cereal products *continued*

Composition of food per 100g edible portion

No.	Food	Description and main data sources	Main data reference	Water g	Total nitrogen g	Protein g	Fat g	Carbo-hydrate g	Energy value kcal	kJ
Breakfast cereals continued										
101	**Muesli**, Swiss style, unfortified	Including Alpen and own brand. Analytical data, 2002[a]	67	7.5	1.58	9.2	6.3	72.6	366	1551
102	Swiss style, no added sugar or salt, unfortified	Including Jordans Natural Muesli and own brands. Analytical data, 2002[a]	67	9.2	1.68	9.8	5.9	70.7	357	1516
103	**Multigrain hoops**, fortified	Including Cheerios and own brands. Industry data, 1999, 2013 and 2014	67	N	1.26	7.9	3.8	80.7[b]	368	1566
104	**Oat cereal, instant**, plain, fortified, raw	Including Ready Brek and own brands. Analytical data, 2002; and industry data, 2013	67	6.7	1.88	11.0	7.3	64.6[b]	352	1491
105	plain, fortified, cooked, made up with semi-skimmed milk	Including Ready Brek and own brands. 40g oat cereal made up with 200g milk. Analytical data, 2002	67	77.5	0.77	4.9	2.5	14.2[b]	95	403
106	flavoured, unfortified, cooked, made up with semi-skimmed milk	Quaker Oat So Simple, including golden syrup, berry and baked apple flavour. 36g sachet made up with 180g milk. Analytical data, 2002; and industry data, 2013	67	75.4	0.69	4.4	2.4	15.6	98	413
107	**Porridge oats**, unfortified	Quaker and other/own brands. Analytical data, 2002	67	9.4	1.87	10.9	8.1	70.7	381	1614
108	unfortified, cooked, made up with semi-skimmed milk	Quaker and other/own brands. Analytical data, 2002	67	79.7	0.73	4.6	2.3	12.1	84	357
109	**Puffed wheat cereal**, unfortified	Including Quaker Puffed Wheat and own brands. Analytical data, 2002	67	3.5	2.26	13.2	2.0	72.0	341	1450
110	honey coated, fortified	Including Sugar Puffs and own brand. Analytical data, 2002; and industry data, 2013	67	2.7	0.80	4.7	1.2	86.8[b]	355	1513

[a] Muesli composition is very variable

[b] Oligosaccharides may be present, but levels are unknown

Cereals and cereal products *continued*

Composition of food per 100g edible portion

No.	Food	Starch	Total sugars	Individual sugars					Dietary fibre		Fatty acids				Cholest-
				Gluc	Fruct	Sucr	Malt	Lact	NSP	AOAC	Satd	Mono-unsatd	Poly-unsatd	Trans	erol
		g	g	g	g	g	g	g	g	g	g	g	g	g	mg

Breakfast cereals continued

No.	Food	Starch	Total sugars	Gluc	Fruct	Sucr	Malt	Lact	NSP	AOAC	Satd	Mono-unsatd	Poly-unsatd	Trans	Cholesterol
101	**Muesli**, Swiss style, unfortified	51.3	21.3	4.9	5.0	7.4	Tr	4.0	6.7	8.8	1.3	3.0	1.7	Tr	2
102	Swiss style, no added sugar or salt, unfortified	57.7	13.0	4.6	5.2	Tr	Tr	3.2	8.4	8.5	1.2	2.8	1.6	Tr	2
103	**Multigrain hoops**, fortified	58.3	22.4	N	N	N	N	0	N	5.7	0.7	N	N	Tr	0
104	**Oat cereal, instant**, plain, fortified, raw	64.1	0.5	Tr	Tr	0.2	0.3	0	8.3	8.5	1.2	2.9	2.8	Tr	Tr
105	plain, fortified, cooked, made up with semi-skimmed milk	10.0	4.2	Tr	Tr	Tr	Tr	4.2	2.0	2.0	1.1	0.8	0.4	0.1	3
106	flavoured, unfortified, cooked, made up with semi-skimmed milk	7.8	7.8	Tr	Tr	4.1	Tr	3.7	0.7	1.0	1.1	0.7	0.4	0.1	3
107	**Porridge oats**, unfortified	70.4	0.3	Tr	Tr	0.3	Tr	0	7.2	7.8	1.3	3.1	3.2	Tr	Tr
108	unfortified, cooked, made up with semi-skimmed milk	8.0	4.1	Tr	Tr	Tr	Tr	4.1	0.9	1.0	1.0	0.7	0.4	0.1	3
109	**Puffed wheat cereal**, unfortified	71.8	0.2	Tr	0.2	Tr	Tr	0	5.8	7.8	0.3	0.3	1.1	Tr	0
110	honey coated, fortified	N	36.8	N	N	N	N	0	2.7	3.1	0.2	0.3	0.5	Tr	0

Cereals and cereal products *continued*

Inorganic constituents per 100g edible portion

No.	Food	mg										µg	
		Na	K	Ca	Mg	P	Fe	Cu	Zn	Cl	Mn	Se	I
Breakfast cereals continued													
101	**Muesli**, Swiss style, unfortified	138	531	93	92	318	2.7	0.39	1.7	277	2.3	5	19
102	Swiss style, no added sugar or salt, unfortified	66	539	78	87	303	2.7	0.41	1.5	188	2.0	5	19
103	**Multigrain hoops**, fortified	330	N	484[a]	N	N	12.8[a]	N	N	N	N	N	N
104	**Oat cereal, instant**, plain, fortified, raw	5	343	1336	104	365	11.9	0.26	2.0	81	3.7	5	5
105	plain, fortified, cooked, made up with semi-skimmed milk	40	199	323	28	145	2.0	Tr	0.7	108	0.6	3	30
106	flavoured, unfortified, cooked, made up with semi-skimmed milk	70	195	115	24	132	0.5	Tr	0.6	N	0.4	2	23
107	**Porridge oats**, unfortified	1	372	50	114	387	3.6	0.37	2.3	87	3.7	3	Tr
108	unfortified, cooked, made up with semi-skimmed milk	39	202	117	28	145	0.6	Tr	0.7	123	0.7	2	23
109	**Puffed wheat cereal**, unfortified	2	410	27	120	356	2.5	0.36	2.7	76	2.3	53	Tr
110	honey coated, fortified	20	188	16	49	148	8.0[a]	0.14	1.1	83	1.1	18	Tr

[a] Value reflects brand leader

64

Vitamins per 100g edible portion

No.	Food	Retinol	Carotene	Vitamin D	Vitamin E	Thiamin	Ribo-flavin	Niacin	Trypt 60	Vitamin B6	Vitamin B12	Folate	Panto-thenate	Biotin	Vitamin C
		µg	µg	µg	mg	mg	mg	mg	mg	mg	µg	µg	mg	µg	mg
Breakfast cereals continued															
101	**Muesli**, Swiss style, unfortified	Tr	Tr	0	0.52	0.17	0.37	6.9	2.3	0.53	0	45	0.6	6	Tr
102	**Muesli**, Swiss style, no added sugar or salt, unfortified	Tr	Tr	0	0.52	0.17	0.37	6.9	2.3	0.53	0	45	0.6	6	Tr
103	**Multigrain hoops**, fortified	0	N	3.0[a,b]	N	0.90[b]	0.90[a]	11.8[a]	N	1.00[a]	2.0[b]	170[b]	3.7[a]	N	48[a,b]
104	**Oat cereal, instant**, plain, fortified, raw	0	0	4.3	0.31	0.90	1.20	13.6	2.7	1.20	2.1	170	0.8	13	Tr
105	plain, fortified, cooked, made up with semi-skimmed milk	16	8	0.7	0.14	0.18	0.27	2.4	1.0	0.34	1.1	36	0.7	4	Tr
106	flavoured, unfortified, cooked, made up with semi-skimmed milk	16	Tr	Tr	0.14	Tr	0.14	0.2	1.2	0.06	Tr	10	0.5	2	Tr
107	**Porridge oats**, unfortified	0	0	0	0.59	1.05	0.05	0.8	2.7	0.34	0	32	0.8	19	0
108	unfortified, cooked, made up with semi-skimmed milk	17	8	Tr	0.20	Tr	0.14	0.2	0.8	0.09	0.4	10	0.6	6	1
109	**Puffed wheat cereal**, unfortified	0	0	0	0.99	Tr	0.03	8.6	2.2	0.11	0	13	0.4	8	0
110	honey coated, fortified	0	0	0	0.57	1.00[a]	1.00[a]	10.0[a]	1.0	0.36	0	13	1.0	5	0

[a] Value reflects brand leader

[b] Value relates to fortified products

65

Cereals and cereal products *continued*

Composition of food per 100g edible portion

No.	Food	Description and main data sources	Main data reference	Water g	Total nitrogen g	Protein g	Fat g	Carbo-hydrate g	Energy value kcal	kJ
Breakfast cereals *continued*										
111	**Rice cereal**, toasted/crisp, fortified	Including Rice Krispies and own brand. Analytical data, 2002; and industry data, 2013	67	3.3	0.97	5.7	1.0	91.2	374	1593
112	chocolate flavoured, fortified	Including Coco Pops and own brand. Analytical data, 2002; and industry data, 2013	67	3.3	0.77	4.6	2.3	89.6	375	1597
113	**Shredded wheat type cereal**, unfortified	Including Shredded Wheat and bitesize and own brand. Analytical data, 2002	67	5.8	1.87	10.9	2.5	71.2	333	1417
114	with fruit, unfortified	Including Raisin Wheats and own brand apricot wheats. Analytical data, 2002; and industry data, 2013	67	9.9	1.43	8.4	1.7	74.0	326	1389
115	**Wheat and multigrain cereal**, chocolate flavoured, fortified	Including Weetos, Nesquik, Coco Shreddies and own brands. Analytical data, 2002; and industry data, 2013	67	3.3	1.12	6.5	4.1	83.2	375	1594
116	**Wheat biscuits**, Weetabix type, fortified	Including Weetabix and own brands. Analytical data, 2002; and industry data, 2013	67	6.0	1.80	10.5	1.9	72.7	332	1412
117	Weetabix type, unfortified	Organic and value products. Analytical data, 2002	67	6.0	1.80	10.5	1.9	72.7	332	1412
Biscuits										
118	**Biscuits, cheese flavoured**	Including Cheddars, Mini Cheddars, Cheese Melts and cheese savouries. Analytical data, 2008	70	3.1	1.84	10.5	28.1	53.2	494	2069
119	**Biscuits, cookies**, chocolate chip, American style	Including milk, plain and white chocolate from instore bakeries and catering outlets. Analytical data, 2008	70	6.9	0.91	5.2	21.3	60.6	440	1845

Composition of food per 100g edible portion

No.	Food	Starch	Total sugars	Individual sugars					Dietary fibre		Fatty acids				Cholest-erol
				Gluc	Fruct	Sucr	Malt	Lact	NSP	AOAC	Satd	Mono-unsatd	Poly-unsatd	Trans	
		g	g	g	g	g	g	g	g	g	g	g	g	g	mg
Breakfast cereals continued															
111	**Rice cereal**, toasted/crisp, fortified	78.8	12.4	0.3	0.5	11.6	Tr	0	0.9	0.7	0.2	0.2	0.3	Tr	0
112	chocolate flavoured, fortified	51.9	37.7	0.5	0.4	36.9	Tr	0	1.5	2.0	1.2	0.7	0.3	Tr	Tr
113	**Shredded wheat type cereal**, unfortified	70.6	0.6	Tr	Tr	0.6	0	0	10.5	12.2	0.3	0.3	1.2	Tr	0
114	with fruit, unfortified	55.3	18.7	4.7	6.0	8.0	0	0	7.8	8.8	0.3	0.2	0.8	Tr	0
115	**Wheat and multigrain cereal**, chocolate flavoured, fortified	52.7	30.5	0.2	0.1	30.0	Tr	0.2	5.8	6.3	1.4	1.6	0.9	Tr	Tr
116	**Wheat biscuits**, Weetabix type, fortified	68.8	3.9	0.7	0.9	1.9	0.4	0	7.3	9.7	0.3	0.2	0.9	Tr	0
117	Weetabix type, unfortified	68.8	3.9	0.7	0.9	1.9	0.4	0	7.3	9.7	0.3	0.2	0.9	Tr	0
Biscuits															
118	**Biscuits, cheese flavoured**	50.5	2.7	Tr	Tr	2.7	Tr	Tr	2.4	4.5	11.7	12.2	2.6	0.1	18
119	**Biscuits, cookies,** chocolate chip, American style	20.0	40.5	Tr	Tr	40.5	Tr	Tr	1.8	2.5	9.6	8.0	2.6	0.1	36

Inorganic constituents per 100g edible portion

No.	Food	Na	K	Ca	Mg	P	Fe	Cu	Zn	Cl	Mn	Se	I
						mg						μg	

Breakfast cereals continued

No.	Food	Na	K	Ca	Mg	P	Fe	Cu	Zn	Cl	Mn	Se	I
111	**Rice cereal**, toasted/crisp, fortified	370	146	9	41	141	11.0	0.24	2.6	540	0.9	2	Tr
112	chocolate flavoured, fortified	320	146	456[a]	41	141	11.0	0.24	2.6	500	0.9	2	Tr
113	**Shredded wheat type cereal**, unfortified	4	340	39	86	271	2.8	0.50	1.8	105	2.2	14	Tr
114	with fruit, unfortified	21	388	34	61	195	3.5	0.39	1.2	105	1.5	14	N
115	**Wheat and multigrain cereal**, chocolate flavoured, fortified	180	355	N[b]	52	143	10.7	0.35	1.0	280	0.9	3	2
116	**Wheat biscuits**, Weetabix type, fortified	260	397	30	83	259	11.9	0.39	1.7	479	1.8	5	Tr
117	Weetabix type, unfortified	278	415	36	107	310	3.5	0.38	2.3	512	2.8	5	Tr

Biscuits

No.	Food	Na	K	Ca	Mg	P	Fe	Cu	Zn	Cl	Mn	Se	I
118	**Biscuits, cheese flavoured**	882	247	263	34	249	2.1	0.16	1.4	650	0.8	5	Tr
119	**Biscuits, cookies**, chocolate chip, American style	422	252	108	36	155	2.5	0.17	0.7	280	0.4	12	6

[a] Value relates to fortified products, non-fortified products contain approximately 9mg per 100g

[b] Products fortified with Ca contain between 267mg and 487mg per 100g

Vitamins per 100g edible portion

No.	Food	Retinol µg	Carotene µg	Vitamin D µg	Vitamin E mg	Thiamin mg	Ribo-flavin mg	Niacin mg	Trypt 60 mg	Vitamin B₆ mg	Vitamin B₁₂ µg	Folate µg	Panto-thenate mg	Biotin µg	Vitamin C mg
	Breakfast cereals continued														
111	**Rice cereal**, toasted/crisp, fortified	0	0	4.6	0.16	1.10	1.40	15.3	1.6	1.50	1.8	180	N[a]	2	0
112	chocolate flavoured, fortified	Tr	Tr	4.6	N	1.10	1.40	15.2	1.2	1.50	1.9	180	N[a]	N	0
113	**Shredded wheat type cereal**, unfortified	0	0	0	0.57	0.15	0.04	5.2	2.7	0.18	0	27	0.7	7	0
114	with fruit, unfortified	0	30	0.1	0.71	0.30	0.28	5.4	1.9	0.74	0	112	0.6	3	Tr
115	**Wheat and multigrain cereal**, chocolate flavoured, fortified	Tr	Tr	N	0.79	1.00	1.20	13.6	1.2	1.40	1.4	170	N[b]	N	N[c]
116	**Wheat biscuits**, Weetabix type, fortified	0	0	0	1.45	1.00	1.20	14.0	2.2	0.22	0	170	0.8	6	0
117	Weetabix type, unfortified	0	0	0	1.45	Tr	0.06	6.4	2.6	0.26	0	36	0.8	8	0
	Biscuits														
118	**Biscuits, cheese flavoured**	49	Tr	Tr	8.71	0.25	0.10	2.1	2.1	0.07	0.2	35	0.8	6	0
119	**Biscuits, cookies**, chocolate chip, American style	Tr	Tr	Tr	2.39	0.07	0.08	0.8	1.1	0.05	0.3	12	0.5	5	0

[a] Products fortified with pantothenate contain 6.0mg per 100g

[b] Products fortified with pantothenate contain between 3.1mg and 5.1mg per 100g

[c] Products fortified with vitamin C contain between 51mg and 62mg per 100g

Cereals and cereal products *continued*

Composition of food per 100g edible portion

Biscuits continued

No.	Food	Description and main data sources	Main data reference	Water g	Total nitrogen g	Protein g	Fat g	Carbohydrate g	Energy value kcal	kJ
120	**Biscuits, cookies**, chocolate chip, standard	Including Maryland, Fox's and own brand. Analytical data, 2008	70	3.6	0.94	5.4	24.9	60.0	471	1973
121	**Biscuits, digestive**, half coated in chocolate	Including milk and plain chocolate. Analytical data, 2008	70	1.8	1.11	6.3	25.7	61.8	488	2047
122	plain	Analytical data, 2008	70	2.8	1.09	6.2	21.3	65.6	463	1943
123	with oats, plain	Including Hobnobs and own brands. Analytical data, 2008	70	3.0	1.09	6.4	22.9	66.4	480	2017
124	**Biscuits, fully coated with chocolate**	Including Breakaway, Rocky and chocolate fingers. Analytical data, 2008	70	1.9	1.12	6.4	27.2	62.8	506	2120
125	with cream	Including Penguin, Club, Classic and own brands. Analytical data, 2008	70	1.6	0.90	5.2	28.2	59.0	496	2075
126	with marshmallow	Including teacakes and Wagon Wheels. Analytical data, 2008	70	9.8	0.78	4.5	19.0	59.9	413	1737
127	**Biscuits, ginger nuts**	Analytical data, 2008	70	3.3	0.84	4.8	15.7	75.3	443	1867
128	**Biscuits, iced**	Including Party Rings and Iced Gems. Analytical data, 2008	70	2.8	0.85	4.8	10.8	77.1	406	1715
129	**Biscuits, jam filled**	Including Jammie Dodgers and own brands. Analytical data, 2008	70	6.5	0.92	5.2	14.4	74.0	428	1806
130	**Biscuits, plain**, reduced fat	Including reduced fat digestives and rich teas. Analytical data, 2008	70	3.1	1.16	6.6	13.5	75.7	432	1823

Composition of food per 100g edible portion

Biscuits continued

No.	Food	Starch	Total sugars	Individual sugars					Dietary fibre		Fatty acids				Cholest-erol
				Gluc	Fruct	Sucr	Malt	Lact	NSP	AOAC	Satd	Mono-unsatd	Poly-unsatd	Trans	
		g	g	g	g	g	g	g	g	g	g	g	g	g	mg
120	**Biscuits, cookies,** chocolate chip, standard	30.0	30.0	Tr	Tr	30.0	Tr	Tr	2.2	3.0	12.2	9.0	2.5	Tr	3
121	**Biscuits, digestive,** half coated in chocolate	37.5	24.3	Tr	Tr	24.3	Tr	Tr	3.1	2.1	12.7	8.9	2.4	Tr	6
122	plain	48.1	17.5	Tr	Tr	17.5	Tr	Tr	2.7	3.8	7.7	10.2	2.3	Tr	2
123	with oats, plain	40.5	25.9	1.2	0.9	23.9	Tr	Tr	4.4	7.2	5.9	12.7	3.1	Tr	10
124	**Biscuits, fully coated with chocolate**	23.5	39.3	Tr	Tr	33.3	Tr	5.9	2.2	1.7	15.1	8.8	1.8	0.1	17
125	with cream	21.6	37.4	Tr	Tr	34.1	Tr	3.3	1.9	3.1	15.8	9.0	2.0	0.1	18
126	with marshmallow	18.5	41.4	6.0	Tr	28.7	6.7	Tr	1.6	2.7	10.6	6.1	1.3	Tr	6
127	**Biscuits, ginger nuts**	44.0	31.3	3.0	2.4	22.6	3.3	Tr	1.5	2.2	7.3	5.9	1.7	Tr	3
128	**Biscuits, iced**	32.5	44.6	Tr	Tr	44.6	Tr	Tr	1.6	0.6	5.0	3.9	1.4	Tr	7
129	**Biscuits, jam filled**	41.0	33.0	6.1	2.1	19.4	5.4	Tr	2.1	1.2	6.8	5.3	1.7	Tr	5
130	**Biscuits, plain,** reduced fat	54.5	21.2	0.9	Tr	20.3	Tr	Tr	2.7	4.4	4.3	6.6	1.9	Tr	2

Inorganic constituents per 100g edible portion

No.	Food	Na	K	Ca	Mg	P	Fe	Cu	Zn	Cl	Mn	Se	I
		mg										μg	

Biscuits continued

No.	Food	Na	K	Ca	Mg	P	Fe	Cu	Zn	Cl	Mn	Se	I
120	**Biscuits, cookies**, chocolate chip, standard	298	217	117	34	132	2.3	0.22	0.7	198	0.6	4	6
121	**Biscuits, digestive**, half coated in chocolate	351	258	100	37	124	2.1	0.32	0.8	280	0.7	3	8
122	plain	561	215	95	31	119	1.8	0.21	0.9	360	0.9	4	Tr
123	with oats, plain	328	248	34	60	214	2.2	0.28	1.4	210	2.2	4	Tr
124	**Biscuits, fully coated with chocolate**	229	344	163	46	204	2.0	0.28	1.0	180	0.7	3	14
125	with cream	174	337	146	42	156	3.0	0.35	0.8	160	0.5	7	14
126	with marshmallow	132	259	102	28	103	1.7	0.26	0.6	121	0.4	3	14
127	**Biscuits, ginger nuts**	429	154	43	18	68	1.5	0.10	0.5	360	0.7	2	Tr
128	**Biscuits, iced**	274	112	74	13	90	1.2	0.12	0.4	230	0.4	5	Tr
129	**Biscuits, jam filled**	164	135	121	14	94	1.1	0.12	0.4	190	0.4	2	Tr
130	**Biscuits, plain**, reduced fat	471	193	102	30	124	2.0	0.18	0.8	302	0.9	4	Tr

Vitamins per 100g edible portion

No.	Food	Retinol µg	Carotene µg	Vitamin D µg	Vitamin E mg	Thiamin mg	Ribo-flavin mg	Niacin mg	Trypt 60 mg	Vitamin B$_6$ mg	Vitamin B$_{12}$ µg	Folate µg	Panto-thenate mg	Biotin µg	Vitamin C mg
	Biscuits continued														
120	**Biscuits, cookies,** chocolate chip, standard	Tr	Tr	0	2.19	0.13	0.08	0.9	1.1	0.03	0	36	0.5	5	0
121	**Biscuits, digestive,** half coated in chocolate	Tr	Tr	Tr	2.35	0.11	0.07	2.2	1.3	0.07	0.1	7	0.6	5	0
122	plain	0	0	0	5.32	0.12	0.02	1.9	1.2	0.07	0	11	0.5	4	0
123	with oats, plain	0	0	0	5.71	0.18	0.13	1.6	1.6	0.14	0	13	0.6	9	0
124	**Biscuits, fully coated with chocolate**	28	Tr	Tr	1.57	0.14	0.19	1.2	1.3	0.09	Tr	14	0.6	3	0
125	with cream	Tr	14	Tr	1.78	0.11	0.13	1.3	1.0	0.06	0.1	9	0.7	5	0
126	with marshmallow	Tr	Tr	Tr	0.83	0.06	0.13	0.6	0.8	0.04	0.2	8	N	N	0
127	**Biscuits, ginger nuts**	0	N	0	2.10	0.10	0.03	0.9	1.1	0.07	0	11	0.5	4	0
128	**Biscuits, iced**	0	151	0	1.21	0.12	0.02	1.3	0.8	0.03	0	7	0.4	2	0
129	**Biscuits, jam filled**	0	Tr	0	2.12	0.09	0.01	0.9	0.9	0.05	0	Tr	Tr	Tr	0
130	**Biscuits, plain,** reduced fat	0	0	0	3.37	0.12	0.02	1.9	1.2	0.07	0	11	0.5	4	0

Composition of food per 100g edible portion

No.	Food	Description and main data sources	Main data reference	Water g	Total nitrogen g	Protein g	Fat g	Carbo-hydrate g	Energy value kcal	kJ
Biscuits continued										
131	**Biscuits, sandwich**, cream	Including custard creams and Bourbons. Analytical data, 2008	70	2.3	0.88	5.0	23.3	65.8	477	2001
132	**Biscuits, semi-sweet**	Including rich tea and Morning Coffee. Analytical data, 2008	70	2.0	1.13	6.4	15.1	75.4	444	1874
133	**Biscuits, short, sweet**	Including malted milk, shortcake and nice. Analytical data, 2008	70	2.9	0.98	5.6	20.9	71.7	479	2016
134	**Biscuits, short or sweet**, half coated in chocolate	Including milk and plain chocolate, shortcake, rich tea, gems and animal shapes. Analytical data, 2008	70	2.2	1.06	6.0	24.2	70.3	506	2124
135	**Breadsticks**	Plain. Analytical data, 2008	70	4.2	1.90	10.9	8.1	72.9	389	1650
136	**Cereal bars**, with fruit and/or nuts, with chocolate, unfortified	Including Cadbury Brunch, Tracker cereal and Alpen cereal bars. Analytical data, 2008	70	6.6	1.03	6.0	18.3	66.0	436	1835
137	with fruit and/or nuts, no chocolate, unfortified	Including Jordans Frusli and Alpen chewy bars. Analytical data, 2008	70	8.9	0.96	5.6	10.7	62.9	354	1497
138	**Cream crackers**	Analytical data, 2008	70	4.9	1.57	8.9	16.4	69.7	445	1874
139	**Cheese straws/twists**	Including cheese straws, twists and crispies. Analytical data, 2008	70	4.7	2.21	14.1	30.3	48.3	510	2133
140	**Crispbread**, rye	Ryvita original and Ryvita dark. Analytical data, 2008	70	7.7	1.47	8.6	1.4	63.4	284	1210
141	**Flapjacks**	Retail. Analytical data, 2008	70	9.3	0.87	5.1	22.8	55.7	434	1821
142	**Minibreads**, toasted	Including bruschettine and crostini. Analytical data, 2008	70	3.0	1.84	10.5	13.6	68.9	423	1784
143	**Oatcakes**, plain	Retail, Nairn's and own brand. Analytical data, 2008	70	4.1	1.60	9.3	20.0	62.8	453	1904

Cereals and cereal products *continued*

Composition of food per 100g edible portion

No.	Food	Starch g	Total sugars g	Individual sugars					Dietary fibre		Fatty acids				Cholest-erol mg
				Gluc g	Fruct g	Sucr g	Malt g	Lact g	NSP g	AOAC g	Satd g	Mono-unsatd g	Poly-unsatd g	Trans g	
Biscuits continued															
131	**Biscuits, sandwich**, cream	36.0	29.9	1.6	Tr	27.2	Tr	1.1	2.3	3.1	13.3	6.8	2.1	Tr	3
132	**Biscuits, semi-sweet**	55.1	20.3	0.6	Tr	19.7	Tr	Tr	1.9	2.7	5.1	7.4	1.9	Tr	5
133	**Biscuits, short, sweet**	48.0	23.8	0.6	0.6	22.0	0.6	Tr	1.6	2.2	10.1	7.5	2.2	0.1	10
134	**Biscuits, short or sweet**, half coated in chocolate	34.9	35.5	Tr	Tr	32.5	Tr	3.0	1.9	1.4	12.5	8.3	2.2	0.1	16
135	**Breadsticks**	69.6	3.3	Tr	Tr	Tr	3.3	Tr	2.1	3.7	6.0	0.8	0.7	Tr	6
136	**Cereal bars**, with fruit and/or nuts, with chocolate, unfortified	25.3	40.7	6.4	6.5	25.9	Tr	1.9	3.0	5.1	8.4	7.2	1.7	Tr	11
137	with fruit and/or nuts, no chocolate, unfortified	28.6	34.3	9.9	9.0	9.5	4.8	1.2	3.7	6.2	3.9	4.5	1.9	Tr	6
138	**Cream crackers**	68.2	1.5	Tr	Tr	Tr	1.5	Tr	3.3	3.9[a]	7.4	6.0	2.2	Tr	5
139	**Cheese straws/twists**	46.6	1.6	Tr	Tr	Tr	1.6	Tr	2.4	2.5	17.5	7.7	1.7	0.8	71
140	**Crispbread**, rye	60.0	3.4	Tr	Tr	2.8	0.6	Tr	14.2	20.0	0.2	0.2	0.6	Tr	0
141	**Flapjacks**	26.5	29.2	4.3	4.2	20.7	Tr	Tr	2.2	5.2	10.3	7.9	3.0	0.2	25
142	**Minibreads**, toasted	65.6	3.3	Tr	Tr	Tr	3.3	Tr	2.9	4.2	3.2	7.8	1.9	Tr	0
143	**Oatcakes**, plain	59.6	3.2	Tr	Tr	1.0	2.2	Tr	8.8	9.4	5.7	9.3	3.9	Tr	5

[a] High fibre varieties contain approximately 7.5g AOAC per 100g

Inorganic constituents per 100g edible portion

No.	Food	Na	K	Ca	Mg	P	Fe	Cu	Zn	Cl	Mn	Se	I
		mg										µg	
Biscuits continued													
131	**Biscuits, sandwich**, cream	188	253	118	29	102	2.2	0.20	0.6	190	0.7	2	8
132	**Biscuits, semi-sweet**	358	168	157	23	99	2.0	0.09	1.0	290	0.8	3	Tr
133	**Biscuits, short, sweet**	403	155	95	20	106	1.6	0.12	0.7	380	0.6	3	Tr
134	**Biscuits, short or sweet**, half coated in chocolate	249	260	123	35	123	2.4	0.27	0.7	190	0.6	4	8
135	**Breadsticks**	817	202	31	30	120	2.0	0.21	0.9	1140	0.6	6	Tr
136	**Cereal bars**, with fruit and/or nuts, with chocolate, unfortified	221	309	73	58	182	1.9	0.32	1.2	300	0.1	2	6
137	with fruit and/or nuts, no chocolate, unfortified	65	308	51	50	177	1.8	0.24	1.0	88	0.2	2	1
138	**Cream crackers**	384	215	93	22	103	2.0	0.17	0.7	430	0.7	3	Tr
139	**Cheese straws/twists**	974	153	233	24	215	1.2	0.14	1.4	1500	0.5	11	9
140	**Crispbread**, rye	264	511	38	89	292	2.5	0.32	2.2	350	0.2	5	Tr
141	**Flapjacks**	194	207	52	47	177	1.9	0.17	1.1	300	1.8	3	Tr
142	**Minibreads**, toasted	865	221	39	26	114	1.4	0.18	0.7	1210	0.6	6	Tr
143	**Oatcakes**, plain	796	359	57	101	383	3.8	0.35	2.0	830	3.8	9	1

Cereals and cereal products *continued*

Vitamins per 100g edible portion

No.	Food	Retinol	Carotene	Vitamin D	Vitamin E	Thiamin	Ribo-flavin	Niacin	Trypt 60	Vitamin B6	Vitamin B12	Folate	Panto-thenate	Biotin	Vitamin C
		µg	µg	µg	mg	mg	mg	mg	mg	mg	µg	µg	mg	µg	mg
Biscuits continued															
131	**Biscuits, sandwich**, cream	Tr	14	0	2.25	0.16	0.05	1.6	1.0	0.06	0	11	0.6	3	0
132	**Biscuits, semi-sweet**	0	0	0	2.85	0.12	0.01	1.4	1.3	0.06	0	12	0.5	4	0
133	**Biscuits, short, sweet**	0	0	0	2.68	0.17	0.02	1.3	1.1	0.05	0	9	0.4	2	0
134	**Biscuits, short or sweet**, half coated in chocolate	22	Tr	Tr	1.84	0.10	0.08	0.9	1.2	0.07	Tr	8	0.4	3	0
135	**Breadsticks**	0	Tr	0	0.18	0.09	0.02	1.5	2.1	0.10	Tr	21	0.6	2	Tr
136	**Cereal bars**, with fruit and/or nuts, with chocolate, unfortified	Tr	Tr	Tr	2.24	0.18	0.08	1.5	1.3	0.07	0.1	10	0.8	6	Tr
137	with fruit and/or nuts, no chocolate, unfortified	Tr	Tr	Tr	1.74	0.18	0.08	1.5	1.3	0.07	Tr	10	0.8	6	2
138	**Cream crackers**	0	0	0	1.68	0.14	0.02	1.5	1.7	0.06	0	19	0.8	4	0
139	**Cheese straws/twists**	173	64	Tr	1.28	0.25	0.10	2.1	2.1	0.07	0.2	35	0.8	6	0
140	**Crispbread**, rye	0	0	0	0.40	0.26	0.04	0.9	1.7	0.10	0	29	0.6	8	0
141	**Flapjacks**	83	16	Tr	2.18	0.15	0.03	0.5	1.2	0.04	Tr	8	0.4	8	0
142	**Minibreads**, toasted	0	Tr	0	2.93	0.09	0.02	1.5	2.1	0.10	Tr	21	0.6	2	0
143	**Oatcakes**, plain	0	0	0	2.52	0.32	0.09	0.7	2.3	0.10	0	26	1.0	17	0

Composition of food per 100g edible portion

No.	Food	Description and main data sources	Main data reference	Water g	Total nitrogen g	Protein g	Fat g	Carbo- hydrate g	Energy value kcal	kJ
Biscuits continued										
144	**Shortbread**	Analytical data, 2008	70	3.5	0.94	5.3	29.0	62.2	515	2158
145	**Wafers**, plain ice cream wafers, not filled	Including cones, cornets and wafers. Analytical data, 2008	70	5.7	1.84	10.5	3.0	79.7	368	1565
Cakes										
146	**Battenberg cake**	Including standard and mini cakes. Analytical data, 2008	70	16.7	0.70	4.4	9.9	65.9	354	1495
147	**Cake bars**, chocolate	Including chocolate chip, Galaxy, Milky Way, Penguin and Crunchie. Analytical data, 2002-2003	65	10.5	0.88	5.0	21.6	57.5[a]	430	1804
148	**Cakes from 'healthy eating' ranges**	Including carrot, lemon and apple slices. Analytical data, 2008; and industry data, 2013	70	24.0	0.57	3.3	2.5	58.8	257	1091
149	**Carrot cake**, iced	Including plain carrot and products with orange and walnuts. Analytical data, 2008; and industry data, 2013	70	20.4	0.74	4.2	20.2	46.8	374	1569
150	**Chocolate cake**, with filling and icing	Including celebration cakes, tray bakes and layer cakes. Analytical data, 2008	70	18.4	0.78	4.5	23.7	48.6	413	1730
151	**Chocolate fudge cake**	Mixture of fresh and frozen. Analytical data, 1998	63	24.7	0.83	5.2	14.3	55.7[a]	358	1509
152	**Crispie cakes**, homemade	Chocolate. Recipe		1.6	0.89	5.5	18.0	73.7	460	1938
153	**Fancy iced cakes**	Including French and fondant fancies, cup cakes, fairy cakes, angel and lemon slices. Analytical data, 2008	70	18.4	0.58	3.3	16.8	57.6	381	1600
154	**Fruit cake**	Including Genoa, sultana and cherry slab, Manor House and country slices. Analytical data, 2008	70	21.8	0.80	4.5	12.1	55.2	334	1408

[a] Includes oligosaccharides

Cereals and cereal products *continued*

Composition of food per 100g edible portion

No.	Food	Starch	Total sugars	Individual sugars					Dietary fibre		Fatty acids				Cholest-erol
				Gluc	Fruct	Sucr	Malt	Lact	NSP	AOAC	Satd	Mono-unsatd	Poly-unsatd	Trans	
		g	g	g	g	g	g	g	g	g	g	g	g	g	mg
Biscuits continued															
144	**Shortbread**	46.5	15.6	Tr	Tr	15.6	Tr	Tr	1.3	2.2	17.5	7.0	1.2	0.7	82
145	**Wafers**, plain ice cream wafers, not filled	76.2	3.5	Tr	Tr	3.5	Tr	Tr	2.1	3.4	0.6	1.0	1.3	Tr	4
Cakes															
146	**Battenberg cake**	9.1	56.8	5.1	0.3	46.7	4.7	Tr	1.1	1.5	3.1	4.1	2.2	Tr	6
147	**Cake bars**, chocolate	15.0	41.5[a]	2.1	1.0	33.3	1.2	4.0	1.6	1.9	9.9	7.9	2.7	0.2	29
148	**Cakes from 'healthy eating' ranges**	11.4	47.4	2.8	1.7	41.9	1.0	Tr	1.7	2.6	1.2	0.7	0.5	Tr	19
149	**Carrot cake**, iced	12.3	34.5	Tr	0.8	31.8	1.9	Tr	1.1	1.9	5.1	8.2	5.6	0.2	53
150	**Chocolate cake**, with filling and icing	12.0	36.6	1.4	Tr	33.2	Tr	2.0	1.8	2.9	9.5	9.5	3.2	0.2	55
151	**Chocolate fudge cake**	11.3	43.5[a]	1.7	0.4	39.1	1.3	1.0	0.9	1.9	4.6	6.4	2.7	0.4	33
152	**Crispie cakes**, homemade	30.7	43.0	0.4	0.4	42.2	Tr	0.1	2.1	N	10.6	5.7	0.7	Tr	4
153	**Fancy iced cakes**	13.5	44.1	1.5	Tr	40.5	2.1	Tr	0.9	1.1	5.9	6.7	3.3	Tr	31
154	**Fruit cake**	15.6	39.6	10.5	11.9	14.0	3.2	Tr	2.4	3.0	4.6	4.7	1.9	0.1	43

[a] Not including oligosaccharides

Inorganic constituents per 100g edible portion

No.	Food	Na	K	Ca	Mg	P	Fe	Cu	Zn	Cl	Mn	Se	I
		mg										µg	
Biscuits continued													
144	**Shortbread**	321	133	138	15	77	1.5	0.08	0.5	530	0.6	6	3
145	**Wafers**, plain ice cream wafers, not filled	192	195	89	28	129	2.3	0.12	1.2	160	0.9	7	Tr
Cakes													
146	**Battenberg cake**	137	174	107	18	134	0.6	0.13	0.4	270	0.2	3	N
147	**Cake bars**, chocolate	235	236	96	34	164	1.6	0.27	0.7	290	0.3	3	14
148	**Cakes from 'healthy eating' ranges**	70	115	103	9	186	0.9	0.17	0.4	80	0.2	4	Tr
149	**Carrot cake**, iced	220	140	101	14	169	0.9	0.16	0.5	240	0.5	4	N
150	**Chocolate cake**, with filling and icing	259	340	144	39	212	3.1	0.35	0.7	268	0.4	3	14
151	**Chocolate fudge cake**	265	357	67	45	156	3.1	0.38	0.8	274	0.4	4	N
152	**Crispie cakes**, homemade[a]	169	232	23	66	123	5.7	0.49	1.3	254	0.6	5	2
153	**Fancy iced cakes**	275	147	72	10	148	0.9	0.06	0.3	180	0.1	3	Tr
154	**Fruit cake**	193	385	74	20	113	1.6	0.21	0.4	200	0.3	4	N[b]

[a] Inorganic content depends on fortification levels of cereal product ingredients

[b] Iodine from erythrosine is present but largely unavailable

Vitamins per 100g edible portion

No.	Food	Retinol	Carotene	Vitamin D	Vitamin E	Thiamin	Ribo-flavin	Niacin	Trypt 60	Vitamin B6	Vitamin B12	Folate	Panto-thenate	Biotin	Vitamin C
		µg	µg	µg	mg	mg	mg	mg	mg	mg	µg	µg	mg	µg	mg
Biscuits continued															
144	**Shortbread**	281	96	0.4	1.30	0.18	0.03	1.1	1.2	0.08	Tr	14	0.5	4	0
145	**Wafers**, plain ice cream wafers, not filled	0	0	0	0.42	0.08	0.02	1.6	2.0	0.04	0	14	0.5	9	0
Cakes															
146	**Battenberg cake**	N	Tr	N	1.14	0.03	0.06	0.4	0.9	0.04	0.1	8	0.2	4	0
147	**Cake bars**, chocolate	37	29	1.3	2.93	0.05	0.17	0.4	0.7	0.01	Tr	4	0.5	3	0
148	**Cakes from 'healthy eating' ranges**	7	2	Tr	0.28	0.06	0.08	0.9	1.1	0.08	0.2	Tr	0.8	5	N
149	**Carrot cake**, iced	70	547	Tr	2.30	0.07	0.08	0.4	1.1	0.09	0.2	9	0.3	4	2
150	**Chocolate cake**, with filling and icing	45	21	0.4	1.14	0.05	0.12	0.6	1.1	0.05	0.2	13	0.6	5	0
151	**Chocolate fudge cake**	30	30	0.4	1.45	0.05	0.06	0.5	1.5	Tr	Tr	7	0.4	3	Tr
152	**Crispie cakes**, homemade[a]	9	33	1.7	0.96	0.43	0.56	6.0	0.8	0.58	0.7	N	N	3	0
153	**Fancy iced cakes**	Tr	Tr	Tr	2.61	0.06	0.07	0.5	0.7	0.03	0.2	7	0.2	3	Tr
154	**Fruit cake**	39	Tr	Tr	1.50	0.09	0.06	1.0	0.9	0.08	0.1	Tr	0.6	5	Tr

[a] Vitamin content depends on fortification levels of cereal product ingredients

Composition of food per 100g edible portion

No.	Food	Description and main data sources	Main data reference	Water g	Total nitrogen g	Protein g	Fat g	Carbo-hydrate g	Energy value kcal	kJ
Cakes continued										
155	**Fruit cake**, rich, iced, homemade	Recipe		15.1	0.63	3.7	9.6	67.0	355	1501
156	**Gateau**, chocolate based, frozen	Including Black Forest gateau. Analytical data, 1993-1994	50	43.1	0.55	3.5	15.7	37.2[a]	295	1236
157	fruit, frozen	Fruit and cream sponge including strawberry, orange and lemon and tropical fruit. Analytical data, 1993-1994	50	51.9	0.50	3.2	12.3	33.3[a]	248	1042
158	**Jaffa cakes**	Including McVities, Lyons and own brands. Analytical data, 2002	65	12.2	0.78	4.4	8.5	69.3[a]	354	1498
159	**Loaf cake**	Including ginger and golden syrup. Analytical data, 2008	70	21.7	0.58	3.3	11.0	56.2	323	1362
160	**Muffins**, American, chocolate	Analytical data, 2002-2003	65	18.6	0.97	5.5	25.4	49.5[a]	436	1825
161	American, not chocolate	Including blueberry, cherry and toffee. Analytical data, 2002-2003; and industry data, 2013	65	24.6	0.87	5.0	19.5	47.8[a]	375	1571
162	**Shortcake**, caramel, chocolate covered	Analytical data, 2008	70	8.5	0.83	4.7	27.3	53.6	466	1948
163	**Sponge cake**, homemade	Recipe		14.6	1.05	6.4	26.4	53.1	463	1935
164	fatless, homemade	Recipe		31.9	1.64	9.9	5.6	53.9	292	1240
165	with dairy cream and jam	Frozen. Analytical data, 1998	63	38.4	0.69	4.3	10.9	43.9[a]	280	1179
166	with jam and butter cream	Including sandwich and Swiss roll. Analytical data, 2008; and industry data, 2013	70	22.2	0.64	3.7	14.8	55.1	354	1492
167	soft iced	Including angel cake, Madeira and lemon drizzle. Analytical data, 2008	70	21.6	0.84	4.8	15.8	55.0	368	1546

[a] Includes oligosaccharides

Cereals and cereal products *continued*

No.	Food	Starch g	Total sugars g	Gluc g	Fruct g	Sucr g	Malt g	Lact g	Dietary fibre NSP g	Dietary fibre AOAC g	Fatty acids Satd g	Fatty acids Mono-unsatd g	Fatty acids Poly-unsatd g	Fatty acids Trans g	Cholesterol mg
Cakes continued															
155	**Fruit cake**, rich, iced, homemade	8.1	58.9	12.9	11.0	32.4	2.6	0.1	1.3	N	4.5	3.3	0.9	0.2	45
156	**Gateau**, chocolate based, frozen	17.6	17.4[a]	2.4	1.8	11.5	0.7	0.9	1.0	N	10.3	3.7	1.2	0.4	56
157	fruit, frozen	17.8	14.9[a]	2.0	1.5	10.1	0.5	0.7	0.9	N	7.9	3.2	1.1	0.3	53
158	**Jaffa cakes**	16.3	51.6[a]	8.5	1.8	35.1	6.0	0.2	1.0	1.5	4.3	2.8	0.9	Tr	9
159	**Loaf cake**	22.7	33.5	10.2	6.8	13.6	2.9	Tr	1.5	1.4	3.2	5.1	2.1	Tr	8
160	**Muffins**, American, chocolate	18.4	30.9[a]	0.6	0.1	28.3	0.4	1.5	0.8	1.0	4.8	13.0	6.5	0.2	45
161	American, not chocolate	19.8	27.7[a]	1.0	0.7	24.3	0.9	0.9	1.0	1.8	2.4	10.3	5.7	0.2	46
162	**Shortcake**, caramel, chocolate covered	17.4	36.2	1.8	2.0	27.8	3.1	1.6	1.3	2.3	15.2	8.4	2.0	0.2	23
163	**Sponge cake**, homemade	22.8	30.3	Tr	Tr	30.1	0	0.2	0.9	1.1	15.7	7.0	1.3	0.8	161
164	fatless, homemade	23.3	30.6	Tr	Tr	30.6	0	0	1.0	1.2	1.6	2.1	0.9	Tr	203
165	with dairy cream and jam	18.6	24.3[a]	3.0	0.7	18.1	1.6	0.9	Tr	2.7	N	N	N	N	59
166	with jam and butter cream	17.5	37.6	3.5	1.0	28.2	4.9	Tr	1.4	1.2	7.0	4.9	1.5	0.3	76
167	soft iced	16.0	39.0	Tr	Tr	35.5	3.5	Tr	1.9	1.3	6.2	5.6	3.1	0.1	36

[a] Not including oligosaccharides

Cereals and cereal products *continued*

Inorganic constituents per 100g edible portion

No.	Food	Na	K	Ca	Mg	P	Fe	Cu	Zn	Cl	Mn	Se	I
		mg										µg	
Cakes continued													
155	**Fruit cake**, rich, iced, homemade	98	351	61	27	73	1.6	0.22	0.5	133	0.3	3	N[a]
156	**Gateau**, chocolate based, frozen	173	189	49	20	153	1.5	0.52	0.6	N	0.2	N	N
157	fruit, frozen	128	107	40	10	110	0.7	0.38	0.7	96	0.2	N	35
158	**Jaffa cakes**	85	133	46	30	98	2.6	0.22	0.7	64	0.3	4	5
159	**Loaf cake**	366	154	34	8	46	0.5	Tr	0.4	564	0.2	4	N
160	**Muffins**, American, chocolate	396	248	70	34	198	3.0	0.31	1.3	317	0.3	5	15
161	American, not chocolate	250	114	64	10	190	1.1	0.12	0.6	200	0.4	5	N
162	**Shortcake**, caramel, chocolate covered	258	254	137	26	125	1.5	0.13	0.7	280	0.4	2	N
163	**Sponge cake**, homemade	430	105	109	12	246	1.0	0.09	0.6	402	0.3	7	25
164	fatless, homemade	91	136	57	15	137	1.6	0.11	0.9	146	0.2	14	29
165	with dairy cream and jam	218	83	33	6	171	0.4	0.04	0.3	179	0.1	4	12
166	with jam and butter cream	220	132	72	8	162	0.7	0.08	0.3	100	0.2	4	7
167	soft iced	251	197	81	14	144	0.9	0.11	0.4	270	0.3	4	Tr

[a] Iodine from erythrosine is present but largely unavailable

Cakes continued

No.	Food	Retinol µg	Carotene µg	Vitamin D µg	Vitamin E mg	Thiamin mg	Ribo-flavin mg	Niacin mg	Trypt 60 mg	Vitamin B$_6$ mg	Vitamin B$_{12}$ µg	Folate µg	Panto-thenate mg	Biotin µg	Vitamin C mg
155	**Fruit cake**, rich, iced, homemade	85	51	0.4	1.28	0.06	0.10	0.5	0.7	0.08	0.3	10	0.2	6	Tr
156	**Gateau**, chocolate based, frozen	102	80	N	1.01	0.05	0.09	0.3	0.5	0.01	0.2	2	0.2	3	Tr
157	fruit, frozen	109	55	Tr	1.06	0.03	0.06	0.4	0.5	0.02	0.2	6	0.1	2	4
158	**Jaffa cakes**	15	10	Tr	0.30	0.13	0.13	1.3	0.6	0.07	0.4	9	0.5	4	2[a]
159	**Loaf cake**	25	7	N	1.69	0.06	0.07	0.4	0.6	0.04	0.2	6	0.3	2	0
160	**Muffins**, American, chocolate	24	N	Tr	3.34	0.03	0.11	0.7	0.8	0.01	0.4	9	0.5	2	0
161	American, not chocolate	25	7	Tr	2.40	0.03	0.10	0.7	0.8	0.01	0.2	9	0.5	2	Tr
162	**Shortcake**, caramel, chocolate covered	79	17	Tr	2.25	0.08	0.14	1.0	1.0	0.05	0.2	9	0.5	3	Tr
163	**Sponge cake**, homemade	309	173	1.2	1.08	0.08	0.15	0.5	1.6	0.07	0.9	9	0.4	6	Tr
164	fatless, homemade	73	Tr	1.9	0.92	0.10	0.26	0.5	2.6	0.10	1.6	16	0.7	12	0
165	with dairy cream and jam	77	40	0.4	N	0.10	0.10	0.4	0.7	0.01	0.3	7	0.3	2	Tr
166	with jam and butter cream	107	55	Tr	1.19	0.05	0.06	0.5	0.8	0.04	0.4	Tr	0.5	4	Tr
167	soft iced	43	12	Tr	1.80	0.06	0.08	0.9	1.1	0.08	0.2	Tr	0.8	5	N

[a] Some 'mini' or 'lunchbox' products may contain added vitamin C

Composition of food per 100g edible portion

No.	Food	Description and main data sources	Main data reference	Water g	Total nitrogen g	Protein g	Fat g	Carbo-hydrate g	Energy value kcal	kJ
Cakes continued										
168	**Swiss rolls**, chocolate covered and filled	Including large, individual and bite-sized rolls. Analytical data, 2008	70	13.4	0.79	4.5	22.7	51.0	414	1733
Pastry										
169	**Filo pastry**, uncooked	Frozen and chilled. Analytical data, 2008; and industry data, 2013	70	26.6	1.33	7.6	2.9	58.9	278	1180
170	cooked	Calculated from uncooked, using weight loss of 23.6%	70	3.9	1.75	10.0	3.8	77.1	363	1544
171	**Flaky/puff pastry**, uncooked	Frozen and chilled, block and ready rolled. Analytical data, 2008	70	31.7	0.93	5.3	26.2	33.7	384	1600
172	cooked	Calculated from uncooked, using weight loss of 21.1%	70	13.4	1.18	6.7	33.2	42.8	486	2027
173	**Shortcrust pastry**, uncooked	Frozen and chilled, block and ready rolled. Analytical data, 2008	70	21.8	1.00	5.7	31.4	39.4	453	1889
174	cooked	Calculated from uncooked, using weight loss of 17.2%	70	5.6	1.21	6.9	37.9	47.5	547	2281
175	cooked, homemade	Recipe		7.9	1.16	6.6	29.9	57.1	509	2131
176	**Wholemeal pastry**, cooked, homemade	Recipe		7.7	1.42	8.3	30.0	48.9	487	2036

No.	Food	Starch	Total sugars	Individual sugars					Dietary fibre		Fatty acids				Cholest-erol
				Gluc	Fruct	Sucr	Malt	Lact	NSP	AOAC	Satd	Mono-unsatd	Poly-unsatd	Trans	
		g	g	g	g	g	g	g	g	g	g	g	g	g	mg
Cakes continued															
168	**Swiss rolls**, chocolate covered and filled	9.8	41.2	4.1	Tr	33.8	3.4	Tr	1.7	3.1	11.7	7.5	1.8	0.2	44
Pastry															
169	**Filo pastry**, uncooked	56.5	2.4	0.2	0.1	Tr	2.1	Tr	1.7	3.4	0.3	1.2	1.2	Tr	2
170	cooked	74.0	3.1	0.2	0.1	Tr	2.7	Tr	2.2	4.5	0.4	1.6	1.6	Tr	2
171	**Flaky/puff pastry**, uncooked	32.2	1.5	Tr	Tr	Tr	1.5	Tr	0.9	2.8	12.6	9.5	2.8	Tr	2
172	cooked	40.8	1.9	Tr	Tr	Tr	1.9	Tr	1.1	3.5	15.9	12.0	3.6	Tr	3
173	**Shortcrust pastry**, uncooked	38.5	0.9	0.3	Tr	Tr	0.5	Tr	1.8	3.4	11.7	13.3	4.8	Tr	2
174	cooked	46.5	1.0	0.4	Tr	Tr	0.6	Tr	2.2	4.1	14.1	16.0	5.8	Tr	2
175	cooked, homemade	56.5	0.6	Tr	Tr	0.4	0.1	0.2	2.4	2.8	18.6	7.5	1.2	1.0	75
176	**Wholemeal pastry**, cooked, homemade	47.8	1.2	Tr	Tr	0.7	0.2	0.2	6.1	7.1	18.4	7.4	1.6	1.0	74

Inorganic constituents per 100g edible portion

No.	Food	Na	K	Ca	Mg	P	Fe	Cu	Zn	Cl	Mn	Se	I
						mg						µg	

Cakes continued

| 168 | **Swiss rolls**, chocolate covered and filled | 259 | 331 | 85 | 44 | 186 | 2.7 | 0.34 | 0.8 | 210 | 0.4 | 3 | 14 |

Pastry

169	**Filo pastry**, uncooked	350	119	108	17	78	1.5	Tr	0.5	500	0.5	5	Tr
170	cooked	460	156	141	23	102	1.9	Tr	0.6	650	0.7	6	Tr
171	**Flaky/puff pastry**, uncooked	337	89	77	10	49	1.1	Tr	0.3	450	0.3	2	Tr
172	cooked	427	112	98	13	61	1.4	Tr	0.4	570	0.4	3	Tr
173	**Shortcrust pastry**, uncooked	224	97	80	10	51	1.0	Tr	0.3	330	0.3	3	Tr
174	cooked	271	118	97	12	61	1.2	Tr	0.4	399	0.4	4	Tr
175	cooked, homemade	258	133	74	17	88	1.4	0.11	0.5	494	0.5	2	13
176	**Wholemeal pastry**, cooked, homemade	257	261	29	59	205	1.7	0.26	1.4	469	1.4	4	13

Cereals and cereal products *continued*

Vitamins per 100g edible portion

No.	Food	Retinol	Carotene	Vitamin D	Vitamin E	Thiamin	Ribo-flavin	Niacin	Trypt 60	Vitamin B_6	Vitamin B_{12}	Folate	Panto-thenate	Biotin	Vitamin C
		µg	µg	µg	mg	mg	mg	mg	mg	mg	µg	µg	mg	µg	mg
Cakes continued															
168	**Swiss rolls**, chocolate covered and filled	45	21	Tr	1.14	0.05	0.12	0.6	1.1	0.05	0.2	13	0.6	5	0
Pastry															
169	**Filo pastry**, uncooked	0	Tr	0	0.30	0.20	0.02	1.0	1.4	0.06	0	11	0.4	2	Tr
170	cooked	0	Tr	0	0.39	0.26	0.03	1.2	1.8	0.08	0	15	0.5	3	Tr
171	**Flaky/puff pastry**, uncooked	0	Tr	0	1.99	0.07	0.01	0.7	1.0	0.04	0	Tr	0.2	2	1
172	cooked	0	Tr	0	2.52	0.09	0.01	0.9	1.3	0.05	0	Tr	0.3	2	Tr
173	**Shortcrust pastry**, uncooked	0	Tr	0	3.26	0.09	0.01	0.8	1.1	0.04	0	6	0.4	2	1
174	cooked	0	Tr	0	3.94	0.10	0.01	1.0	1.3	0.05	0	8	0.5	2	Tr
175	cooked, homemade	337	214	0.3	1.06	0.15	0.05	1.1	1.4	0.09	0.1	6	0.3	1	Tr
176	**Wholemeal pastry**, cooked, homemade	334	212	0.3	1.13	0.19	0.08	3.3	2.1	0.26	0.1	9	0.5	5	Tr

Composition of food per 100g edible portion

No.	Food	Description and main data sources	Main data reference	Water g	Total nitrogen g	Protein g	Fat g	Carbo-hydrate g	Energy value kcal	Energy value kJ
Buns and pastries										
177	**Bakewell tarts**, iced	Including large, slices and individual cherry bakewells. Analytical data, 2008	70	14.9	0.55	3.1	16.8	65.9	411	1729
178	**Cream filled pastries**	Including fresh cream slices and horns. Analytical data, 2008	70	29.8	0.57	3.3	27.4	41.4	415	1731
179	**Custard tarts**, individual	Analytical data, 2008	70	49.5	1.07	6.7	14.3	28.7	263	1102
180	**Danish pastries**	Assorted shapes and flavours. Analytical data, 2008	70	20.0	0.85	4.9	29.2	43.6	446	1861
181	**Doughnuts**, with jam	Branded and own brand. Analytical data, 2008	70	28.9	0.95	5.4	13.1	48.4	321	1352
182	ring, iced	Branded and own brand. Analytical data, 2008	70	21.3	1.03	5.8	25.7	42.3	413	1728
183	**Eccles cakes**	Analytical data, 2008	70	17.6	0.77	4.4	18.3	48.8	365	1532
184	**Eclairs**, chocolate, cream filled	Analytical data, 2008	70	34.5	0.97	6.1	28.5	28.2	387	1609
185	**Greek pastries**, baklava	Assorted baklava. Analytical data, 2008	70	10.8	1.18	6.7	25.1	54.1	456	1909
186	**Iced buns**	Analytical data, 2008	70	24.4	1.05	6.0	7.8	60.8	322	1364
187	**Jam tarts**	Analytical data, 2008	70	16.9	0.56	3.2	13.5	58.2	353	1485
188	**Mince pies**	Analytical data, 2008	70	18.5	0.68	3.8	14.9	60.7	377	1588
189	**Scones**, fruit	Analytical data, 1998; and industry data, 2013	61	24.5	1.10	6.5	11.2	56.2	338	1424
190	plain	Analytical data, 2008	70	23.2	1.25	7.2	12.3	55.2	346	1459
191	plain, homemade	Recipe		23.5	1.23	7.2	12.7	55.9	352	1484
192	**Scotch pancakes**	Analytical data, 1998	61	39.7	1.00	5.6	9.6	43.0	270	1138

Buns and pastries

No.	Food	Starch g	Total sugars g	Individual sugars					Dietary fibre		Fatty acids				Cholest-erol mg
				Gluc g	Fruct g	Sucr g	Malt g	Lact g	NSP g	AOAC g	Satd g	Mono-unsatd g	Poly-unsatd g	Trans g	
177	**Bakewell tarts**, iced	20.7	45.2	3.5	1.1	35.5	5.2	Tr	1.1	1.1	6.9	6.4	2.6	Tr	4
178	**Cream filled pastries**	14.1	27.3	2.7	1.0	20.8	1.6	1.2	0.9	2.9	16.1	7.4	1.6	0.4	52
179	**Custard tarts**, individual	14.5	14.2	0.9	Tr	11.2	2.0	Tr	1.0	1.1	5.9	5.6	2.0	0.1	91
180	**Danish pastries**	26.3	17.3	3.3	2.7	9.6	1.7	Tr	1.5	2.1	11.8	11.5	4.4	0.1	19
181	**Doughnuts**, with jam	28.2	20.3	11.4	5.5	Tr	3.4	Tr	1.4	1.7	5.0	5.1	2.2	0.1	7
182	ring, iced	26.2	16.2	1.7	0.8	13.7	Tr	Tr	1.4	2.7	14.1	7.9	2.3	0.1	9
183	**Eccles cakes**	14.7	34.0	10.8	15.4	3.3	4.5	Tr	2.0	3.6	9.4	6.0	1.7	0.2	23
184	**Eclairs**, chocolate, cream filled	4.2	24.0	2.7	Tr	18.4	Tr	2.9	1.0	1.4	13.6	9.7	2.8	0.4	136
185	**Greek pastries**, baklava	25.1	29.0	9.7	8.6	9.0	1.7	Tr	1.6	2.0	9.7	10.1	3.8	0.2	20
186	**Iced buns**	35.0	25.8	6.4	7.0	11.4	1.0	Tr	3.2	2.5	3.6	2.5	1.3	Tr	5
187	**Jam tarts**	26.2	32.1	9.4	3.7	10.9	8.2	Tr	1.3	1.4	5.5	5.4	1.9	Tr	3
188	**Mince pies**	25.2	35.5[a]	16.6	11.9	3.4	2.7	0.4	1.7	2.6	6.0	5.8	2.2	0.1	12
189	**Scones**, fruit	37.3	18.9	3.0	2.7	9.9	0.4	2.8	2.0	2.9	6.3	3.4	0.8	N	6
190	plain	42.5	12.7	0.9	Tr	10.4	Tr	1.5	2.3	2.2	6.4	3.5	1.2	0.2	35
191	plain, homemade	50.5	5.4	Tr	Tr	3.5	0.1	1.8	2.1	2.4	4.4	5.4	1.9	0.1	4
192	**Scotch pancakes**	21.5	21.5	2.0	1.6	14.1	Tr	3.8	1.5	1.9	0.7	3.5	2.1	0.1	21

[a] Includes galactose

Inorganic constituents per 100g edible portion

No.	Food	mg										µg	
		Na	K	Ca	Mg	P	Fe	Cu	Zn	Cl	Mn	Se	I
Buns and pastries													
177	**Bakewell tarts**, iced	132	117	69	12	73	0.6	0.12	0.3	180	0.2	2	Tr
178	**Cream filled pastries**	205	94	68	10	86	0.5	Tr	0.3	250	0.2	3	10
179	**Custard tarts**, individual	114	138	92	14	101	0.7	0.09	0.5	342	0.2	8	20
180	**Danish pastries**	233	136	52	17	74	0.8	0.12	0.7	310	0.4	4	Tr
181	**Doughnuts**, with jam	404	121	72	15	135	1.2	Tr	0.6	320	0.4	3	15
182	ring, iced	326	202	55	22	154	1.0	Tr	0.6	260	0.4	6	Tr
183	**Eccles cakes**	221	428	75	22	77	1.5	0.22	0.4	359	0.4	1	8
184	**Eclairs**, chocolate, cream filled	125	161	83	22	120	1.8	0.10	0.6	200	0.2	6	12
185	**Greek pastries**, baklava	163	180	48	49	119	1.6	0.35	1.0	205	0.6	5	N
186	**Iced buns**	228	130	294	18	96	1.6	0.12	0.6	245	0.4	5	Tr
187	**Jam tarts**	26	68	22	6	27	0.3	Tr	Tr	100	0.3	2	Tr
188	**Mince pies**	101	211	66	16	65	1.2	Tr	0.3	140	0.4	2	N
189	**Scones**, fruit	400	220	150	24	360	1.5	0.22	0.8	290	0.4	N	N
190	plain	592	270	131	20	476	1.3	0.12	0.6	130	0.4	4	7
191	plain, homemade	635	173	156	19	467	1.2	0.09	0.7	285	0.4	2	12
192	**Scotch pancakes**	418	233	84	20	240	1.0	0.10	0.4	351	0.3	3	10

Cereals and cereal products *continued*

Vitamins per 100g edible portion

No.	Food	Retinol	Carotene	Vitamin D	Vitamin E	Thiamin	Ribo-flavin	Niacin	Trypt 60	Vitamin B$_6$	Vitamin B$_{12}$	Folate	Panto-thenate	Biotin	Vitamin C
		µg	µg	µg	mg	mg	mg	mg	mg	mg	µg	µg	mg	µg	mg
Buns and pastries															
177	**Bakewell tarts**, iced	Tr	Tr	Tr	2.03	0.06	0.04	0.6	0.7	0.03	0.1	6	0.3	3	1
178	**Cream filled pastries**	183	136	Tr	1.66	0.05	0.05	0.4	0.7	0.03	0.2	6	0.2	2	1
179	**Custard tarts**, individual	55	100	Tr	1.27	0.14	0.16	0.5	1.4	0.03	Tr	13	0.5	6	0
180	**Danish pastries**	191	81	Tr	3.98	0.08	0.03	0.8	0.9	0.04	0.1	21	0.3	4	0
181	**Doughnuts**, with jam	Tr	Tr	N	1.75	0.08	0.03	1.3	1.1	0.04	0.1	21	0.3	5	N
182	ring, iced	Tr	Tr	N	2.43	0.08	0.06	0.9	1.1	0.03	Tr	17	0.4	4	0
183	**Eccles cakes**	57	39	0.8	0.90	0.09	0.03	0.6	0.6	0.07	Tr	3	0.1	2	Tr
184	**Eclairs**, chocolate, cream filled	240	90	0.3	1.25	0.10	0.19	0.3	1.2	0.03	0.3	11	0.3	5	Tr
185	**Greek pastries**, baklava	N	N	N	3.03	0.09	0.04	1.0	1.0	N	N	9	0.2	6	N
186	**Iced buns**	0	N	0	0.77	0.14	0.03	1.3	1.2	0.05	0	22	0.8	5	Tr
187	**Jam tarts**	Tr	81	0	2.32	0.06	0.01	0.6	0.6	0.03	0	5	0.1	Tr	Tr
188	**Mince pies**	25	16	Tr	2.06	0.11	0.01	1.0	0.7	0.04	Tr	14	0.2	2	Tr
189	**Scones**, fruit	Tr	Tr	Tr	0.11	0.22	0.10	1.2	1.5	0.05	Tr	6	N	N	Tr
190	plain	84	23	Tr	0.92	0.11	0.05	1.9	1.5	0.06	0.1	6	0.5	5	1
191	plain, homemade	N	107	N	N	0.14	0.12	1.0	1.5	0.10	0.4	7	0.4	2	1
192	**Scotch pancakes**	102	Tr	0.6	1.35	0.16	0.08	0.8	1.5	0.08	Tr	6	0.3	1	Tr

Composition of food per 100g edible portion

No.	Food	Description and main data sources	Main data reference	Water g	Total nitrogen g	Protein g	Fat g	Carbo-hydrate g	Energy value kcal	kJ
Puddings										
193	**Apple pie**, pastry, double crust	Chilled and frozen. Analytical data, 1998	63	46.8	0.61	3.8	12.9	30.3[a]	245	1026
194	**Christmas pudding**	CCP Supplement, 1988; and industry data, 2013	7	29.1	0.53	3.0	6.9	56.3[b]	285	1207
195	**Crumble**, fruit	Frozen and chilled, including apple, blackberry and rhubarb. Analytical data, 1998	63	49.1	0.38	2.4	8.3	36.0[a]	219	924
196	fruit, wholemeal, homemade	Apple, gooseberry, plum and rhubarb. Recipe		54.2	0.41	2.5	7.3	32.7	198	834
197	**Fruit pie**, individual	Including apple, apple and blackcurrant and cherry. Analytical data, 2008	70	23.5	0.55	3.1	13.7	60.0	361	1520
198	one crust, homemade	Apple, gooseberry, plum and rhubarb. Recipe		59.1	0.36	2.1	9.1	26.7	190	800
199	pastry top and bottom, homemade	Apple, gooseberry, plum and rhubarb. Recipe		48.7	0.53	3.1	15.1	30.4	262	1099
200	**Lemon meringue pie**	Fresh and frozen. Analytical data, 1998	63	42.1	0.46	2.9	8.5	43.5[a]	251	1060
201	**Sevyian**, homemade	Dessert made from vermicelli and milk. Analytical data, 2007	69	69.6	0.61	3.8	3.1	20.2	119	503
202	**Sponge pudding**, canned	CCP Supplement, 1988	7	35.3	0.54	3.1	9.1	45.4	265	1116
Savouries										
203	**Cheese and onion rolls**, pastry	Retail. Analytical data, 1995; and industry data, 2013	57	39.6	1.31	8.2	20.0	30.4[a]	327	1366
204	**Dumplings**, homemade	Recipe		59.8	0.47	2.7	11.7	25.4	211	886
205	**Pancakes**, savoury, made with semi-skimmed milk, homemade	Recipe		58.1	1.14	6.9	8.4	26.6	203	855
206	**Papadums**, takeaway	Analytical data, 1997	53	3.9	1.84	11.5	38.8	28.3	501	2084

[a] Includes oligosaccharides

[b] Oligosaccharides may be present, but levels are unknown

Cereals and cereal products *continued*

Composition of food per 100g edible portion

No.	Food	Starch g	Total sugars g	Individual sugars					Dietary fibre		Fatty acids				Cholesterol mg
				Gluc g	Fruct g	Sucr g	Malt g	Lact g	NSP g	AOAC g	Satd g	Mono-unsatd g	Poly-unsatd g	Trans g	erol mg
Puddings															
193	**Apple pie**, pastry, double crust	23.2	7.0[a]	1.1	1.3	4.6	Tr	Tr	1.0	2.6	4.0	6.0	2.2	Tr	Tr
194	**Christmas pudding**	10.1	46.2	20.3	20.8	3.5	1.5	0.1	N	4.0	3.6	2.4	0.4	Tr	21
195	**Crumble**, fruit	14.0	21.8[a]	4.1	4.2	11.3	2.2	Tr	1.3	2.3	4.0	3.1	0.8	Tr	13
196	fruit, wholemeal, homemade	11.4	21.3	1.3	1.6	18.2	Tr	Tr	2.6	N	4.4	1.8	0.4	0.2	18
197	**Fruit pie**, individual	28.9	31.0	8.3	2.4	17.1	2.6	0.7	1.6	4.3	4.9	5.9	2.3	Tr	Tr
198	one crust, homemade	11.0	15.7	1.4	1.6	12.6	0.1	Tr	1.6	N	3.3	3.8	1.4	Tr	1
199	pastry top and bottom, homemade	18.5	12.0	1.1	1.2	9.4	0.2	Tr	1.7	N	5.6	6.4	2.3	Tr	1
200	**Lemon meringue pie**	13.6	29.3[a]	4.5	3.4	20.0	1.0	0.4	0.7	N	3.1	3.5	1.5	0.5	12
201	**Sevyian**, homemade	6.6	13.6	0.5	0.5	8.3	0	4.3	Tr	1.0	1.9	0.8	0.2	0.1	23
202	**Sponge pudding**, canned	19.6	25.8	4.6	3.8	14.9	2.0	0.6	0.8	N	5.0	3.0	0.5	N	32
Savouries															
203	**Cheese and onion rolls**, pastry	24.2	3.0[a]	0.4	0.4	0.3	1.4	0.6	1.2	2.9	9.0	7.1	2.2	0.6	26
204	**Dumplings**, homemade	25.2	0.2	0	0	0.1	0	0	1.0	1.2	6.6	4.0	0.4	0.5	11
205	**Pancakes**, savoury, made with semi-skimmed milk, homemade	22.8	3.8	Tr	Tr	0.1	0	3.7	1.0	1.1	2.0	2.0	3.8	0.1	49
206	**Papadums**, takeaway	28.3	Tr	Tr	Tr	Tr	Tr	Tr	5.8	6.3	8.0	16.5	12.5	0.1	2

[a] Not including oligosaccharides

Inorganic constituents per 100g edible portion

No.	Food	mg										µg	
		Na	K	Ca	Mg	P	Fe	Cu	Zn	Cl	Mn	Se	I
Puddings													
193	**Apple pie**, pastry, double crust	158	97	66	10	71	0.3	0.02	0.3	257	0.2	2	N
194	**Christmas pudding**	100	340	35	18	92	1.2	0.14	0.7	190	0.5	N	N
195	**Crumble**, fruit	82	82	41	6	27	0.3	Tr	0.2	130	0.1	2	4
196	fruit, wholemeal, homemade	63	200	31	19	62	0.6	0.12	0.4	127	0.4	1	3
197	**Fruit pie**, individual	115	117	33	11	53	0.6	0.07	0.2	180	0.3	2	N
198	one crust, homemade	66	162	46	8	28	0.5	0.05	0.1	110	0.2	1	Tr
199	pastry top and bottom, homemade	109	146	56	9	34	0.6	0.04	0.2	170	0.2	1	Tr
200	**Lemon meringue pie**	113	70	38	6	40	Tr	0.04	0.2	237	0.1	2	8
201	**Sevyian**, homemade	40	177	106	14	89	0.3	Tr	0.4	61	N	N	N
202	**Sponge pudding**, canned	340	160	50	13	170	1.2	0.31	0.4	220	0.2	N	4
Savouries													
203	**Cheese and onion rolls**, pastry	310	169	121	19	119	1.3	0.08	0.8	460	0.3	4	19
204	**Dumplings**, homemade	138	52	41	7	132	0.6	0.04	0.2	42	0.2	1	1
205	**Pancakes**, savoury, made with semi-skimmed milk, homemade	53	190	127	16	129	0.8	0.05	0.7	132	0.2	5	30
206	**Papadums**, takeaway	N	609	N	121	196	4.4	0.36	1.7	N	1.0	15	N

Vitamins per 100g edible portion

No.	Food	Retinol µg	Carotene µg	Vitamin D µg	Vitamin E mg	Thiamin mg	Ribo-flavin mg	Niacin mg	Trypt 60 mg	Vitamin B_6 mg	Vitamin B_{12} µg	Folate µg	Panto-thenate mg	Biotin µg	Vitamin C mg
Puddings															
193	**Apple pie**, pastry, double crust	35	20	Tr	1.25	0.09	Tr	0.7	0.4	0.03	Tr	3	0.2	1	37
194	**Christmas pudding**	N	N	N	N	Tr	0.03	0.4	0.6	0.07	Tr	9	N	N	Tr
195	**Crumble**, fruit	47	35	0.7	0.74	0.08	0.02	0.5	0.7	0.05	0	10	0.1	Tr	3
196	fruit, wholemeal, homemade	80	144	0.1	0.51	0.06	0.03	1.0	0.6	0.08	0	3	0.2	2	5
197	**Fruit pie**, individual	Tr	Tr	0	2.17	0.08	0.01	0.7	0.6	0.03	0	6	0.2	2	8
198	one crust, homemade	0	91	0	1.17	0.04	0.02	0.4	0.4	0.03	0	2	0.2	1	5
199	pastry top and bottom, homemade	0	67	0	1.74	0.05	0.01	0.5	0.6	0.03	0	2	0.2	1	4
200	**Lemon meringue pie**	46	10	Tr	0.96	0.08	0.04	0.4	0.7	0.02	Tr	6	0.2	1	5
201	**Sevyian**, homemade	N	N	1.1	N	0.02	0.05	0.1	N	N	0.1	N	0.3	2	Tr
202	**Sponge pudding**, canned	N	N	N	0.59	0.05	0.16	0.4	0.6	0.09	Tr	3	0.2	1	0
Savouries															
203	**Cheese and onion rolls**, pastry	Tr	17	1.0	N	0.15	0.08	1.0	1.5	0.06	0.5	9	0.3	2	Tr
204	**Dumplings**, homemade	7	10	Tr	0.37	0.06	0.01	0.5	0.6	0.04	Tr	2	0.1	1	0
205	**Pancakes**, savoury, made with semi-skimmed milk, homemade	30	7	0.4	1.60	0.09	0.22	0.6	1.5	0.09	1.0	10	0.6	5	2
206	**Papadums**, takeaway	N	N	0	3.70	0.35	0.09	0.6	1.8	0.05	0	23	0.7	5	0

Composition of food per 100g edible portion

No.	Food	Description and main data sources	Main data reference	Water g	Total nitrogen g	Protein g	Fat g	Carbo-hydrate g	Energy value kcal	kJ
Savouries continued										
207	**Prawn crackers**, takeaway	Analytical data, 1997	53	2.8	0.05	0.3	39.0	58.2	570	2379
208	**Pot savouries**, made up	MSF Supplement, 1994; and industry data, 2013	14	74.2	0.53	3.3	3.1	16.7[a]	103	437
209	**Stuffing mix**, dried, assorted flavours, made up	MW5, 1991	10	76.4	0.45	2.8	1.5	19.3	97	412
210	**Stuffing**, sage and onion, homemade	Recipe		49.0	0.94	5.6	13.3	29.4[a]	253	1060
211	**Yorkshire pudding**, made with semi-skimmed milk, homemade	Recipe		58.1	1.10	6.7	8.3	25.6	197	830
Pizzas										
212	**Pizza base**, raw	Average of ambient and chilled. Analytical data, 1994; and industry data, 2013	49	30.1	1.37	7.8	4.8	57.5	290	1229
213	**Pizza**, cheese and tomato, retail	Frozen and chilled, all bases, not stuffed crust. Analytical data, 2010	72	38.1	1.95	12.2	9.8	36.1	272	1148
214	chicken topped, retail	Includes thin base and deep pan. Analytical data, 1994; and industry data, 2013	49	50.8	2.15	13.4	8.3	31.3	246	1036
215	fish topped, takeaway	Prawn and tuna toppings, includes thin base and deep pan. Analytical data, 1994; and industry data, 2013	49	50.1	2.13	13.3	7.5	28.2	226	955
216	ham and pineapple, retail	Includes thin base and deep pan. Analytical data, 1994; and industry data, 2013	49	43.3	2.16	13.5	8.6	34.4	260	1098

[a] Includes oligosaccharides

No.	Food	Starch g	Total sugars g	Individual sugars					Dietary fibre		Fatty acids				Cholest-erol mg
				Gluc g	Fruct g	Sucr g	Malt g	Lact g	NSP g	AOAC g	Satd g	Mono-unsatd g	Poly-unsatd g	Trans g	
Savouries continued															
207	**Prawn crackers**, takeaway	56.0	2.2	Tr	Tr	1.9	0.3	0	1.2	0.9	3.6	22.4	11.0	0.1	Tr
208	**Pot savouries**, made up	13.3	2.3ᵃ	0.4	0.5	1.1	0.2	0.1	N	N	N	N	N	N	0
209	**Stuffing mix**, dried, assorted flavours, made up	18.0	1.3	0.2	0.5	0.6	0	0	1.3	N	0.8	0.5	Tr	N	1
210	**Stuffing**, sage and onion, homemade	22.8	5.4ᵃ	1.5	1.3	1.4	1.2	Tr	N	N	4.2	5.7	2.1	Tr	50
211	**Yorkshire pudding**, made with semi-skimmed milk, homemade	22.1	3.5	Tr	Tr	0.1	0	3.3	0.9	1.1	1.9	2.0	3.7	0.1	52
Pizzas															
212	**Pizza base**, raw	54.1	3.4	0.3	0.3	Tr	2.8	Tr	2.1	2.5	N	N	N	N	N
213	**Pizza**, cheese and tomato, retail	32.2	3.9	0.8	0.9	Tr	2.1	Tr	1.7	2.9	4.1	3.7	1.4	0.1	19
214	chicken topped, retail	29.2	2.1	0.5	0.7	Tr	1.0	Tr	N	2.7	N	N	N	N	N
215	fish topped, takeaway	26.2	2.0	0.3	0.4	Tr	1.1	0.1	N	N	3.2	2.5	1.3	0.1	25
216	ham and pineapple, retail	31.3	3.1	0.7	0.8	Tr	1.4	0.2	N	2.5	N	N	N	N	N

ᵃ Not including oligosaccharides

99

Inorganic constituents per 100g edible portion

No.	Food	Na	K	Ca	Mg	P	Fe	Cu	Zn	Cl	Mn	Se	I
						mg						µg	
Savouries *continued*													
207	**Prawn crackers**, takeaway	767	17	21	5	6	1.6	0.12	0.1	1000	1.5	3	N
208	**Pot savouries**, made up	210	180	51	22	59	1.2	0.10	0.4	40	0.3	N	N
209	**Stuffing mix**, dried, assorted flavours, made up	420	69	280	12	37	1.5	0.05	0.2	810	0.3	N	N
210	**Stuffing**, sage and onion, homemade	263	173	68	18	81	1.1	0.13	0.6	441	0.4	N	N
211	**Yorkshire pudding**, made with semi-skimmed milk, homemade	52	181	119	16	124	0.8	0.05	0.7	127	0.2	5	29
Pizzas													
212	**Pizza base**, raw	400	124	86	18	85	1.6	0.09	0.7	N	0.5	N	N
213	**Pizza**, cheese and tomato, retail	397	223	217	24	179	1.1	0.10	1.3	630	0.4	4	17
214	chicken topped, retail	380	270	217	27	190	1.3	0.12	1.6	N	0.3	N	N
215	fish topped, takeaway	400	179	173	24	170	1.2	0.10	1.3	1370	0.3	10	59
216	ham and pineapple, retail	400	226	221	23	210	1.3	0.10	1.5	N	0.5	N	N

Cereals and cereal products *continued*

Vitamins per 100g edible portion

No.	Food	Retinol µg	Carotene µg	Vitamin D µg	Vitamin E mg	Thiamin mg	Ribo-flavin mg	Niacin mg	Trypt 60 mg	Vitamin B$_6$ mg	Vitamin B$_{12}$ µg	Folate µg	Panto-thenate mg	Biotin µg	Vitamin C mg
Savouries continued															
207	**Prawn crackers**, takeaway	0	Tr	0	5.77	Tr	Tr	0.1	N	0.43	0	2	Tr	Tr	0
208	**Pot savouries**, made up	0	N	0	N	N	N	N	N	N	0	N	N	N	0
209	**Stuffing mix**, dried, assorted flavours, made up	0	0	0	N	0.31	0.22	0.5	0.5	N	0	N	N	N	0
210	**Stuffing**, sage and onion, homemade	N	126	N	N	0.19	0.10	0.7	1.3	0.08	0.4	10	N	N	1
211	**Yorkshire pudding**, made with semi-skimmed milk, homemade	30	6	0.4	3.07	0.08	0.21	0.5	1.5	0.08	1.0	9	0.6	5	2
Pizzas															
212	**Pizza base**, raw	N	N	N	N	0.41	0.03	1.7	N	0.03	0	8	N	N	0
213	**Pizza**, cheese and tomato, retail	119	91	Tr	1.68	0.15	0.15	1.0	2.8	Tr	0.4	4	0.2	4	2
214	chicken topped, retail	N	N	N	N	0.28	0.14	2.9	N	0.07	0.4	9	N	N	3
215	fish topped, takeaway	N	N	N	N	0.15	0.10	2.3	2.5	0.05	1.1	5	0.3	3	2
216	ham and pineapple, retail	N	N	N	N	0.28	0.16	2.3	2.4	0.05	0.5	6	N	N	0

101

Composition of food per 100g edible portion

Pizzas continued

No.	Food	Description and main data sources	Main data reference	Water g	Total nitrogen g	Protein g	Fat g	Carbo-hydrate g	Energy value kcal	kJ
217	**Pizza**, meat topped, retail and takeaway	Including pepperoni, spicy beef, spicy pork. Includes frozen, chilled and takeaway, thin base and deep pan. Analytical data, 1994; and industry data, 2013	49	44.9	2.11	13.2	10.3	29.1	255	1071
218	vegetarian, retail and takeaway	Includes chilled and takeaway, thin base and deep pan Analytical data, 1994; and industry data, 2013	49	51.1	1.72	10.8	6.9	29.6[a]	216	913

[a] Includes oligosaccharides

Composition of food per 100g edible portion

No.	Food	Starch	Total sugars	Individual sugars					Dietary fibre		Fatty acids				Cholest-erol
				Gluc	Fruct	Sucr	Malt	Lact	NSP	AOAC	Satd	Mono-unsatd	Poly-unsatd	Trans	
		g	g	g	g	g	g	g	g	g	g	g	g	g	mg

Pizzas continued

No.	Food	Starch	Total sugars	Gluc	Fruct	Sucr	Malt	Lact	NSP	AOAC	Satd	Mono-unsatd	Poly-unsatd	Trans	Cholesterol
217	**Pizza**, meat topped, retail and takeaway	27.3	1.8	0.4	0.5	Tr	0.9	Tr	N	2.0	4.0	3.7	1.5	N	19
218	vegetarian, retail and takeaway	26.9	2.4[a]	0.6	0.7	Tr	1.0	0.2	1.9	3.1	N	N	N	N	N

[a] Not including oligosaccharides

Inorganic constituents per 100g edible portion

No.	Food	Na	K	Ca	Mg	P	Fe	Cu	Zn	Cl	Mn	Se	I
						mg						μg	

Pizzas continued

| 217 | **Pizza**, meat topped, retail and takeaway | 440 | 196 | 203 | 23 | 190 | 1.2 | 0.10 | 1.6 | N | 0.3 | 7 | N |
| 218 | vegetarian, retail and takeaway | 330 | 192 | 196 | 22 | 160 | 1.2 | 0.11 | 1.3 | 1040 | 0.3 | N | 34 |

Vitamins per 100g edible portion

No.	Food	Retinol	Carotene	Vitamin D	Vitamin E	Thiamin	Ribo-flavin	Niacin	Trypt 60	Vitamin B_6	Vitamin B_{12}	Folate	Panto-thenate	Biotin	Vitamin C
		µg	µg	µg	mg	mg	mg	mg	mg	mg	µg	µg	mg	µg	mg
Pizzas continued															
217	**Pizza**, meat topped, retail and takeaway	N	N	N	0.93	0.23	0.13	1.9	2.3	0.05	0.8	7	3.2	4	0
218	vegetarian, retail and takeaway	42	114	N	1.52	0.23	0.11	1.4	2.1	0.05	Tr	7	N	N	4

Milk and milk products

Section 2.2

Milk and milk products

The majority of the data in this section of the Tables have been taken from analytical studies undertaken during the mid to late 1990s[51,59,60,62,63] and were previously published in the sixth summary edition[18]. However, a few new foods (e.g. 1% milk, fermented drinks, and some additional cheeses[62] and yogurts[60]) have been included and some values for ice cream products[72] have been updated based on new analytical data. Values for many foods, particularly fat and sodium values for cheese, have been reviewed, and, where necessary, updated based on data from manufacturers.

Variation of milk composition by season is pertinent to this section due to seasonal differences in cattle feeding practices (e.g. carotenes, iodine). Where summer and winter values are given separately, summer is June-September and winter is January-March. Recipe calculations use the average of the values for summer and winter milks. Values for whole milk refer to standardised milk, which has a minimum fat content of 3.5% fat. Some loss of vitamins is inevitable when milk is stored and exposed to sunlight.

As many products are sold or measured by volume, typical specific gravities (densities) of some of these products are given below, and in the appropriate analytical reports (see general introduction). For the majority of purposes, the values are given on a weight basis and may be regarded as the same as those expressed by volume, with the exception of ice creams which have a much lower specific gravity.

Specific gravities of selected dairy products			
Skimmed milk	1.04	Single cream	1.00
Semi-skimmed milk	1.03	Whipping cream	0.96
Whole milk	1.03	Double cream	0.94
Evaporated milk	1.07	Yogurt, low fat, fruit	1.08
		Ice creams:	
		vanilla, dairy	0.61
		vanilla, non dairy	0.51

Losses of labile vitamins assigned on recipe calculation were estimated using figures in Section 4.3.

Composition of food per 100g edible portion

Milk[a]

No.	Food	Description and main data sources	Main data reference	Water g	Total nitrogen g	Protein g	Fat g	Carbo-hydrate g	Energy value kcal	Energy value kJ
219	**Channel Islands milk**, whole, pasteurised	Breakfast milk, average of summer and winter milk. Analytical data, 1996-1997	59	86.6	0.56	3.5	4.7	4.3	72	302
220	**Milk, 1% fat**, pasteurised	Estimated from skimmed and semi-skimmed milk; and industry data, 2013		90.1	0.55	3.5	1.0	4.8	41	173
221	**Semi-skimmed milk**, pasteurised, average	Average of summer/autumn and winter/spring milk. Analytical data, 1995-1996	51	89.4	0.54	3.5	1.7	4.7	46	195
222	pasteurised, summer and autumn	Analytical data, 1995-1996	51	89.5	0.55	3.5	1.7	4.5	46	194
223	pasteurised, winter and spring	Analytical data, 1996	51	89.5	0.54	3.4	1.7	4.9	47	196
224	UHT	Average of summer and winter milk. Analytical data, 1996-1997	59	90.9	0.50	3.3	1.6	4.9	46	194
225	**Skimmed milk**, pasteurised, average	Average of summer and winter milk. Analytical data, 1996	51	90.8	0.55	3.5	0.3	4.8	34	144
226	UHT	Average of summer and winter milk, unfortified. Analytical data, 1996-1997	59	91.3	0.53	3.4	0.1	4.9	33	140
227	**Whole milk**[b], pasteurised, average	Average of summer/autumn and winter/spring milk. Analytical data, 1995-1996; and industry data, 2014	51	87.6	0.53	3.4	3.6[c]	4.6	63	265
228	pasteurised, summer and autumn	Analytical data, 1995-1996; and industry data, 2014	51	87.7	0.54	3.4	3.6[c]	4.1	61	257
229	pasteurised, winter and spring	Analytical data, 1996; and industry data, 2014	51	87.5	0.52	3.3	3.6[c]	5.0	64	270
230	UHT	Average of summer and winter milk. Analytical data, 1996-1997; and industry data, 2014	59	90.2	0.50	3.2	3.6[c]	4.8	63	264

[a] All the values for pasteurised milk are equally applicable to unpasteurised milk

[b] Whole milk values are for milk standardised to a minimum 3.5% fat content

[c] Whole milk that is not standardised contains 3.9g fat per 100g

Milk and milk products

Composition of food per 100g edible portion

Milk

No.	Food	Starch g	Total sugars g	Gluc g	Fruct g	Sucr g	Malt g	Lact g	NSP g	AOAC g	Satd g	Mono-unsatd g	Poly-unsatd g	Trans g	Cholesterol mg
					Individual sugars				Dietary fibre		Fatty acids				
219	**Channel Islands milk**, whole, pasteurised	0	4.3	0	0	0	0	4.3	0	0	3.0	1.1	0.2	0.2	16
220	**Milk, 1% fat**, pasteurised	0	4.8	0	0	0	0	4.8	0	0	0.6	0.2	Tr	Tr	5
221	**Semi-skimmed milk**, pasteurised, average	0	4.7	0	0	0	0	4.7	0	0	1.1	0.4	Tr	0.1	6
222	pasteurised, summer and autumn	0	4.5	0	0	0	0	4.5	0	0	1.0	0.4	0.1	0.1	6
223	pasteurised, winter and spring	0	4.9	0	0	0	0	4.9	0	0	1.0	0.4	0.1	0.1	6
224	UHT	0	4.9	0	0	0	0	4.9	0	0	1.1	0.4	Tr	Tr	7
225	**Skimmed milk**, pasteurised, average	0	4.8	0	0	0	0	4.8	0	0	0.1	0.1	Tr	Tr	4
226	UHT	0	4.9	0	0	0	0	4.9	0	0	N	N	Tr	Tr	2
227	**Whole milk**[a], pasteurised, average	0	4.6	0	0	0	0	4.6	0	0	2.3	1.0	0.1	0.1	12
228	pasteurised, summer and autumn	0	4.1	0	0	0	0	4.1	0	0	2.3	1.0	0.1	0.1	12
229	pasteurised, winter and spring	0	5.0	0	0	0	0	5.0	0	0	2.3	1.0	0.1	0.1	12
230	UHT	0	4.8	0	0	0	0	4.8	0	0	2.2	1.0	0.1	0.1	13

[a] Whole milk values are for milk standardised to a minimum 3.5% fat content

109

Inorganic constituents per 100g edible portion

Milk

No.	Food	mg												µg	
		Na	K	Ca	Mg	P	Fe	Cu	Zn	Cl	Mn	Se	I
219	**Channel Islands milk**, whole, pasteurised	39	131	129	12	106	Tr	0.01	0.4	100	Tr	1	29
220	**Milk, 1% fat**, pasteurised	44	159	123	11	95	Tr	Tr	0.5	87	Tr	1	30
221	**Semi-skimmed milk**, pasteurised, average	43	156	120	11	94	0.02	Tr	0.4	87	Tr	1	30
222	pasteurised, summer and autumn	43	152	118	11	93	0.02	Tr	0.4	85	Tr	Tr	20
223	pasteurised, winter and spring	43	161	123	11	96	0.02	Tr	0.5	89	Tr	1	41
224	UHT	50	150	110	11	90	0.17	Tr	0.4	100	Tr	1	31
225	**Skimmed milk**, pasteurised, average	44	162	125	11	96	0.03	Tr	0.5	87	Tr	1	30[a]
226	UHT	40	148	102	10	92	Tr	0.01	0.3	102	Tr	2	25
227	**Whole milk**[b], pasteurised, average	42	157	120	11	96	0.02	Tr	0.5	89	Tr	1	31
228	pasteurised, summer and autumn	45	160	123	12	95	0.02	Tr	0.5	90	Tr	1	20
229	pasteurised, winter and spring	40	154	116	11	98	0.02	Tr	0.5	88	Tr	1	41
230	UHT	55	140	110	11	87	0.23	0.01	0.4	93	Tr	1	31

[a] The iodine content of summer and winter skimmed milk is 20µg and 39µg per 100g respectively

[b] Whole milk values are for milk standardised to a minimum 3.5% fat content

Vitamins per 100g edible portion

No.	Food	Retinol	Carotene	Vitamin D	Vitamin E	Thiamin	Ribo-flavin	Niacin	Trypt 60	Vitamin B₆	Vitamin B₁₂	Folate	Panto-thenate	Biotin	Vitamin C
		µg	µg	µg	mg	mg	mg	mg	mg	mg	µg	µg	mg	µg	mg
Milk															
219	**Channel Islands milk**, whole, pasteurised	35	41	0.1	0.17	0.04	0.22	0.1	0.6	0.03	0.8	6	0.38	1.9	1
220	**Milk, 1% fat**, pasteurised	8	5	Tr	0.02	0.03	0.23	0.1	0.7	0.06	0.9	9	0.59	2.8	2
221	**Semi-skimmed milk**, pasteurised, average	19	9	Tr	0.04	0.03	0.24	0.1	0.6	0.06	0.9	9	0.68	3.0	2
222	pasteurised, summer and autumn	15	7	Tr	0.05	0.03	0.24	0.2	0.6	0.06	0.8	7	0.57	2.9	2
223	pasteurised, winter and spring	22	11	Tr	0.03	0.03	0.24	0.1	0.7	0.06	0.9	11	0.80	3.0	2
224	UHT	20	11	Tr	0.03	0.04	0.18	0.1	0.8	0.05	0.2	2	0.33	1.8	Tr
225	**Skimmed milk**, pasteurised, average	1	Tr	Tr	Tr	0.03	0.22	0.1	0.7	0.06	0.8	9	0.50	2.5	1
226	UHT	Tr	Tr	Tr	0.02	0.04	0.17	0.1	0.8	0.02	0.6	1	0.41	1.8	Tr
227	**Whole milk**ᵃ, pasteurised, average	36	14	Tr	0.06	0.03	0.23	0.2	0.6	0.06	0.9	8	0.58	2.5	2
228	pasteurised, summer and autumn	46	22	Tr	0.08	0.03	0.24	0.2	0.5	0.06	0.9	6	0.57	2.3	2
229	pasteurised, winter and spring	27	6	Tr	0.05	0.03	0.22	0.2	0.7	0.07	0.8	9	0.60	2.8	2
230	UHT	50	29	0	0.07	0.04	0.18	0.1	0.8	0.04	0.2	1	0.32	1.8	Tr

ᵃ Whole milk values are for milk standardised to a minimum 3.5% fat content

Composition of food per 100g edible portion

No.	Food	Description and main data sources	Main data reference	Water g	Total nitrogen g	Protein g	Fat g	Carbo-hydrate g	Energy value kcal	kJ
Processed milks										
231	**Condensed milk**, sweetened	MPE Supplement, 1989; and industry data, 2013	8	29.1	1.16	7.4	8.0	55.5	310	1310
232	**Dried skimmed milk**	MPE Supplement, 1989; and industry data, 2013	8	3.0	5.70	36.1	0.6	52.9	348	1482
233	**Evaporated milk**, whole	MPE Supplement, 1989; and industry data, 2013	8	69.1	1.32	8.4	9.4	12.7	166	694
234	light	Analytical data, 1996	59	75.9	1.22	7.8	4.1	10.3	107	449
235	**Flavoured milk**, pasteurised, strawberry, banana	Including low fat and semi-skimmed. Analytical data, 1996-1997	59	83.9	0.57	3.6	1.5	9.6[a]	64	270
236	pasteurised, chocolate	Including low fat and semi-skimmed. Analytical data, 1996-1997; and industry data, 2013	59	82.8	0.56	3.6	1.5	11.7[a]	72	305
237	**Milkshake**, thick, takeaway	Including chocolate, vanilla, and banana. Analytical data, 1996	59	73.2	0.58	3.7	1.8	15.3[a]	88	374
Other milks										
238	**Goats milk**, pasteurised	MPE Supplement, 1989	8	88.9	0.49	3.1	3.7	4.4	62	260
239	**Human milk**, mature	Literature sources, 1977. Reviewed 2010[b]	97	87.1	0.31[c]	1.3[d]	4.1	7.2	69	289
240	**Sheeps milk**, raw	MPE Supplement, 1989	8	83.0	0.85	5.4	5.8	5.1	93	388
241	**Soya, non-dairy alternative to milk**, sweetened, fortified	Analytical data, 1996; and industry data, 2013	59	90.1	0.55	3.1	2.4	2.5[a]	43	182
242	unsweetened, fortified	Analytical data, 1996; and industry data, 2013	59	93.0	0.42	2.4	1.6	0.5[a]	26	108

[a] Includes oligosaccharides

[b] White R. & Allen R. Department of Health, Composition of breast milk review (2010). Published as Annex D in Diet and Nutrition Survey of Infants and Young Children, 2011

[c] 35 per cent of this nitrogen is non-protein nitrogen

[d] (Total N - non-protein N) x 6.38

Milk and milk products *continued*

Composition of food per 100g edible portion

No.	Food	Starch	Total sugars	Individual sugars					Dietary fibre		Fatty acids				Cholest-erol
				Gluc	Fruct	Sucr	Malt	Lact	NSP	AOAC	Satd	Mono-unsatd	Poly-unsatd	Trans	
		g	g	g	g	g	g	g	g	g	g	g	g	g	mg
Processed milks															
231	**Condensed milk**, sweetened	0	55.5	0	0	43.2	0	12.3	0	0	5.0	2.3	0.2	N	29
232	**Dried skimmed milk**	0	52.9	0	0	0	0	52.9	0	0	0.4	0.2	Tr	Tr	12
233	**Evaporated milk**, whole	0	12.7	0	0	0	0	12.7	0	0	5.9	2.7	0.3	N	34
234	light	0	10.3	0	0	0	0	10.3	0	0	2.5	1.1	0.2	0.2	17
235	**Flavoured milk**, pasteurised, strawberry, banana	0.2	8.9[a]	Tr	Tr	3.9	0.1	4.9	0	0	1.0	0.3	0.1	Tr	7
236	pasteurised, chocolate	0.3	11.0[a]	Tr	1.7	2.8	1.1	5.5	0	0	1.0	0.4	0.1	0.1	7
237	**Milkshake**, thick, takeaway	0.3	11.1[a]	0.3	4.2	1.4	0.7	4.5	Tr	Tr	1.2	0.4	0.1	0.1	11
Other milks															
238	**Goats milk**, pasteurised	0	4.4	0	0	0	0	4.4	0	0	2.4	0.9	0.2	0.1	11
239	**Human milk**, mature	0	7.2	0	0	0	0	7.2	0	0	1.9	1.5	0.5	N	16
240	**Sheeps milk**, raw	0	5.1	0	0	0	0	5.1	0	0	3.6	1.5	0.3	0.4	12
241	**Soya, non-dairy alternative to milk**, sweetened, fortified	0	2.2[a]	0.3	1.2	0.7	0	0	0.2	0.5	0.4	0.5	1.4	Tr	0
242	unsweetened, fortified	0	0.2[a]	0	0	0.2	0	0	0.2	0.5	0.2	0.3	1.1	Tr	0

[a] Not including oligosaccharides

Inorganic constituents per 100g edible portion

No.	Food	mg										µg	
		Na	K	Ca	Mg	P	Fe	Cu	Zn	Cl	Mn	Se	I
Processed milks													
231	**Condensed milk**, sweetened	90	360	290	29	240	0.23	Tr	1.0	150	Tr	3	74
232	**Dried skimmed milk**	550	1590	1280	130	970	0.27	Tr	4.0	1070	Tr	11	150
233	**Evaporated milk**, whole	180	360	290	29	260	0.26	0.02	0.9	250	Tr	3	11
234	light	115	336	260	25	233	Tr	Tr	1.0	222	Tr	3	47
235	**Flavoured milk**, pasteurised, strawberry, banana	52	168	120	12	102	0.13	Tr	0.4	110	Tr	N	N
236	pasteurised, chocolate	45	206	115	19	107	0.62	0.06	0.5	110	0.1	N	N
237	**Milkshake**, thick, takeaway	57	171	129	13	120	Tr	Tr	0.1	111	Tr	2	37
Other milks													
238	**Goats milk**, pasteurised	42	170	100	13	90	0.12	0.03	0.5	150	Tr	N	N
239	**Human milk**, mature	15	58	34	3	15	0.07	0.04	0.3	42	Tr	1	7
240	**Sheeps milk**, raw	44	120	170	18	150	0.03	0.10	0.7	82	Tr	N	N
241	**Soya, non-dairy alternative to milk,** sweetened, fortified	56	119	130	18	89	0.31	0.09	0.3	3	0.2	4	1
242	unsweetened, fortified	Tr	74	120	15	48	0.43	0.09	0.3	3	0.3	4	1

Milk and milk products *continued*

Vitamins per 100g edible portion

No.	Food	Retinol µg	Carotene µg	Vitamin D µg	Vitamin E mg	Thiamin mg	Ribo-flavin mg	Niacin mg	Trypt 60 mg	Vitamin B$_6$ mg	Vitamin B$_{12}$ µg	Folate µg	Panto-thenate mg	Biotin µg	Vitamin C mg
Processed milks															
231	**Condensed milk**, sweetened	110	70	Tr	0.19	0.09	0.46	0.3	2.0	0.07	0.7	15	0.85	3.9	4
232	**Dried skimmed milk**	550[a]	5[a]	1.5[a]	0.01	0.38	1.63	1.0	8.6	0.60	2.6	51	3.28	20.1	13
233	**Evaporated milk**, whole	105	100	2.7[b]	0.19	0.07	0.42	0.2	2.0	0.07	0.1	11	0.75	4.0	1
234	light	50	21	3.1[c]	0.11	0.07	0.42	0.2	2.0	0.04	0.2	8	0.75	4.0	1
235	**Flavoured milk**, pasteurised, strawberry, banana	20	8	Tr	0.03	0.03	0.17	0.1	0.8	0.03	0.1	2	0.30	2.2	Tr
236	pasteurised, chocolate	20	8	Tr	0.03	0.03	0.17	0.1	0.8	0.03	0.1	2	0.30	2.2	Tr
237	**Milkshake**, thick, takeaway	35	11	Tr	0.10	0.03	0.23	0.1	0.7	0.03	0.5	4	0.31	2.0	1
Other milks															
238	**Goats milk**, pasteurised	44	Tr	0.1	0.03	0.03	0.04	0.1	0.7	0.06	0.1	1	0.41	3.0	1
239	**Human milk**, mature	58	24	N	0.34	0.02	0.03	0.2	0.5	0.01	Tr	5	0.25	0.7	4
240	**Sheeps milk**, raw	83	Tr	0.2	0.11	0.08	0.32	0.4	1.3	0.08	0.6	5	0.45	2.5	5
241	**Soya, non-dairy alternative to milk**, sweetened, fortified	0	Tr	0.8	0.32[d]	0.06	0.20	0.1	0.7	0.03	0.4	9	Tr	1.0	1
242	unsweetened, fortified	Tr	Tr	0.8	0.32[d]	0.06	0.20	0.1	0.7	0.03	0.4	14	Tr	1.0	0

[a] Unfortified skimmed milk powder contains approximately 8µg retinol, 3µg carotene and Tr vitamin D per 100g

[b] Value is for fortified products. Unfortified evaporated milk contains approximately 0.09µg vitamin D per 100g

[c] Value is for fortified products

[d] Value is for unfortified products. Some brands have added vitamin E

115

Composition of food per 100g edible portion

No.	Food	Description and main data sources	Main data reference	Water g	Total nitrogen g	Protein g	Fat g	Carbo-hydrate g	Energy value kcal	kJ
Fresh creams (pasteurised)										
243	**Cream**, fresh, single	Average of summer and winter cream. Analytical data, 1996-1997	59	77.0	0.52	3.3	19.1	2.2	193	798
244	fresh, whipping	Average of summer and winter cream. Analytical data, 1996-1997	59	54.5	0.31	2.0	40.3	2.7	381	1568
245	fresh, double, including Jersey cream	Average of summer and winter cream. Analytical data, 1996-1997	59	46.9	0.25	1.6	53.7[a,b]	1.7[a]	496[a]	2041[a]
246	fresh, clotted	MPE Supplement, 1989	8	32.2	0.25	1.6	63.5	2.3	586	2413
247	**Creme fraiche**	Plain. Analytical data, 1996	59	55.8	0.34	2.2	40.0	2.4	378	1556
248	half fat	Plain. Analytical data, 1996	59	76.5	0.42	2.7	15.0	4.4	162	671
249	**Cream**, dairy, extra thick, 24% fat	Average of summer and winter cream. Analytical data, 1997	59	69.0	0.45	2.9	23.5	3.4	236	973
UHT creams										
250	**Cream, dairy, UHT**, canned spray, 85% cream	Analytical data, 1996-1997	59	63.6	0.30	1.9	24.2[c]	7.2	252	1043
251	half fat, canned spray	Anchor Light. Analytical data, 1996; and estimated from 85% fat canned spray	59	71.9	0.44	2.8	17.3	7.6[d]	196	811
Cream substitutes										
252	**Cream substitute**, single	Including Elmlea. Analytical data, 1996	59	76.8	0.49	3.1	14.5	4.0	158	654

[a] Double cream with added alcohol contains 39.7g fat, 10.3g carbohydrate (8.0g sucrose, 2.0g lactose, 0.3 maltodextrins), 5.0g alcohol, 531kcal and 2186kJ energy per 100g

[b] The average fat content of double cream excluding Jersey cream is approximately 48g

[c] The average fat content is variable and dependent on the percentage of cream in the product

[d] Includes oligosaccharides

Milk and milk products *continued*

Composition of food per 100g edible portion

No.	Food	Starch	Total sugars	Individual sugars					Dietary fibre		Fatty acids				Cholest-erol
				Gluc	Fruct	Sucr	Malt	Lact	NSP	AOAC	Satd	Mono-unsatd	Poly-unsatd	Trans	
		g	g	g	g	g	g	g	g	g	g	g	g	g	mg
Fresh creams (pasteurised)															
243	**Cream**, fresh, single	0	2.2	0	0	0	0	2.2	0	0	12.2	5.1	0.6	0.7	55
244	fresh, whipping	0	2.7	0	0	0	0	2.7	0	0	25.2	11.7	1.1	N	105
245	fresh, double, including Jersey cream	0	1.7	0	0	0	0	1.7	0	0	33.4	13.8	1.9	1.8	137
246	fresh, clotted	0	2.3	0	0	0	0	2.3	0	0	39.7	18.4	1.8	N	170
247	**Creme fraiche**	0.3	2.1	0	0	0	0	2.1	0	0	27.1	8.6	1.1	0.8	113
248	half fat	1.4	3.0	0	0	0	0	3.0	0	0	10.2	3.2	0.4	0.3	N
249	**Cream**, dairy, extra thick, 24% fat	0	3.4	0	0	0	0	3.4	0	0	15.3	6.0	0.8	0.8	74
UHT creams															
250	**Cream, dairy, UHT**, canned spray, 85% cream	0	7.2	0	0	3.9	0	3.3	0	0	15.2	6.1	0.8	0.8	68
251	half fat, canned spray	0	7.4[a]	0	0	3.8	0	3.6	0	0	10.9	4.3	0.6	0.6	46
Cream substitutes															
252	**Cream substitute**, single	0	4.0	0	0	0	0	4.0	N[b]	N[b]	9.2	3.2	1.3	0.4	4

[a] Not including oligosaccharides

[b] Carob and guar gums are added as thickeners

Inorganic constituents per 100g edible portion

No.	Food	Na	K	Ca	Mg	P	Fe	Cu	Zn	Cl	Mn	Se	I
						mg						µg	
Fresh creams (pasteurised)													
243	**Cream, fresh, single**	29	104	89	8	79	Tr	Tr	0.3	80	Tr	N	N
244	fresh, whipping	25	86	58	6	59	Tr	Tr	0.2	59	Tr	N	N
245	fresh, double, including Jersey cream	22	65	49	5	52	0.06	Tr	0.2	36	Tr	3	35
246	fresh, clotted	18	55	37	5	40	0.10	0.09	0.2	40	Tr	Tr	N
247	**Creme fraiche**	22	81	58	6	58	0.11	Tr	0.2	55	Tr	0	8
248	half fat	36	122	95	9	81	0.10	Tr	0.3	N	Tr	4	8
249	**Cream, dairy, extra thick, 24% fat**	29	100	95	8	81	0.05	0.01	0.3	N	Tr	N	N
UHT creams													
250	**Cream, dairy, UHT**, canned spray, 85% cream	31	107	54	7	57	Tr	Tr	0.2	66	Tr	1	11
251	half fat, canned spray	35	110	87	9	77	Tr	Tr	0.3	66	Tr	1	11
Cream substitutes													
252	**Cream substitute, single**	61	139	96	10	88	0.12	Tr	0.3	N	Tr	2	N

Milk and milk products *continued*

Vitamins per 100g edible portion

No.	Food	Retinol µg	Carotene µg	Vitamin D µg	Vitamin E mg	Thiamin mg	Ribo-flavin mg	Niacin mg	Trypt 60 mg	Vitamin B_6 mg	Vitamin B_{12} µg	Folate µg	Panto-thenate mg	Biotin µg	Vitamin C mg
Fresh creams (pasteurised)															
243	**Cream, fresh, single**	291	169	0.3	0.47	0.03	0.19	0.1	0.5	0.03	0.4	5	0.30	2.8	1
244	fresh, whipping	399	247	0.3	1.32	0.02	0.17	Tr	0.5	0.04	0.2	7	0.22	1.4	1
245	fresh, double, including Jersey cream	779[a]	483[a]	0.3	1.64[a]	0.02	0.19	Tr	0.3	0.01	0.6	7	0.23	0.9	1
246	fresh, clotted	705	685	0.3	1.48	0.02	0.16	Tr	0.4	0.03	0.1	6	0.14	1.0	Tr
247	**Creme fraiche**	388	143	0.3	0.72	0.02	0.21	0.1	N	0.01	0.2	3	N	N	N
248	half fat	300	21	Tr	0.42	0.02	0.21	0.1	N	0.01	0.2	3	N	N	N
249	**Cream, dairy, extra thick, 24% fat**	435	384	0.3	0.80	0.03	0.19	0.1	0.5	0.03	0.4	5	0.30	2.8	1
UHT creams															
250	**Cream, dairy, UHT**, canned spray, 85% cream	279	111	0.3	0.79	0.03	0.26	0.1	0.5	0.02	0.1	6	0.19	1.7	0
251	half fat, canned spray	147	39	Tr	0.46	0.03	0.26	0.1	0.5	0.02	0.1	6	0.19	1.7	0
Cream substitutes															
252	**Cream substitute**, single	11	166	Tr	0.84	N	N	N	0.7	N	N	N	N	N	N

[a] Double cream with added alcohol contains 390µg retinol, 187µg carotene and 1.08mg vitamin E

Composition of food per 100g edible portion

No.	Food	Description and main data sources	Main data reference	Water g	Total nitrogen g	Protein g	Fat g	Carbo-hydrate g	Energy value kcal	kJ
Cream substitutes continued										
253	**Cream substitute**, double	Including Elmlea. Analytical data, 1996	59	55.8	0.41	2.6	35.7	3.6	345	1423
Cheeses										
254	**Brie**	Excluding rind. Analytical data, 1998	62	48.7	3.18	20.3	29.1	Tr	343	1422
255	**Camembert**	Analytical data, 1998	62	54.4	3.37	21.5	22.7	Tr	290	1205
256	**Cheddar**, English	Including mild and mature, spring and autumn. Analytical data, 1998	62	36.6	3.98	25.4	34.9	0.1	416	1725
257	**Cheddar type**, '30% less fat'	Industry data, 2013; and analytical data, 1998 (cheddar type, half fat)	62	45.9	4.37	27.9	22.1	0.8	314	1305
258	**Cheese spread**, plain	Portions and tubs. Analytical data, 1998; and industry data, 2013	62	58.1	1.77	11.3	18.6	6.5	237	984
259	plain, reduced fat	Portions and tubs. Analytical data, 1995; and industry data, 2013	48	61.4	2.35	15.0	7.2	7.9	154	648
260	**Cottage cheese**, plain	Analytical data, 1998; and industry data, 2013	62	83.5	1.47	9.4	6.0	3.1	103	431
261	plain, reduced fat	Analytical data, 1998; and industry data, 2013	62	84.1	1.66	10.6	1.5	3.3	68	289
262	**Danish blue**	Analytical data, 1998	62	46.3	3.22	20.5	28.9	Tr	342	1418
263	**Double Gloucester**	Sampled in spring and autumn. Analytical data, 1998	62	37.9	3.83	24.4	35.0	0.1	413	1711
264	**Edam**	Analytical data, 1998	62	43.8	4.18	26.7	26.0	Tr	341	1416
265	**Feta**	Made from sheeps and goats milk. MPE Supplement, 1989; and industry data, 2013	8	56.5	2.45	15.6	20.2	1.5	250	1037

No.	Food	Starch	Total sugars	Individual sugars					Dietary fibre		Fatty acids				Cholest-erol
				Gluc	Fruct	Sucr	Malt	Lact	NSP	AOAC	Satd	Mono-unsatd	Poly-unsatd	Trans	
		g	g	g	g	g	g	g	g	g	g	g	g	g	mg
Cream substitutes continued															
253	**Cream substitute**, double	0	3.6	0	0	0	0	3.6	0.1[a]	0.2[a]	24.3	6.5	2.8	0.9	11
Cheeses															
254	**Brie**	0	Tr	0	0	0	0	Tr	0	0	18.2	6.7	0.6	1.3	93
255	**Camembert**	0	Tr	0	0	0	0	Tr	0	0	14.2	6.6	0.7	N	72
256	**Cheddar**, English	0	0.1	0	0	0	0	0.1	0	0	21.7	9.4	1.1	1.4	97
257	**Cheddar type**, '30% less fat'	0.7	0.1	0	0	0	0	0.1	0	0	13.8	6.5	0.6	N	60
258	**Cheese spread**, plain	0	6.5	0	0	0	0	6.5	0	0	12.9	4.8	0.7	0.9	55
259	plain, reduced fat	0.6	7.3	0	0	0	0	7.3	0	0	4.6	1.7	0.2	0.3	N
260	**Cottage cheese**, plain	0	3.1	0	0	0	0	3.1	0	0	3.2	1.7	0.2	0.3	22
261	plain, reduced fat	0	3.3	0	0	0	0	3.3	0	0	1.0	0.4	Tr	Tr	5
262	**Danish blue**	0	Tr	0	0	0	0	Tr	0	0	19.1	7.5	1.0	1.1	75
263	**Double Gloucester**	0	0.1	0	0	0	0	0.1	0	0	21.9	10.2	1.0	1.4	100
264	**Edam**	0	Tr	0	0	0	0	Tr	0	0	15.8	5.2	0.4	0.7	71
265	**Feta**	0	1.5[b]	0	0	0	0	1.4	0	0	13.7	4.1	0.6	N	70

[a] Carob and guar gums are added as thickeners

[b] Contains galactose

121

Inorganic constituents per 100g edible portion

No.	Food	mg										µg	
		Na	K	Ca	Mg	P	Fe	Cu	Zn	Cl	Mn	Se	I
Cream substitutes continued													
253	**Cream substitute**, double	47	109	79	8	73	0.22	Tr	0.3	N	N	2	N
Cheeses													
254	**Brie**	556	91	256	15	232	Tr	Tr	2.0	900	Tr	5	16
255	**Camembert**	605	104	235	14	241	Tr	Tr	2.1	1120	Tr	7	N
256	**Cheddar**, English	723	75	739	29	505	0.30	0.03	4.1	1040	Tr	6	30
257	**Cheddar type**, '30% less fat'	720	110	840	39	620	0.20	0.05	2.8	1190	Tr	11	N
258	**Cheese spread**, plain	730	219	498	24	835	Tr	Tr	1.8	560	Tr	4	29
259	plain, reduced fat	750	235	485	24	850	0.29	0.05	1.7	562	Tr	4	29
260	**Cottage cheese**, plain	250	161	127	13	171	Tr	Tr	0.6	400	Tr	4	24
261	plain, reduced fat	210	161	127	13	171	Tr	Tr	0.6	340	Tr	4	24
262	**Danish blue**	1220	88	488	20	344	Tr	Tr	3.0	1950	Tr	7	12
263	**Double Gloucester**	673	79	660	23	460	0.40	0.03	1.8	970	Tr	12	46
264	**Edam**	996	89	795	34	508	0.30	Tr	3.8	1570	Tr	7	13
265	**Feta**	1000	95	360	20	280	0.20	0.07	0.9	1630	Tr	5	N

Vitamins per 100g edible portion

No.	Food	Retinol µg	Carotene µg	Vitamin D µg	Vitamin E mg	Thiamin mg	Ribo-flavin mg	Niacin mg	Trypt 60 mg	Vitamin B6 mg	Vitamin B12 µg	Folate µg	Panto-thenate mg	Biotin µg	Vitamin C mg
Cream substitutes continued															
253	**Cream substitute**, double	10	363	Tr	1.33	N	N	N	0.6	N	N	N	N	N	N
Cheeses															
254	**Brie**	297	192	0.2	0.81	0.03[a]	0.33	0.5	4.6	0.14	0.6	55	0.50	3.6	Tr
255	**Camembert**	230	315	0.1	0.65	0.05	0.52	0.9	4.9	0.23	1.1	83	0.80	7.5	Tr
256	**Cheddar**, English	364	141	0.3	0.52	0.03	0.39	0.1	6.8	0.15	2.4	31	0.50	4.4	Tr
257	**Cheddar type**, '30% less fat'	266	169	0.1	0.66	0.03	0.53	0.1	7.4	0.13	1.3	56	0.51	3.8	Tr
258	**Cheese spread**, plain	214	119	0.2	0.24	0.05	0.36	0.1	3.2	0.08	0.6	19	0.51	3.6	Tr
259	plain, 'reduced fat'	119	90	N	0.40	0.06	0.53	0.1	3.1	0.07	2.0	7	0.42	3.0	Tr
260	**Cottage cheese**, plain	64	13	0	0.14	0.05	0.24	0.2	3.4	0.05	0.6	22	0.30	5.1	Tr
261	plain, reduced fat	16	4	0	0.03	0.05	0.24	0.2	3.4	0.05	0.6	22	0.30	5.1	Tr
262	**Danish blue**	244	283	0.2	0.71	0.03	0.41	0.6	5.5	0.10	1.3	55	0.53	2.7	Tr
263	**Double Gloucester**	335	203	0.3	0.64	0.03	0.45	0.1	5.8	0.11	1.3	30	0.32	3.1	Tr
264	**Edam**	188	182	0.2	0.48	0.03	0.35	0.1	6.1	0.09	2.1	36	0.38	1.8	Tr
265	**Feta**	220	33	0.5	0.37	0.04	0.21	0.2	3.5	0.07	1.1	23	0.36	2.4	Tr

[a] The rind alone contains 0.05mg thiamin per 100g

Composition of food per 100g edible portion

No.	Food	Description and main data sources	Main data reference	Water g	Total nitrogen g	Protein g	Fat g	Carbo-hydrate g	Energy value kcal	kJ
	Cheeses continued									
266	**Goats milk cheese**, soft, white rind	English and French. Analytical data, 1998	62	50.8	3.30	21.1	25.8	1.0	320	1329
267	**Gouda**	Analytical data, 1998	62	40.4	3.97	25.3	30.6	Tr	377	1562
268	**Halloumi**	Sampled in spring and autumn. Analytical data, 1998; and industry data, 2013	62	50.9	3.75	23.9	23.5	1.7	313	1303
269	**Mascarpone**	Sampled in spring and autumn. Analytical data, 1998	62	46.2	0.72	4.6	44.5	4.3	435	1794
270	**Mozzarella**, fresh	Soft, not grated. Analytical data, 1998	62	57.4	2.91	18.6	20.3	Tr	257	1067
271	**Paneer**	Sampled in spring and autumn. Analytical data, 1998	62	46.8	4.07	26.0	24.5	0.9	328	1363
272	**Parmesan**, fresh	Wedges/freshly grated. Analytical data, 1998; and industry data, 2013	62	27.6	5.67	36.2	29.7	0.9	415	1729
273	**Processed cheese**, plain	Analytical data, 1998; and industry data, 2013	62	47.4	2.79	17.8	23.0	5.0	297	1234
274	slices, reduced fat	Industry data, 2013		61.9	2.62	16.7	9.6	9.7	190	794
275	**Red Leicester**	Sampled in spring and autumn. Analytical data, 1998	62	37.5	3.92	25.0	33.6	0.1	403	1670
276	**Spreadable cheese**, soft white, low fat	Extra light soft cheese spreads. Industry data, 2013	62	78.4	1.87	11.9	3.6	5.0	99	416
277	soft white, medium fat	Including Philadelphia light and own brands. Analytical data, 1998; and industry data, 2013	62	74.4	1.54	9.8	11.2	3.5	153	637
278	soft white, full fat	Including Philadelphia and own brands. Analytical data, 1998; and industry data, 2013	62	66.3	0.83	5.3	24.4	3.0	252	1041
279	**Stilton**, blue	Analytical data, 1998	62	38.0	3.72	23.7	35.0	0.1	410	1698
280	**Wensleydale**	Sampled in spring and autumn. Analytical data, 1998	62	41.6	3.72	23.7	31.8	0.1	381	1581

Milk and milk products *continued*

Composition of food per 100g edible portion

Cheeses continued

No.	Food	Starch g	Total sugars g	Gluc g	Fruct g	Sucr g	Malt g	Lact g	Dietary fibre NSP g	AOAC g	Fatty acids Satd g	Mono-unsatd g	Poly-unsatd g	Trans g	Cholesterol mg
266	**Goats milk cheese**, soft, white rind	0	1.0[a]	0	0	0	0	0.9	0	0	17.9	6.1	1.0	1.0	93
267	**Gouda**	0	Tr	0	0	0	0	Tr	0	0	20.3	7.4	0.9	1.1	85
268	**Halloumi**	0	1.7[a]	0	0	0	0	1.5	0	0	16.6	5.7	1.1	0.8	63
269	**Mascarpone**	0	4.3	0	0	0	0	4.3	0	0	29.5	11.7	1.9	1.8	123
270	**Mozzarella**, fresh	0	Tr	0	0	0	0	Tr	0	0	13.8	5.0	0.8	0.8	58
271	**Paneer**	0	0.9	0	0	0	0	0.9	0	0	15.4	7.1	1.1	1.3	N
272	**Parmesan**, fresh	0	0.9	0	0	0	0	0.9	0	0	19.3	7.7	1.1	1.1	93
273	**Processed cheese**, plain	0	5.0	0	0	0	0	5.0	0	0	14.3	6.3	0.8	1.1	85
274	slices, reduced fat	2.1	7.6	0	0	0	0	7.6	0	0	5.9	2.6	0.3	0.3	35
275	**Red Leicester**	0	0.1	0	0	0	0	0.1	0	0	21.1	9.8	1.0	1.4	100
276	**Spreadable cheese**, soft white, low fat	0	5.0	0	0	0	0	5.0	0	0	2.4	0.9	0.1	0.1	11
277	soft white, medium fat	0	3.5	0	0	0	0	3.5	0	0	7.4	2.8	0.3	0.5	33
278	soft white, full fat	0	3.0	0	0	0	0	3.0	0	0	16.0	6.1	0.8	0.9	72
279	**Stilton**, blue	0	0.1	0	0	0	0	0.1	0	0	23.0	9.2	1.2	1.5	95
280	**Wensleydale**	0	0.1	0	0	0	0	0.1	0	0	19.7	9.1	0.9	1.4	90

[a] Contains galactose

Milk and milk products *continued*

Inorganic constituents per 100g edible portion

No.	Food	Na	K	Ca	Mg	P	Fe	Cu	Zn	Cl	Mn	Se	I
						mg						μg	

Cheeses continued

No.	Food	Na	K	Ca	Mg	P	Fe	Cu	Zn	Cl	Mn	Se	I
266	**Goats milk cheese**, soft, white rind	601	132	133	14	229	Tr	0.06	1.0	1060	Tr	6	51
267	**Gouda**	925	82	773	32	498	0.30	Tr	3.9	1440	Tr	8	N
268	**Halloumi**	1200	88	794	40	517	Tr	Tr	3.7	1730	0.1	12	60
269	**Mascarpone**	70	137	161	11	116	Tr	Tr	0.7	110	Tr	2	14
270	**Mozzarella**, fresh	395	51	362	15	267	Tr	Tr	2.7	650	Tr	6	18
271	**Paneer**	19	69	537	23	383	Tr	Tr	3.2	N	Tr	N	N
272	**Parmesan**, fresh	660	152	1025	41	680	0.80	0.84	5.1	1100	Tr	12	72
273	**Processed cheese**, plain	1000	178	610	27	768	0.50	Tr	2.6	800	Tr	5	27
274	slices, reduced fat	810	148	642	25	513	0.27	0.06	2.4	630	Tr	6	22
275	**Red Leicester**	665	76	723	29	495	0.30	0.05	4.0	961	Tr	11	46
276	**Spreadable cheese**, soft white, low fat	260	141	121	11	154	Tr	Tr	1.1	440	Tr	5	17
277	soft white, medium fat	270	120	99	10	129	Tr	Tr	0.7	460	Tr	4	11
278	soft white, full fat	260	89	76	7	97	Tr	Tr	0.7	440	Tr	3	11
279	**Stilton**, blue	788	96	326	15	314	0.20	0.04	2.9	1230	Tr	7	40
280	**Wensleydale**	440	89	560	19	410	0.30	0.11	3.4	710	Tr	11	46

Cheeses continued

No.	Food	Retinol	Carotene	Vitamin D	Vitamin E	Thiamin	Ribo-flavin	Niacin	Trypt 60	Vitamin B₆	Vitamin B₁₂	Folate	Panto-thenate	Biotin	Vitamin C
		µg	µg	µg	mg	mg	mg	mg	mg	mg	µg	µg	mg	µg	mg
266	**Goats milk cheese**, soft, white rind	333	Tr	0.5	0.63	0.03	0.39	0.7	6.0	0.10	0.5	22	0.40	5.1	Tr
267	**Gouda**	258	139	0.2	0.57	0.03	0.30	0.1	7.0	0.08	1.7	43	0.32	1.4	Tr
268	**Halloumi**	288	201	0.2	0.60	0.03	0.39	0.1	6.1	0.10	0.5	40	0.40	5.1	Tr
269	**Mascarpone**	376	214	0.3	1.14	0.04	0.22	0.1	1.7	0.04	0.6	11	0.27	1.6	Tr
270	**Mozzarella**, fresh	258	152	0.2	0.31	0.03	0.40	0.1	5.0	0.10	1.7	20	0.25	2.2	Tr
271	**Paneer**	248	34	N	0.41	N	0.20	0.1	7.7	N	N	25	N	N	Tr
272	**Parmesan**, fresh	371	233	0.3	0.76	0.03	0.32	0.1	9.0	0.11	3.3	12	0.43	3.3	Tr
273	**Processed cheese**, plain	270	95	N	0.55	0.06	0.25	0.1	4.7	0.07	1.2	15	0.60	5.6	Tr
274	slices, reduced fat	113	142	N	0.39	0.05	0.20	0.1	3.8	0.06	1.0	12	0.48	4.5	Tr
275	**Red Leicester**	290	300	0.3	0.38	0.03	0.44	0.1	5.7	0.11	1.2	30	0.38	3.0	Tr
276	**Spreadable cheese**, soft white, low fat	39	158	N	N	0.05	0.41	0.1	4.3	0.02	0.5	36	0.32	8.1	Tr
277	soft white, medium fat	134	175	0.1	0.08	0.04	0.34	0.1	3.5	0.01	0.4	30	0.26	6.7	Tr
278	soft white, full fat	203	199	0.1	0.19	0.03	0.26	0.1	2.7	0.01	0.3	23	0.20	5.1	Tr
279	**Stilton**, blue	360	182	0.2	0.60	0.03	0.47	0.7	5.9	0.13	1.2	78	0.90	3.3	Tr
280	**Wensleydale**	345	280	0.2	0.45	0.03	0.46	0.1	5.5	0.09	1.1	43	0.30	4.0	Tr

Composition of food per 100g edible portion

Yogurts and fromage frais

No.	Food	Description and main data sources	Main data reference	Water g	Total nitrogen g	Protein g	Fat g	Carbohydrate g	Energy value kcal	kJ
281	**Fermented milk drink** with probiotics	Including Yakult, Danone, Muller and own brand yogurt drinks. Industry data, 2013		83.0	0.47	3.0	1.2	12.7	70	299
282	**Fromage frais**, fruit, children's, fortified	Industry data, 2013; and estimated from previous values for fromage frais (analytical data, 1998)	60	77.9	0.91	5.8	2.9	13.2	99	417
283	virtually fat free, fruit	Including strawberry, raspberry, apricot and black cherry flavour. Analytical data, 1997	60	86.7	1.07	6.8	0.2	5.6	50	213
284	virtually fat free, natural	Analytical data, 1997	60	87.2	1.20	7.7	0.1	4.6	49	208
285	**Lassi**, sweetened	Takeaway and retail. Analytical data, 1996	59	83.3	0.41	2.6	0.9	12.3[a]	65	274
286	**Yogurt, Greek style**, fruit	Including peach, apricot, strawberry and blackcurrant, made with whole milk. Analytical data, 1997	60	73.5	0.76	4.8	8.4	11.2	137	572
287	plain	Made with whole milk. Analytical data, 1997	60	78.2	0.90	5.7	10.2	4.8	133	551
288	**Yogurt, low fat**, fruit	Including French set. Analytical data, 1997	60	78.9	0.66	4.2	1.1	13.7	78	331
289	hazelnut	Analytical data, 1997	60	77.4	0.70	4.4	1.5	16.0	91	387
290	plain	Analytical data, 1997	60	87.2	0.75	4.8	1.0	7.8	57	243
291	toffee	Analytical data, 1997	60	76.0	0.60	3.8	0.9	18.0	91	386
292	**Yogurt, soya**, non-dairy alternative to yogurt, fruit, fortified	Analytical data, 1997; and industry data, 2013	60	82.7	0.58	3.3	2.0	11.0	72	306
293	**Yogurt, whole milk**, fruit	Assorted flavours including bio varieties. Analytical data, 1997	60	76.0	0.63	4.0	3.0	17.7	109	463

[a] Includes oligosaccharides

Milk and milk products *continued*

Composition of food per 100g edible portion

No.	Food	Starch	Total sugars	Gluc	Fruct	Sucr	Malt	Lact	Dietary fibre		Fatty acids				Cholest-erol
									NSP	AOAC	Satd	Mono-unsatd	Poly-unsatd	Trans	
		g	g	g	g	g	g	g	g	g	g	g	g	g	mg
281	**Fermented milk drink** with probiotics	0.4	12.3	N	N	N	N	N	N	0.1	0.8	N	N	N	N
	Yogurts and fromage frais														
282	**Fromage frais**, fruit, children's, fortified	1.4	11.8	N	N	N	N	N	N	0.2	1.9	N	N	N	N
283	virtually fat free, fruit	0.7	4.9[a]	0.7	0.9	0.2	0	2.9	0.4	0.7	0.1	0.1	Tr	Tr	1
284	virtually fat free, natural	0.2	4.4[a]	0.2	0	0	0	4.1	0	0	0.1	Tr	Tr	Tr	1
285	**Lassi**, sweetened	0.2	11.9[a,b]	0.1	0.1	2.3	0.1	8.6	0	0	0.6	0.2	Tr	N	N
286	**Yogurt, Greek style**, fruit	0.7	10.5[a]	Tr	1.0	3.8	0.4	4.0	Tr	Tr	5.6	2.2	0.2	0.2	14
287	plain	0.3	4.5[a]	0.1	Tr	Tr	Tr	3.5	0	0	6.8	2.5	0.3	0.2	17
288	**Yogurt, low fat**, fruit	1.0	12.7[a]	Tr	1.0	6.1	0.3	4.4	0.2	0.3	0.8	0.3	Tr	Tr	6
289	hazelnut	1.1	14.9[a]	Tr	0.8	7.9	0.2	5.1	0.2	0.9	0.6	0.8	0.1	0	2
290	plain	0.3	7.5[a]	0	0	0	0	4.6	N	N	0.7	0.2	Tr	Tr	1
291	toffee	1.2	16.8	Tr	0.5	10.4	0.3	5.6	0	0	0.6	0.2	Tr	Tr	1
292	**Yogurt, soya**, non-dairy alternative to yogurt, fruit, fortified	0.3	10.7	2.3	1.7	6.7	0	0	N	1.0	0.3	0.4	1.2	0	0
293	**Yogurt, whole milk**, fruit	1.1	16.6[a]	3.3	2.2	6.2	0.2	4.0	N	N	2.0	0.7	0.1	0.1	3

[a] Contains galactose

[b] Not including oligosaccharides

Inorganic constituents per 100g edible portion

Yogurts and fromage frais

No.	Food	Na	K	Ca	Mg	P	Fe	Cu	Zn	Cl	Mn	Se	I
						mg						μg	
281	**Fermented milk drink** with probiotics	20	N	N	N	N	N	N	N	N	N	N	N
282	**Fromage frais**, fruit, children's, fortified	60	143	140ᵃ	11	123	0.06	0.03	0.4	230	Tr	Tr	17
283	virtually fat free, fruit	33	110	87	8	110	0.10	0.01	0.3	89	Tr	2	N
284	virtually fat free, natural	37	155	127	12	120	0.06	0.03	0.6	137	Tr	3	23
285	**Lassi**, sweetened	45	109	92	9	74	Tr	Tr	0.3	85	Tr	N	N
286	**Yogurt, Greek style**, fruit	64	218	141	14	136	0.16	Tr	0.6	159	Tr	3	39
287	plain	66	184	126	13	138	0.11	Tr	0.5	159	Tr	3	39
288	**Yogurt, low fat**, fruit	62	204	140	15	120	0.11	Tr	0.5	130	Tr	2	48
289	hazelnut	58	215	160	18	141	0.17	0.02	0.6	151	0.1	2	46
290	plain	63	228	162	16	143	0.08	0.03	0.6	235	Tr	2	34
291	toffee	67	220	159	16	132	0.11	Tr	0.6	250	Tr	2	34
292	**Yogurt, soya**, non-dairy alternative to yogurt, fruit, fortified	24	94	120	15	72	0.45	Tr	0.2	22	0.2	2	10
293	**Yogurt, whole milk**, fruit	58	170	122	13	96	0.12	Tr	0.4	179	Tr	2	27

ᵃValue is for fortified products

Milk and milk products *continued*

Vitamins per 100g edible portion

No.	Food	Retinol	Carotene	Vitamin D	Vitamin E	Thiamin	Ribo-flavin	Niacin	Trypt 60	Vitamin B6	Vitamin B12	Folate	Panto-thenate	Biotin	Vitamin C
		µg	µg	µg	mg	mg	mg	mg	mg	mg	µg	µg	mg	µg	mg
	Yogurts and fromage frais														
281	**Fermented milk drink** with probiotics	N	N	N	N	N	N	N	N	N	N	N	N	N	N
282	**Fromage frais**, fruit, children's, fortified	82	Tr	N[a]	0.15	0.11	0.29	0.1	0.1	Tr	0.5	15	0.38	0.6	Tr
283	virtually fat free, fruit	3	Tr	Tr	Tr	0.03	0.37	0.1	1.8	0.07	1.4	15	N	N	Tr
284	virtually fat free, natural	3	Tr	Tr	Tr	0.13	0.20	0.1	1.2	0.01	1.0	15	0.47	Tr	Tr
285	**Lassi**, sweetened	9	Tr	Tr	N	N	0.21	N	N	N	N	N	N	N	N
286	**Yogurt, Greek style**, fruit	115	Tr	0.1	0.39	0.12	0.13	0.1	1.5	Tr	0	6	N	N	Tr
287	plain	115	Tr	0.1	0.38	0.12	0.13	0.1	1.0	0.01	0.2	18	0.56	1.5	Tr
288	**Yogurt, low fat**, fruit	10	Tr	Tr	0.28	0.12	0.21	0.1	1.0	Tr	0.3	16	0.33	2.3	1
289	hazelnut	8	Tr	0.1	0.28	0.12	0.22	0.1	1.0	0.01	0.3	18	0.56	1.5	1
290	plain	8	Tr	0.1	Tr	0.12	0.22	0.1	1.0	0.01	0.3	18	0.56	1.5	1
291	toffee	8	Tr	0.1	Tr	0.12	0.33	0.1	1.0	0.01	0.3	18	0.56	1.5	1
292	**Yogurt, soya**, non-dairy alternative to yogurt, fruit, fortified	N	3	0.8[b]	N	0.11	0.21[b]	N	0.7	Tr	0.4[b]	N	0.12	1.0	N
293	**Yogurt, whole milk**, fruit	36	Tr	0.1	0.18	0.12	0.16	0.1	0.7	0.01	0.3	10	0.40	1.1	1

[a] Some products are fortified with vitamin D

[b] Values are for fortified products. Unfortified products contain 0µg of vitamin D and B12 and 0.02mg riboflavin per 100g

Composition of food per 100g edible portion

No.	Food	Description and main data sources	Main data reference	Water g	Total nitrogen g	Protein g	Fat g	Carbo-hydrate g	Energy value kcal	kJ
	Yogurts and fromage frais continued									
294	**Yogurt, whole milk**, infant, fruit flavour	No fruit pieces. Analytical data, 1997; and industry data, 2013	60	78.4	0.59	3.8	3.7	11.1	90	378
295	plain	MPE Supplement, 1989	8	81.9	0.89	5.7	3.0	7.8	79	333
296	twin pot, not fruit	With biscuit pieces and chocolate-coated cereal pieces. Industry data, 2013		68.4	0.66	4.2	5.6	21.5	148	623
297	twin pot, thick and creamy with fruit	Various flavours. Analytical data, 1995	48	74.7	0.71	4.1	3.2	16.2	106	446
298	**Yogurt, virtually fat free/diet**, fruit	Including bio varieties, flavours include strawberry, raspberry, black cherry and rhubarb. Analytical data, 1997	60	85.4	0.75	4.8	0.2	10.1	59	250
299	plain	Including bio varieties. Analytical data, 1997	60	86.9	0.84	5.4	0.2	8.2	54	230
	Ice creams									
300	**Chocolate nut sundae**	Recipe		48.5	0.43	2.6	15.0	33.5[a]	271	1136
301	**Cornetto type ice cream cone**	Analytical data, 2010	72	41.9	0.56	3.5[b]	14.4[b]	39.6[b]	292	1225
302	**Frozen ice cream desserts**	Including Viennetta, Romantica, After Eight. Analytical data, 1998	63	51.4	0.56	3.5	17.6	21.0[a]	251	1047
303	**Ice cream bars/choc ices**, chocolate coated, luxury	Including Magnum and Galaxy. Analytical data, 2010	72	40.4	0.60	3.9	21.1	34.9[a]	336	1405

[a] Includes oligosaccharides

[b] Strawberry flavour contains 2.5g protein, 11.0g fat, 39.0g carbohydrate (29.0g sugar)

Composition of food per 100g edible portion

No.	Food	Starch	Total sugars	Individual sugars					Dietary fibre		Fatty acids				Cholesterol
				Gluc	Fruct	Sucr	Malt	Lact	NSP	AOAC	Satd	Mono-unsatd	Poly-unsatd	Trans	erol
		g	g	g	g	g	g	g	g	g	g	g	g	g	mg
Yogurts and fromage frais *continued*															
294	**Yogurt, whole milk**, infant, fruit flavour	0.7	10.4[a]	Tr	1.5	4.5	0.1	3.6	0.1	0.2	2.5	0.9	0.1	0.1	4
295	plain	0	7.8[a]	0	0	0	0	4.7	0	0	1.9	0.8	0.1	0.1	11
296	twin pot, not fruit	3.3	18.2	N	N	N	N	N	N	0.3	3.2	N	N	N	N
297	twin pot, thick and creamy with fruit	0.6[b]	15.6[a]	2.3	2.2	6.9	0.2	3.5	0.5	1.0	N	N	N	N	N
298	**Yogurt, virtually fat free/diet**, fruit	0.7	9.4[a]	1.3	0.5	2.1	0.1	4.4	Tr	0.4	0.1	0.1	Tr	Tr	N
299	plain	0.3	7.9[a]	1.6	Tr	0.1	Tr	4.6	0	0	0.1	0.1	Tr	Tr	N
Ice creams															
300	**Chocolate nut sundae**	N	29.9[c]	9.7	8.8	7.9	0.7	2.8	N	N	8.9	4.2	0.8	0.4	39
301	**Cornetto type ice cream cone**	11.7	27.9	2.0	1.5	19.1	2.0	3.3	1.1	1.2	11.0	2.0	0.6	Tr	6
302	**Frozen ice cream desserts**	0.7	19.7[c]	0.5	Tr	13.8	1.3	4.1	Tr	Tr	14.2	2.2	0.5	0.2	4
303	**Ice cream bars/choc ices**, chocolate coated, luxury	Tr	32.9[c]	1.4	1.5	23.9	Tr	6.2	Tr	N	14.2	5.1	0.6	0.1	19

[a] Includes galactose

[b] Includes oligosaccharides

[c] Not including oligosaccharides

Milk and milk products *continued*

Inorganic constituents per 100g edible portion

No.	Food	Na	K	Ca	Mg	P	Fe	Cu	Zn	Cl	Mn	Se	I
						mg						μg	
Yogurts and fromage frais *continued*													
294	**Yogurt, whole milk**, infant, fruit flavour	46	176	120	12	114	0.21	0.02	0.5	179	Tr	2	27
295	plain	80	280	200	19	170	0.10	Tr	0.7	170	Tr	2	63
296	twin pot, not fruit	100	N	136	N	N	N	N	N	N	N	N	N
297	twin pot, thick and creamy with fruit	53	175	130	13	106	0.16	Tr	0.4	N	Tr	N	N
298	**Yogurt, virtually fat free/diet**, fruit	62	204	140	15	120	0.10	Tr	0.5	102	Tr	1	N
299	plain	71	247	160	16	151	0.13	0.03	0.6	252	Tr	2	53
Ice creams													
300	**Chocolate nut sundae**	36	131	65	18	71	0.36	0.07	0.3	61	0.1	1	21
301	**Cornetto type ice cream cone**	90	212	62	33	88	1.53	0.13	0.4	140	0.3	1	17
302	**Frozen ice cream desserts**	62	234	93	21	94	0.19	0.13	0.4	110	0.1	N	20
303	**Ice cream bars/choc ices**, chocolate coated, luxury	64	250	121	27	119	1.20	0.15	0.5	140	0.1	3	23

Milk and milk products *continued*

Vitamins per 100g edible portion

No.	Food	Retinol µg	Carotene µg	Vitamin D µg	Vitamin E mg	Thiamin mg	Ribo-flavin mg	Niacin mg	Trypt 60 mg	Vitamin B$_6$ mg	Vitamin B$_{12}$ µg	Folate µg	Panto-thenate mg	Biotin µg	Vitamin C mg
Yogurts and fromage frais continued															
294	**Yogurt, whole milk**, infant, fruit flavour	36	Tr	0.1[a]	0.18	0.12	0.15	0.1	0.7	0.01	0.3	10	0.40	1.1	Tr
295	plain	28	21	0	0.05	0.06	0.27	0.2	1.3	0.10	0.2	18	0.50	2.6	1
296	twin pot, not fruit	N	N	N	N	N	N	N	N	N	N	N	N	N	N
297	twin pot, thick and creamy with fruit	20	15	Tr	0.12	0.06	0.19	0.2	0.9	0.08	0.2	13	0.36	2.0	2
298	**Yogurt, virtually fat free/diet**, fruit	Tr	Tr	Tr	0.03	0.12	0.21	0.1	1.0	Tr	0.3	8	N	N	1
299	plain	Tr	Tr	Tr	Tr	0.12	0.22	0.1	1.0	0.01	0.3	18	0.56	1.5	1
Ice creams															
300	**Chocolate nut sundae**	185	109	0.3	0.86	0.08	0.18	0.4	0.6	0.03	0.4	7	0.61	3.0	1
301	**Cornetto type ice cream cone**	27	15	N	0.06	0.07	0.18	0.4	0.9	0.03	0.7	9	0.47	2.5	N
302	**Frozen ice cream desserts**	2	5	0.3	Tr	0.04	0.20	0.2	0.8	0.06	0.4	3	N	N	0
303	**Ice cream bars/choc ices**, chocolate coated, luxury	470	189	Tr	0.71	0.10	0.17	0.1	0.7	0.13	0.3	7	0.50	1.9	0

[a] Some products are fortified with vitamin D

135

Composition of food per 100g edible portion

No.	Food	Description and main data sources	Main data reference	Water g	Total nitrogen g	Protein g	Fat g	Carbohydrate g	Energy value kcal	kJ
	Ice creams continued									
304	**Ice cream bars/choc ices**, non-dairy, with chocolate flavoured coating	Analytical data, 1998	63	44.4	0.51	3.2	21.7	23.2[a]	295	1229
305	**Ice cream**, dairy, vanilla, soft scoop	Including Wall's, Mackies and own brands. Analytical data, 2010	72	64.9	0.51	3.2	8.2	22.0	169	711
306	dairy, luxury, with chocolate/caramel	Including Ben & Jerry's, Häagen-Dazs and own brands. Analytical data, 2010	72	48.4	0.66	4.2	13.9	32.2[a]	262	1100
307	non-dairy, vanilla, soft scoop	Including Wall's, Carte D'or and own brands. Analytical data, 2010	72	65.6	0.41	2.6	7.7	29.8[a]	192	807
308	**Lollies**, containing ice-cream	Analytical data, 1992	34	75.2	0.19	1.4	3.8	20.9	118	499
309	with real fruit juice	Assorted flavours. Analytical data, 1998	63	77.8	0.02	0.1	0.3	18.6[a]	73	310
310	**Sorbet**, fruit	Assorted flavours. Analytical data, 1998	63	68.9	0.03	0.2	0.3	24.8[a]	97	411
	Puddings and chilled desserts									
311	**Banoffee pie**	Including Mississippi mud pies. Analytical data, 1998	63	41.4	0.61	3.8	20.0	32.9[a]	319	1331
312	**Cheesecake**, fruit, frozen	Assorted flavours, fruit topping. Analytical data, 1998	63	43.6	0.64	4.0	16.2	35.2[a]	294	1231
313	fruit, individual	Including strawberry, apricot, blackcurrant and cherry. Analytical data, 1997; and industry data, 2013	60	46.6	0.97	6.1	12.3	34.5	264	1111
314	**Chocolate dairy desserts**	Including milk chocolate and caramel and white chocolate dessert pots, chilled. Analytical data, 1995	48	58.8	0.68	4.3	10.7	26.7	214	896

[a] Includes oligosaccharides

Composition of food per 100g edible portion

No.	Food	Starch	Total sugars	Individual sugars					Dietary fibre		Fatty acids				Cholest-erol
				Gluc	Fruct	Sucr	Malt	Lact	NSP	AOAC	Satd	Mono-unsatd	Poly-unsatd	Trans	
		g	g	g	g	g	g	g	g	g	g	g	g	g	mg
Ice creams continued															
304	**Ice cream bars/choc ices**, non-dairy, with chocolate flavoured coating	0.7	20.5[a]	0.3	Tr	13.1	2.4	4.7	Tr	Tr	18.4	1.9	0.4	0.1	7
305	**Ice cream**, dairy, vanilla, soft scoop	Tr	22.0	2.7	0.9	11.9	1.5	5.1	Tr[b]	0.2	5.2	2.1	0.3	0.2	29
306	dairy, luxury, with chocolate/caramel	2.9	28.4[a]	1.2	1.2	22.2	Tr	3.8	0.9	1.3	9.0	3.4	0.6	0.2	58
307	non-dairy, vanilla, soft scoop	0	23.5[a]	5.0	0.8	11.4	1.1	5.3	Tr[b]	0.2	5.0	1.9	0.4	Tr	13
308	**Lollies**, containing ice-cream	0	20.9	2.9	0.4	12.6	0	5.0	Tr	Tr	2.1	1.2	0.3	Tr	4
309	with real fruit juice	0	17.8[a]	1.0	0.9	15.9	0	0	Tr	Tr	N	N	N	N	N
310	**Sorbet**, fruit	0	23.3[a]	3.6	1.6	17.2	0.8	0	Tr	1.0	N	N	N	N	0
Puddings and chilled desserts															
311	**Banoffee pie**	11.4	20.9[a]	1.4	1.3	15.0	0.8	2.4	2.5	1.8	11.2	6.9	1.1	N	N
312	**Cheesecake**, fruit, frozen	10.0	25.0[a]	1.8	1.6	19.4	0.9	1.3	0.8	1.0	9.4	5.0	0.8	0.7	92
313	fruit, individual	9.1	25.4	2.3	2.0	18.1	0.4	2.6	1.0	1.6	7.5	3.5	0.5	0.2	15
314	**Chocolate dairy desserts**	2.7	24.0	0.4	0.2	17.3	0.7	5.4	Tr	Tr	6.3	3.3	0.4	0.5	21

[a] Not including oligosaccharides

[b] Gums and cellulose derivatives are added as stabilisers

137

Inorganic constituents per 100g edible portion

No.	Food	mg										µg	
		Na	K	Ca	Mg	P	Fe	Cu	Zn	Cl	Mn	Se	I
Ice creams continued													
304	**Ice cream bars/choc ices**, non-dairy, with chocolate flavoured coating	70	189	84	22	87	0.27	0.10	0.3	N	0.1	N	N
305	**Ice cream**, dairy, vanilla, soft scoop	63	163	104	13	85	0.06	0.02	0.3	110	Tr	1	30
306	dairy, luxury, with chocolate/caramel	75	249	108	27	110	1.41	0.15	0.6	160	0.2	3	17
307	non-dairy, vanilla, soft scoop	76	178	80	12	68	0.35	Tr	0.2	130	Tr	1	22
308	**Lollies**, containing ice-cream	31	69	49	6	39	0.20	Tr	0.1	53	Tr	Tr	8
309	with real fruit juice	11	28	5	2	3	Tr	Tr	Tr	114	Tr	Tr	Tr
310	**Sorbet**, fruit	10	41	8	4	4	0.09	0.04	0	16	0.2	1	Tr
Puddings and chilled desserts													
311	**Banoffee pie**	164	163	84	15	89	0.34	0.08	0.4	N	0.2	N	N
312	**Cheesecake**, fruit, frozen	146	96	56	9	64	0.46	0.06	0.4	220	0.2	2	9
313	fruit, individual	90	165	78	13	100	0.40	Tr	0.5	150	0.1	2	26
314	**Chocolate dairy desserts**	74	195	135	20	125	0.44	0.07	0.5	N	0.1	1	26

Vitamins per 100g edible portion

No.	Food	Retinol µg	Carotene µg	Vitamin D µg	Vitamin E mg	Thiamin mg	Ribo-flavin mg	Niacin mg	Trypt 60 mg	Vitamin B6 mg	Vitamin B12 µg	Folate µg	Panto-thenate mg	Biotin µg	Vitamin C mg
Ice creams continued															
304	**Ice cream bars/choc ices**, non-dairy, with chocolate flavoured coating	Tr	Tr	Tr	0.27	N	N	N	0.8	N	N	N	N	N	N
305	**Ice cream**, dairy, vanilla, soft scoop	91	45	0.5	0.49	0.10	0.28	0.2	0.9	0.04	0.5	6	1.05	2.2	1
306	dairy, luxury, with chocolate/caramel	139	52	Tr	0.49	0.02	0.80	0.3	0.9	Tr	0.2	4	0.36	1.3	1
307	non-dairy, vanilla, soft scoop	1	5	Tr	0.60	0.14	0.26	0.2	0.7	Tr	0.7	8	0.43	3.0	1
308	**Lollies**, containing ice-cream	14	9	0.5	0.51	0.02	0.09	0.1	0.4	0.04	0.2	8	0.30	3.0	Tr
309	with real fruit juice	Tr	Tr	Tr	Tr	0.04	N	N	N	Tr	Tr	N	N	N	7
310	**Sorbet**, fruit	Tr	95	0	Tr	0.04	Tr	0.2	0.2	Tr	Tr	5	0.08	0.4	12
Puddings and chilled desserts															
311	**Banoffee pie**	105	70	N	1.11	0.09	0.12	0.5	0.8	Tr	0.3	5	N	N	N
312	**Cheesecake**, fruit, frozen	97	50	0.2	1.19	0.07	0.09	0.5	0.9	0.02	0.5	7	N	N	6
313	fruit, individual	N	Tr	N	1.29	0.12	0.14	0.5	0.8	0.04	Tr	7	0.35	1.4	Tr
314	**Chocolate dairy desserts**	83	52	Tr	0.52	0.04	0.28	0.2	1.0	0.03	0.6	1	0.50	1.9	Tr

Puddings and chilled desserts continued

No.	Food	Description and main data sources	Main data reference	Water g	Total nitrogen g	Protein g	Fat g	Carbohydrate g	Energy value kcal	Energy value kJ
315	**Creme caramel**	MPE Supplement, 1989	8	72.0	0.47	3.0	1.6	20.6	104	440
316	**Custard,** made up with semi-skimmed milk	Recipe		77.4	0.63	4.0	2.0	16.4	95	403
317	ready to eat	Canned and tetra-pak; ambient. Analytical data, 1997; and industry data, 2013	60	77.5	0.43	2.7	2.9	16.3	98	414
318	**Jelly,** made with water	MPE Supplement, 1989	8	84.0	0.21	1.2	0	15.1	61	260
319	sugar free, made with water	Industry data, 2013; and estimated from standard jelly		98.4	0.26	1.6	0	Tr[a]	6	27
320	**Meringue,** homemade	Without cream. Recipe		1.2	1.01	6.3	Tr	96.0	385	1643
321	**Mousse,** chocolate, low fat	Analytical data, 1997	60	69.0	0.86	5.5	3.7	18.0	123	518
322	fruit	MPE Supplement, 1989	8	71.7	0.71	4.5	6.4	18.0	143	601
323	**Pavlova,** with fruit and cream	Including raspberry, strawberry and tropical fruits, frozen. Analytical data, 1998; and industry data, 2013	63	44.9	0.43	2.7	8.3	42.2[a]	244	1028
324	toffee/chocolate, no fruit	Analytical data, 1998; and industry data, 2013	63	26.0	0.61	3.8	19.7	47.4[a]	370	1552
325	**Profiteroles** with sauce	Analytical data, 1998	63	39.6	0.88	5.5	25.7	24.6[a]	346	1438
326	**Rice pudding,** canned	Analytical data, 1993-1994	50	79.2	0.53	3.3	1.3	16.1[a]	85	362
327	canned, low fat	Analytical data, 1993	50	79.6	0.56	3.5	0.8	16.0[a]	81	345
328	made with semi-skimmed milk, homemade	Recipe		72.1	0.67	4.2	4.4	19.0	127	535
329	**Torte,** fruit	Including lemon, raspberry and passion fruit. Analytical data, 1993-1994	50	53.0	0.60	3.8	15.5	27.7[a]	258	1080

[a] Includes oligosaccharides

Composition of food per 100g edible portion

Puddings and chilled desserts continued

No.	Food	Starch	Total sugars	Individual sugars					Dietary fibre		Fatty acids				Cholest-erol
				Gluc	Fruct	Sucr	Malt	Lact	NSP	AOAC	Satd	Mono-unsatd	Poly-unsatd	Trans	
		g	g	g	g	g	g	g	g	g	g	g	g	g	mg
315	**Creme caramel**	2.6	18.0[a]	2.3	1.3	10.3	0.5	3.5	N	N	0.9	0.5	0.1	0.2	N
316	**Custard**, made up with semi-skimmed milk	5.1	11.2	Tr	0	5.9	0	5.4	Tr	Tr	1.2	0.5	Tr	0.1	7
317	ready to eat	3.5	12.8	Tr	Tr	8.2	Tr	4.6	Tr	Tr	1.9	0.8	0.1	0.1	2
318	**Jelly**, made with water	0	15.1	3.5	1.7	8.6	1.3	0	0	0	0	0	0	0	0
319	sugar free, made with water	0	0	0	0	0	0	0	0	0	0	0	0	0	0
320	**Meringue**, homemade	0	96.0	Tr	0	96.0	0	0	0	0	Tr	Tr	Tr	Tr	0
321	**Mousse**, chocolate, low fat	2.2	15.8	Tr	6.3	3.8	Tr	5.7	N	N	2.5	0.9	0.1	0	1
322	fruit	Tr	18.0[a]	3.1	2.9	7.6	0.3	3.7	N	N	4.1	1.8	0.1	0.7	N
323	**Pavlova**, with fruit and cream	1.1	41.0[b]	2.5	1.7	35.9	Tr	0.9	N	1.9	4.6	2.9	0.4	0.6	19
324	toffee/chocolate, no fruit	0.3	45.3[b]	2.1	0.8	40.1	1.1	1.1	N	1.1	10.8	6.8	1.0	1.3	45
325	**Profiteroles** with sauce	6.4	17.0[b]	1.8	0.8	11.7	1.2	1.5	1.0	1.4	14.0	8.7	1.7	1.3	N
326	**Rice pudding**, canned	7.3	8.7[b]	Tr	Tr	4.9	Tr	3.9	0.1	N	0.8	0.3	0.1	Tr	9
327	canned, low fat	7.2	8.7[b]	Tr	Tr	4.9	Tr	3.9	0.1	0.1	0.5	0.2	0.1	Tr	N
328	made with semi-skimmed milk, homemade	8.7	10.3	0	0	5.3	0	4.9	0.1	0.1	2.8	1.1	0.1	0.2	13
329	**Torte**, fruit	9.9	17.4[b]	1.3	0.6	13.0	0.7	1.8	0.5	1.2	9.4	4.7	1.2	0.6	42

[a] Contains galactose

[b] Not including oligosaccharides

Milk and milk products *continued*

Inorganic constituents per 100g edible portion

Puddings and chilled desserts continued

No.	Food	mg										µg	
		Na	K	Ca	Mg	P	Fe	Cu	Zn	Cl	Mn	Se	I
315	**Creme caramel**	70	150	94	9	77	Tr	Tr	0.3	100	Tr	N	33
316	**Custard**, made up with semi-skimmed milk	67	184	140	13	111	0.11	0.01	0.5	127	N	1	35
317	ready to eat	41	129	91	9	83	0.05	Tr	0.3	137	Tr	1	26
318	**Jelly**, made with water	5	5	7	Tr	1	0.40	0.01	N	6	N	N	N
319	sugar free, made with water	5	5	7	Tr	1	0.40	0.01	N	6	N	N	N
320	**Meringue**, homemade	113	92	13	9	8	0.19	0.12	0.1	93	Tr	5	2
321	**Mousse**, chocolate, low fat	69	301	126	33	133	1.21	0.12	0.8	191	0.1	2	66
322	fruit	62	150	120	12	96	Tr	Tr	0.4	110	Tr	N	N
323	**Pavlova**, with fruit and cream	41	80	26	6	27	0.25	Tr	0.1	N	0.1	N	N
324	toffee/chocolate, no fruit	67	133	44	15	48	0.53	0.11	0.3	N	0.3	N	N
325	**Profiteroles** with sauce	130	190	58	25	114	1.52	0.18	0.6	209	0.2	5	12
326	**Rice pudding**, canned	43	130	88	12	86	0.10	0.13	0.5	93	0.1	N	28
327	canned, low fat	43	130	88	12	86	0.10	0.13	0.5	93	0.1	N	28
328	made with semi-skimmed milk, homemade	67	175	128	14	111	0.05	0.03	0.6	131	0.1	1	33
329	**Torte**, fruit	88	116	66	10	77	0.30	0.34	0.5	N	0.1	N	N

Vitamins per 100g edible portion

No.	Food	Retinol µg	Carotene µg	Vitamin D µg	Vitamin E mg	Thiamin mg	Ribo-flavin mg	Niacin mg	Trypt 60 mg	Vitamin B$_6$ mg	Vitamin B$_{12}$ µg	Folate µg	Panto-thenate mg	Biotin µg	Vitamin C mg
	Puddings and chilled desserts continued														
315	**Creme caramel**	37	8	0.1	0.03	0.03	0.20	0.1	0.7	0.03	0.3	8	N	N	0
316	**Custard**, made up with semi-skimmed milk	21	10	Tr	0.04	0.03	0.25	0.2	0.7	0.06	0.9	8	0.71	3.4	1
317	ready to eat	36	376	Tr	0.29	0.12	0.19	0.1	0.3	0.01	0.2	2	0.43	1.3	0
318	**Jelly**, made with water	0	0	0	0	0	0	0	0	0	0	0	0	0	0
319	sugar free, made with water	0	0	0	0	0	0	0	0	0	0	0	0	0	0
320	**Meringue**, homemade	0	0	0	0	0.01	0.21	Tr	1.6	0.02	0.2	3	0.12	3.3	0
321	**Mousse**, chocolate, low fat	N	Tr	Tr	0.79	0.12	0.26	0.2	0.8	0.01	0	0	0.74	2.1	0
322	fruit	36	16	0.1	0.39	0.04	0.23	0.2	1.1	0.05	0.2	6	N	N	Tr
323	**Pavlova**, with fruit and cream	75	44	N	0.21	0.03	0.18	0.2	1.0	Tr	Tr	10	0.38	1.3	5
324	toffee/chocolate, no fruit	155	50	Tr	1.00	0.06	0.12	0.2	0.8	Tr	Tr	8	N	N	0
325	**Profiteroles** with sauce	114	90	0.3	1.18	0.07	0.14	0.3	1.2	0.02	0.3	9	0.63	3.7	Tr
326	**Rice pudding**, canned	16	10	Tr	0.16	0.01	0.13	0.2	0.7	0.01	Tr	Tr	0.30	2.0	Tr
327	canned, low fat	16	10	Tr	0.10	0.01	0.13	0.2	0.7	0.01	Tr	Tr	0.30	2.0	Tr
328	made with semi-skimmed milk, homemade	49	28	Tr	0.09	0.03	0.21	0.3	0.8	0.06	0.9	5	0.57	3.3	2
329	**Torte**, fruit	99	77	Tr	1.43	0.03	0.09	0.2	0.5	0.02	Tr	3	N	N	Tr

Composition of food per 100g edible portion

No.	Food	Description and main data sources	Main data reference	Water g	Total nitrogen g	Protein g	Fat g	Carbo-hydrate g	Energy value kcal	Energy value kJ

Puddings and chilled desserts continued

No.	Food	Description and main data sources	Main data reference	Water g	Total nitrogen g	Protein g	Fat g	Carbo-hydrate g	Energy value kcal	Energy value kJ
330	**Trifle**, fruit	Analytical data, 1997	60	67.9	0.41	2.6	9.0	19.5	164	689
331	**Tiramisu**	Analytical data, 1998; and industry data, 2013	63	51.2	0.66	4.2	14.0	27.1[a]	244	1021

[a] Includes oligosaccharides

Composition of food per 100g edible portion

No.	Food	Starch	Total sugars	Individual sugars					Dietary fibre		Fatty acids				Cholest-
				Gluc	Fruct	Sucr	Malt	Lact	NSP	AOAC	Satd	Mono-unsatd	Poly-unsatd	Trans	erol
		g	g	g	g	g	g	g	g	g	g	g	g	g	mg

Puddings and chilled desserts continued

No.	Food	Starch	Total sugars	Gluc	Fruct	Sucr	Malt	Lact	NSP	AOAC	Satd	Mono-unsatd	Poly-unsatd	Trans	Cholesterol
330	Trifle, fruit	4.2	15.3	1.8	4.6	6.2	Tr	2.7	2.1	2.4	5.6	2.5	0.4	0.2	13
331	Tiramisu	4.5	21.1[a]	2.3	1.4	13.5	2.4	1.5	N	1.0	8.6	3.8	0.8	1.0	45

[a] Not including oligosaccharides

Inorganic constituents per 100g edible portion

No.	Food	Na	K	Ca	Mg	P	Fe	Cu	Zn	Cl	Mn	Se	I
						mg						µg	
	Puddings and chilled desserts continued												
330	**Trifle**, fruit	65	137	73	10	84	0.24	0.02	0.3	95	Tr	2	37
331	**Tiramisu**	67	105	59	10	86	0.40	Tr	0.3	194	Tr	3	30

Vitamins per 100g edible portion

No.	Food	Retinol	Carotene	Vitamin D	Vitamin E	Thiamin	Ribo-flavin	Niacin	Trypt 60	Vitamin B_6	Vitamin B_{12}	Folate	Panto-thenate	Biotin	Vitamin C
		µg	µg	µg	mg	mg	mg	mg	mg	mg	µg	µg	mg	µg	mg

Puddings and chilled desserts continued

No.	Food	Retinol	Carotene	Vitamin D	Vitamin E	Thiamin	Ribo-flavin	Niacin	Trypt 60	Vitamin B_6	Vitamin B_{12}	Folate	Panto-thenate	Biotin	Vitamin C
330	**Trifle**, fruit	N	Tr	N	0.66	0.12	0.08	0.1	0.5	0.01	0.2	8	0.29	0.7	Tr
331	**Tiramisu**	69	25	N	0.61	0.06	0.12	0.3	0.8	0.03	0.4	10	0.57	2.0	Tr

147

Eggs and egg dishes

Section 2.3

Eggs and egg dishes

New analytical values for eggs (2012)[71] have been incorporated into this section.

The nutrient content of eggs may vary by rearing method (e.g. enriched cage, barn, free range, organic) and by the type of feed used (e.g. for vitamin D). The new values are based on composite samples that included eggs produced using all the different methods in proportion to their prevalence on the market, as well as eggs of different sizes. Nutrient composition data for eggs is broadly similar to data from analyses carried out in the late 1980s[30], although levels of fat soluble vitamins D and E, and selenium appear to be higher. Discussion of the impact of changes in hens feed and egg size on the new nutrient values was published in 2012 (Benelam *et al.*, 2012)[81].

Losses of labile vitamins assigned on recipe calculation were estimated using the figures in Section 4.3.

Composition of food per 100g edible portion

No.	Food	Description and main data sources	Main data reference	Water g	Total nitrogen g	Protein g	Fat g	Carbo-hydrate g	Energy value kcal	kJ
Eggs										
332	**Eggs, chicken**, whole, raw	Including enriched cage, barn, free-range and organic. Analytical data, 2011[a]	71	76.8	2.02	12.6	9.0	Tr	131	547
333	white, raw	Including enriched cage, barn, free-range and organic. Analytical data, 2011	71	87.3	1.73	10.8	Tr	Tr	43	184
334	yolk, raw	Including enriched cage, barn, free-range and organic. Analytical data, 2011	71	48.8	2.62	16.4	31.3	Tr	347	1437
335	whole, boiled	Mixture of soft- and hard-boiled eggs. Including enriched cage, barn, free-range and organic. Analytical data, 2011	71	75.4	2.26	14.1	9.6	Tr	143	595
336	white, boiled	Mixture of soft- and hard-boiled eggs. Including enriched cage, barn, free-range and organic. Analytical data, 2011	71	85.8	2.08	13.0	Tr	Tr	52	221
337	yolk, boiled	Mixture of soft- and hard-boiled eggs. Including enriched cage, barn, free-range and organic. Analytical data, 2011	71	47.2	2.67	16.7	32.6	Tr	360	1490
338	whole, fried in sunflower oil	Including enriched cage, barn, free-range and organic. Analytical data, 2011	71	68.0	2.35	14.7	15.7	Tr	200	831
339	whole, poached	Poached in water and in a poacher. Including enriched cage, barn, free-range and organic. Analytical data, 2011	71	75.3	2.13	13.3	10.6	Tr	149	618
340	scrambled, with semi-skimmed milk	Recipe		65.1	1.76	11.0	21.2	0.7	237	981

[a] An average egg is composed of approximately 25% yolk, 60% white and 15% shell

Composition of food per 100g edible portion

No.	Food	Starch	Total sugars	Individual sugars					Dietary fibre		Fatty acids				Cholest-
				Gluc	Fruct	Sucr	Malt	Lact	NSP	AOAC	Satd	Mono-unsatd	Poly-unsatd	Trans	erol
		g	g	g	g	g	g	g	g	g	g	g	g	g	mg
Eggs															
332	**Eggs, chicken**, whole, raw	0	Tr	Tr	0	0	0	0	0	0	2.5	3.4	1.4	Tr	350
333	white, raw	0	Tr	Tr	0	0	0	0	0	0	Tr	Tr	Tr	Tr	0
334	yolk, raw	0	Tr	Tr	0	0	0	0	0	0	8.8	12.0	5.0	0.1	1255
335	whole, boiled	0	Tr	Tr	0	0	0	0	0	0	2.7	3.7	1.5	Tr	360
336	white, boiled	0	Tr	Tr	0	0	0	0	0	0	Tr	Tr	Tr	Tr	0
337	yolk, boiled	0	Tr	Tr	0	0	0	0	0	0	9.2	12.5	5.2	0.1	1175
338	whole, fried in sunflower oil	0	Tr	Tr	0	0	0	0	0	0	3.4	5.4	4.2	Tr	371
339	whole, poached	0	Tr	Tr	0	0	0	0	0	0	3.0	4.0	1.7	Tr	423
340	scrambled, with semi-skimmed milk	Tr	0.7	Tr	0	Tr	0	0.7	Tr	0.1	10.8	6.3	1.7	0.5	325

Inorganic constituents per 100g edible portion

No.	Food	mg										µg	
		Na	K	Ca	Mg	P	Fe	Cu	Zn	Cl	Mn	Se	I
Eggs													
332	**Eggs, chicken**, whole, raw	154	145	46	13	179	1.7	0.05	1.1	180	Tr	23	50
333	white, raw	185	149	6	12	12	Tr	0.02	Tr	159	Tr	8	4
334	yolk, raw	52	124	149	12	600	6.2	0.16	4.0	163	0.1	59	130
335	whole, boiled	150	141	55	14	205	2.0	0.07	1.3	179	Tr	27	52
336	white, boiled	151	123	8	12	13	0.1	0.04	0.1	164	Tr	11	4
337	yolk, boiled	52	119	147	12	600	6.2	0.15	3.9	180	0.1	64	137
338	whole, fried in sunflower oil	172	164	53	14	209	2.0	0.06	1.3	188	Tr	27	58
339	whole, poached	121	117	50	12	195	1.9	0.08	1.3	138	Tr	28	54
340	scrambled, with semi-skimmed milk	253	150	58	13	164	1.5	0.05	1.0	345	0.1	19	51

Vitamins per 100g edible portion

No.	Food	Retinol µg	Carotene µg	Vitamin D µg	Vitamin E mg	Thiamin mg	Ribo-flavin mg	Niacin mg	Trypt 60 mg	Vitamin B$_6$ mg	Vitamin B$_{12}$ µg	Folate µg	Panto-thenate mg	Biotin µg	Vitamin C mg
Eggs															
332	**Eggs, chicken,** whole, raw	126	Tr	3.2	1.29	0.08	0.50	0.1	3.4	0.13	2.7	47	1.35	19.5	0
333	white, raw	0	0	0	0	0.02	0.42	Tr	2.8	0.04	0.3	10	0.28	5.6	0
334	yolk, raw	447	Tr	12.8	5.21	0.20	0.59	Tr	2.8	0.35	8.2	122	4.53	63.6	0
335	whole, boiled	120	Tr	3.2	1.63	0.08	0.47	0.1	3.6	0.10	2.0	30	1.25	16.7	0
336	white, boiled	0	0	0	0	0.03	0.20	0.1	4.0	0.03	0.5	4	0.22	3.2	0
337	yolk, boiled	410	Tr	12.6	4.78	0.19	0.58	Tr	3.0	0.31	7.2	101	3.72	50.0	0
338	whole, fried in sunflower oil	190	Tr	1.9	3.84	0.06	0.46	0.1	3.5	0.12	1.0	25	1.22	18.2	0
339	whole, poached	150	Tr	2.9	1.82	0.09	0.41	0.1	3.2	0.11	1.8	49	1.30	15.1	0
340	scrambled, with semi-skimmed milk	264	103	2.8	1.38	0.07	0.37	0.1	2.9	0.10	2.4	28	1.03	16.5	Tr

Composition of food per 100g edible portion

No.	Food	Description and main data sources	Main data reference	Water g	Total nitrogen g	Protein g	Fat g	Carbo- hydrate g	Energy value kcal	kJ
Egg dishes										
341	**Omelette**, plain	Recipe		69.1	1.75	10.9	16.4	Tr	191	793
342	cheese	Recipe		58.0	2.51	15.9	22.7	Tr	268	1113
343	**Quiche**, cheese and egg, homemade	Recipe, containing retail pastry		48.7	2.01	12.5	22.3	14.6	305	1270
344	cheese and egg, wholemeal, homemade	Recipe, containing homemade pastry		48.1	2.08	13.0	20.4	15.6	294	1226
345	Lorraine with shortcrust pastry	Retail, with bacon and cheese. Analytical data, 2010	72	52.5	1.45	9.1	17.6	19.7	269	1121

Composition of food per 100g edible portion

No.	Food	Starch	Total sugars	Individual sugars					Dietary fibre		Fatty acids				Cholest-
				Gluc	Fruct	Sucr	Malt	Lact	NSP	AOAC	Satd	Mono-unsatd	Poly-unsatd	Trans	erol
		g	g	g	g	g	g	g	g	g	g	g	g	g	mg

Egg dishes

No.	Food	Starch	Total sugars	Gluc	Fruct	Sucr	Malt	Lact	NSP	AOAC	Satd	Mono-unsatd	Poly-unsatd	Trans	Cholesterol
341	**Omelette**, plain	0	Tr	Tr	0	0	0	0	0	0	3.2	4.8	6.7	Tr	303
342	cheese	0	Tr	Tr	0	0	0	Tr	0	0	9.6	6.4	4.8	0.5	232
343	**Quiche**, cheese and egg, homemade	13.1	1.6	0.1	Tr	Tr	0.2	1.3	0.6	1.2	10.4	7.9	2.3	0.4	116
344	cheese and egg, wholemeal, homemade	14.0	1.6	Tr	Tr	0.2	0.1	1.3	1.8	2.1	11.8	5.6	1.1	0.7	137
345	Lorraine with shortcrust pastry	16.5	3.2	0.4	0.3	0.3	0.7	1.5	0.9	1.3	8.3	6.5	1.8	0.2	80

Inorganic constituents per 100g edible portion

No.	Food	Na	K	Ca	Mg	P	Fe	Cu	Zn	Cl	Mn	Se	I
						mg						µg	
Egg dishes													
341	**Omelette**, plain	136	128	41	11	158	1.5	0.05	1.0	159	Tr	20	44
342	cheese	337	110	280	17	277	1.1	0.04	2.1	461	Tr	15	39
343	**Quiche**, cheese and egg, homemade	310	130	259	17	216	0.9	0.02	1.5	445	0.1	9	28
344	cheese and egg, wholemeal, homemade	310	173	240	31	259	1.0	0.10	1.8	471	0.4	9	32
345	Lorraine with shortcrust pastry	339	155	147	15	177	0.6	0.03	1.0	450	0.1	7	16

Eggs and egg dishes *continued*

Vitamins per 100g edible portion

No.	Food	Retinol	Carotene	Vitamin D	Vitamin E	Thiamin	Ribo-flavin	Niacin	Trypt 60	Vitamin B6	Vitamin B12	Folate	Panto-thenate	Biotin	Vitamin C
		µg	µg	µg	mg	mg	mg	mg	mg	mg	µg	µg	mg	µg	mg
Egg dishes															
341	**Omelette**, plain	109	Tr	2.8	5.38	0.07	0.35	Tr	2.9	0.10	2.3	28	0.99	16.9	0
342	cheese	196	48	1.9	3.71	0.06	0.36	Tr	4.2	0.12	2.3	29	0.82	12.6	Tr
343	**Quiche**, cheese and egg, homemade	130	38	0.9	1.55	0.05	0.25	0.3	3.1	0.08	1.5	12	0.59	7.5	1
344	cheese and egg, wholemeal, homemade	227	100	1.0	0.80	0.10	0.27	1.1	3.4	0.17	1.5	17	0.70	8.3	Tr
345	Lorraine with shortcrust pastry	103	35	N	2.08	0.13	0.18	1.2	1.8	0.04	0.5	9	0.69	4.6	Tr

Fats and oils

Section 2.4

Fats and oils

The data on oils in this section are derived from the *Miscellaneous Foods* (1994)[14] supplement. However, the values for most cooking and spreading fats are new for this edition, largely based on new analytical data collected in 2009/10[72], with categories based on the range of products now available. In addition, there are a few new values obtained from manufacturers to reflect reformulated products, including changes to nutrients added to spreading fats. The range and levels of added nutrients change·with time and also vary by brand. Users requiring details of possible recent changes in fortification practices and brand-specific information should contact manufacturers directly.

Most oils show a wide range of fatty acid composition depending on the variety, growing conditions and maturity of the seed. In addition, the blend of fats and oils used in many of the foods included in this section can frequently be adjusted by manufacturers and this will alter the fatty acid composition. If accurate fatty acid data are required for specific products, and analytical facilities are not available, it is advisable to contact the manufacturer directly. Nutrient values for oils are presented on a weight basis; the specific gravity (density) of most vegetable oils is in the range 0.910-0.925[127].

Sunflower oil has been used for recipe calculations that include vegetable oil as an ingredient. Vegetable oils that do not specify a plant source are usually rapeseed oil so the nutrient profile of 'vegetable oil, average' is as for rapeseed oil. This profile has been included to aid recipe calculation where unidentified oil has been used.

Composition of food per 100g edible portion

No.	Food	Description and main data sources	Main data reference	Water g	Total nitrogen g	Protein g	Fat g	Carbo-hydrate g	Energy value kcal	kJ
Spreading fats										
346	**Butter**, salted	Analytical data, 1996-1997; and industry data, 2013	59	14.9	0.10	0.6	82.2	0.6	744	3059
347	unsalted	Analytical data, 1996-1997	59	14.9	0.10	0.6	82.2	0.6	744	3059
348	spreadable (75-80% fat)	Containing butter and vegetable oil, including Anchor, Lurpak, Country Life and own brand equivalents. Analytical data, 2010	72	18.7	0.06	0.4	79.1	0.5	715	2941
349	spreadable, light (60% fat)	Containing butter and vegetable oil, including Anchor Lighter, Lurpak Lighter, Country Life Lighter and own brand equivalents. Analytical data, 2010	72	37.3	0.08	0.5	60.2	0.8	547	2248
350	**Fat spread**, reduced fat (62-75%), polyunsaturated	Including Flora buttery spread and Pure sunflower, dairy free. MSF Supplement, 1994; and industry data, 2013	14	29.0	0.06	0.4	68.5	0.6	620	2551
351	reduced fat (62-75%), not polyunsaturated	Including Clover and own brands. Analytical data, 2010	72	24.6	0.04	0.3	73.2	Tr	660	2713
352	reduced fat (41-62%), not polyunsaturated	Including I Can't Believe It's Not Butter, Utterly Butterly and own brands. Analytical data, 2010	72	37.4	0.07	0.4	60.6	1.3	552	2270
353	reduced fat (41-62%), not polyunsaturated, with olive oil	Including Bertolli Spread and own brands. Analytical data, 2010	72	38.8	0.03	0.2	59.1	1.1	537	2208
354	reduced fat (41-62%), polyunsaturated	Including Flora Original, Vitalite Sunflower Spread, and own brands. Analytical data, 2010	72	40.0	Tr	Tr	59.2	Tr	533	2190

Spreading fats

No.	Food	Starch g	Total sugars g	Gluc g	Fruct g	Sucr g	Malt g	Lact g	Dietary fibre NSP g	Dietary fibre AOAC g	Fatty acids Satd g	Fatty acids Mono-unsatd g	Fatty acids Poly-unsatd g	Fatty acids Trans g	Cholesterol mg
346	**Butter**, salted	0	0.6	0	0	0	0	0.6	0	0	52.1	20.9	2.8	2.9	213
347	unsalted	0	0.6	0	0	0	0	0.6	0	0	52.1	20.9	2.8	2.9	213
348	spreadable (75-80% fat)	0	0.5	0	0	0	0	0.5	0	0	34.2	29.5	10.0	1.4	153
349	spreadable, light (60% fat)	0	0.8	0	0	0	0	0.8	0	0	25.7	22.7	7.8	1.0	111
350	**Fat spread**, reduced fat (62-75%), polyunsaturated	0	0.6	0	0	0	0	0.6	0	0	15.0	19.5	32.0	0.3	Tr
351	reduced fat (62-75%), not polyunsaturated	0	Tr	0	0	0	0	Tr	0	0	24.4	33.4	11.8	0.1	10
352	reduced fat (41-62%), not polyunsaturated	0	1.3	0	0	0	0	1.3	0	0	15.6	30.0	11.9	0.2	5
353	reduced fat (41-62%), not polyunsaturated, with olive oil	0	1.1	0	0	0	0	1.1	0	0	13.2	31.4	11.5	0.1	3
354	reduced fat (41-62%), polyunsaturated	0	Tr	0	0	0	0	Tr	0	0	13.2	17.7	25.2	0.1	Tr

Inorganic constituents per 100g edible portion

No.	Food	Na	K	Ca	Mg	P	Fe	Cu	Zn	Cl	Mn	Se	I
						mg						µg	
Spreading fats													
346	**Butter**, salted	730[a]	27	18	2	23	Tr	0.01	0.1	1120	Tr	Tr	38
347	unsalted	8	27	18	2	23	Tr	0.01	0.1	18	Tr	Tr	38
348	spreadable (75-80% fat)	484	16	11	1	12	Tr	Tr	0.1	720	Tr	Tr	4
349	spreadable, light (60% fat)	467	26	17	Tr	15	0.3	Tr	0.1	680	Tr	1	8
350	**Fat spread**, reduced fat (62-75%), polyunsaturated	600	N	N	N	N	Tr	Tr	N	920	Tr	Tr	N
351	reduced fat (62-75%), not polyunsaturated	747	17	10	1	9	Tr	Tr	Tr	1070	Tr	Tr	N
352	reduced fat (41-62%), not polyunsaturated	689	43	14	2	12	Tr	0.01	0.1	990	Tr	Tr	N
353	reduced fat (41-62%), not polyunsaturated, with olive oil	551	46	7	1	7	Tr	Tr	Tr	800	Tr	Tr	N
354	reduced fat (41-62%), polyunsaturated	600	21	3	Tr	1	Tr	0.01	Tr	870	Tr	1	N

[a] Slightly salted butters contain approximately 500mg Na per 100g

Vitamins per 100g edible portion

No.	Food	Retinol μg	Carotene[a] μg	Vitamin D μg	Vitamin[b] E mg	Thiamin mg	Ribo-flavin mg	Niacin mg	Trypt 60 mg	Vitamin B₆ mg	Vitamin B₁₂ μg	Folate μg	Panto-thenate mg	Biotin μg	Vitamin C mg
	Spreading fats														
346	**Butter**, salted	958	608	0.9	1.85	Tr	0.07	Tr	0.1	Tr	0.3	Tr	0.05	0.2	Tr
347	unsalted	958	608	0.9	1.85	Tr	0.07	Tr	0.1	Tr	0.3	Tr	0.05	0.2	Tr
348	spreadable (75-80% fat)	521	243	0.6	10.50	Tr	0.04	Tr	0.1	Tr	0.1	Tr	0.03	0.1	Tr
349	spreadable, light (60% fat)	380	342	0.4	8.27	Tr	0.03	Tr	Tr	Tr	0.1	Tr	0.02	0.1	Tr
350	**Fat spread**, reduced fat (62-75%), polyunsaturated	N	N	7.5[c]	N[d]	Tr	Tr	Tr	Tr	Tr	N[d]	Tr	Tr	Tr	0
351	reduced fat (62-75%), not polyunsaturated	N	680	N	N	Tr	0.07	Tr	Tr	Tr	0.1	1	0.02	0.3	0
352	reduced fat (41-62%), not polyunsaturated	N[e]	N[a]	N[e]	12.40	Tr	N	Tr	Tr	Tr	Tr	Tr	Tr	Tr	0
353	reduced fat (41-62%), not polyunsaturated, with olive oil	734[e,f]	495	4.2[e,f]	12.50	Tr	N	Tr	Tr	Tr[g]	Tr[g]	Tr[g]	Tr	Tr	0
354	reduced fat (41-62%), polyunsaturated	606[f,h]	461	5.8[f,h]	26.30	Tr	N	N	Tr	N	N	N	Tr	Tr	0

[a] Some brands may not contain β-carotene

[b] In foods containing oil, the vitamin E content will vary according to the type of oil used

[c] Value relates to fortified products

[d] Fortified products contain 38.00mg vitamin E and 5.0μg vitamin B12 per 100g

[e] Fortified products contain 800μg retinol and approximately 6.0μg vitamin D per 100g

[f] Value relates to a mixture of fortified and unfortified products

[g] Some brands may contain added vitamin B₆, vitamin B₁₂ and folate

[h] Fortified products contain approximately 800μg retinol and 7.5μg vitamin D per 100g

Fats and oils *continued*

Composition of food per 100g edible portion

No.	Food	Description and main data sources	Main data reference	Water g	Total nitrogen g	Protein g	Fat g	Carbohydrate g	Energy value kcal	Energy value kJ
Spreading fats continued										
355	**Fat spread**, low fat (26-39%), not polyunsaturated, including dairy type	Vegetable oil/dairy blend, including I Can't Believe It's Not Butter Light and own brands. Analytical data, 2010; and industry data, 2013	72	57.5	0.02	0.2	39.0	0.7	354	1457
356	low fat (26-39%), not polyunsaturated, with olive oil	Including Bertolli Light Spread and own brands. Analytical data, 2010	72	58.9	0.02	0.1	38.9	0.5	353	1450
357	low fat (26-39%), polyunsaturated	Including Flora Light and own brands. Analytical data, 2010	72	52.5	Tr	Tr	36.9	1.8	339	1394
Cooking fats										
358	**Baking fat and margarine** (75-90% fat), hard block	Including Stork and own brands. Analytical data, 2010; and industry data 2013	72	22.2	Tr	Tr	76.4	0	688	2827
359	**Compound cooking fat**, not polyunsaturated	Including Cookeen, Trex and Crisp 'n' Dry Solid Vegetable Oil. Analytical data, 2010	72	0.2	Tr	Tr	100.0	0	900	3700
360	**Dripping**, beef	MW1, 1940; and FA Supplement, 1998	1, 17	1.0	Tr	Tr	99.0	Tr	891	3663
361	**Ghee**, butter	Retail and homemade. Analytical data, 2007	69	0.4	0.02	0.1	97.6	Tr	878	3611
362	made from vegetable oil	Analytical data, 2010	72	Tr	0.02	0.1	100.0	0	900	3702
363	**Lard**	MW1, 1940; and MSF Supplement, 1994	1, 14	1.0	Tr	Tr	99.0	0	891	3663
364	**Suet**, shredded	Beef. MW4, 1978	4	1.5	Tr	Tr	86.7	12.1	826	3402
365	vegetable, reduced fat	Industry data, 2013		2.1	0.40	2.5	65.7	31.1	718	2971

Composition of food per 100g edible portion

No.	Food	Starch g	Total sugars g	Individual sugars					Dietary fibre		Fatty acids				Cholest-erol mg
				Gluc g	Fruct g	Sucr g	Malt g	Lact g	NSP g	AOAC g	Satd g	Mono-unsatd g	Poly-unsatd g	Trans g	
Spreading fats continued															
355	**Fat spread**, low fat (26-39%), not polyunsaturated, including dairy type	0.3	0.4	0	0	0	0	0.4	0	0	9.8	17.4	9.8	0.1	Tr
356	low fat (26-39%), not polyunsaturated, with olive oil	Tr	0.5	0	0	0	0	0.5	0	0	8.9	21.7	6.4	0.1	5
357	low fat (26-39%), polyunsaturated	0.6	1.3	0	0	0	0	1.3	0	0	8.6	11.5	15.0	0.1	Tr
Cooking fats															
358	**Baking fat and margarine** (75-90% fat), hard block	0	0	0	0	0	0	0	0	0	26.4	34.0	12.2	0.1	15
359	**Compound cooking fat**, not polyunsaturated	0	0	0	0	0	0	0	0	0	42.3	40.1	12.8	0.1	8
360	**Dripping**, beef	0	0	0	0	0	0	0	0	0	50.6	38.0	2.4	4.4	94
361	**Ghee**, butter	0	Tr	0	0	0	0	Tr	0	0	58.4	25.7	4.6	2.1	246
362	made from vegetable oil	0	0	0	0	0	0	0	0	0	46.7	38.9	9.5	0.1	0
363	**Lard**	0	0	0	0	0	0	0	0	0	40.3	43.4	10.0	Tr	93
364	**Suet**, shredded	11.9	0.2	0.1	0.1	Tr	Tr	0	0.5	N	49.9	30.4	2.2	4.0	82
365	vegetable, reduced fat	29.7	1.4	0.7	0.7	Tr	Tr	0	N	1.3	32.8	22.8	7.2	Tr	0

Inorganic constituents per 100g edible portion

No.	Food	Na	K	Ca	Mg	P	Fe	Cu	Zn	Cl	Mn	Se	I
		mg									µg		
Spreading fats *continued*													
355	**Fat spread**, low fat (26-39%), not polyunsaturated, including dairy type	692	61	12	2	9	Tr	Tr	Tr	970	Tr	Tr	15
356	low fat (26-39%), not polyunsaturated, with olive oil	488	48	9	1	6	Tr	Tr	Tr	690	Tr	Tr	N
357	low fat (26-39%), polyunsaturated	482	31	4	Tr	4	Tr	0.01	Tr	770	Tr	Tr	N
Cooking fats													
358	**Baking fat and margarine** (75-90% fat), hard block	600	Tr	1	Tr	Tr	0.1	Tr	Tr	1220	Tr	Tr	Tr
359	**Compound cooking fat**, not polyunsaturated	Tr	Tr	Tr	Tr	Tr	Tr	Tr	Tr	Tr	Tr	Tr	Tr
360	**Dripping**, beef	5	4	1	Tr	13	0.2	N	N	2	Tr	Tr	5
361	**Ghee**, butter	1	Tr	1	Tr	Tr	Tr	Tr	Tr	28	Tr	Tr	44
362	made from vegetable oil	1	1	Tr	Tr	Tr	Tr	0.14	Tr	Tr	Tr	Tr	Tr
363	**Lard**	2	1	1	1	3	0.1	0.02	N	4	Tr	Tr	Tr
364	**Suet**, shredded	Tr	Tr	Tr	Tr	Tr	Tr	Tr	Tr	Tr	Tr	Tr	5
365	vegetable, reduced fat	10	Tr	Tr	Tr	Tr	Tr	Tr	Tr	N	Tr	Tr	Tr

Fats and oils *continued*

Vitamins per 100g edible portion

No.	Food	Retinol µg	Carotene[a] µg	Vitamin D µg	Vitamin[b] E mg	Thiamin mg	Ribo-flavin mg	Niacin mg	Trypt 60 mg	Vitamin B6 mg	Vitamin B12 µg	Folate µg	Panto-thenate mg	Biotin µg	Vitamin C mg
Spreading fats continued															
355	**Fat spread**, low fat (26-39%), not polyunsaturated, including dairy type	750[c,d]	859	3.0[c,d]	12.50	Tr	0.07	Tr	Tr	Tr	0.1	1	0.02	0.3	0
356	low fat (26-39%), not polyunsaturated, with olive oil	787[c,e]	630	4.5[c,e]	13.00	Tr	Tr	Tr	Tr.	Tr[f]	Tr[f]	Tr[f]	Tr	Tr	0
357	low fat (26-39%), polyunsaturated	811[c,g]	903	8.4[c,g]	10.10	Tr	Tr	Tr	Tr	Tr[f]	Tr[f]	Tr[f]	Tr	Tr	0
Cooking fats															
358	**Baking fat and margarine** (75-90% fat), hard block	796	655	8.8	12.20	Tr	Tr	Tr	Tr	Tr	0	Tr	Tr	Tr	0
359	**Compound cooking fat**, not polyunsaturated	0	0	0	Tr	0	0	0	0	0	0	0	0	0	0
360	**Dripping**, beef	N	N	Tr	0.40	Tr	Tr	Tr	Tr	Tr	Tr	Tr	Tr	Tr	0
361	**Ghee**, butter	922	1860	1.1	5.76	0	Tr	Tr	Tr	Tr	Tr	0	Tr	Tr	0
362	made from vegetable oil	0	Tr	0	8.70	0	0	Tr	Tr	Tr	0	0	Tr	Tr	0
363	**Lard**	Tr	0	N	1.00	Tr	Tr	Tr	Tr	Tr	Tr	Tr	Tr	Tr	0
364	**Suet**, shredded	52	73	Tr	1.50	Tr	Tr	Tr	Tr	Tr	Tr	Tr	Tr	Tr	0
365	vegetable, reduced fat	0	0	0	13.43	Tr	Tr	Tr	Tr	Tr	0	Tr	Tr	Tr	0

[a] Some brands may not contain β-carotene

[b] In foods containing oil, the vitamin E content will vary according to the type of oil used

[c] Value relates to a mixture of fortified and unfortified products

[d] Fortified products contain approximately 800µg retinol and 6.0µg vitamin D per 100g

[e] Fortified products contain 800µg retinol and 5.0µg vitamin D per 100g

[f] Some brands may contain added vitamin B6, vitamin B12 and folate

[g] Fortified products contain approximately 800µg retinol and 7.5µg vitamin D per 100g

Composition of food per 100g edible portion

Oils

No.	Food	Description and main data sources	Main data reference	Water g	Total nitrogen g	Protein g	Fat g	Carbo-hydrate g	Energy value kcal	kJ
366	Coconut oil	MSF Supplement, 1994	14	Tr	Tr	Tr	99.9	0	899	3696
367	Cod liver oil	MSF Supplement, 1994	14	Tr	Tr	Tr	99.9	0	899	3696
368	Corn oil	MSF Supplement, 1994	14	Tr	Tr	Tr	99.9	0	899	3696
369	Evening primrose oil	MSF Supplement, 1994	14	Tr	Tr	Tr	99.9	0	899	3696
370	Grapeseed oil	MSF Supplement, 1994	14	Tr	Tr	Tr	99.9	0	899	3696
371	Olive oil	Including virgin and extra virgin olive oil. MSF Supplement, 1994	14	Tr	Tr	Tr	99.9	0	899	3696
372	Palm oil	MSF Supplement, 1994	14	Tr	Tr	Tr	99.9	0	899	3696
373	Peanut (groundnut) oil	MSF Supplement, 1994	14	Tr	Tr	Tr	99.9	0	899	3696
374	Rapeseed oil	MSF Supplement, 1994	14	Tr	Tr	Tr	99.9	0	899	3696
375	Sesame oil	Literature sources, 1972; and MSF Supplement, 1994	176, 14	0.1	0.03	0.2	99.7	0	898	3692
376	Soya oil	MSF Supplement, 1994	14	Tr	Tr	Tr	99.9	0	899	3696
377	Sunflower oil	MSF Supplement, 1994	14	Tr	Tr	Tr	99.9	0	899	3696
378	Vegetable oil, average	Based on rapeseed oil[a]. MSF Supplement, 1994	14	Tr	Tr	Tr	99.9	0	899	3696
379	Walnut oil	MSF Supplement, 1994	14	Tr	Tr	Tr	99.9	0	899	3696

[a] Most vegetable oils are made from rapeseed oil

Composition of food per 100g edible portion

No.	Food	Starch	Total sugars	Individual sugars					Dietary fibre		Fatty acids				Cholest-
				Gluc	Fruct	Sucr	Malt	Lact	NSP	AOAC	Satd	Mono-unsatd	Poly-unsatd	Trans	erol
		g	g	g	g	g	g	g	g	g	g	g	g	g	mg
Oils															
366	Coconut oil	0	0	0	0	0	0	0	0	0	86.5	6.0	1.5	Tr	0
367	Cod liver oil	0	0	0	0	0	0	0	0	0	21.1	44.6	30.5	Tr	570
368	Corn oil	0	0	0	0	0	0	0	0	0	14.4	29.9	51.3	Tr	0
369	Evening primrose oil	0	0	0	0	0	0	0	0	0	7.8	10.6	76.6	Tr	0
370	Grapeseed oil	0	0	0	0	0	0	0	0	0	11.1	15.8	68.2	Tr	0
371	Olive oil	0	0	0	0	0	0	0	0	0	14.3	73.0	8.2	Tr	0
372	Palm oil	0	0	0	0	0	0	0	0	0	47.8	37.1	10.4	Tr	0
373	Peanut (groundnut) oil	0	0	0	0	0	0	0	0	0	20.0	44.4	31.0	Tr	0
374	Rapeseed oil	0	0	0	0	0	0	0	0	0	6.6	59.3	29.3	Tr	0
375	Sesame oil	0	0	0	0	0	0	0	0	0	14.6	37.5	43.4	Tr	0
376	Soya oil	0	0	0	0	0	0	0	0	0	15.6	21.3	58.8	Tr	0
377	Sunflower oil	0	0	0	0	0	0	0	0	0	12.0	20.5	63.3	Tr	0
378	Vegetable oil, average	0	0	0	0	0	0	0	0	0	6.6	59.3	29.3	Tr	0
379	Walnut oil	0	0	0	0	0	0	0	0	0	9.1	16.5	69.9	Tr	0

Inorganic constituents per 100g edible portion

No.	Food	Na	K	Ca	Mg	P	Fe	Cu	Zn	Cl	Mn	Se	I
					mg							µg	
Oils													
366	Coconut oil	Tr	Tr	Tr	Tr	Tr	Tr	Tr	Tr	Tr	Tr	Tr	Tr
367	Cod liver oil	Tr	Tr	Tr	Tr	Tr	Tr	Tr	Tr	Tr	Tr	Tr	Tr
368	Corn oil	Tr	Tr	Tr	Tr	Tr	0.1	0.01	Tr	Tr	Tr	Tr	Tr
369	Evening primrose oil	Tr	Tr	Tr	Tr	Tr	Tr	Tr	Tr	Tr	Tr	Tr	Tr
370	Grapeseed oil	Tr	Tr	Tr	Tr	Tr	Tr	Tr	Tr	Tr	Tr	Tr	Tr
371	Olive oil	Tr	Tr	Tr	Tr	Tr	0.4	0.01	Tr	Tr	Tr	Tr	Tr
372	Palm oil	Tr	Tr	Tr	Tr	Tr	0.4	Tr	Tr	Tr	Tr	Tr	Tr
373	Peanut (groundnut) oil	Tr	Tr	Tr	Tr	Tr	Tr	Tr	Tr	Tr	Tr	Tr	Tr
374	Rapeseed oil	Tr	Tr	Tr	Tr	Tr	0.1	0.01	Tr	Tr	Tr	Tr	Tr
375	Sesame oil	2	20	10	Tr	N	0.1	Tr	Tr	N	Tr	Tr	Tr
376	Soya oil	Tr	Tr	Tr	Tr	Tr	0.1	0.01	Tr	Tr	Tr	Tr	Tr
377	Sunflower oil	Tr	Tr	Tr	Tr	Tr	0.1	0.01	Tr	Tr	Tr	Tr	Tr
378	Vegetable oil, average	Tr	Tr	Tr	Tr	Tr	0.1	0.01	Tr	Tr	Tr	Tr	Tr
379	Walnut oil	Tr	Tr	Tr	Tr	Tr	Tr	Tr	Tr	Tr	Tr	Tr	Tr

Vitamins per 100g edible portion

No.	Food	Retinol	Carotene	Vitamin D	Vitamin E	Thiamin	Ribo-flavin	Niacin	Trypt/60	Vitamin B$_6$	Vitamin B$_{12}$	Folate	Panto-thenate	Biotin	Vitamin C
		µg	µg	µg	mg	mg	mg	mg	mg	mg	µg	µg	mg	µg	mg
Oils															
366	**Coconut oil**	0	Tr	0	0.66	Tr	Tr	Tr	Tr	Tr	0	Tr	Tr	Tr	0
367	**Cod liver oil**	18000[a]	Tr	210[a]	20.00[a]	Tr	Tr	Tr	Tr	Tr	Tr	Tr	Tr	Tr	0
368	**Corn oil**	0	Tr	0	17.24	Tr	Tr	Tr	Tr	Tr	0	Tr	Tr	Tr	0
369	**Evening primrose oil**	0	Tr	0	N	Tr	Tr	Tr	Tr	Tr	0	Tr	Tr	Tr	0
370	**Grapeseed oil**	0	Tr	0	N	Tr	Tr	Tr	Tr	Tr	0	Tr	Tr	Tr	0
371	**Olive oil**	0	N	0	5.10	Tr	Tr	Tr	Tr	Tr	0	Tr	Tr	Tr	0
372	**Palm oil**	0	Tr[b]	0	33.12	Tr	Tr	Tr	Tr	Tr	0	Tr	Tr	Tr	0
373	**Peanut (groundnut) oil**	0	Tr	0	15.16	Tr	Tr	Tr	Tr	Tr	0	Tr	Tr	Tr	0
374	**Rapeseed oil**	0	Tr	0	22.21	Tr	Tr	Tr	Tr	Tr	0	Tr	Tr	Tr	0
375	**Sesame oil**	0	Tr	0	N	0.01	0.07	0.1	Tr	Tr	0	Tr	Tr	Tr	0
376	**Soya oil**	0	Tr	0	16.06	Tr	Tr	Tr	Tr	Tr	0	Tr	Tr	Tr	0
377	**Sunflower oil**	0	Tr	0	49.22	Tr	Tr	Tr	Tr	Tr	0	Tr	Tr	Tr	0
378	**Vegetable oil,** average	0	Tr	0	22.21	Tr	Tr	Tr	Tr	Tr	0	Tr	Tr	Tr	0
379	**Walnut oil**	0	Tr	0	N	Tr	Tr	Tr	Tr	Tr	0	Tr	Tr	Tr	0

[a] Content will vary as some products contain added vitamin A, D and E

[b] Unrefined palm oil contains approximately 30000µg β- and 24000µg α- carotene per 100g

171

Meat and meat products

Section 2.5

Meat and meat products

This section of the Tables is largely based on the *Meat, Poultry and Game* (1995)[15] and *Meat Products and Dishes* (1996)[16] supplements, which are based on analytical data from the early and mid 1990s[32,36,37,41,42,45,46]. New analytical data (2010)[72] for a few processed poultry products, meat pies, pastries and meat dishes have been included. In addition, values for processed meats and meat products have been reviewed using data from manufacturers, particularly fat and sodium values, and have been updated where necessary to reflect reformulation work.

The nutrient values for carcase meat and poultry were constructed from the separable fat and lean in meat (and meat and skin for poultry) analysed following dissection into lean meat, separable fat and inedible matter (or meat, skin and inedible matter for poultry). Since it was not possible to analyse all samples for all nutrients, some values for minerals and vitamins were interpolated from analytical values from similar cuts and cooking methods, usually in proportion to the protein content of the samples.

The major source of variation in meat composition is the proportion of lean to fat, as a result of husbandry techniques and trimming practices - both at retail level and in the home. This affects levels of most other nutrients, which are distributed differently in the two fractions.

Users should note that all values are expressed per 100g edible portion. Guidance for calculating nutrient content 'as purchased' or 'as served' (e.g. including rind or bone) is given in Section 4.2. For weight loss on cooking and calculation of the cooked edible proportion obtained from raw meat see Section 4.3.

Losses of labile vitamins assigned to cooked dishes and food were estimated using figures in Section 4.3. Taxonomic names for foods in this part of the Tables can be found in Section 4.5.

Composition of food per 100g edible portion

Bacon and ham

No.	Food	Description and main data sources	Main data reference	Water g	Total nitrogen g	Protein g	Fat g	Carbo-hydrate g	Energy value kcal	kJ
380	**Bacon rashers, back**, raw	Smoked and unsmoked; loose and prepacked; British, Danish and Dutch bacon. Analytical data, 1994; and industry data, 2013	41	63.9	2.64	16.5	16.5	0	215	891
381	dry-fried	Smoked and unsmoked; loose and prepacked; British, Danish and Dutch bacon. Analytical data, 1994; and calculated from raw 2013 data	41	49.7	3.87	24.2	22.0	0	295	1225
382	grilled	Smoked and unsmoked; loose and prepacked; British, Danish and Dutch bacon. Analytical data, 1994; and calculated from raw 2013 data	41	50.4	3.71	23.2	21.6	0	287	1194
383	grilled crispy	Smoked and unsmoked; loose and prepacked; British, Danish and Dutch bacon. Analytical data, 1994; and calculated from raw 2013 data	41	37.8	5.76	36.0	18.8	0	313	1308
384	microwaved	Smoked and unsmoked; loose and prepacked; British, Danish and Dutch bacon. Analytical data, 1994; and calculated from raw 2013 data	41	45.5	3.87	24.2	23.3	0	307	1274
385	fat trimmed, grilled	Smoked and unsmoked; loose and prepacked; British, Danish and Dutch bacon. Analytical data, 1994; and calculated from raw 2013 data	41	56.2	4.11	25.7	12.3	0	214	892

Composition of food per 100g edible portion

No.	Food	Starch	Total sugars	Individual sugars					Dietary fibre		Fatty acids				Cholest-
				Gluc	Fruct	Sucr	Malt	Lact	NSP	AOAC	Satd	Mono-unsatd	Poly-unsatd	Trans	erol
		g	g	g	g	g	g	g	g	g	g	g	g	g	mg
Bacon and ham															
380	**Bacon rashers, back**, raw	0	0	0	0	0	0	0	0	0	6.2	6.9	2.2	0.1	53
381	dry-fried	0	0	0	0	0	0	0	0	0	8.3	9.2	2.8	0.1	65
382	grilled	0	0	0	0	0	0	0	0	0	8.1	9.0	2.8	Tr	75
383	grilled crispy	0	0	0	0	0	0	0	0	0	7.1	7.9	2.4	0.1	68
384	microwaved	0	0	0	0	0	0	0	0	0	8.8	9.8	3.0	0.1	84
385	fat trimmed, grilled	0	0	0	0	0	0	0	0	0	4.6	5.2	1.6	0.1	44

Inorganic constituents per 100g edible portion

No.	Food	Na	K	Ca	Mg	P	Fe	Cu	Zn	Cl	Mn	Se	I
						mg						μg	
	Bacon and ham												
380	**Bacon rashers, back,** raw	1140	300	5	17	150	0.4	0.06	1.2	1740	0.01	8	5
381	dry-fried	1410	300	6	21	180	0.6	0.06	1.9	2600	0.01	18	7
382	grilled	1390	340	7	21	180	0.6	0.05	1.7	2060	0.01	12	7
383	grilled crispy	2000	510	10	32	300	1.1	0.10	3.1	2600	0.01	18	11
384	microwaved	1730	360	8	23	200	0.7	0.06	2.0	1750	0.01	12	7
385	fat trimmed, grilled	1430	360	8	23	210	0.7	0.07	2.2	1850	0.01	13	8

Vitamins per 100g edible portion

No.	Food	Retinol µg	Carotene µg	Vitamin D µg	Vitamin E mg	Thiamin mg	Ribo-flavin mg	Niacin mg	Trypt 60 mg	Vitamin B6 mg	Vitamin B12 µg	Folate µg	Panto-thenate mg	Biotin µg	Vitamin C mg
Bacon and ham															
380	**Bacon rashers, back**, raw	Tr	Tr	0.3	0.02	0.63	0.11	5.6	2.6	0.46	Tr	3	1.00	2	1
381	dry-fried	Tr	Tr	0.6	0.07	0.86	0.14	6.8	4.4	0.53	1	2	1.26	5	Tr
382	grilled	Tr	Tr	0.6	0.07	1.16	0.15	7.2	3.8	0.52	1	5	1.24	3	Tr
383	grilled crispy	Tr	Tr	1.0	0.10	1.38	0.24	10.8	6.6	0.71	1	4	1.34	5	Tr
384	microwaved	Tr	Tr	0.6	0.07	1.10	0.16	7.9	4.4	0.55	1	2	1.26	5	Tr
385	fat trimmed, grilled	Tr	Tr	0.7	0.07	0.98	0.17	7.7	4.7	0.50	1	3	1.34	5	Tr

Composition of food per 100g edible portion

Bacon and ham continued

No.	Food	Description and main data sources	Main data reference	Water g	Total nitrogen g	Protein g	Fat g	Carbo-hydrate g	Energy value kcal	kJ
386	**Bacon rashers, middle**, grilled	Smoked and unsmoked; loose and prepacked; British, Danish and Dutch bacon. Analytical data, 1994; and calculated from raw 2013 data	41	47.8	3.97	24.8	23.1	0	307	1276
387	**Bacon rashers, streaky**, fried in corn oil	Smoked and unsmoked; loose and prepacked; British, Danish and Dutch bacon. Analytical data, 1994	41	45.1	3.81	23.8	26.6	0	335	1389
388	grilled	Smoked and unsmoked; loose and prepacked; British, Danish and Dutch bacon. Analytical data, 1994	41	44.0	3.81	23.8	26.9	0	337	1400
389	**Bacon, fat only**, average, cooked	MW4, 1978; and industry data, 2013	4	13.8	1.48	9.3	72.8	0	692	2852
390	**Ham**	Loose and prepacked including honey roast and smoked ham. Added water 10-15%. Analytical data, 1994; and industry data, 2013	44	73.2	2.94	18.4	3.3	1.0	107	451
391	**Ham, gammon joint**, raw	Smoked and unsmoked, prepacked British and Danish gammon. Analytical data, 1994	41	68.6	2.80	17.5	7.5	0	138	575
392	boiled	Smoked and unsmoked, prepacked British and Danish gammon. Analytical data, 1994	41	61.2	3.73	23.3	12.3	0	204	851
393	**Ham, gammon rashers,** grilled	Unsmoked British gammon. Analytical data, 1994; and industry data, 2013	41	58.2	4.40	27.5	9.9	0	199	834

Composition of food per 100g edible portion

No.	Food	Starch g	Total sugars g	Gluc g	Fruct g	Sucr g	Malt g	Lact g	Dietary fibre NSP g	AOAC g	Fatty acids Satd g	Mono- unsatd g	Poly- unsatd g	Trans g	Cholest- erol mg
Bacon and ham continued															
386	**Bacon rashers, middle,** grilled	0	0	0	0	0	0	0	0	0	8.4	10.0	3.0	0.1	83
387	**Bacon rashers, streaky,** fried in corn oil	0	0	0	0	0	0	0	0	0	9.1	11.1	4.5	0.1	78
388	grilled	0	0	0	0	0	0	0	0	0	9.8	11.5	3.7	0.1	90
389	**Bacon, fat only,** average, cooked	0	0	0	0	0	0	0	0	0	28.5	32.9	7.6	N	270
390	**Ham**	0	1.0	N	N	N	N	0	0	0.1	1.1	1.4	0.5	Tr	58
391	**Ham, gammon joint,** raw	0	0	0	0	0	0	0	0	0	2.5	3.3	1.2	Tr	23
392	boiled	0	0	0	0	0	0	0	0	0	4.1	5.4	1.9	Tr	83
393	**Ham, gammon rashers,** grilled	0	0	0	0	0	0	0	0	0	3.4	4.1	1.7	0.1	83

Inorganic constituents per 100g edible portion

No.	Food	Na	K	Ca	Mg	P	Fe	Cu	Zn	Cl	Mn	Se	I
						mg						µg	

Bacon and ham continued

No.	Food	Na	K	Ca	Mg	P	Fe	Cu	Zn	Cl	Mn	Se	I
386	**Bacon rashers, middle**, grilled	1390	350	8	21	220	0.7	0.07	2.2	2060	0.01	11	8
387	**Bacon rashers, streaky**, fried in corn oil	1680	350	7	21	200	0.7	0.07	2.1	2630	0.01	10	7
388	grilled	1680	330	9	20	180	0.8	0.15	2.5	2630	0.01	11	6
389	**Bacon, fat only**, average, cooked	740	130	7	10	90	0.8	0.09	0.8	1140	Tr	2	11
390	**Ham**	800	340	7	24	340	0.7	0.12	1.8	980	0.01	11	5
391	**Ham, gammon joint**, raw	880	190	7	17	130	0.6	0.08	1.5	1980	0.01	11	7
392	boiled	1180	250	9	18	170	0.8	0.10	2.1	2640	0.01	12	9
393	**Ham, gammon rashers**, grilled	1360	380	8	26	230	0.8	0.09	2.2	2090	0.02	14	8

Meat and meat products *continued*

Vitamins per 100g edible portion

No.	Food	Retinol µg	Carotene µg	Vitamin D µg	Vitamin E mg	Thiamin mg	Ribo-flavin mg	Niacin mg	Trypt 60 mg	Vitamin B$_6$ mg	Vitamin B$_{12}$ µg	Folate µg	Panto-thenate mg	Biotin µg	Vitamin C mg
	Bacon and ham continued														
386	**Bacon rashers, middle**, grilled	Tr	Tr	0.6	0.13	0.77	0.17	7.5	5.1	0.42	1	3	1.27	6	Tr
387	**Bacon rashers, streaky**, fried in corn oil	Tr	Tr	0.6	N	0.75	0.14	7.1	4.4	0.47	1	1	1.24	5	Tr
388	grilled	Tr	Tr	0.7	0.07	0.70	0.17	6.3	4.3	0.40	1	3	1.22	4	Tr
389	**Bacon, fat only**, average, cooked	Tr	Tr	N	0.36	N	N	N	1.7	N	Tr	Tr	N	Tr	0
390	**Ham**	Tr	Tr	N	0.04	0.80	0.17	6.5	3.1	0.61	1	19	1.03	3	Tr
391	**Ham, gammon joint**, raw	Tr	Tr	0.6	0.06	0.44	0.13	5.3	2.9	0.43	Tr	4	1.07	2	Tr
392	boiled	Tr	Tr	0.8	0.08	0.58	0.16	5.4	3.9	0.42	Tr	3	1.43	2	Tr
393	**Ham, gammon rashers**, grilled	Tr	Tr	0.8	0.08	1.16	0.18	6.4	5.5	0.16	1	3	1.43	6	Tr

Composition of food per 100g edible portion

No.	Food	Description and main data sources	Main data reference	Water g	Total nitrogen g	Protein g	Fat g	Carbo-hydrate g	Energy value kcal	Energy value kJ
Beef and veal										
394	**Beef, fat**, average, raw	Average of 10 different cuts, trimmed of lean. Analytical data, 1993	36	35.0	3.02	18.9	53.6	0	558	2305
395	average, cooked	Average of 8 different cuts. Analytical data, 1993	36	33.6	2.48	15.5	52.3	0	533	2199
396	**Beef, lean**, average, raw	Average of 10 different cuts, trimmed of fat. Analytical data, 1993	36	71.9	3.60	22.5	4.3	0	129	542
397	**Braising steak**, braised, lean only	Analytical data, 1993	36	55.5	5.50	34.4	9.7	0	225	944
398	braised, lean and fat	Calculated from 90% lean and 9% fat. Analytical data, 1993	36	53.1	5.26	32.9	12.7	0	246	1029
399	**Mince**, raw	Analytical data, 1993	36	62.0[a]	3.15	19.7	16.2[b]	0	225	934
400	microwaved	Analytical data, 1993	36	55.3	4.22	26.4	17.5	0	263	1096
401	stewed	Analytical data, 1993	36	64.4	3.49	21.8	13.5	0	209	870
402	**Mince, extra lean**, stewed	Analytical data, 1993; and industry data, 2013	36	71.1	3.95	24.7	4.2	0	137	575
403	**Rump steak**, raw, lean and fat	Calculated from 88% lean and 11% fat. Analytical data, 1993	36	68.2	3.31	20.7	10.1	0	174	726
404	barbecued, lean	Analytical data, 1993	36	62.4	4.99	31.2	5.7	0	176	741
405	fried in corn oil, lean only	Analytical data, 1993	36	61.7	4.94	30.9	6.6	0	183	770
406	fried in corn oil, lean and fat	Calculated from 87% lean and 12% fat. Analytical data, 1993	36	57.2	4.54	28.4	12.7	0	228	953
407	grilled, lean only	Analytical data, 1993	36	62.9	4.96	31.0	5.9	0	177	745
408	from steakhouse, lean only	Analytical data, 1993	36	63.0	4.77	29.8	4.7	0	162	681

[a] Water typically varies from 57.3g to 70.0g per 100g

[b] Fat typically varies from 7.8g to 26.5g per 100g

Composition of food per 100g edible portion

No.	Food	Starch g	Total sugars g	Individual sugars					Dietary fibre		Fatty acids				Cholest-erol mg
				Gluc g	Fruct g	Sucr g	Malt g	Lact g	NSP g	AOAC g	Satd g	Mono-unsatd g	Poly-unsatd g	Trans g	
Beef and veal															
394	**Beef, fat**, average, raw	0	0	0	0	0	0	0	0	0	24.9	24.2	1.7	2.4	72
395	average, cooked	0	0	0	0	0	0	0	0	0	24.3	23.4	1.8	2.4	97
396	**Beef, lean**, average, raw	0	0	0	0	0	0	0	0	0	1.7	1.9	0.2	0.1	58
397	**Braising steak**, braised, lean only	0	0	0	0	0	0	0	0	0	4.1	4.1	0.6	0.4	100
398	braised, lean and fat	0	0	0	0	0	0	0	0	0	5.3	5.2	0.8	0.5	100
399	**Mince**, raw	0	0	0	0	0	0	0	0	0	6.9	6.9	0.5	0.8	60
400	microwaved	0	0	0	0	0	0	0	0	0	7.6	7.7	0.7	0.8	80
401	stewed	0	0	0	0	0	0	0	0	0	5.7	5.7	0.6	0.7	79
402	**Mince, extra lean**, stewed	0	0	0	0	0	0	0	0	0	1.8	1.8	0.2	0.2	36
403	**Rump steak**, raw, lean and fat	0	0	0	0	0	0	0	0	0	4.3	4.4	0.6	0.3	60
404	barbecued, lean	0	0	0	0	0	0	0	0	0	2.4	2.4	0.4	0.2	76
405	fried in corn oil, lean only	0	0	0	0	0	0	0	0	0	2.4	2.5	0.9	0.2	86
406	fried in corn oil, lean and fat	0	0	0	0	0	0	0	0	0	4.9	5.2	1.6	0.4	84
407	grilled, lean only	0	0	0	0	0	0	0	0	0	2.5	2.5	0.5	0.2	76
408	from steakhouse, lean only	0	0	0	0	0	0	0	0	0	2.0	2.0	0.3	0.1	73

Inorganic constituents per 100g edible portion

No.	Food	Na	K	Ca	Mg	P	Fe	Cu	Zn	Cl	Mn	Se	I
						mg						µg	
Beef and veal													
394	**Beef, fat**, average, raw	26	140	5	9	79	0.7	0.02	1.1	28	Tr	2	10
395	average, cooked	35	200	6	12	110	1.0	0.01	1.5	39	0.01	3	14
396	**Beef, lean**, average, raw	63	350	5	22	200	2.7	0.03	4.1	51	0.01	7	10
397	**Braising steak**, braised, lean only	62	340	8	23	220	2.7	Tr	9.5	62	Tr	11	15
398	braised, lean and fat	60	330	8	22	210	2.6	Tr	8.7	61	Tr	10	15
399	**Mince**, raw	80	260	9	17	160	1.4	Tr	3.9	76	Tr	7	9
400	microwaved	91	290	12	20	190	2.0	Tr	5.2	110	0.02	9	16
401	stewed	73	210	20	15	150	2.7	0.10	5.0	63	0.02	7	14
402	**Mince, extra lean**, stewed	75	280	14	18	170	2.3	0.08	5.6	61	Tr	8	10
403	**Rump steak**, raw, lean and fat	56	350	4	22	200	2.7	0.04	3.5	38	Tr	7	11
404	barbecued, lean	78	460	8	29	270	3.2	0.10	5.1	61	0.04	10	11
405	fried in corn oil, lean only	78	390	5	25	240	3.0	0.02	5.2	50	0.02	10	9
406	fried in corn oil, lean and fat	71	360	5	23	220	2.7	0.02	4.7	47	0.02	9	9
407	grilled, lean only	74	430	7	29	260	3.6	0.04	5.6	62	0.02	10	12
408	from steakhouse, lean only	72	410	7	28	250	2.4	0.04	5.4	60	0.02	10	11

Meat and meat products *continued*

Vitamins per 100g edible portion

Beef and veal

No.	Food	Retinol µg	Carotene µg	Vitamin D µg	Vitamin E mg	Thiamin mg	Ribo-flavin mg	Niacin mg	Trypt 60 mg	Vitamin B$_6$ mg	Vitamin B$_{12}$ µg	Folate µg	Panto-thenate mg	Biotin µg	Vitamin C mg
394	**Beef, fat**, average, raw	Tr	Tr	Tr	0.06	0.04	0.13	1.2	1.7	0.17	1	18	0.43	1	0
395	average, cooked	Tr	Tr	Tr	0.08	0.05	0.18	1.6	1.8	0.23	2	26	0.60	2	0
396	**Beef, lean**, average, raw	Tr	Tr	0.5	0.13	0.10	0.21	5.0	4.7	0.53	2	19	0.75	1	0
397	**Braising steak**, braised, lean only	Tr	8	0.8	0.02	0.05	0.26	5.2	8.0	0.34	3	54	0.55	2	0
398	braised, lean and fat	Tr	7	0.7	0.03	0.05	0.26	4.9	7.5	0.33	3	52	0.57	2	0
399	**Mince**, raw	Tr	Tr	0.7	0.17	0.06	0.13	5.8	3.6	0.37	2	14	0.49	1	0
400	microwaved	Tr	8	0.6	0.31	0.08	0.31	8.0	4.3	0.38	3	17	0.53	2	0
401	stewed	Tr	8	0.8	0.34	0.03	0.19	4.6	4.4	0.28	2	17	0.36	5	0
402	**Mince, extra lean**, stewed	Tr	8	0.6	0.30	0.03	0.13	4.8	4.5	0.16	3	20	0.36	2	0
403	**Rump steak**, raw, lean and fat	Tr	Tr	0.4	0.04	0.09	0.23	4.9	4.5	0.61	2	5	0.65	1	0
404	barbecued, lean	Tr	8	0.7	0.20	0.15	0.32	6.8	7.0	0.36	3	10	0.78	2	0
405	fried in corn oil, lean only	Tr	8	0.7	0.18	0.14	0.29	5.9	6.7	0.63	2	5	0.74	2	0
406	fried in corn oil, lean and fat	Tr	7	0.6	N	0.13	0.27	5.3	6.0	0.57	2	5	0.70	2	0
407	grilled, lean only	Tr	8	0.4	0.07	0.13	0.28	6.8	7.0	0.65	3	5	0.91	2	0
408	from steakhouse, lean only	Tr	8	0.7	N	0.13	0.27	6.5	6.7	0.63	2	17	0.88	2	0

Meat and meat products *continued*

Composition of food per 100g edible portion

No.	Food	Description and main data sources	Main data reference	Water g	Total nitrogen g	Protein g	Fat g	Carbo-hydrate g	Energy value kcal	kJ
409	**Rump steak**, strips, stir-fried in corn oil, lean	Analytical data, 1993	36	57.9	5.17	32.3	8.8	0	208	875

Beef and veal continued

No.	Food	Description and main data sources	Main data reference	Water g	Total nitrogen g	Protein g	Fat g	Carbo-hydrate g	Energy value kcal	kJ
410	**Stewing steak**, raw, lean	Analytical data, 1993	36	73.4	3.62	22.6	3.5	0	122	514
411	raw, lean and fat	Calculated from 90% lean and 9% fat. Analytical data, 1993	36	70.1	3.54	22.1	6.4	0	146	613
412	stewed, lean only	Analytical data, 1993	36	61.6	5.12	32.0	6.3	0	185	777
413	stewed, lean and fat	Calculated from 84% lean and 14% fat. Analytical data, 1993	36	59.4	4.67	29.2	9.6	0	203	852
414	**Topside**, roasted medium-rare, lean only	Analytical data, 1993	36	62.2	5.15	32.2	5.1	0	175	736
415	roasted medium-rare, lean and fat	Calculated from 87% lean and 12% fat. Analytical data, 1993	36	57.6	4.78	29.9	11.4	0	222	930
416	**Veal**, escalope, fried in corn oil	Analytical data, 1993	36	58.7	5.39	33.7	6.8	0	196	825

Lamb

No.	Food	Description and main data sources	Main data reference	Water g	Total nitrogen g	Protein g	Fat g	Carbo-hydrate g	Energy value kcal	kJ
417	**Lamb, fat**, average, raw	Average of 8 different cuts, trimmed of lean. Analytical data, 1994	42	34.7	2.13	13.3	51.6	0	518	2135
418	average, cooked	Average of 8 different cuts, trimmed of lean. Analytical data, 1994	42	28.3	2.64	15.4	56.3	0	568	2345
419	**Lamb, lean only**, average, raw	Average of 8 different cuts. Analytical data, 1994	42	70.6	3.23	20.2	8.0	0	153	639

Meat and meat products *continued*

Composition of food per 100g edible portion

No.	Food	Starch	Total sugars	Individual sugars					Dietary fibre		Fatty acids				Cholest-
				Gluc	Fruct	Sucr	Malt	Lact	NSP	AOAC	Satd	Mono-unsatd	Poly-unsatd	Trans	erol
		g	g	g	g	g	g	g	g	g	g	g	g	g	mg
Beef and veal continued															
409	**Rump steak**, strips, stir-fried in corn oil, lean	0	0	0	0	0	0	0	0	0	3.3	3.5	1.2	0.3	92
410	**Stewing steak**, raw, lean	0	0	0	0	0	0	0	0	0	1.4	1.6	0.2	0.1	67
411	raw, lean and fat	0	0	0	0	0	0	0	0	0	2.6	2.9	0.4	0.2	69
412	stewed, lean only	0	0	0	0	0	0	0	0	0	2.3	2.6	0.8	0.2	91
413	stewed, lean and fat	0	0	0	0	0	0	0	0	0	3.7	4.2	0.9	0.3	91
414	**Topside**, roasted medium-rare, lean only	0	0	0	0	0	0	0	0	0	2.1	2.3	0.2	0.2	68
415	roasted medium-rare, lean and fat	0	0	0	0	0	0	0	0	0	4.8	5.2	0.5	0.4	71
416	**Veal**, escalope, fried in corn oil	0	0	0	0	0	0	0	0	0	1.8	2.5	1.9	0.1	110
Lamb															
417	**Lamb, fat**, average, raw	0	0	0	0	0	0	0	0	0	26.3	19.5	2.3	4.8	92
418	average, cooked	0	0	0	0	0	0	0	0	0	28.4	21.6	2.4	5.2	100
419	**Lamb, lean only**, average, raw	0	0	0	0	0	0	0	0	0	3.5	3.1	0.5	0.6	74

Inorganic constituents per 100g edible portion

No.	Food	Na	K	Ca	Mg	P	Fe	Cu	Zn	Cl	Mn	Se	I
						mg						µg	
	Beef and veal continued												
409	**Rump steak**, strips, stir-fried in corn oil, lean	78	450	7	30	270	2.6	0.04	5.8	64	0.02	11	12
410	**Stewing steak**, raw, lean	69	360	5	21	190	2.1	0.04	5.7	69	Tr	7	12
411	raw, lean and fat	66	340	5	20	180	2.0	0.04	5.3	66	Tr	7	13
412	stewed. lean only	54	270	17	21	200	2.6	0.04	8.6	32	0.01	11	12
413	stewed, lean and fat	51	250	15	19	180	2.3	0.04	7.5	33	0.01	10	12
414	**Topside**, roasted medium-rare, lean only	66	390	5	25	230	2.5	0.07	5.6	56	0.02	10	9
415	roasted medium-rare, lean and fat	62	360	5	23	210	2.3	0.06	5.1	54	0.02	9	10
416	**Veal**, escalope, fried in corn oil	86	460	6	32	300	0.9	Tr	3.1	77	0.02	11	8
	Lamb												
417	**Lamb, fat**, average, raw	36	140	9	9	86	0.7	0.03	0.9	43	0.01	2	6
418	average, cooked	72	260	11	18	160	1.1	0.05	1.5	67	0.01	4	6
419	**Lamb, lean only**, average, raw	70	330	12	22	190	1.4	0.08	3.3	74	0.01	4	6

Meat and meat products *continued*

Vitamins per 100g edible portion

No.	Food	Retinol	Carotene	Vitamin D	Vitamin E	Thiamin	Ribo-flavin	Niacin	Trypt 60	Vitamin B$_6$	Vitamin B$_{12}$	Folate	Panto-thenate	Biotin	Vitamin C
		µg	µg	µg	mg	mg	mg	mg	mg	mg	µg	µg	mg	µg	mg
Beef and veal continued															
409	**Rump steak**, strips, stir-fried in corn oil, lean	Tr	8	0.7	0.06	0.21	0.30	6.8	7.2	0.73	3	5	0.94	2	0
410	**Stewing steak**, raw, lean	Tr	Tr	0.8	0.20	0.07	0.27	4.2	4.5	0.45	2	5	0.65	1	0
411	raw, lean and fat	Tr	Tr	0.7	0.20	0.07	0.26	4.0	4.3	0.42	2	6	0.65	1	0
412	stewed, lean only	Tr	8	0.7	0.19	0.02	0.15	2.6	7.2	0.23	3	8	0.31	2	0
413	stewed, lean and fat	Tr	7	0.6	0.17	0.03	0.15	2.4	6.2	0.23	2	11	0.30	2	0
414	**Topside**, roasted medium-rare, lean only	Tr	Tr	0.4	0.04	0.06	0.32	5.4	6.6	0.54	2	14	0.55	2	0
415	roasted medium-rare, lean and fat	Tr	Tr	0.4	0.05	0.06	0.30	4.9	5.9	0.50	2	15	0.55	2	0
416	**Veal**, escalope, fried in corn oil	6	Tr	1.3	0.39	0.08	0.25	7.8	7.6	0.70	4	17	1.02	5	0
Lamb															
417	**Lamb, fat**, average, raw	29	Tr	0.5	0.14	0.07	0.12	2.2	1.3	0.10	1	4	0.47	1	0
418	average, cooked	29	Tr	0.5	0.28	0.09	0.17	3.6	2.0	0.20	1	4	0.74	1	0
419	**Lamb, lean only**, average, raw	6	Tr	0.4	0.09	0.09	0.20	5.4	3.9	0.30	2	6	0.92	2	0

Meat and meat products *continued*

Composition of food per 100g edible portion

420 to 431

Lamb continued

No.	Food	Description and main data sources	Main data reference	Water g	Total nitrogen g	Protein g	Fat g	Carbo-hydrate g	Energy value kcal	kJ
420	**Breast**, roasted, lean only	Analytical data, 1994	42	54.4	4.27	26.7	18.5	0	273	1138
421	roasted, lean and fat	Calculated from 62% lean and 36% fat. Analytical data, 1994	42	45.5	3.59	22.4	29.9	0	359	1487
422	**Leg**, average, raw, lean and fat	Calculated from 83% lean and 17% fat. Analytical data, 1994	42	67.4	3.05	19.0	12.3	0	187	778
423	half knuckle, pot-roasted, lean and fat	Calculated from 89% lean and 11% fat. Analytical data, 1994	42	58.1	4.49	28.1	13.8	0	237	988
424	whole, roasted, lean only	Analytical data, 1994	42	60.5	4.75	29.7	9.4	0	203	853
425	whole, roasted, lean and fat	Calculated from 89% lean and 11% fat. Analytical data, 1994	42	57.3	4.50	28.1	14.2	0	240	1003
426	**Loin chops**, raw, lean and fat	Calculated from 72% lean and 28% fat. Analytical data, 1994	42	59.3	2.81	17.6	23.0	0	277	1150
427	grilled, lean only	Analytical data, 1994	42	59.6	4.67	29.2	10.7	0	213	892
428	grilled, lean and fat	Calculated from 76% lean and 24% fat. Analytical data, 1994	42	50.5	4.24	26.5	22.1	0	305	1268
429	microwaved, lean and fat	Calculated from 72% lean and 28% fat. Analytical data, 1994	42	45.3	4.39	27.5	26.9	0	352	1463
430	roasted, lean only	Analytical data, 1994	42	52.1	5.50	34.4	13.3	0	257	1077
431	roasted, lean and fat	Calculated from 73% lean and 27% fat. Analytical data, 1994	42	43.8	4.66	29.1	26.9	0	359	1490

Composition of food per 100g edible portion

No.	Food	Starch g	Total sugars g	Gluc g	Fruct g	Sucr g	Malt g	Lact g	NSP g	AOAC g	Satd g	Mono- unsatd g	Poly- unsatd g	Trans g	Cholest- erol mg
						Individual sugars			Dietary fibre			Fatty acids			

Lamb continued

No.	Food	Starch g	Total sugars g	Gluc g	Fruct g	Sucr g	Malt g	Lact g	NSP g	AOAC g	Satd g	Mono- unsatd g	Poly- unsatd g	Trans g	Cholest- erol mg
420	**Breast**, roasted, lean only	0	0	0	0	0	0	0	0	0	8.6	7.0	0.9	1.6	95
421	roasted, lean and fat	0	0	0	0	0	0	0	0	0	14.3	11.4	1.4	2.7	93
422	**Leg**, average, raw, lean and fat	0	0	0	0	0	0	0	0	0	5.4	4.9	0.7	0.9	78
423	half knuckle, pot-roasted, lean and fat	0	0	0	0	0	0	0	0	0	6.0	5.6	0.8	1.1	105
424	whole, roasted, lean only	0	0	0	0	0	0	0	0	0	3.8	3.9	0.6	0.7	100
425	whole, roasted, lean and fat	0	0	0	0	0	0	0	0	0	5.9	6.1	0.8	1.2	100
426	**Loin chops**, raw, lean and fat	0	0	0	0	0	0	0	0	0	10.8	8.8	1.2	1.8	79
427	grilled, lean only	0	0	0	0	0	0	0	0	0	4.9	4.0	0.6	0.9	96
428	grilled, lean and fat	0	0	0	0	0	0	0	0	0	10.5	8.4	1.3	1.9	100
429	microwaved, lean and fat	0	0	0	0	0	0	0	0	0	12.8	10.2	1.5	2.3	110
430	roasted, lean only	0	0	0	0	0	0	0	0	0	6.1	5.0	0.8	1.1	120
431	roasted, lean and fat	0	0	0	0	0	0	0	0	0	12.8	10.2	1.5	2.3	115

Meat and meat products *continued*

Inorganic constituents per 100g edible portion

No.	Food	Na	K	Ca	Mg	P	Fe	Cu	Zn	Cl	Mn	Se	I
		mg										µg	
	Lamb continued												
420	**Breast**, roasted, lean only	93	330	8	22	200	1.6	0.07	5.1	67	0.01	4	6
421	roasted, lean and fat	85	300	9	21	180	1.4	0.06	3.7	67	0.01	4	6
422	**Leg**, average, raw, lean and fat	58	320	7	22	190	1.4	0.08	2.8	59	0.01	2	2
423	half knuckle, pot-roasted, lean and fat	60	300	11	24	200	2.0	0.10	4.3	74	0.01	4	6
424	whole, roasted, lean only	63	360	7	26	220	1.8	0.11	4.6	67	0.02	4	3
425	whole, roasted, lean and fat	64	340	7	25	210	1.7	0.10	4.3	67	0.02	4	3
426	**Loin chops**, raw, lean and fat	63	280	13	19	170	1.3	0.07	2.0	65	0.01	3	7
427	grilled, lean only	80	400	22	28	240	2.1	0.10	3.6	73	0.02	4	6
428	grilled, lean and fat	81	370	20	27	230	1.9	0.09	3.1	74	0.02	4	6
429	microwaved, lean and fat	74	310	17	24	200	1.8	0.09	3.3	76	0.01	4	6
430	roasted, lean only	91	410	23	30	260	2.5	0.13	5.8	86	0.01	4	6
431	roasted, lean and fat	85	370	20	27	230	2.1	0.11	4.6	80	0.01	4	6

Meat and meat products *continued*

Vitamins per 100g edible portion

No.	Food	Retinol µg	Carotene µg	Vitamin D µg	Vitamin E mg	Thiamin mg	Ribo-flavin mg	Niacin mg	Trypt 60 mg	Vitamin B6 mg	Vitamin B12 µg	Folate µg	Panto-thenate mg	Biotin µg	Vitamin C mg
Lamb continued															
420	**Breast**, roasted, lean only	Tr	Tr	0.6	0.11	0.08	0.19	5.7	5.6	0.16	3	6	1.30	2	0
421	roasted, lean and fat	10	Tr	0.5	0.17	0.09	0.18	4.9	4.2	0.16	2	5	1.09	2	0
422	**Leg**, average, raw, lean and fat	9	Tr	0.7	0.05	0.14	0.23	5.1	3.7	0.33	1	11	1.25	2	0
423	half knuckle, pot-roasted, lean and fat	Tr	Tr	0.6	0.04	0.11	0.23	5.8	5.7	0.30	3	3	1.33	2	0
424	whole, roasted, lean only	Tr	Tr	0.7	0.03	0.12	0.29	6.2	5.8	0.34	2	2	1.50	3	0
425	whole, roasted, lean and fat	Tr	Tr	0.6	0.05	0.12	0.28	5.9	5.4	0.32	2	2	1.41	2	0
426	**Loin chops**, raw, lean and fat	12	Tr	0.8	0.07	0.13	0.22	5.0	3.6	0.23	1	3	0.86	1	0
427	grilled, lean only	Tr	Tr	0.6	0.02	0.17	0.26	8.3	6.1	0.52	3	6	1.40	3	0
428	grilled, lean and fat	7	Tr	0.3	0.09	0.16	0.25	7.3	5.2	0.44	3	6	1.28	2	0
429	microwaved, lean and fat	8	Tr	0.6	0.14	0.14	0.20	5.5	5.4	0.27	3	3	1.34	2	0
430	roasted, lean only	Tr	Tr	0.6	0.06	0.16	0.38	6.9	7.2	0.34	3	6	1.60	3	0
431	roasted, lean and fat	8	Tr	0.6	0.11	0.14	0.31	6.0	5.7	0.29	3	5	1.35	2	0

Meat and meat products *continued*

Composition of food per 100g edible portion

No.	Food	Description and main data sources	Main data reference	Water g	Total nitrogen g	Protein g	Fat g	Carbo-hydrate g	Energy value kcal	kJ
Lamb continued										
432	**Mince**, raw	Analytical data, 1994	42	67.1[a]	3.06	19.1	13.3[b]	0	196	817
433	stewed	Analytical data, 1994	42	62.8	3.90	24.4	12.3	0	208	870
434	**Neck fillet**, strips, stir-fried in corn oil, lean only	Analytical data, 1994	42	55.3	3.90	24.4	20.0	0	278	1155
435	**Shoulder**, diced, kebabs, grilled, lean and fat	Calculated from 85% lean and 15% fat. Analytical data, 1994	42	52.1	4.56	28.5	19.3	0	288	1199
436	whole, roasted, lean only	Analytical data, 1994	42	56.9	4.35	27.2	12.1	0	218	910
437	whole, roasted, lean and fat	Calculated from 78% lean and 22% fat. Analytical data, 1994	42	50.5	3.96	24.7	22.1	0	298	1238
438	**Stewing lamb**, stewed, lean only	Analytical data, 1994	42	58.9	4.26	26.6	14.8	0	240	1000
439	stewed, lean and fat	Calculated from 85% lean and 15% fat. Analytical data, 1994	42	56.1	3.91	24.4	20.1	0	279	1159
Pork										
440	**Pork, fat**, average, raw	Average of 8 different cuts, trimmed of lean. Analytical data, 1992-1993	37	33.6	1.62	10.1	56.4	0	548	2259
441	average, cooked	Average of 5 different cuts. Analytical data, 1992-1993	37	33.1	2.27	14.2	50.9	0	515	2125
442	**Pork, lean**, average, raw	Average of 8 different cuts, trimmed of fat. Analytical data, 1992-1993	37	74.0	3.49	21.8	4.0	0	123	519

[a] Water typically varies from 63.0g to 71.6g per 100g

[b] Fat typically varies from 8.1g to 22.8g per 100g

Meat and meat products *continued*

Composition of food per 100g edible portion

No.	Food	Starch g	Total sugars g	Individual sugars					Dietary fibre		Fatty acids				Cholest- erol mg
				Gluc g	Fruct g	Sucr g	Malt g	Lact g	NSP g	AOAC g	Satd g	Mono- unsatd g	Poly- unsatd g	Trans g	
Lamb continued															
432	**Mince**, raw	0	0	0	0	0	0	0	0	0	6.2	5.3	0.6	1.1	77
433	stewed	0	0	0	0	0	0	0	0	0	5.9	4.9	0.6	0.9	96
434	**Neck fillet**, strips, stir-fried in corn oil, lean only	0	0	0	0	0	0	0	0	0	8.2	7.6	2.2	1.3	86
435	**Shoulder**, diced, kebabs, grilled, lean and fat	0	0	0	0	0	0	0	0	0	9.0	7.5	1.0	1.5	110
436	whole, roasted, lean only	0	0	0	0	0	0	0	0	0	5.5	4.7	0.6	0.9	105
437	whole, roasted, lean and fat	0	0	0	0	0	0	0	0	0	10.4	8.7	1.0	1.7	105
438	**Stewing lamb**, stewed, lean only	0	0	0	0	0	0	0	0	0	6.5	5.6	1.0	1.0	94
439	stewed, lean and fat	0	0	0	0	0	0	0	0	0	9.2	7.7	1.3	1.5	92
Pork															
440	**Pork, fat**, average, raw	0	0	0	0	0	0	0	0	0	20.4	23.7	9.5	0.3	71
441	average, cooked	0	0	0	0	0	0	0	0	0	17.9	21.5	8.9	0.3	98
442	**Pork, lean**, average, raw	0	0	0	0	0	0	0	0	0	1.4	1.5	0.7	Tr	63

Inorganic constituents per 100g edible portion

No.	Food	Na	K	Ca	Mg	P	Fe	Cu	Zn	Cl	Mn	Se	I
		mg										µg	
Lamb continued													
432	**Mince**, raw	69	310	17	21	190	1.6	0.08	3.5	68	0.01	2	6
433	stewed	59	270	15	20	180	2.1	0.11	4.6	46	0.02	3	5
434	**Neck fillet**, strips, stir-fried in corn oil, lean only	68	360	7	23	210	1.8	0.08	5.2	61	0.02	4	6
435	**Shoulder**, diced, kebabs, grilled, lean and fat	87	420	14	28	240	1.8	0.12	5.6	76	0.03	4	6
436	whole, roasted, lean only	80	330	8	23	210	1.8	0.10	5.8	81	0.01	6	6
437	whole, roasted, lean and fat	80	320	9	22	190	1.6	0.09	5.0	79	0.01	5	7
438	**Stewing lamb**, stewed, lean only	49	160	37	16	140	1.9	0.09	6.1	67	0.01	4	6
439	stewed, lean and fat	50	170	33	16	140	1.7	0.08	5.4	65	0.01	4	6
Pork													
440	**Pork, fat**, average, raw	47	160	9	9	91	0.4	0.04	0.6	51	Tr	7	5
441	average, cooked	69	240	10	14	140	0.6	0.05	0.9	67	Tr	9	5
442	**Pork, lean**, average, raw	63	380	7	24	190	0.7	0.05	2.1	51	0.01	13	5

Meat and meat products *continued*

Vitamins per 100g edible portion

No.	Food	Retinol µg	Carotene µg	Vitamin D µg	Vitamin E mg	Thiamin mg	Ribo-flavin mg	Niacin mg	Trypt 60 mg	Vitamin B6 mg	Vitamin B12 µg	Folate µg	Panto-thenate mg	Biotin µg	Vitamin C mg
Lamb continued															
432	**Mince**, raw	5	Tr	0.8	0.18	0.12	0.18	4.8	3.7	0.20	2	2	0.90	2	0
433	stewed	5	Tr	0.5	0.11	0.09	0.21	5.2	5.3	0.21	2	9	0.90	4	0
434	**Neck fillet**, strips, stir-fried in corn oil, lean only	Tr	Tr	0.6	0.59	0.17	0.20	4.6	5.1	0.20	2	7	1.20	2	0
435	**Shoulder**, diced, kebabs, grilled, lean and fat	Tr	Tr	0.6	0.19	0.12	0.25	6.8	5.7	0.21	3	7	1.40	2	0
436	whole, roasted, lean only	Tr	Tr	0.8	0.06	0.11	0.23	5.3	5.6	0.21	2	4	1.10	2	0
437	whole, roasted, lean and fat	6	Tr	0.7	0.15	0.10	0.21	5.0	4.8	0.20	2	4	0.99	2	0
438	**Stewing lamb**, stewed, lean only	Tr	Tr	0.6	0.20	0.04	0.12	2.3	5.5	0.11	3	2	1.30	2	0
439	stewed, lean and fat	Tr	Tr	0.6	0.20	0.05	0.12	2.4	4.9	0.11	2	2	1.19	2	0
Pork															
440	**Pork, fat**, average, raw	Tr	Tr	1.3	0.03	0.20	0.13	2.1	1.1	0.11	1	2	0.61	5	0
441	average, cooked	Tr	Tr	2.1	0.05	0.37	0.16	3.8	1.5	0.16	Tr	2	0.86	8	0
442	**Pork, lean**, average, raw	Tr	Tr	0.5	0.05	0.98	0.24	6.9	4.5	0.54	1	3	1.46	2	0

Meat and meat products *continued*

443 to 453

Composition of food per 100g edible portion

Pork continued

No.	Food	Description and main data sources	Main data reference	Water g	Total nitrogen g	Protein g	Fat g	Carbohydrate g	Energy value kcal	kJ
443	**Belly joint/slices**, grilled, lean and fat	58% lean and 42% fat. Analytical data, 1992-1993	37	48.6	4.38	27.4	23.4	0	320	1332
444	**Diced**, casseroled, lean only	Analytical data, 1992-1993	37	62.2	5.07	31.7	6.4	0	184	776
445	**Fillet strips**, stir-fried in corn oil, lean	Analytical data, 1992-1993	37	59.6	5.14	32.1	5.9	0	182	764
446	**Leg joint**, raw, lean and fat	Calculated from 79% lean and 21% fat. Analytical data, 1992-1993	37	64.4	3.04	19.0	15.2	0	213	885
447	roast, lean only	Analytical data, 1992-1993	37	61.1	5.28	33.0	5.5	0	182	765
448	roast, lean and fat	Calculated from 83% lean and 17% fat. Analytical data, 1992-1993	37	58.3	4.94	30.9	10.2	0	215	903
449	**Loin chops**, raw, lean and fat	Calculated from 70% lean and 30% fat. Analytical data, 1992-1993	37	59.8	2.98	18.6	21.7	0	270	1119
450	barbecued, lean and fat	Calculated from 82% lean and 18% fat. Analytical data, 1992-1993	37	55.0	4.53	28.3	15.8	0	255	1066
451	grilled, lean only	Loin and pork chops. Analytical data, 1992-1993	37	61.2	5.06	31.6	6.4	0	184	774
452	grilled, lean and fat	Calculated from 80% lean and 20% fat. Analytical data, 1992-1993	37	54.6	4.64	29.0	15.7	0	257	1074
453	microwaved, lean and fat	Calculated from 82% lean and 18% fat. Analytical data, 1992-1993	37	55.4	4.83	30.2	14.1	0	248	1035

Pork continued

No.	Food	Starch g	Total sugars g	Gluc g	Fruct g	Sucr g	Malt g	Lact g	NSP g	AOAC g	Satd g	Mono- unsatd g	Poly- unsatd g	Trans g	Cholest- erol mg
443	**Belly joint/slices**, grilled, lean and fat	0	0	0	0	0	0	0	0	0	8.2	9.5	4.0	0.1	97
444	**Diced**, casseroled, lean only	0	0	0	0	0	0	0	0	0	1.9	2.3	1.6	Tr	99
445	**Fillet strips**, stir-fried in corn oil, lean	0	0	0	0	0	0	0	0	0	1.3	1.8	2.2	Tr	90
446	**Leg joint**, raw, lean and fat	0	0	0	0	0	0	0	0	0	5.1	6.4	2.5	0.1	63
447	roast, lean only	0	0	0	0	0	0	0	0	0	1.9	2.3	0.7	Tr	100
448	roast, lean and fat	0	0	0	0	0	0	0	0	0	3.6	4.4	1.4	Tr	100
449	**Loin chops**, raw, lean and fat	0	0	0	0	0	0	0	0	0	8.0	8.5	3.6	0.1	61
450	barbecued, lean and fat	0	0	0	0	0	0	0	0	0	5.7	6.3	2.6	0.1	87
451	grilled, lean only	0	0	0	0	0	0	0	0	0	2.2	2.6	1.0	Tr	75
452	grilled, lean and fat	0	0	0	0	0	0	0	0	0	5.6	6.5	2.5	0.1	86
453	microwaved, lean and fat	0	0	0	0	0	0	0	0	0	4.9	5.7	2.5	0.1	100

Pork continued

No.	Food	mg									µg	
		Na	K	Ca	Mg	P	Fe	Cu	Zn	Cl	Mn	Se	I
443	**Belly joint/slices**, grilled, lean and fat	97	350	20	23	220	0.9	0.12	2.9	96	0.02	17	5
444	**Diced**, casseroled, lean only	37	220	12	21	180	1.0	0.13	3.6	39	0.02	20	5
445	**Fillet strips**, stir-fried in corn oil, lean	71	540	8	35	320	1.4	0.14	2.6	70	0.02	20	3
446	**Leg joint**, raw, lean and fat	60	330	6	21	180	0.7	0.02	1.9	50	Tr	12	5
447	roast, lean only	69	400	10	27	250	1.1	0.06	3.2	67	Tr	21	3
448	roast, lean and fat	70	380	10	26	240	1.0	0.06	2.9	67	Tr	20	3
449	**Loin chops**, raw, lean and fat	53	300	10	19	170	0.4	0.06	1.3	56	0.01	11	8
450	barbecued, lean and fat	68	400	21	26	240	0.8	0.08	2.3	64	0.02	17	5
451	grilled, lean only	66	410	14	28	250	0.7	0.08	2.4	70	0.02	18	3
452	grilled, lean and fat	70	390	14	26	230	0.7	0.08	2.2	73	0.02	17	3
453	microwaved, lean and fat	58	330	19	24	220	0.7	0.07	2.4	65	0.02	19	5

Meat and meat products *continued*

Vitamins per 100g edible portion

Pork continued

No.	Food	Retinol µg	Carotene µg	Vitamin D µg	Vitamin E mg	Thiamin mg	Ribo-flavin mg	Niacin mg	Trypt 60 mg	Vitamin B$_6$ mg	Vitamin B$_{12}$ µg	Folate µg	Panto-thenate mg	Biotin µg	Vitamin C mg
443	**Belly joint/slices**, grilled, lean and fat	Tr	Tr	1.1	0.03	0.60	0.18	7.0	4.9	0.38	1	8	1.77	4	0
444	**Diced**, casseroled, lean only	Tr	Tr	0.8	0.05	0.48	0.25	4.2	6.6	0.36	1	3	0.94	5	0
445	**Fillet strips**, stir-fried in corn oil, lean	Tr	Tr	0.8	0.19	1.53	0.41	10.1	6.6	0.78	1	4	2.20	5	0
446	**Leg joint**, raw, lean and fat	Tr	Tr	0.9	0.07	0.68	0.18	5.8	3.9	0.42	1	1	1.32	3	0
447	roast, lean only	Tr	Tr	0.7	0.02	0.73	0.25	9.7	6.7	0.50	1	4	2.90	5	0
448	roast, lean and fat	Tr	Tr	1.0	0.03	0.71	0.24	9.2	6.1	0.47	1	4	2.67	5	0
449	**Loin chops**, raw, lean and fat	Tr	Tr	0.9	0.11	0.81	0.18	4.9	3.3	0.62	1	1	0.97	3	0
450	barbecued, lean and fat	Tr	Tr	1.0	0.02	1.03	0.17	8.6	5.6	0.32	1	1	1.82	6	0
451	grilled, lean only	Tr	Tr	0.8	0.01	0.78	0.16	9.1	6.2	0.56	1	7	1.22	4	0
452	grilled, lean and fat	Tr	Tr	1.1	0.02	0.70	0.17	8.2	5.3	0.49	1	6	1.20	5	0
453	microwaved, lean and fat	Tr	Tr	1.0	0.03	0.92	0.17	7.0	6.0	0.37	1	4	1.93	5	0

Composition of food per 100g edible portion

No.	Food	Description and main data sources	Main data reference	Water g	Total nitrogen g	Protein g	Fat g	Carbohydrate g	Energy value kcal	kJ
Pork continued										
454	**Loin chops**, roasted, lean and fat	Calculated from 78% lean and 22% fat. Analytical data, 1992-1993	37	49.1	5.10	31.9	19.3	0	301	1256
455	**Steaks**, grilled, lean only	Pork and leg steaks. Analytical data, 1992-1993	37	61.5	5.42	33.9	3.7	0	169	713
456	grilled, lean and fat	Calculated from 92% lean and 8% fat. Analytical data, 1992-1993	37	59.1	5.19	32.4	7.6	0	198	832
Chicken										
457	**Dark meat**, raw	Fresh and frozen. Analytical data, 1995	45	75.8	3.34	20.9	2.8	0	109	459
458	roasted	Fresh and frozen. Analytical data, 1995	45	63.9	3.90	24.4	10.9	0	196	819
459	**Light meat**, raw	Fresh and frozen. Analytical data, 1995	45	74.2	3.84	24.0	1.1	0	106	449
460	roasted	Fresh and frozen. Analytical data, 1995	45	66.9	4.83	30.2	3.6	0	153	645
461	**Meat, average**, raw	Calculated from 44% light meat and 56% dark meat. Analytical data, 1995	45	75.1	3.57	22.3	2.1	0	108	457
462	roasted	Calculated from 46% light meat and 54% dark meat. Analytical data, 1995	45	65.3	4.37	27.3	7.5	0	177	742
463	**Breast**, casseroled, meat only	Fresh and frozen. Analytical data, 1995	45	67.7	4.54	28.4	5.2	0	160	675
464	grilled without skin, meat only	Analytical data, 1995	45	66.6	5.11	32.0	2.2	0	148	626
465	strips, stir-fried in corn oil	Skinless. Analytical data, 1995	45	65.9	4.76	29.7	4.6	0	161	677
466	**Drumsticks**, casseroled, meat and skin	Fresh and frozen, calculated from 85% dark meat and 15% skin. Analytical data, 1995	45	63.7	3.57	22.3	14.2	0	217	905

No.	Food	Starch g	Total sugars g	Gluc g	Fruct g	Sucr g	Malt g	Lact g	Dietary fibre NSP g	AOAC g	Satd g	Mono-unsatd g	Poly-unsatd g	Trans g	Cholest-erol mg
												Fatty acids			

Pork continued

No.	Food	Starch g	Total sugars g	Gluc g	Fruct g	Sucr g	Malt g	Lact g	NSP g	AOAC g	Satd g	Mono-unsatd g	Poly-unsatd g	Trans g	Cholest-erol mg
454	**Loin chops**, roasted, lean and fat	0	0	0	0	0	0	0	0	0	7.0	7.8	3.1	0.1	110
455	**Steaks**, grilled, lean only	0	0	0	0	0	0	0	0	0	1.3	1.4	0.6	Tr	99
456	grilled, lean and fat	0	0	0	0	0	0	0	0	0	2.7	3.0	1.2	Tr	100
Chicken															
457	**Dark meat**, raw	0	0	0	0	0	0	0	0	0	0.8	1.3	0.6	Tr	105
458	roasted	0	0	0	0	0	0	0	0	0	2.9	5.1	2.2	0.1	120
459	**Light meat**, raw	0	0	0	0	0	0	0	0	0	0.3	0.5	0.2	Tr	70
460	roasted	0	0	0	0	0	0	0	0	0	1.0	1.6	0.7	0.1	82
461	**Meat, average**, raw	0	0	0	0	0	0	0	0	0	0.6	1.0	0.4	Tr	90
462	roasted	0	0	0	0	0	0	0	0	0	2.1	3.4	1.5	0.1	105
463	**Breast**, casseroled, meat only	0	0	0	0	0	0	0	0	0	1.5	2.4	1.0	0.1	90
464	grilled without skin, meat only	0	0	0	0	0	0	0	0	0	0.6	1.0	0.4	Tr	94
465	strips, stir-fried in corn oil	0	0	0	0	0	0	0	0	0	N	N	N	N	87
466	**Drumsticks**, casseroled, meat and skin	0	0	0	0	0	0	0	0	0	3.8	6.6	2.8	0.2	125

Inorganic constituents per 100g edible portion

No.	Food	Na	K	Ca	Mg	P	Fe	Cu	Zn	Cl	Mn	Se	I
						mg						µg	
Pork continued													
454	**Loin chops**, roasted, lean and fat	68	360	19	25	230	0.8	0.09	2.4	70	0.02	20	5
455	**Steaks**, grilled, lean only	76	480	8	33	300	1.1	0.10	2.9	67	0.02	21	5
456	grilled, lean and fat	76	460	8	32	280	1.1	0.10	2.7	68	0.02	20	5
Chicken													
457	**Dark meat**, raw	90	390	7	24	110	0.8	0.02	1.7	110	0.01	14	6
458	roasted	100	300	17	23	200	0.8	0.08	2.2	88	0.02	17	6
459	**Light meat**, raw	60	370	5	29	220	0.5	0.05	0.7	77	0.01	12	6
460	roasted	60	360	7	30	250	0.4	0.17	0.8	62	0.01	14	7
461	**Meat, average**, raw	77	380	6	26	160	0.7	0.03	1.2	95	0.01	13	6
462	roasted	80	330	11	26	220	0.7	0.10	1.5	75	0.02	16	7
463	**Breast**, casseroled, meat only	60	270	9	25	210	0.5	0.06	1.1	60	0.01	13	8
464	grilled without skin, meat only	55	460	6	36	310	0.4	0.04	0.8	67	0.01	16	7
465	strips, stir-fried in corn oil	61	420	6	33	280	0.5	0.08	0.8	63	0.01	15	7
466	**Drumsticks**, casseroled, meat and skin	75	200	30	18	170	1.1	0.07	1.9	70	0.02	15	7

Vitamins per 100g edible portion

No.	Food	Retinol	Carotene	Vitamin D	Vitamin E	Thiamin	Ribo-flavin	Niacin	Trypt 60	Vitamin B$_6$	Vitamin B$_{12}$	Folate	Panto-thenate	Biotin	Vitamin C
		µg	µg	µg	mg	mg	mg	mg	mg	mg	µg	µg	mg	µg	mg
Pork continued															
454	**Loin chops**, roasted, lean and fat	Tr	Tr	1.1	0.03	0.77	0.16	8.4	6.3	0.42	1	2	2.05	6	0
455	**Steaks**, grilled, lean only	Tr	Tr	0.8	0.02	1.55	0.28	9.5	7.0	0.72	1	9	2.19	5	0
456	grilled, lean and fat	Tr	Tr	0.9	0.02	1.45	0.27	9.1	6.6	0.68	1	8	2.09	5	0
Chicken															
457	**Dark meat**, raw	20	Tr	0.1	0.17	0.14	0.22	5.6	4.1	0.28	1	9	1.09	3	0
458	roasted	24	Tr	0.1	0.23	0.07	0.11	6.2	5.3	0.27	1	10	1.34	4	0
459	**Light meat**, raw	Tr	Tr	0.2	0.13	0.14	0.14	10.7	4.7	0.51	Tr	14	1.26	2	0
460	roasted	Tr	Tr	0.3	0.31	0.07	0.23	12.6	5.5	0.54	Tr	10	1.38	2	0
461	**Meat, average**, raw	11	Tr	0.1	0.15	0.14	0.18	7.8	4.3	0.38	Tr	19	1.16	2	0
462	roasted	11	Tr	0.2	0.23	0.07	0.16	9.2	5.3	0.36	Tr	10	1.39	3	0
463	**Breast**, casseroled, meat only	Tr	Tr	0.1	0.07	0.06	0.13	8.8	5.6	0.36	Tr	6	1.34	2	0
464	grilled without skin, meat only	Tr	Tr	0.3	0.17	0.14	0.13	15.8	6.2	0.63	Tr	6	1.67	2	0
465	strips, stir-fried in corn oil	Tr	Tr	0.2	N	0.11	0.16	14.4	5.8	0.44	Tr	5	1.56	2	0
466	**Drumsticks**, casseroled, meat and skin	27	Tr	0.2	0.35	0.05	0.12	5.0	4.2	0.21	Tr	8	1.08	3	0

Composition of food per 100g edible portion

No.	Food	Description and main data sources	Main data reference	Water g	Total nitrogen g	Protein g	Fat g	Carbohydrate g	Energy value kcal	kJ
Chicken *continued*										
467	**Drumsticks**, roasted, meat and skin	Fresh and frozen, calculated from 89% dark meat and 11% skin. Analytical data, 1995	45	63.0	4.14	25.8	9.1	0	185	775
468	**Skin**, dry roasted/grilled	Crisp skin. Analytical data, 1995	45	31.1	3.45	21.5	46.1	0	501	2070
469	**Whole chicken**, roasted, meat and skin	Fresh and frozen, Calculated from 40% light meat, 47% dark meat and 13% skin. Analytical data, 1995	45	61.3	4.21	26.3	12.5	0	218	910
Turkey										
470	**Dark meat**, raw	Analytical data, 1995	45	75.8	3.26	20.4	2.5	0	104	439
471	roasted	Including self-basting turkey. Analytical data, 1995	45	64.3	4.71	29.4	6.6	0	177	745
472	**Light meat**, raw	Analytical data, 1995	45	74.9	3.90	24.4	0.8	0	105	444
473	roasted	Analytical data, 1995	45	65.1	5.39	33.7	2.0	0	153	648
474	**Meat, average**, raw	Calculated from 56% light meat and 44% dark meat. Analytical data, 1995	45	75.3	3.62	22.6	1.6	0	105	443
475	roasted	Including self-basting turkey. Fresh and frozen, calculated from 51% light meat and 49% dark meat. Analytical data, 1995	45	64.6	4.99	31.2	4.6	0	166	701
476	**Breast**, fillet, grilled, meat only	Skinless. Analytical data, 1995	45	63.0	5.60	35.0	1.7	0	155	658
477	strips, stir-fried in corn oil	Skinless. Analytical data, 1995	45	64.4	4.96	31.0	4.5	0	164	692
478	**Skin**, dry, roasted	Crisp skin. Analytical data, 1995	45	29.5	3.06	29.9	40.2	0	481	1995
479	**Thighs**, diced, casseroled, meat only	Skinless. Analytical data, 1995	45	64.5	4.54	28.3	7.5	0	181	760

Composition of food per 100g edible portion

No.	Food	Starch	Total sugars	Individual sugars					Dietary fibre		Fatty acids				Cholest-
				Gluc	Fruct	Sucr	Malt	Lact	NSP	AOAC	Satd	Mono-unsatd	Poly-unsatd	Trans	erol
		g	g	g	g	g	g	g	g	g	g	g	g	g	mg
Chicken continued															
467	**Drumsticks**, roasted, meat and skin	0	0	0	0	0	0	0	0	0	2.5	4.3	1.8	0.1	135
468	**Skin**, dry roasted/grilled	0	0	0	0	0	0	0	0	0	12.9	22.5	7.7	0.6	170
469	**Whole chicken**, roasted, meat and skin	0	0	0	0	0	0	0	0	0	3.4	5.7	2.4	0.1	110
Turkey															
470	**Dark meat**, raw	0	0	0	0	0	0	0	0	0	0.8	1.0	0.6	Tr	86
471	roasted	0	0	0	0	0	0	0	0	0	2.0	2.4	1.7	0.1	120
472	**Light meat**, raw	0	0	0	0	0	0	0	0	0	0.3	0.3	0.2	Tr	57
473	roasted	0	0	0	0	0	0	0	0	0	0.7	0.7	0.5	Tr	82
474	**Meat, average**, raw	0	0	0	0	0	0	0	0	0	0.5	0.6	0.4	Tr	70
475	roasted	0	0	0	0	0	0	0	0	0	1.4	1.7	1.1	0.1	100
476	**Breast**, fillet, grilled, meat only	0	0	0	0	0	0	0	0	0	0.6	0.6	0.3	Tr	74
477	strips, stir-fried in corn oil	0	0	0	0	0	0	0	0	0	N	N	N	N	72
478	**Skin**, dry, roasted	0	0	0	0	0	0	0	0	0	13.2	15.6	8.8	0.6	290
479	**Thighs**, diced, casseroled, meat only	0	0	0	0	0	0	0	0	0	2.5	2.7	1.8	0.1	120

Meat and meat products *continued*

Inorganic constituents per 100g edible portion

No.	Food	Na	K	Ca	Mg	P	Fe	Cu	Zn	Cl	Mn	Se	I
						mg						µg	
Chicken continued													
467	**Drumsticks**, roasted, meat and skin	130	280	15	25	210	1.0	0.09	2.3	90	0.02	17	7
468	**Skin**, dry roasted/grilled	80	260	16	26	210	1.3	0.05	1.2	N	0.03	N	N
469	**Whole chicken**, roasted, meat and skin	80	320	11	26	220	0.7	0.09	1.5	80	0.02	15	7
Turkey													
470	**Dark meat**, raw	90	310	7	22	200	1.0	0.04	3.1	73	Tr	15	5
471	roasted	110	330	17	25	260	1.2	0.11	3.4	86	0.02	17	8
472	**Light meat**, raw	50	360	4	27	230	0.3	0.01	1.0	39	Tr	10	6
473	roasted	50	400	6	30	260	0.5	0.05	1.4	52	0.01	14	8
474	**Meat, average**, raw	68	340	5	25	220	0.6	0.02	1.9	54	Tr	13	6
475	roasted	90	350	11	27	260	0.8	0.09	2.5	85	0.01	17	8
476	**Breast**, fillet, grilled, meat only	90	550	5	42	380	0.6	0.08	1.7	85	0.01	17	8
477	strips, stir-fried in corn oil	60	420	5	32	280	0.4	0.04	1.3	75	0.01	15	7
478	**Skin**, dry, roasted	110	330	20	33	250	1.6	0.07	1.8	N	0.03	N	N
479	**Thighs**, diced, casseroled, meat only	65	230	12	23	210	2.0	0.20	5.4	84	0.02	19	8

Meat and meat products *continued*

Vitamins per 100g edible portion

No.	Food	Retinol	Carotene	Vitamin D	Vitamin E	Thiamin	Ribo-flavin	Niacin	Trypt 60	Vitamin B$_6$	Vitamin B$_{12}$	Folate	Panto-thenate	Biotin	Vitamin C
		µg	µg	µg	mg	mg	mg	mg	mg	mg	µg	µg	mg	µg	mg
Chicken continued															
467	**Drumsticks**, roasted, meat and skin	24	Tr	0.2	0.21	0.09	0.14	5.5	4.9	0.19	1	12	1.31	3	0
468	**Skin**, dry roasted/grilled	N	Tr	1.0	N	N	N	N	N	N	N	N	N	N	0
469	**Whole chicken**, roasted, meat and skin	18	Tr	0.3	0.21	0.07	0.15	8.7	4.9	0.34	Tr	9	1.29	3	0
Turkey															
470	**Dark meat**, raw	Tr	Tr	0.4	Tr	0.08	0.31	4.6	4.0	0.35	2	28	0.75	2	0
471	roasted	Tr	Tr	0.3	Tr	0.05	0.25	7.2	5.7	0.44	2	20	1.06	3	0
472	**Light meat**, raw	Tr	Tr	0.3	Tr	0.06	0.15	10.7	4.3	0.81	1	9	0.66	1	0
473	roasted	Tr	Tr	0.1	0.02	0.05	0.16	12.9	6.8	0.47	1	18	0.97	2	0
474	**Meat, average**, raw	Tr	Tr	0.3	0.01	0.07	0.22	8.0	4.4	0.61	2	17	0.70	2	0
475	roasted	Tr	Tr	0.3	0.06	0.06	0.19	10.3	6.2	0.49	1	17	0.98	2	0
476	**Breast**, fillet, grilled, meat only	Tr	Tr	0.4	0.02	0.07	0.15	14.0	6.8	0.63	1	7	0.95	2	0
477	strips, stir-fried in corn oil	Tr	Tr	0.3	N	0.07	0.12	13.5	6.1	0.69	1	8	0.84	2	0
478	**Skin**, dry, roasted	N	Tr	N	N	N	N	N	N	N	N	N	N	N	0
479	**Thighs**, diced, casseroled, meat only	Tr	Tr	0.5	Tr	0.07	0.22	6.0	5.5	0.41	2	21	1.04	3	0

Meat and meat products *continued*

Composition of food per 100g edible portion

No.	Food	Description and main data sources	Main data reference	Water g	Total nitrogen g	Protein g	Fat g	Carbo-hydrate g	Energy value kcal	kJ
Other poultry and game										
480	**Duck**, raw, meat only	Meat from dressed carcase. Analytical data, 1984, 1992	22, 40	74.8	3.15	19.7	6.5	0	137	575
481	crispy, Chinese style, meat and skin	Seasoned roasted duck. Analytical data, 1997	53	44.0	4.46	27.9	24.2	0.3[a]	331	1375
482	roasted, meat only	Analytical data, 1984	22	62.1	4.05	25.3	10.4	0	195	815
483	roasted, meat, fat and skin	Analytical data, 1984	22	42.6	3.20	20.0	38.1	0	423	1750
484	**Goose**, roasted, meat, fat and skin	Analytical data, 1984	22	51.1	4.40	27.5	21.2	0	301	1252
485	**Pheasant**, roasted, meat only	Meat from carcase. Analytical data, 1984	22	59.4	4.46	27.9	12.0	0	220	918
486	**Rabbit**, raw, meat only	Loin and leg. Analytical data, 1984	22	71.5	3.50	21.9	5.5	0	137	576
487	stewed, meat only	Loin and leg. Analytical data, 1984	22	70.7	3.39	21.2	3.2	0	114	479
488	**Venison**, roasted	Calculated from raw, including diced and steaks. Analytical data, 1984	22	60.4	5.70	35.6	2.5	0	165	698
Offal										
489	**Heart**, lamb, roasted	Fat and valves removed. Analytical data, 1983	20	58.8	4.05	25.3	13.9	0	226	944
490	**Kidney**, lamb, fried in corn oil	Skin and core removed. Analytical data, 1983	20	62.8	3.79	23.7	10.3	0	188	784
491	ox, stewed	Skin and core removed. Analytical data, 1983	20	69.2	3.92	24.5	4.4	0	138	579
492	**Liver**, calf, fried in corn oil	Analytical data, 1983	20	64.5	3.57	22.3	9.6	Tr	176	734
493	chicken, fried in corn oil	Analytical data, 1983	20	65.9	3.54	22.1	8.9	Tr	169	705
494	lamb, fried in corn oil	Analytical data, 1983	20	53.9	4.82	30.1	12.9	Tr	237	989
495	ox, stewed	Coated in seasoned flour. MW4, 1978	4	62.6	3.96	24.8	9.5	3.6	198	831

[a] Includes oligosaccharides

Composition of food per 100g edible portion

No.	Food	Starch g	Total sugars g	Individual sugars					Dietary fibre		Fatty acids				Cholest-erol mg
				Gluc g	Fruct g	Sucr g	Malt g	Lact g	NSP g	AOAC g	Satd g	Mono-unsatd g	Poly-unsatd g	Trans g	
Other poultry and game															
480	**Duck,** raw, meat only	0	0	0	0	0	0	0	0	0	2.0	3.2	1.0	0.1	110
481	crispy, Chinese style, meat and skin	0	0	0	0	0	0	0	0	0	7.2	12.3	3.4	0.2	63
482	roasted, meat only	0	0	0	0	0	0	0	0	0	3.3	5.2	1.3	0.1	115
483	roasted, meat, fat and skin	0	0	0	0	0	0	0	0	0	11.4	19.3	5.3	0.4	99
484	**Goose,** roasted, meat, fat and skin	0	0	0	0	0	0	0	0	0	6.6	9.9	2.4	Tr	91
485	**Pheasant,** roasted, meat only	0	0	0	0	0	0	0	0	0	4.1	5.6	1.6	0.1	220
486	**Rabbit,** raw, meat only	0	0	0	0	0	0	0	0	0	2.1	1.3	1.8	0.1	53
487	stewed, meat only	0	0	0	0	0	0	0	0	0	1.7	0.7	0.6	0.1	49
488	**Venison,** roasted	0	0	0	0	0	0	0	0	0	N	N	N	Tr	N
Offal															
489	**Heart,** lamb, roasted	0	0	0	0	0	0	0	0	0	N	N	N	Tr	260
490	**Kidney,** lamb, fried	0	0	0	0	0	0	0	0	0	N	N	N	Tr	610
491	ox, stewed	0	0	0	0	0	0	0	0	0	1.4	1.0	0.9	0.1	460
492	**Liver,** calf, fried	0	0	0	0	0	0	0	0	0	N	N	N	Tr	330
493	chicken, fried	0	0	0	0	0	0	0	0	0	N	N	N	Tr	350
494	lamb, fried	0	0	0	0	0	0	0	0	0	N	N	N	Tr	400
495	ox, stewed	3.6	Tr	Tr	Tr	Tr	Tr	0	0	0	3.5	1.5	2.0	Tr	240

Inorganic constituents per 100g edible portion

No.	Food	Na	K	Ca	Mg	P	Fe	Cu	Zn	Cl	Mn	Se	I
						mg						µg	

Other poultry and game

No.	Food	Na	K	Ca	Mg	P	Fe	Cu	Zn	Cl	Mn	Se	I
480	**Duck**, raw, meat only	110	290	12	19	200	2.4	0.34	1.9	98	Tr	22	N
481	crispy, Chinese style, meat and skin	453	292	22	25	257	4.0	0.30	2.8	396	0.10	22	N
482	roasted, meat only	96	270	13	20	200	2.7	0.31	2.6	96	Tr	22	N
483	roasted, meat, fat and skin	87	220	22	17	180	1.7	0.23	2.2	76	0.20	22	N
484	**Goose**, roasted, meat, fat and skin	80	320	10	23	220	3.3	0.15	2.6	80	0.01	N	N
485	**Pheasant**, roasted, meat only	66	360	28	26	220	2.2	0.10	1.3	170	0.02	14	N
486	**Rabbit**, raw, meat only	67	360	22	25	220	1.0	0.06	1.4	74	0.01	17	N
487	stewed, meat only	48	200	39	18	150	1.1	0.06	1.7	45	0.02	16	N
488	**Venison**, roasted	52	290	6	27	240	5.1	0.36	3.9	59	0.04	14	N

Offal

No.	Food	Na	K	Ca	Mg	P	Fe	Cu	Zn	Cl	Mn	Se	I
489	**Heart**, lamb, roasted	84	210	7	21	240	6.0	0.66	2.8	100	0.03	N	N
490	**Kidney**, lamb, fried	230	280	14	21	350	11.2	0.58	3.6	410	0.13	209	N
491	ox, stewed	150	210	17	19	290	9.0	0.63	3.0	190	0.14	210	N
492	**Liver**, calf, fried	70	350	8	24	380	12.2	23.86	15.9	110	0.29	27	N
493	chicken, fried	79	300	9	23	350	11.3	0.52	3.8	110	0.35	N	N
494	lamb, fried	82	340	8	25	500	7.7	13.54	5.9	140	0.45	62	N
495	ox, stewed	110	250	11	19	380	7.8	2.30	4.3	120	0.44	50	N

Meat and meat products *continued*

Vitamins per 100g edible portion

No.	Food	Retinol	Carotene	Vitamin D	Vitamin E	Thiamin	Ribo- flavin	Niacin	Trypt 60	Vitamin B$_6$	Vitamin B$_{12}$	Folate	Panto- thenate	Biotin	Vitamin C
		µg	µg	µg	mg	mg	mg	mg	mg	mg	µg	µg	mg	µg	mg
Other poultry and game															
480	**Duck**, raw, meat only	24	Tr	N	0.02	0.36	0.45	5.3	4.2	0.34	3	25	1.60	6	0
481	crispy, Chinese style, meat and skin	9	Tr	1.0	2.17	0.09	0.39	3.5	4.2	0.15	3	15	1.50	4	0
482	roasted, meat only	N	N	N	0.02	0.26	0.47	5.1	5.4	0.25	3	10	1.50	4	0
483	roasted, meat, fat and skin	N	N	N	N	0.18	0.51	3.8	4.2	0.31	2	15	2.60	7	0
484	**Goose**, roasted, meat, fat and skin	21	Tr	N	N	0.12	0.51	4.6	5.5	0.42	2	12	1.40	3	0
485	**Pheasant**, roasted, meat only	N	N	N	N	0.02	0.29	9.2	6.0	0.57	3	20	0.96	N	0
486	**Rabbit**, raw, meat only	N	N	N	0.13	0.10	0.19	8.4	4.1	0.50	10	5	0.80	1	0
487	stewed, meat only	N	N	N	N	0.02	0.16	6.2	5.1	0.29	3	5	0.80	1	0
488	**Venison**, roasted	N	N	N	N	0.16	0.69	5.5	6.5	0.65	1	6	N	N	0
Offal															
489	**Heart**, lamb, roasted	Tr	Tr	0.1	N	0.24	1.37	3.8	5.6	0.26	6	2	3.80	8	2
490	**Kidney**, lamb, fried	110	Tr	0.6	0.41	0.52	3.10	9.1	5.3	0.48	54	70	4.60	73	5
491	ox, stewed	45	N	N	0.42	0.24	3.29	6.2	5.5	0.57	38	130	3.10	79	5
492	**Liver**, calf, fried	25200	100	0.3	0.50	0.61	2.89	13.6	5.8	0.89	58	110	4.10	50	19
493	chicken, fried	10500	Tr	N	0.34	0.63	2.72	12.9	4.4	0.55	45	1350	5.90	216	23
494	lamb, fried	19700	60	0.9	0.32	0.38	5.65	19.9	4.9	0.53	83	207	8.00	33	19
495	ox, stewed	17300	1540	1.1	0.44	0.18	3.60	10.3	5.3	0.52	110	290	5.70	50	15

Composition of food per 100g edible portion

No.	Food	Description and main data sources	Main data reference	Water g	Total nitrogen g	Protein g	Fat g	Carbo-hydrate g	Energy value kcal	kJ
Offal continued										
496	**Liver**, pig, stewed	Coated in seasoned flour. MW4, 1978	4	62.1	4.09	25.6	8.1	3.6	189	793
Burgers										
497	**Beefburgers**, 98-99% beef, raw	Chilled and frozen. Analytical data, 1990; and industry data, 2013	32	56.1	2.74	17.1	24.7	0.1	291	1206
498	98-99% beef, fried in vegetable oil	Chilled and frozen. Analytical data, 1990; and industry data, 2013	32	46.2	4.56	28.5	23.9	0.1	329	1370
499	98-99% beef, grilled	Chilled and frozen. Analytical data, 1990; and industry data, 2013	32	47.9	4.24	26.5	24.4	0.1	326	1355
500	62-85% beef, grilled	Frozen and chilled. Analytical data, 1990; and industry data, 2013	32	57.1	2.93	18.3	13.8	8.5	229	958
501	**Big Mac**, takeaway	Includes two beefburgers, bun, sauce, cheese, lettuce, onions and pickles. Industry data (McDonald's), 2013		N	2.09	13.1	11.2	20.9	232	972
502	**Cheeseburger**, takeaway	Includes beefburger, bun, cheese, mustard, ketchup, onions and pickles. Industry data 1998, 2013; and calculated from ingredients		47.0	2.18	13.6	10.4	28.3	254	1069
503	**Chicken burger**, takeaway	Includes chicken burger, bun, lettuce and mayonnaise. MPD Supplement, 1996	16	N	2.00	12.5	10.8	23.4	235	987
504	**Chicken/turkey burger**, coated, baked	Retail, breaded and battered. Analytical data, 2010	72	48.3	2.27	14.2	15.5	18.7	266	1113

Composition of food per 100g edible portion

No.	Food	Starch g	Total sugars g	Individual sugars					Dietary fibre		Fatty acids				Cholest-erol mg
				Gluc g	Fruct g	Sucr g	Malt g	Lact g	NSP g	AOAC g	Satd g	Mono-unsatd g	Poly-unsatd g	Trans g	
Offal continued															
496	**Liver**, pig, stewed	3.6	0	0	0	0	0	0	0	0	2.5	1.3	2.2	Tr	290
Burgers															
497	**Beefburgers**, 98-99% beef, raw	Tr	0.1	0.1	0	0	0	0	N	0.5	10.7	11.4	0.5	1.4	76
498	98-99% beef, fried in vegetable oil	Tr	0.1	0.1	0	0	0	0	N	0.7	10.7	10.8	0.8	0.8	96
499	98-99% beef, grilled	Tr	0.1	0.1	0	0	0	0	N	0.7	10.9	11.2	0.7	1.4	75
500	62-85% beef, grilled	6.4	2.1	N	N	N	0	0	N	0.6	5.2	6.2	1.4	0.5	60
501	**Big Mac**, takeaway	17.0	3.9	N	N	N	N	N	N	1.9	4.7	4.6	1.7	0.1	23
502	**Cheeseburger**, takeaway	22.6	5.7	N	N	N	N	N	0.7	1.4	4.9	N	N	N	32
503	**Chicken burger**, takeaway	N	N	N	N	N	N	N	1.0	1.3	N	N	N	N	N
504	**Chicken/turkey burger**, coated, baked	17.7	0.9	0.2	Tr	0.2	0.5	Tr	1.1	0.8	2.6	7.6	4.5	Tr	36

Inorganic constituents per 100g edible portion

No.	Food	Na	K	Ca	Mg	P	Fe	Cu	Zn	Cl	Mn	Se	I
						mg						µg	

Offal continued

No.	Food	Na	K	Ca	Mg	P	Fe	Cu	Zn	Cl	Mn	Se	I
496	**Liver**, pig, stewed	130	250	11	22	390	17.0	2.50	8.2	150	0.40	50	N

Burgers

No.	Food	Na	K	Ca	Mg	P	Fe	Cu	Zn	Cl	Mn	Se	I
497	**Beefburgers**, 98-99% beef, raw	290	290	7	16	150	1.7	0.12	3.8	350	0.02	8	8
498	98-99% beef, fried in vegetable oil	470	420	12	26	240	2.8	0.13	6.3	570	0.02	10	13
499	98-99% beef, grilled	400	380	10	22	210	2.5	0.13	6.1	520	0.02	9	12
500	62-85% beef, grilled	440	270	40	25	200	2.5	0.15	1.2	660	0.25	N	N
501	**Big Mac**, takeaway	390	142	68	22	142	0.9	N	N	N	N	N	N
502	**Cheeseburger**, takeaway	560	210	85	27	230	1.1	0.13	3.0	760	0.23	15	15
503	**Chicken burger**, takeaway	560	190	19	N	N	0.4	N	N	N	Tr	9	N
504	**Chicken/turkey burger**, coated, baked	383	337	41	23	160	1.0	0.09	0.8	610	0.20	9	3

Vitamins per 100g edible portion

No.	Food	Retinol	Carotene	Vitamin D	Vitamin E	Thiamin	Ribo-flavin	Niacin	Trypt 60	Vitamin B6	Vitamin B12	Folate	Panto-thenate	Biotin	Vitamin C
		µg	µg	µg	mg	mg	mg	mg	mg	mg	µg	µg	mg	µg	mg
Offal continued															
496	**Liver**, pig, stewed	22600	Tr	1.1	0.16	0.21	3.10	11.5	5.5	0.64	26	110	4.60	34	9
Burgers															
497	**Beefburgers**, 98-99% beef, raw	Tr	Tr	1.2	0.28	0.01	0.15	3.5	2.5	0.28	2	9	0.78	1	0
498	98-99% beef, fried in vegetable oil	Tr	Tr	1.9	0.54	Tr	0.22	5.5	4.3	0.31	3	8	0.85	2	0
499	98-99% beef, grilled	Tr	Tr	1.8	0.39	0.01	0.20	5.1	4.0	0.31	3	10	0.84	2	0
500	62-85% beef, grilled	5	Tr	N	N	0.07	0.07	3.8	N	0.17	2	24	N	N	Tr
501	**Big Mac**, takeaway	2	N	0.3	0.23	0.05	0.11	N	N	0.01	N	N	N	N	1
502	**Cheeseburger**, takeaway	24	23	0.3	0.26	0.17	0.18	2.2	2.8	0.19	2	23	0.46	1	N
503	**Chicken burger**, takeaway	N	N	N	N	0.26	0.07	4.3	N	0.28	N	N	N	N	N
504	**Chicken/turkey burger**, coated, baked	Tr	Tr	Tr	2.47	0.10	0.11	7.2	4.2	0.42	3	21	1.23	1	0

Composition of food per 100g edible portion

No.	Food	Description and main data sources	Main data reference	Water g	Total nitrogen g	Protein g	Fat g	Carbo-hydrate g	Energy value kcal	kJ
Burgers *continued*										
505	**Hamburger**, takeaway	Includes bun, beefburger, mustard, ketchup, onions and pickles. Industry data, 2013		45.2	2.16	13.5	8.3	31.2	246	1036
506	**Quarter Pounder with cheese**, takeaway	Includes a quarter pound beefburger, bun, ketchup, mustard, onions, pickles and slice of cheese. Industry data (McDonald's), 2013		N	2.61	16.3	13.2	21.2	263	1102
507	**Whopper burger**, takeaway	Includes bun, beefburger, mayonnaise, lettuce, tomato, ketchup, onions and pickles. Industry data (Burger King), 2013		55.8	1.66	10.4	12.1	19.2	223	932
Meat products										
508	**Beef pie, puff or shortcrust pastry**, family size	Including steak and mushroom and steak and ale. Analytical data, 2010	72	58.1	1.42	8.9	13.0	18.1	220	921
509	individual	Including beef and onion. Analytical data, 2010	72	44.1	1.47	9.2	17.7	25.5	292	1220
510	**Black pudding**, dry-fried	Analytical data, 1990	32	44.3	1.65	10.3	21.5	16.6	297	1236
511	**Chicken breast/steak**, coated, baked	Breaded and battered. Analytical data, 2010	72	51.6	2.83	17.7	11.6	15.8	234	982
512	**Chicken pie**, individual, baked	Chilled and frozen, including chicken, chicken and ham, chicken and mushroom and chicken and vegetable pies. 10-25% meat. Analytical data, 1994; and industry data, 2013	44	45.6	1.44	9.0	17.7	24.6	288	1202

Composition of food per 100g edible portion

| No. | Food | Starch g | Total sugars g | Individual sugars | | | | | Dietary fibre | | Fatty acids | | | | Cholest- erol mg |
				Gluc g	Fruct g	Sucr g	Malt g	Lact g	NSP g	AOAC g	Satd g	Mono- unsatd g	Poly- unsatd g	Trans g	
Burgers continued															
505	**Hamburger**, takeaway	24.6	6.6	N	N	N	N	N	0.8	1.8	3.5	3.6	0.7	0.2	35
506	**Quarter Pounder with cheese**, takeaway	15.6	5.5	N	N	N	N	N	N	1.6	6.8	5.6	0.9	0.1	33
507	**Whopper burger**, takeaway	15.0	4.2	N	N	N	N	N	0.8	1.2	3.3	6.3	2.0	0.3	25
Meat products															
508	**Beef pie, puff or shortcrust pastry**, family size	16.8	1.2	0.2	0.2	0.4	0.5	Tr	2.0	2.0	5.5	5.3	1.5	0.1	16
509	individual	24.3	1.2	0.2	0.1	0.2	0.7	Tr	1.3	2.1	7.9	6.9	1.9	0.1	24
510	**Black pudding**, dry-fried	16.4	0.2	0.1	Tr	0.1	Tr	Tr	0.2	N	8.5	8.1	3.6	N	68
511	**Chicken breast/steak**, coated, baked	14.6	1.1	0.3	Tr	0.3	0.6	Tr	1.1	0.8	1.8	6.3	2.9	Tr	48
512	**Chicken pie**, individual, baked	23.0	1.6	0.1	0.1	0.2	0.9	0.3	0.8	1.7	7.0	7.4	2.4	N	32

Inorganic constituents per 100g edible portion

No.	Food	Na	K	Ca	Mg	P	Fe	Cu	Zn	Cl	Mn	Se	I
		mg										µg	
Burgers continued													
505	**Hamburger**, takeaway	480	210	40	28	170	1.2	0.12	3.0	700	0.25	16	13
506	**Quarter Pounder with cheese**, takeaway	463	168	110	22	141	1.0	N	N	354	N	N	N
507	**Whopper burger**, takeaway	357	230	50	20	130	1.8	0.09	2.2	N	0.21	12	13
Meat products													
508	**Beef pie, puff or shortcrust pastry,** family size	332	150	41	12	91	1.1	0.07	1.7	510	0.18	3	3
509	individual	346	163	49	15	83	1.2	0.07	1.5	560	0.30	4	3
510	**Black pudding**, dry-fried	940	110	120	16	80	12.3	0.11	0.7	1560	N	6	5
511	**Chicken breast/steak**, coated, baked	466	300	30	26	203	0.7	0.07	0.6	580	0.16	7	3
512	**Chicken pie**, individual, baked	270	140	60	15	90	0.8	0.06	0.6	450	0.23	N	N

Vitamins per 100g edible portion

No.	Food	Retinol	Carotene	Vitamin D	Vitamin E	Thiamin	Ribo-flavin	Niacin	Trypt 60	Vitamin B_6	Vitamin B_{12}	Folate	Panto-thenate	Biotin	Vitamin C
		µg	µg	µg	mg	mg	mg	mg	mg	mg	µg	µg	mg	µg	mg
Burgers continued															
505	**Hamburger**, takeaway	N	Tr	0.3	0.22	0.19	0.12	2.5	2.7	0.18	1	24	0.48	1	N
506	**Quarter Pounder with cheese**, takeaway	Tr	N	0.2	0.14	0.04	0.12	N	N	0.06	N	N	N	N	Tr
507	**Whopper burger**, takeaway	7	94	0.2	1.80	0.15	0.11	2.4	2.0	0.13	1	25	0.40	1	2
Meat products															
508	**Beef pie, puff or shortcrust pastry,** family size	Tr	44	Tr	0.77	0.04	0.14	1.1	1.5	0.04	Tr	3	0.15	1	N
509	individual	N	32	Tr	1.50	0.08	0.15	2.1	1.8	0.20	1	2	0.16	2	N
510	**Black pudding**, dry-fried	41	Tr	0.7	0.24	0.09	0.07	1.0	2.8	0.04	1	5	0.60	2	0
511	**Chicken breast/steak**, coated, baked	Tr	Tr	Tr	2.47	0.10	0.11	7.2	4.2	0.42	3	21	1.23	1	0
512	**Chicken pie**, individual, baked	Tr	Tr	N	N	0.41	0.09	1.5	1.6	0.12	Tr	8	0.64	4	N

Composition of food per 100g edible portion

No.	Food	Description and main data sources	Main data reference	Water g	Total nitrogen g	Protein g	Fat g	Carbo-hydrate g	Energy value kcal	Energy value kJ
	Meat products continued									
513	**Chicken pieces**, coated, takeaway	Including chicken nuggets. Analytical data, 2010	72	44.5	2.96	18.5	14.1	17.6	267	1118
514	**Chicken/turkey pieces**, coated, baked	Breaded and battered, including chicken nuggets. Analytical data, 2010	72	46.9	2.30	14.4	13.9	19.6	256	1073
515	**Chicken portions**, battered, deep fried, takeaway	From fast food outlets, including KFC. Analytical data, 2010	72	54.5	3.97	24.8	12.8	4.8	233	972
516	**Chicken slices**	Including smoked and wafer thin chicken breast, 80-100% meat. Analytical data, 1995; and industry data, 2013	46	71.8	3.71	23.2	1.5	2.0[a]	114	482
517	**Chicken/turkey pasties/slices**, puff pastry	Including chicken and mushroom and chicken and bacon. Analytical data, 2010	72	48.4	1.29	8.1	18.5	23.9	289	1205
518	**Chorizo**	Industry data, 2013	16	N	3.84	24.0	32.2	2.4	395	1638
519	**Corned beef**, canned	MPD Supplement, 1996	16	59.5	4.14	25.9	10.9	1.0	205	860
520	**Cornish pasty**	Analytical data, 2010	72	47.3	1.12	7.0	17.8	24.0	278	1161
521	**Frankfurter**	Continental style frankfurters, 75-90% meat. Analytical data, 1990; and industry data, 2013	32	54.2	2.17	13.6	25.4	1.1	287	1189
522	**Haggis**, boiled	MW4, 1978	4	46.2	1.71	10.7	21.7	19.2	310	1292
523	**Liver sausage**	MPD Supplement, 1996	16	58.4	2.14	13.4	16.7	6.0	226	942
524	**Meat spread**	Analytical data, 1990; and industry data, 2013	32	64.6	2.51	15.7	13.4	2.3	192	800
525	**Meat samosas**, takeaway	From Indian restaurants. Analytical data, 1997	53	44.5	1.82	11.4	17.3	18.9[a]	272	1136
526	**Pate**, liver	Including canned. MPD Supplement, 1996	16	47.6	2.02	12.6	32.7	1.2	349	1443

[a] Includes oligosaccharides

Meat and meat products continued

Composition of food per 100g edible portion

No.	Food	Starch g	Total sugars g	Gluc g	Fruct g	Sucr g	Malt g	Lact g	NSP g	AOAC g	Satd g	Mono-unsatd g	Poly-unsatd g	Trans g	Cholesterol mg
									Dietary fibre		Fatty acids				
Meat products continued															
513	**Chicken pieces**, coated, takeaway	17.6	Tr	Tr	Tr	Tr	Tr	0	1.1	1.3	2.3	7.2	3.8	Tr	45
514	**Chicken/turkey pieces**, coated, baked	18.5	1.1	0.2	Tr	0.4	0.5	Tr	1.1	2.3	2.1	7.2	3.9	Tr	4
515	**Chicken portions**, battered, deep fried, takeaway	4.8	0	0	0	0	0	0	0.8	2.9	3.1	6.6	2.4	0.1	90
516	**Chicken slices**	1.5	0.2[a]	0	0	0.2	0	0	N	0.3	0.4	0.7	0.3	0	63
517	**Chicken/turkey pasties/slices**, puff pastry	22.8	1.2	0.2	0.1	0.2	0.7	Tr	1.0	2.9	9.2	6.5	1.9	0.1	24
518	**Chorizo**	1.3	1.1	0	0	Tr	0	1.1	N	1.0	12.0	14.5	4.9	N	N
519	**Corned beef**, canned	0	1.0	0.1	0	0.9	0	0	0	0	5.7	4.3	0.3	0.7	84
520	**Cornish pasty**	21.9	2.1	0.5	0.4	0.4	0.9	Tr	1.1	2.9	8.5	6.8	1.5	0.1	13
521	**Frankfurter**	Tr	1.1	0.2	Tr	Tr	Tr	0.9	0.1	0.1	9.2	11.5	3.0	0.1	76
522	**Haggis**, boiled	19.2	Tr	Tr	Tr	Tr	Tr	Tr	0.2	N	7.6	6.9	1.4	N	91
523	**Liver sausage**	5.0	1.0	1.0	0	0	0	0	0.7	N	5.3	5.7	2.3	Tr	115
524	**Meat spread**	2.1	0.2	0.1	0	0.1	0	0	N	2.2	5.5	5.8	1.2	0.2	62
525	**Meat samosas**, takeaway	16.8	1.9[a]	Tr	0.5	Tr	1.4	Tr	2.4	N	4.5	7.0	4.8	0.2	20
526	**Pate**, liver	0.8	0.4	0.4	0	0	0	0	Tr	0.6	9.5	11.8	3.0	Tr	170

[a] Not including oligosaccharides

223

Inorganic constituents per 100g edible portion

No.	Food	Na	K	Ca	Mg	P	Fe	Cu	Zn	Cl	Mn	Se	I
						mg						µg	
Meat products continued													
513	**Chicken pieces**, coated, takeaway	535	350	28	27	218	0.7	0.07	0.6	700	0.21	8	3
514	**Chicken/turkey pieces**, coated, baked	360	278	31	24	169	1.1	0.08	0.8	510	0.20	7	3
515	**Chicken portions**, battered, deep fried, takeaway	477	338	20	28	204	0.9	0.06	1.4	660	0.07	15	3
516	**Chicken slices**	580	360	13	28	350	0.4	0.08	0.8	730	0.02	11	5
517	**Chicken/turkey pasties/slices**, puff pastry	360	169	36	15	81	0.7	0.07	0.5	570	0.23	4	6
518	**Chorizo**	1400	240	N	N	N	N	N	N	N	N	N	N
519	**Corned beef**, canned	860	140	27	15	130	2.4	0.18	5.5	1560	0.02	8	14
520	**Cornish pasty**	470	200	47	16	69	1.0	0.08	1.0	720	0.34	3	3
521	**Frankfurter**	730	170	12	11	200	1.1	0.11	1.4	1020	0.02	8	18
522	**Haggis**, boiled	770	170	29	36	160	4.8	0.44	1.9	1200	N	N	N
523	**Liver sausage**	810	180	20	14	260	6.0	0.91	2.6	1150	0.19	N	N
524	**Meat spread**	580	220	15	14	140	4.7	0.13	3.3	1100	0.09	N	N
525	**Meat samosas**, takeaway	409	258	64	26	138	2.6	0.15	2.3	631	0.45	N	N
526	**Pate**, liver	750	150	16	11	450	5.9	0.46	2.8	880	0.16	N	N

Meat products continued

No.	Food	Retinol µg	Carotene µg	Vitamin D µg	Vitamin E mg	Thiamin mg	Ribo-flavin mg	Niacin mg	Trypt 60 mg	Vitamin B6 mg	Vitamin B12 µg	Folate µg	Panto-thenate mg	Biotin µg	Vitamin C mg
513	Chicken pieces, coated, takeaway	Tr	Tr	Tr	2.70	0.09	0.12	7.4	4.9	0.45	2	8	1.15	1	0
514	Chicken/turkey pieces, coated, baked	Tr	Tr	Tr	2.75	0.07	0.17	7.1	3.1	0.39	Tr	27	0.61	3	0
515	Chicken portions, battered, deep fried, takeaway	28	Tr	Tr	1.65	0.09	0.25	8.4	5.9	0.42	Tr	4	1.25	1	0
516	Chicken slices	Tr	Tr	0.2	0.24	0.05	0.18	9.7	4.2	0.42	Tr	8	1.06	2	Tr
517	Chicken/turkey pasties/slices, puff pastry	Tr	Tr	Tr	1.38	0.08	0.15	1.8	1.1	0.07	Tr	3	0.34	1	N
518	Chorizo	N	N	N	N	N	N	N	N	N	N	N	N	N	N
519	Corned beef, canned	Tr	Tr	1.3	0.78	Tr	0.20	2.6	6.5	0.18	2	5	0.40	2	0
520	Cornish pasty	Tr	21	Tr	0.85	0.09	0.06	1.3	1.7	0.19	Tr	5	0.60	1	Tr
521	Frankfurter	Tr	Tr	N	0.63	0.32	0.15	2.8	2.2	0.12	1	3	0.75	2	N
522	Haggis, boiled	1800	Tr	0.1	0.41	0.16	0.35	1.5	2.0	0.07	2	8	0.50	12	Tr
523	Liver sausage	2600	N	0.6	0.10	0.36	1.16	3.7	2.4	0.25	10	36	1.50	7	Tr
524	Meat spread	Tr	Tr	N	0.49	0.07	0.19	3.4	1.8	0.13	3	6	0.75	4	0
525	Meat samosas, takeaway	2	28	0.3	0.55	0.21	0.09	2.3	2.2	0.15	1	6	0.75	2	Tr
526	Pate, liver	7300	130	1.2	N	0.10	1.17	1.9	2.8	0.25	8	99	2.10	14	N

Meat and meat products *continued*

Composition of food per 100g edible portion

Meat products continued

No.	Food	Description and main data sources	Main data reference	Water g	Total nitrogen g	Protein g	Fat g	Carbo-hydrate g	Energy value kcal	Energy value kJ
527	**Pate**, meat, reduced fat	Assorted types; pork meat and liver based, 70-80% meat. MW5, 1991	10	65.0	2.88	18.0	12.0	3.0	191	798
528	**Pork pie**, individual	Analytical data, 2010	72	32.1	1.58	9.9	26.0	25.7	370	1542
529	**Salami**	Analytical data, 1990; and industry data, 2013	32	33.7	3.34	20.9[a]	39.2[a]	0.5[a]	438[a]	1814[a]
530	**Salami snack**	Peperami and own brand equivalents. Industry data, 2013		23.5	4.02	25.1	44.0	1.9	504	2085
531	**Sausages**, beef, grilled	Approx 60-81% meat. Analytical data, 2003; and industry data, 2013	64	51.3	2.75	17.2	17.2	11.0	265	1105
532	pork, raw	Frozen and chilled; thick and thin; 65-70% meat. Analytical data, 1990; and industry data, 2013	32	49.4	1.91	11.9	25.0	9.6	309	1282
533	pork, fried in vegetable oil	Analytical data, 1990; and industry data, 2013	32	46.4	2.22	13.9	23.9	9.9	308	1279
534	pork, grilled	Analytical data, 1990; and industry data, 2013	32	45.9	2.32	14.5	22.1	9.8	294	1221
535	pork, reduced fat, grilled	Frozen and chilled, 65-68% meat. Analytical data, 1990, 2003; and industry data, 2013	32, 64	63.2	2.58	16.2	6.1	10.7	160	672
536	premium, grilled	Calculation from raw. Analytical data, 1990; and industry data, 2013	32	54.8	2.69	19.0	21.1	2.3	275	1141
537	**Sausage roll**, flaky pastry, ready-to-eat	Mini and large. Analytical data, 2010	72	36.5	1.35	8.4	24.1	27.0	352	1467
538	**Scotch eggs**	MW5, 1991; and industry data, 2013	10	54.0	1.92	12.0	16.0	13.1	241	1006
539	**Steak and kidney pie**, single crust, homemade	Recipe		51.5	2.76	17.0	13.1	15.3	243	1019

[a] Values for protein, fat, carbohydrate and energy can vary between products from different countries

Meat products continued

No.	Food	Starch	Total sugars	Individual sugars					Dietary fibre		Fatty acids				Cholesterol
				Gluc	Fruct	Sucr	Malt	Lact	NSP	AOAC	Satd	Mono-unsatd	Poly-unsatd	Trans	erol
		g	g	g	g	g	g	g	g	g	g	g	g	g	mg
527	**Pate**, meat, reduced fat	1.7	1.3	1.1	0	0.1	0	0.1	Tr	0.8	3.5	3.9	1.5	0.1	160
528	**Pork pie**, individual	24.2	1.5	0.2	Tr	0.1	1.2	Tr	1.2	2.9	10.1	11.0	3.6	0.1	35
529	**Salami**	Tr	0.5	0.1	0	0	0	0.4	0.1	0.4	14.6	17.7	4.4	0.2	83
530	**Salami snack**	Tr	1.9	1.9	0	0	0	0	N	0.5	16.8	19.9	4.4	0.3	N
531	**Sausages**, beef, grilled	8.6	2.4	0.4	0.2	0.7	1.0	0.1	1.7	1.6	8.0	7.9	0.6	0.5	42
532	pork, raw	6.8	2.8	1.1	Tr	Tr	1.6	Tr	1.6	2.8	9.2	11.2	3.4	0.2	60
533	pork, fried in vegetable oil	8.4	1.6	0.4	Tr	0.2	0.9	0.1	0.7	2.1	8.5	10.3	3.5	0.1	53
534	pork, grilled	8.3	1.5	0.4	Tr	0.2	0.8	0.1	0.7	2.3	8.0	9.6	3.0	0.1	53
535	pork, reduced fat, grilled	7.3	3.4	1.2	0	0.1	2.0	0.1	1.5	2.5	2.2	2.4	1.2	0.1	24
536	premium, grilled	1.4	0.9	0.7	0	0.1	0	0.1	N	0.6	8.0	8.4	3.6	0.2	72
537	**Sausage roll**, flaky pastry, ready-to-eat	25.6	1.3	0.2	Tr	0.2	1.0	Tr	2.7	3.4	10.4	9.4	3.1	Tr	N
538	**Scotch eggs**	13.1	Tr	Tr	0	0	0	0	N	1.7	4.3	6.8	2.8	0.2	165
539	**Steak and kidney pie**, single crust, homemade	14.7	0.6	Tr	Tr	0	0.6	Tr	0.4	1.2	6.1	4.8	1.4	0.1	107

Inorganic constituents per 100g edible portion

No.	Food	Na	K	Ca	Mg	P	Fe	Cu	Zn	Cl	Mn	Se	I
		mg										µg	
	Meat products continued												
527	**Pate**, meat, reduced fat	710	190	14	14	240	6.4	0.46	2.7	1180	0.16	N	N
528	**Pork pie**, individual	542	153	53	7	23	2.9	0.04	0.5	830	0.07	1	2
529	**Salami**	1530[a]	320	11	18	170	1.3	0.12	3.0	2780	0.04	7	15
530	**Salami snack**	1600	330	11	19	180	2.2	0.11	3.9	2380	0.18	N	N
531	**Sausages**, beef, grilled	500	246	103	19	259	1.8	0.14	2.6	680	0.27	5	8
532	pork, raw	470	160	103	13	175	0.9	0.07	0.9	675	0.17	5	7
533	pork, fried in vegetable oil	640	180	110	15	220	1.1	0.12	1.1	880	0.19	6	8
534	pork, grilled	640	190	110	15	220	1.1	0.11	1.4	980	0.20	6	8
535	pork, reduced fat, grilled	720	260	130	19	230	1.3	0.08	1.7	960	0.24	7	9
536	premium, grilled	570	220	180	16	180	1.2	0.07	1.4	620	0.16	N	N
537	**Sausage roll**, flaky pastry, ready-to-eat	577	129	61	14	89	1.2	Tr	0.7	880	0.31	5	2
538	**Scotch eggs**	330	130	50	15	170	1.8	0.23	1.2	480	0.20	N	17
539	**Steak and kidney pie**, single crust, homemade	209	273	38	19	177	2.8	0.17	3.4	277	0.17	N	N

[a] Danish salami contains 1840mg Na; French 1700mg; German 1500mg; Italian 1335mg per 100g

Vitamins per 100g edible portion

No.	Food	Retinol µg	Carotene µg	Vitamin D µg	Vitamin E mg	Thiamin mg	Ribo-flavin mg	Niacin mg	Trypt 60 mg	Vitamin B6 mg	Vitamin B12 µg	Folate µg	Panto-thenate mg	Biotin µg	Vitamin C mg
	Meat products continued													
527	**Pate**, meat, reduced fat	5930	N	N	0.77	0.46	1.12	7.1	2.2	0.35	12	31	2.68	27	18
528	**Pork pie**, individual	Tr	Tr	Tr	2.11	0.08	0.11	1.7	1.7	0.18	Tr	2	0.24	1	4
529	**Salami**	Tr	Tr	N	0.23	0.60	0.23	5.6	2.8	0.36	2	3	1.66	7	N
530	**Salami snack**	Tr	Tr	N	1.77	0.27	0.16	5.5	2.2	0.27	2	1	1.19	6	N
531	**Sausages**, beef, grilled	Tr	Tr	N	0.59	Tr	0.14	3.2	2.3	0.14	1	9	0.83	4	N[a]
532	pork, raw	Tr	Tr	0.9	0.93	0.03	0.11	2.5	1.5	0.12	1	13	0.77	5	7
533	pork, fried in vegetable oil	Tr	Tr	1.1	0.86	0.01	0.13	3.1	2.0	0.09	1	3	0.85	5	5
534	pork, grilled	Tr	Tr	1.1	0.92	Tr	0.13	3.1	2.0	0.12	1	4	0.93	5	5
535	pork, reduced fat, grilled	Tr	Tr	N	0.13	Tr	0.13	2.8	2.0	0.11	1	32	1.04	3	N
536	premium, grilled	Tr	Tr	N	0.80	0.05	0.10	2.7	1.5	0.14	1	8	0.76	3	8
537	**Sausage roll**, flaky pastry, ready-to-eat	Tr	Tr	Tr	2.11	0.08	0.11	1.7	1.7	0.18	Tr	2	0.24	1	2
538	**Scotch eggs**	30	Tr	0.7	N	0.08	0.21	1.0	2.9	0.13	1	42	1.10	9	N
539	**Steak and kidney pie**, single crust, homemade	23	Tr	N	0.98	0.12	0.55	3.6	3.4	0.30	4	2	1.13	9	1

[a] Ascorbic acid is added as an antioxidant. Measurable levels may be present

Composition of food per 100g edible portion

No.	Food	Description and main data sources	Main data reference	Water g	Total nitrogen g	Protein g	Fat g	Carbo-hydrate g	Energy value kcal	Energy value kJ
	Meat products continued									
540	**Turkey slices**	Including honey roast and wafer thin turkey breast, 78-100% meat. Analytical data, 1995; and industry data, 2013	46	72.6	3.68	23.0	1.9	1.2[a]	114	481
	Meat Dishes									
541	**Beef bourguignon**, homemade	Recipe		71.4	2.26	13.8	6.2	2.5[a]	140	587
542	**Beef casserole**, made with cook-in sauce	Recipe		71.0	2.41	15.0	6.6	4.8	137	576
543	**Beef chow mein**, reheated	Noodles with beef and vegetables in sauce. Analytical data, 1997; and industry data, 2013	53	71.7	1.07	6.7	6.0	14.7	136	571
544	**Beef curry**, reheated	Meat and sauce only. Analytical data, 1990; and industry data, 2013	32	69.5	2.16	13.5	6.6	6.3	137	575
545	reheated, with rice	Calculated from 57% retail beef curry and 43% retail, ready cooked, plain white rice		65.2	1.53	9.5	4.6	18.2	147	621
546	reduced fat, homemade	Recipe		70.5	3.01	18.8	7.1	1.3[a]	139	583
547	**Beef stew**, homemade	Recipe		76.3	1.91	11.9	4.6	4.8[a]	105	441
548	**Beef, stir-fried with green peppers**, homemade	Recipe		71.2	1.89	11.8	8.0	6.1	145	607
549	**Bolognese sauce (with meat)**, homemade	Recipe		70.5	1.89	11.8	11.6	2.8[a]	161	668

[a] Includes oligosaccharides

Composition of food per 100g edible portion

No.	Food	Starch	Total sugars	Individual sugars					Dietary fibre		Fatty acids				Cholest-
				Gluc	Fruct	Sucr	Malt	Lact	NSP	AOAC	Satd	Mono-unsatd	Poly-unsatd	Trans	erol
		g	g	g	g	g	g	g	g	g	g	g	g	g	mg
Meat products continued															
540	**Turkey slices**	0.4	0.4[a]	N	N	N	Tr	0	0	Tr	0.6	0.7	0.4	0	62
Meat Dishes															
541	**Beef bourguignon**, homemade	1.4	0.9[a]	0.3	0.3	0.2	0	0	0.4	0.4	2.1	2.5	1.2	0.1	42
542	**Beef casserole**, made with cook-in sauce	2.0	2.7	0.8	0.9	0.9	0	0	0.7	0.7	2.8	2.9	0.6	0.3	44
543	**Beef chow mein**, reheated	12.3	2.4	N	0	1.2	0	0	N	1.8	1.3	3.1	1.4	N	N
544	**Beef curry**, reheated	1.8	4.5	1.5	1.6	0.7	0	0.7	1.2	2.4	3.1	2.5	-0.6	N	32
545	reheated, with rice	15.6	2.6	0.9	0.9	0.4	0	0.4	0.7	1.8	1.9	1.6	0.7	N	18
546	reduced fat, homemade	0.2	0.7[a]	0.3	0.2	0.2	0	0	0.1	1.0	2.3	2.7	1.5	0.2	53
547	**Beef stew**, homemade	2.5	2.0[a]	0.5	0.4	1.1	0	0	0.6	1.1	1.5	1.8	1.0	0.1	35
548	**Beef, stir-fried with green peppers**, homemade	2.2	3.8	0.8	0.9	2.1	0	0	0.8	N	2.7	2.9	1.9	0.2	33
549	**Bolognese sauce (with meat)**, homemade	0.1	2.6[a]	1.1	1.1	0.4	0	0	0.6	0.7	4.2	4.4	1.9	0.5	33

[a] Not including oligosaccharides

Inorganic constituents per 100g edible portion

No.	Food	Na	K	Ca	Mg	P	Fe	Cu	Zn	Cl	Mn	Se	I
						mg						μg	
Meat products continued													
540	**Turkey slices**	590	330	6	25	310	0.4	0.13	1.1	810	0.01	11	5
Meat Dishes													
541	**Beef bourguignon**, homemade	238	331	13	19	135	1.6	0.11	3.2	339	0.08	7	8
542	**Beef casserole**, made with cook-in sauce	302	317	18	19	139	1.3	0.03	4.0	478	0.07	5	12
543	**Beef chow mein**, reheated	200	N	N	N	N	1.3	N	N	310	N	N	N
544	**Beef curry**, reheated	190	340	N	N	N	N	N	N	290	N	N	N
545	reheated, with rice	173	216	N	N	N	N	N	N	264	N	N	N
546	reduced fat, homemade	64	338	27	27	174	2.1	0.04	5.2	63	0.10	6	14
547	**Beef stew**, homemade	259	233	15	14	104	1.2	0.05	2.7	383	0.05	4	7
548	**Beef, stir-fried with green peppers**, homemade	212	274	10	19	122	1.9	0.04	2.0	298	0.07	4	6
549	**Bolognese sauce (with meat)**, homemade	180	288	16	16	104	1.1	0.05	2.3	280	0.07	4	6

Meat and meat products continued

Vitamins per 100g edible portion

No.	Food	Retinol µg	Carotene µg	Vitamin D µg	Vitamin E mg	Thiamin mg	Ribo- flavin mg	Niacin mg	Trypt 60 mg	Vitamin B$_6$ mg	Vitamin B$_{12}$ µg	Folate µg	Panto- thenate mg	Biotin µg	Vitamin C mg
Meat products continued															
540	**Turkey slices**	Tr	Tr	0.2	0.24	0.05	0.18	9.6	4.2	0.41	Tr	8	1.05	2	Tr
Meat Dishes															
541	**Beef bourguignon**, homemade	Tr	19	0.4	0.77	0.09	0.17	2.4	2.7	0.24	1	6	0.67	3	1
542	**Beef casserole**, made with cook-in sauce	Tr	173	0.4	0.66	0.09	0.16	2.5	3.1	0.26	1	20	0.45	2	1
543	**Beef chow mein**, reheated	Tr	Tr	N	0.43	0.03	0.03	N	1.1	N	Tr	N	N	N	Tr
544	**Beef curry**, reheated	Tr	Tr	N	0.62	0.05	0.16	2.4	1.6	0.20	N	N	0.71	3	Tr
545	reheated, with rice	Tr	Tr	N	0.51	0.06	0.09	2.4	1.4	0.15	N	N	0.62	2	Tr
546	reduced fat, homemade	Tr	81	0.4	0.99	0.07	0.20	3.0	3.9	0.32	1	22	0.42	1	1
547	**Beef stew**, homemade	Tr	1784	0.4	0.70	0.06	0.11	1.7	2.3	0.19	1	3	0.31	1	Tr
548	**Beef, stir-fried with green peppers,** homemade	Tr	165	0.2	1.54	0.05	0.11	2.3	2.6	0.38	1	11	0.32	N	38
549	**Bolognese sauce (with meat),** homemade	Tr	694	0.4	1.97	0.09	0.08	3.0	2.1	0.22	1	7	0.28	1	3

Composition of food per 100g edible portion

No.	Food	Description and main data sources	Main data reference	Water g	Total nitrogen g	Protein g	Fat g	Carbo-hydrate g	Energy value kcal	kJ
Meat Dishes continued										
550	**Bolognese sauce (with meat)**, homemade, with extra lean minced beef	Recipe		76.9	2.08	13.0	4.9	2.8[b]	108	452
551	reheated[a]	Chilled and frozen, 10-18% meat. Analytical data, 1994; and industry data, 2013	44	76.9	1.49	9.3	5.7	5.3	108	454
552	**Chicken balti**	Chilled, frozen and ambient. Analytical data, 2007; and industry data, 2013	69	75.8	1.68	10.5	5.0	4.8	105	441
553	**Chicken chow mein**, takeaway	Analytical data, 1997	53	69.0	1.36	8.5	7.2	12.7[b]	147	614
554	**Chicken curry**, average, takeaway	Including korma, tikka masala, dhansak, jalfrezi and dopiaza; meat and sauce only. Analytical data, 1997	53	70.2	1.88	11.7	9.8	2.5[b]	145	603
555	reheated	Chilled and frozen, korma and masala varieties. Analytical data, 1990; and industry data, 2013	32	68.7	1.94	12.1	8.9	5.4	149	621
556	reheated, with rice	Calculated from 55% retail chicken curry and 45% retail, ready cooked, plain white rice		64.6	1.38	8.5	5.8	18.2	154	648
557	made with cook-in sauce	Recipe		67.7	2.99	18.6	5.4	5.5	144	604
558	Thai green, takeaway and restaurant	Usual sauce ingredients include coconut milk, lemongrass, ginger and peppers. Analytical data, 1997	53	74.7	1.41	8.8	8.7	1.5	119	496
559	**Chicken fajita**, meat only, takeaway and restaurant	Analytical data, 1997	53	72.6	2.69	16.8	6.3	0.3	125	524
560	**Chicken satay**, takeaway	Analytical data, 1997	53	60.5	3.47	21.7	10.3	3.0	191	798

[a] The publication number for Spaghetti Bolognese is 587

[b] Includes oligosaccharides

Composition of food per 100g edible portion

Meat Dishes continued

No.	Food	Starch g	Total sugars g	Gluc g	Fruct g	Sucr g	Malt g	Lact g	NSP g	AOAC g	Satd g	Mono- unsatd g	Poly- unsatd g	Trans g	Cholest- erol mg
				Individual sugars					**Dietary fibre**		**Fatty acids**				
550	**Bolognese sauce (with meat)**, homemade, with extra lean minced beef	0.1	2.6[a]	1.1	1.1	0.4	0	0	0.6	0.6	1.5	1.7	1.7	0.1	21
551	reheated	2.3	3.0	1.1	1.3	0.6	0	0	0.9	N	2.3	2.5	0.5	0.2	N
552	**Chicken balti**	1.3	3.5	N	N	N	Tr	Tr	N	2.0	0.9	2.4	1.4	Tr	29
553	**Chicken chow mein**, takeaway	6.6	0.3[a]	Tr	0.3	Tr	Tr	Tr	1.1	1.5	1.2	3.9	1.9	0	13
554	**Chicken curry**, average, takeaway	1.2	1.2[a]	0.4	0.5	0	0	0.3	2.0	2.2	2.9	4.0	2.5	0.1	37
555	reheated	1.0	4.4	1.5	1.6	0.7	0	0.7	1.3	1.5	4.0	2.9	1.5	N	51
556	reheated, with rice	15.8	2.4	0.8	0.9	0.4	0	0.4	0.7	1.3	2.3	1.8	1.2	N	28
557	made with cook-in sauce	1.6	3.9	1.2	1.4	1.3	0	Tr	0.9	1.5	1.0	1.9	2.2	Tr	N
558	Thai green, takeaway and restaurant	1.0	0.5	Tr	0.5	Tr	Tr	Tr	2.4	2.6	5.3	2.0	1.1	Tr	26
559	**Chicken fajita**, meat only, takeaway and restaurant	0.2	Tr	Tr	Tr	Tr	Tr	Tr	1.0	0.8	2.1	2.3	1.6	Tr	48
560	**Chicken satay**, takeaway	1.4	1.6	0.5	1.1	Tr	Tr	Tr	2.2	2.0	3.0	4.3	2.5	0	57

[a] Not including oligosaccharides

Meat Dishes continued

Inorganic constituents per 100g edible portion

| No. | Food | mg | | | | | | | | | | µg | |
		Na	K	Ca	Mg	P	Fe	Cu	Zn	Cl	Mn	Se	I
550	**Bolognese sauce (with meat)**, homemade, with extra lean minced beef	186	305	16	17	115	1.2	0.08	2.5	286	0.07	4	8
551	reheated	290	290	21	18	85	1.3	0.08	1.5	450	0.15	1	N
552	**Chicken balti**	258	333	39	26	105	0.9	0.12	0.5	367	N	7	N
553	**Chicken chow mein**, takeaway	466	90	46	11	64	1.0	0.05	0.4	720	0.15	N	N
554	**Chicken curry**, average, takeaway	356	218	41	22	112	2.3	0.08	0.6	515	0.24	7	7
555	reheated	240	300	N	N	N	N	N	N	340	N	N	N
556	reheated, with rice	200	188	N	N	N	N	N	N	290	N	N	N
557	made with cook-in sauce	246	448	25	32	147	1.2	0.08	1.1	395	0.19	11	6
558	Thai green, takeaway and restaurant	550	224	23	25	87	1.3	0.07	0.5	800	0.51	7	7
559	**Chicken fajita**, meat only, takeaway and restaurant	334	316	37	25	176	2.9	Tr	0.6	480	Tr	10	18
560	**Chicken satay**, takeaway	613	363	30	43	223	1.0	0.14	0.9	690	0.39	12	23

Vitamins per 100g edible portion

Meat Dishes continued

No.	Food	Retinol µg	Carotene µg	Vitamin D µg	Vitamin E mg	Thiamin mg	Ribo-flavin mg	Niacin mg	Trypt 60 mg	Vitamin B₆ mg	Vitamin B₁₂ µg	Folate µg	Panto-thenate mg	Biotin µg	Vitamin C mg
550	**Bolognese sauce (with meat)**, homemade, with extra lean minced beef	Tr	693	0.3	1.97	0.09	0.08	3.3	2.3	0.24	1	8	0.31	1	3
551	reheated	Tr	N	N	N	N	N	N	N	N	N	N	N	N	Tr
552	**Chicken balti**	N	210	N	2.37	0.04	0.14	3.3	N	0.14	Tr	14	0.33	4	3
553	**Chicken chow mein**, takeaway	Tr	110	N	0.96	0.05	0.03	1.8	1.3	0.08	Tr	4	0.47	2	Tr
554	**Chicken curry**, average, takeaway	15	119	0.3	2.12	0.05	0.07	2.5	1.8	0.19	Tr	N	0.66	2	Tr
555	reheated	N	370	N	1.30	0.20	0.14	3.8	2.3	0.24	N	N	1.02	3	1
556	reheated, with rice	N	204	N	0.88	0.15	0.08	3.1	1.8	0.17	N	N	0.79	2	1
557	made with cook-in sauce	9	236	0.1	2.40	0.11	0.13	5.5	3.5	0.29	Tr	14	0.93	3	2
558	Thai green, takeaway and restaurant	2	386	0.3	0.99	0.02	0.05	2.5	1.5	0.14	Tr	7	0.49	2	1
559	**Chicken fajita**, meat only, takeaway and restaurant	27	22	0.3	1.90	0.07	0.10	7.0	2.7	0.27	Tr	N	0.90	1	7
560	**Chicken satay**, takeaway	5	23	N	1.41	0.07	0.07	11.0	3.2	0.22	Tr	27	0.93	6	Tr

Meat and meat products *continued*

Composition of food per 100g edible portion

No.	Food	Description and main data sources	Main data reference	Water g	Total nitrogen g	Protein g	Fat g	Carbo-hydrate g	Energy value kcal	kJ
	Meat Dishes continued									
561	**Chicken tandoori**, reheated	95-96% meat. Analytical data, 1990; and industry data, 2013	32	56.4	4.38	27.4	10.8	2.0	214	897
562	**Chicken tikka masala**, reheated	Chilled and frozen. Analytical data, 1994; and industry data, 2013	44	69.2	2.00	12.4	9.8	4.9	156	652
563	**Chicken wings**, marinated, barbecued	Including American and Chinese style and hot and spicy wings. Analytical data, 1995; and industry data, 2013	48	50.5	4.38	27.4	16.6	4.1	274	1146
564	**Chicken, stir-fried with rice and vegetables**, reheated	Frozen, 10-13% meat. Fried in corn oil. Analytical data, 1995	46	67.9	1.04	6.5	4.6	17.1[a]	132	554
565	**Chilli con carne**, homemade	Recipe		74.3	1.48	9.2	7.5	4.4[a]	120	500
566	reheated, with rice	Calculated from 60% retail chilli con carne and 40% boiled white rice.		72.6	0.94	5.8	2.7	18.1	116	491
567	**Coq au vin**, homemade	Recipe		68.7	1.79	11.0	11.0	3.3	188	783
568	**Coronation chicken**, homemade	Recipe		47.4	2.66	16.6	31.4	3.5	362	1500
569	**Cottage/Shepherd's pie**, reheated	Including beef and lamb, chilled and frozen, 11-25% meat. Analytical data, 1994; and industry data, 2013	44	73.1	0.72	4.5	5.4	11.9	111	467
570	**Doner kebab**, meat only	Takeaway. Analytical data, 1994	42	42.0	3.76	23.5	31.4	0	377	1561
571	in pitta bread with salad	Calculated from 50% doner kebab, 22% pitta bread and 28% salad.		54.8	2.29	14.1	16.0	12.5	248	1033
572	**Faggots in gravy**, reheated	Chilled and frozen. Analytical data, 1995	46	69.6	1.31	8.2	7.5	12.6[a]	148	619
573	**Irish stew**, homemade	Recipe		76.4	1.18	7.3	6.2	9.4[a]	119	501

[a] Includes oligosaccharides

Composition of food per 100g edible portion

No.	Food	Starch	Total sugars	Gluc	Fruct	Sucr	Malt	Lact	Dietary fibre NSP	AOAC	Fatty acids Satd	Mono-unsatd	Poly-unsatd	Trans	Cholest-erol
		g	g	g	g	g	g	g	g	g	g	g	g	g	mg
Meat Dishes continued															
561	**Chicken tandoori**, reheated	1.0	1.0	0.3	0.2	0.1	0	0.5	N	0.8	3.3	5.0	2.0	0.1	120
562	**Chicken tikka masala**, reheated	1.3	3.6	0.7	0.9	0.8	Tr	1.2	1.0	1.4	3.3	4.0	2.1	0.3	46
563	**Chicken wings**, marinated, barbecued	0.5	3.6	0.5	0.6	2.5	0	0	N	0.5	4.6	7.5	3.3	0.2	120
564	**Chicken, stir-fried with rice and vegetables**, reheated	12.6	3.9[a]	1.8	1.1	1.0	0	0	1.3	N	N	N	N	N	N
565	**Chilli con carne**, homemade	1.3	2.9[a]	1.1	1.1	0.6	0	0	1.1	N	2.9	3.0	0.9	0.3	24
566	reheated, with rice	16.5	1.6	N	N	N	0	0	0.8	N	1.2	1.2	0.2	0.1	N
567	**Coq au vin**, homemade	2.9	0.4	0.1	0.1	0.1	0	0	0.3	0.2	4.2	4.5	1.6	0.2	67
568	**Coronation chicken**, homemade	0.1	3.4	1.1	0.7	1.3	0.3	Tr	N	0.2	3.3	18.2	8.0	0.1	82
569	**Cottage/Shepherd's pie**, reheated	10.3	1.6	0.3	0.2	0.3	0	0.8	0.9	1.2	2.4	2.2	0.4	0.3	16
570	**Doner kebab**, meat only	0	0	0	0	0	0	0	0	0	15.0	11.8	1.9	2.6	94
571	in pitta bread with salad	11.5	1.1	0.3	0.3	Tr	0.4	0	0.9	0.9	7.5	5.9	1.1	1.3	47
572	**Faggots in gravy**, reheated	10.8	1.7[a]	0.5	0.3	0.3	0.6	0	0.2	N	2.5	2.9	1.0	0.1	45
573	**Irish stew**, homemade	7.2	1.9[a]	0.6	0.5	0.9	0	0	0.7	1.5	2.9	2.4	0.3	0.5	27

[a] Not including oligosaccharides

Inorganic constituents per 100g edible portion

Meat Dishes continued

No.	Food	Na	K	Ca	Mg	P	Fe	Cu	Zn	Cl	Mn	Se	I
						mg						μg	
561	**Chicken tandoori**, reheated	N	470	58	36	280	1.8	0.12	1.5	N	0.18	16	7
562	**Chicken tikka masala**, reheated	220	310	60	25	140	1.3	0.10	0.7	340	0.20	7	7
563	**Chicken wings**, marinated, barbecued	390	350	42	27	200	1.3	0.09	1.6	610	0.15	17	6
564	**Chicken, stir-fried with rice and vegetables**, reheated	N	180	22	13	95	1.1	0.10	2.0	N	0.08	N	N
565	**Chilli con carne**, homemade	101	263	21	17	90	1.1	0.05	1.7	166	0.10	3	5
566	reheated, with rice	188	187	33	15	70	0.9	0.11	1.0	317	0.21	3	N
567	**Coq au vin**, homemade	154	286	14	19	88	1.0	0.08	0.9	239	0.10	9	6
568	**Coronation chicken**, homemade	122	208	10	17	134	0.7	0.07	0.9	228	0.03	9	7
569	**Cottage/Shepherd's pie**, reheated	240	240	20	14	65	0.7	0.04	0.9	410	0.08	N	N
570	**Doner kebab**, meat only	N	350	23	25	210	2.1	0.11	4.0	N	0.06	6	4
571	in pitta bread with salad	N	276	49	20	133	1.5	0.09	2.2	N	0.17	3	2
572	**Faggots in gravy**, reheated	540	120	32	10	80	1.7	0.30	0.9	830	0.15	N	N
573	**Irish stew**, homemade	115	306	14	16	78	0.7	0.06	1.4	206	0.11	1	3

Meat and meat products *continued*

Vitamins per 100g edible portion

No.	Food	Retinol	Carotene	Vitamin D	Vitamin E	Thiamin	Ribo- flavin	Niacin	Trypt 60	Vitamin B_6	Vitamin B_{12}	Folate	Panto- thenate	Biotin	Vitamin C
		µg	µg	µg	mg	mg	mg	mg	mg	mg	µg	µg	mg	µg	mg
	Meat Dishes continued														
561	**Chicken tandoori**, reheated	Tr	210	0.2	1.49	0.12	0.19	10.2	5.8	0.61	1	16	2.25	5	2
562	**Chicken tikka masala**, reheated	49	104	0.3	1.57	0.08	0.14	4.2	1.9	0.29	1	21	0.98	6	Tr
563	**Chicken wings**, marinated, barbecued	24	N	0.1	0.23	0.07	0.11	6.2	5.3	0.27	1	10	1.34	4	Tr
564	**Chicken, stir-fried with rice and vegetables**, reheated	Tr	565	N	N	0.09	0.09	1.9	1.3	0.22	Tr	21	0.50	4	2
565	**Chilli con carne**, homemade	Tr	246	0.3	1.15	0.10	0.07	2.3	1.6	0.20	1	9	0.21	1	7
566	reheated, with rice	39	59	N	N	0.06	0.07	1.2	1.1	0.13	1	11	0.34	3	N
567	**Coq au vin**, homemade	50	28	0.3	0.18	0.10	0.15	2.6	2.0	0.15	Tr	5	0.63	3	1
568	**Coronation chicken**, homemade	34	Tr	0.1	7.98	0.04	0.13	5.5	3.2	0.24	Tr	9	0.88	2	Tr
569	**Cottage/Shepherd's pie**, reheated	17	110	0.1	0.28	0.15	0.10	1.3	0.8	0.19	1	14	0.39	1	1
570	**Doner kebab**, meat only	Tr	Tr	0.6	0.56	0.11	0.25	5.8	4.9	0.20	2	7	1.10	2	0
571	in pitta bread with salad	Tr	17	0.3	0.46	0.17	0.16	3.5	3.0	0.11	1	25	0.60	1	0
572	**Faggots in gravy**, reheated	1100	55	0.5	0.33	0.10	0.56	2.0	N	0.13	6	19	N	N	Tr
573	**Irish stew**, homemade	3	1625	0.1	0.07	0.12	0.05	1.3	1.4	0.11	1	4	0.40	1	3

Composition of food per 100g edible portion

Meat Dishes continued

No.	Food	Description and main data sources	Main data reference	Water g	Total nitrogen g	Protein g	Fat g	Carbo-hydrate g	Energy value kcal	kJ
574	**Lamb curry**, made with cook-in sauce	Recipe		60.3	2.48	15.5	17.7	5.5	242	1008
575	**Lamb kheema**, homemade	Recipe		69.3	1.76	11.0	13.4	4.0[a]	178	740
576	**Lamb/beef hot pot with potatoes**, reheated	Chilled and frozen,10-32% meat. Analytical data, 1995; and industry data, 2013	46	74.4	1.15	7.2	4.4	10.6	108	455
577	**Lasagne**, reheated	Chilled and frozen, 10-20% beef. Analytical data, 1994; and industry data, 2013	44	68.1	1.18	7.4	6.1	15.7	143	603
578	homemade	Beef. Recipe		63.3	1.57	9.6	9.6	15.2[a]	180	756
579	homemade, with extra lean minced beef	Recipe		65.7	1.65	10.1	7.0	15.2[a]	160	671
580	**Moussaka**, reheated	Beef/lamb, chilled/frozen/ambient, 20-23% meat. Analytical data, 1994; and industry data, 2013	46	70.6	1.33	8.3	8.3	8.6[a]	140	586
581	**Pasta with meat and tomato sauce**, homemade	Recipe		65.9	1.11	6.6	4.1	20.4	140	590
582	**Pork casserole**, made with cook-in sauce	Recipe		69.6	2.73	17.0	7.9	4.0	154	646
583	**Pork spare ribs, 'barbecue style'**, reheated	Including American and Chinese style and hot and spicy ribs, chilled/frozen, 80-90% meat. Analytical data, 1995	48	49.6	4.21	26.3	17.1	5.8	281	1173
584	**Sausage casserole**, homemade	Recipe		68.6	1.91	11.9	10.9	5.2[a]	165	685
585	**Shish kebab**, meat only	Takeaway. Analytical data, 1994	42	59.4	4.64	29.0	10.0	0	206	863

[a] Includes oligosaccharides

Meat and meat products *continued*

Composition of food per 100g edible portion

Meat Dishes continued

No.	Food	Starch g	Total sugars g	Gluc g	Fruct g	Sucr g	Malt g	Lact g	NSP g	AOAC g	Satd g	Mono-unsatd g	Poly-unsatd g	Trans g	Cholesterol mg
574	**Lamb curry**, made with cook-in sauce	1.6	3.9	1.2	1.4	1.3	0	Tr	0.9	1.5	7.1	6.5	2.6	1.2	63
575	**Lamb kheema**, homemade	1.1	2.4[a]	0.6	0.6	1.3	0	0	1.0	1.5	3.8	4.0	4.5	0.5	38
576	**Lamb/beef hot pot with potatoes**, reheated	9.6	1.0	0.3	0.3	0.4	0	0	0.9	1.9	1.7	1.9	0.5	0.4	N
577	**Lasagne**, reheated	12.7	3.0	0.6	0.7	0.4	0	1.3	0.7	1.7	2.8	2.2	0.7	0.3	18
578	homemade	12.3	2.8[a]	0.5	0.4	0.3	0.2	1.4	0.9	1.0	4.2	3.4	1.1	0.3	25
579	homemade, with extra lean minced beef	12.3	2.8[a]	0.5	0.4	0.3	0.2	1.4	0.9	1.0	3.1	2.3	1.1	0.2	20
580	**Moussaka**, reheated	6.5	2.0[a]	0.4	0.6	0	0	1.0	0.8	1.9	2.9	3.6	1.1	0.4	26
581	**Pasta with meat and tomato sauce**, homemade	18.5	1.9	0.7	0.7	0.2	0.3	0	2.0	2.1	1.4	1.7	0.5	0.2	11
582	**Pork casserole**, made with cook-in sauce	1.7	2.3	0.7	0.8	0.7	0	0	0.5	0.7	2.7	3.2	1.5	0.1	50
583	**Pork spare ribs**, 'barbecue style', reheated	1.4	4.4	N	N	N	0	0	Tr	0.6	6.2	6.8	2.7	0.1	160
584	**Sausage casserole**, homemade	2.9	2.0[a]	0.6	0.3	0.9	0.3	Tr	1.1	1.6	3.7	4.5	2.1	Tr	40
585	**Shish kebab**, meat only	0	0	0	0	0	0	0	0	0	3.9	4.3	0.8	0.6	90

[a] Not including oligosaccharides

243

Inorganic constituents per 100g edible portion

No.	Food	Na	K	Ca	Mg	P	Fe	Cu	Zn	Cl	Mn	Se	I
						mg						µg	
Meat Dishes continued													
574	**Lamb curry**, made with cook-in sauce	231	392	24	26	155	1.6	0.11	3.2	373	0.19	2	6
575	**Lamb kheema**, homemade	37	271	30	23	123	1.8	0.10	2.0	65	0.16	1	4
576	**Lamb/beef hot pot with potatoes**, reheated	200	260	17	16	80	0.8	0.07	1.3	310	0.08	N	N
577	**Lasagne**, reheated	210	230	80	19	120	1.0	0.10	1.4	325	0.22	N	N
578	homemade	235	220	104	19	143	0.8	0.08	1.5	375	0.15	7	15
579	homemade, with extra lean minced beef	237	227	105	19	147	0.8	0.09	1.6	377	0.15	7	16
580	**Moussaka**, reheated	280	250	75	77	110	0.6	0.12	0.1	430	0.13	N	N
581	**Pasta with meat and tomato sauce**, homemade	90	158	24	20	81	0.8	0.14	1.1	167	0.25	5	4
582	**Pork casserole**, made with cook-in sauce	183	374	17	22	177	0.8	0.04	1.4	274	0.05	11	4
583	**Pork spare ribs**, 'barbecue style', reheated	440	380	70	27	220	1.6	0.15	3.1	640	0.16	25	4
584	**Sausage casserole**, homemade	443	247	32	18	136	0.8	0.10	1.2	596	0.12	6	4
585	**Shish kebab**, meat only	510	420	7	29	250	2.6	0.14	6.1	N	0.03	4	6

Vitamins per 100g edible portion

No.	Food	Retinol µg	Carotene µg	Vitamin D µg	Vitamin E mg	Thiamin mg	Ribo-flavin mg	Niacin mg	Trypt 60 mg	Vitamin B6 mg	Vitamin B12 µg	Folate µg	Panto-thenate mg	Biotin µg	Vitamin C mg
Meat Dishes continued															
574	**Lamb curry**, made with cook-in sauce	6	236	0.3	2.33	0.11	0.12	3.0	2.9	0.18	1	7	0.74	3	2
575	**Lamb kheema**, homemade	2	236	0.4	3.58	0.18	0.10	2.5	2.0	0.14	1	7	0.39	1	4
576	**Lamb/beef hot pot with potatoes**, reheated	N	N	N	N	0.43	0.09	1.5	N	0.29	1	25	N	N	Tr
577	**Lasagne**, reheated	Tr	N	N	N	0.33	0.12	1.4	1.3	0.14	1	11	0.38	4	N
578	homemade	N	509	N	N	0.07	0.13	1.6	1.9	0.13	1	9	0.49	2	2
579	homemade, with extra lean minced beef	N	509	N	N	0.07	0.14	1.8	2.0	0.13	1	9	0.51	2	2
580	**Moussaka**, reheated	40	235	0.3	N	0.05	0.19	1.5	1.5	0.15	1	8	0.48	2	N
581	**Pasta with meat and tomato sauce**, homemade	Tr	148	0.1	0.97	0.02	0.04	1.7	1.4	0.12	Tr	6	0.32	1	Tr
582	**Pork casserole**, made with cook-in sauce	Tr	144	0.5	0.66	0.59	0.15	4.6	3.4	0.37	1	3	1.02	3	1
583	**Pork spare ribs**, 'barbecue style', reheated	7	220	1.7	0.05	0.82	0.38	7.0	7.3	0.30	1	7	2.64	4	Tr
584	**Sausage casserole**, homemade	Tr	12	0.5	0.65	0.35	0.10	2.7	2.2	0.21	1	7	0.59	2	1
585	**Shish kebab**, meat only	Tr	Tr	0.6	0.67	0.14	0.28	7.0	6.0	0.26	3	9	1.40	3	0

Composition of food per 100g edible portion

Meat Dishes continued

No.	Food	Description and main data sources	Main data reference	Water g	Total nitrogen g	Protein g	Fat g	Carbo-hydrate g	Energy value kcal	kJ
586	**Shish kebab**, in pitta bread with salad	Calculated from 37% shish kebab, 27% pitta bread and 36% salad.		65.1	2.22	13.6	4.1	15.4	149	629
587	**Spaghetti bolognese**[a], reheated, with spaghetti	Calculated as 56% white spaghetti and 44% retail meat and sauce.		70.2	1.09	6.6	2.8	20.0	126	536
588	**Spring rolls**, meat, takeaway	Analytical data, 1997	53	54.9	1.04	6.5	16.4	18.2[b]	242	1009
589	**Sweet and sour chicken**, takeaway	Analytical data, 1997	53	59.2	1.21	7.6	10.0	19.7[b]	194	814
590	**Sweet and sour pork**, homemade	Recipe		65.5	2.03	12.7	8.3	11.6[b]	176	736

[a] The publication number for Bolognese sauce (with meat), reheated is 551

[b] Includes oligosaccharides

Composition of food per 100g edible portion

No.	Food	Starch	Total sugars	Individual sugars					Dietary fibre		Fatty acids				Cholest-
				Gluc	Fruct	Sucr	Malt	Lact	NSP	AOAC	Satd	Mono- unsatd	Poly- unsatd	Trans	erol
		g	g	g	g	g	g	g	g	g	g	g	g	g	mg

Meat Dishes continued

No.	Food	Starch	Total sugars	Gluc	Fruct	Sucr	Malt	Lact	NSP	AOAC	Satd	Mono-unsatd	Poly-unsatd	Trans	Cholesterol
586	**Shish kebab**, in pitta bread with salad	14.1	1.3	0.4	0.4	Tr	0.5	0	1.1	1.2	1.5	1.6	0.5	0.2	33
587	**Spaghetti bolognese**, reheated, with spaghetti	18.1	1.9	0.5	0.6	0.3	0.5	0	1.2	N	1.1	1.1	0.4	0.1	N
588	**Spring rolls**, meat, takeaway	12.0	1.8[a]	0.4	0.6	0.5	0.3	Tr	1.9	2.0	3.8	7.1	4.8	Tr	7
589	**Sweet and sour chicken**, takeaway	8.8	10.7[a]	3.4	3.2	4.1	Tr	Tr	N	N	1.3	5.2	3.0	Tr	24
590	**Sweet and sour pork**, homemade	3.5	7.8[a]	1.2	1.1	5.5	0	0	0.5	N	2.0	2.6	3.2	Tr	49

[a] Not including oligosaccharides

Inorganic constituents per 100g edible portion

Meat Dishes continued

No.	Food	Na	K	Ca	Mg	P	Fe	Cu	Zn	Cl	Mn	Se	I
						mg						μg	
586	**Shish kebab**, in pitta bread with salad	300	283	48	20	127	1.5	0.09	2.6	N	0.19	2	3
587	**Spaghetti bolognese**, reheated, with spaghetti	182	151	24	20	74	0.9	0.04	0.9	308	0.25	5	N
588	**Spring rolls**, meat, takeaway	485	117	32	13	64	1.2	0.06	0.6	750	0.24	N	N
589	**Sweet and sour chicken**, takeaway	259	142	35	13	114	2.4	0.04	0.4	400	0.19	6	N
590	**Sweet and sour pork**, homemade	282	311	15	21	141	0.8	0.08	1.3	408	0.07	8	5

Meat and meat products *continued*

Vitamins per 100g edible portion

No.	Food	Retinol	Carotene	Vitamin D	Vitamin E	Thiamin	Ribo-flavin	Niacin	Trypt 60	Vitamin B$_6$	Vitamin B$_{12}$	Folate	Panto-thenate	Biotin	Vitamin C
		µg	µg	µg	mg	mg	mg	mg	mg	mg	µg	µg	mg	µg	mg
	Meat Dishes continued														
586	**Shish kebab**, in pitta bread with salad	Tr	22	0.2	0.48	0.19	0.14	3.4	2.8	0.10	1	30	0.59	1	Tr
587	**Spaghetti bolognese**, reheated, with spaghetti	Tr	N	N	N	N	N	N	N	N	N	N	N	N	Tr
588	**Spring rolls**, meat, takeaway	Tr	175	N	1.47	0.10	0.07	1.0	1.0	0.06	Tr	3	0.33	3	Tr
589	**Sweet and sour chicken**, takeaway	2	135	0.6	2.14	0.04	0.06	2.1	1.3	0.12	Tr	2	0.39	2	Tr
590	**Sweet and sour pork**, homemade	4	129	0.5	2.27	0.48	0.14	3.3	2.7	0.29	1	9	0.71	2	14

Fish and fish products

Section 2.6

Fish and fish products

New analytical data (2011/2012)[73] for a range of commonly consumed fish and fish products have been incorporated into this section. These include cod[73], haddock[73], prawns[73], canned fish[73] and breaded and battered fish[72,73], together with fish and fish products that have become more widely consumed, e.g. Alaskan pollock[73], pangasius[73] and sushi[65]. Values for less commonly consumed fish and fish products are largely based on data in the *Fish and Fish Products* (1993)[13] supplement, which are based on analytical data, mainly from the 1980s. In addition, values for processed fish and fish products have been reviewed using data from manufacturers, particularly fat and sodium values, and have been updated where necessary to reflect reformulation.

Fish are mainly drawn from a wild population, which means that their composition is probably more variable than that of foods drawn from domesticated inbred stock whose nutrition has been closely controlled. There is considerable variation in composition within one species and this variation could be greater than that between species.

The fat content of many fish show considerable seasonal changes and it is difficult to assign typical values. The actual fat content of fish normally landed and consumed shows less variation because the fish tend to be caught during a limited part of the cycle; the values used are therefore based on the fat content of the fish during the period when the major landings of the species are made.

In fish with fine bones it is often difficult to remove the bones completely, whether before analysis or before consumption. The calcium and phosphorus content of these fish is more variable than in a fish which can be boned easily. The values in the tables are based on samples which have been prepared for consumption in the normal way and so may contain a few bones.

The crustaceans and molluscs tend to accumulate many cations from their environment, and the concentration of iron, copper and zinc reported in these fish shows very wide variation, depending on the source of the samples and the metallic contamination to which they have been exposed.

Users should note that all values are expressed per 100g edible portion. Guidance for calculating nutrient content 'as purchased' or 'as served' (e.g. including bone or shells) is given in Section 4.2. For weight loss on cooking and calculation of the cooked edible portion obtainable from raw fish see Section 4.3. Losses of labile vitamins assigned to cooked dishes or foods were estimated from figures found in Section 4.3. Taxonomic names for foods in this part of the Tables can be found in Section 4.5.

Fish and fish products

Composition of food per 100g edible portion

No.	Food	Description and main data sources	Main data reference	Water g	Total nitrogen g	Protein g	Fat g	Carbo-hydrate g	Energy value kcal	Energy value kJ
White fish										
591	**Cod**, raw	Flesh only, frozen and chilled. Analytical data, 2010–2011	73	81.6	2.80	17.5	0.6	0	75	320
592	baked	Flesh only, frozen and chilled. Analytical data, 2010–2011	73	76.9	3.82	23.9	0.5	0	100	425
593	microwaved	Flesh only, frozen and chilled. Analytical data, 2010–2011	73	77.2	3.76	23.5	0.4	0	98	414
594	in batter, baked	Frozen and chilled. Analytical data, 2010; and industry data, 2013	72	56.0	1.97	12.3	11.8	19.7	229	961
595	in batter, fried in rapeseed oil[a]	Calculated from baked using analysed water and fat values	73	49.2	2.02	12.6	17.9	19.5	285	1189
596	in batter, fried, takeaway	Fried in beef fat or commercial vegetable oil. Analytical data, 2010	72	57.3	2.69	16.8	14.7	10.7	240	1001
597	in breadcrumbs, baked	Analytical data, 2010	72	55.5	2.19	13.7	8.3	19.8	204	858
598	**Coley**, raw	Flesh only, frozen and chilled. Analytical data, 2010–2011	73	81.9	2.88	18.0	1.1	0	82	347
599	baked	Flesh only, frozen and chilled. Calculated from raw using weight loss on cooking	73	75.5	3.90	24.4	1.5	0	111	469
600	**Haddock**, raw	Flesh only, frozen and chilled. Analytical data, 2010–2011	73	81.7	2.85	17.8	0.4	0	75	317
601	grilled	Flesh only, frozen and chilled. Analytical data, 2010–2011	73	75.9	3.82	23.9	0.3	0	98	417
602	steamed	Flesh only, frozen and chilled. Analytical data, 2010–2011	73	78.2	3.49	21.8	0.6	0	93	393
603	smoked, poached	Flesh only, frozen and chilled. Analytical data, 2010–2011	73	76.0	3.49	21.8	0.5	0	92	389
604	**Lemon sole**, raw	Flesh only, frozen and chilled. Analytical data, 2010–2011	73	82.7	2.67	16.7	0.7	0	73	310
605	grilled	Flesh only, frozen and chilled. Analytical data, 2010–2011	73	76.8	3.44	21.5	0.6	0	91	388
606	**Pangasius**, raw	Flesh only, frozen and chilled. Also known as Vietnamese river cobbler and basa. Analytical data, 2010–2011	73	83.7	2.38	14.9	1.6	0	74	313

[a] Most unspecified vegetable oils are made from rapeseed oil

Fish and fish products

Composition of food per 100g edible portion

No.	Food	Starch	Total sugars	Individual sugars					Dietary fibre		Fatty acids				Cholest-erol
				Gluc	Fruct	Sucr	Malt	Lact	NSP	AOAC	Satd	Mono-unsatd	Poly-unsatd	Trans	
		g	g	g	g	g	g	g	g	g	g	g	g	g	mg
White fish															
591	**Cod**, raw	0	0	0	0	0	0	0	0	0	0.2	0.1	0.1	Tr	52
592	baked	0	0	0	0	0	0	0	0	0	0.1	0.1	0.2	Tr	43
593	microwaved	0	0	0	0	0	0	0	0	0	0.1	0.1	0.1	Tr	35
594	in batter, baked	17.7	2.0	N	Tr	N	Tr	N	0.8	1.5	1.7	6.6	2.8	Tr	37
595	in batter, fried in rapeseed oil	18.1	1.4	N	Tr	N	Tr	N	0.8	1.5	2.1	10.3	4.5	Tr	37
596	in batter, fried, takeaway	9.7	1.0	0.1	0.2	0.3	0.3	Tr	0.5	0.5	7.6	5.4	0.9	0.3	60
597	in breadcrumbs, baked	18.9	0.9	0.2	Tr	0.1	0.6	Tr	1.7	1.9	1.3	4.6	1.9	Tr	36
598	**Coley**, raw	0	0	0	0	0	0	0	0	0	0.2	0.3	0.3	Tr	47
599	baked	0	0	0	0	0	0	0	0	0	0.3	0.4	0.4	Tr	64
600	**Haddock**, raw	0	0	0	0	0	0	0	0	0	0.1	0.1	0.1	Tr	49
601	grilled	0	0	0	0	0	0	0	0	0	0.1	0.1	0.1	Tr	41
602	steamed	0	0	0	0	0	0	0	0	0	0.1	0.1	0.2	Tr	74
603	smoked, poached	0	0	0	0	0	0	0	0	0	0.1	0.1	0.2	Tr	65
604	**Lemon sole**, raw	0	0	0	0	0	0	0	0	0	0.2	0.1	0.2	Tr	47
605	grilled	0	0	0	0	0	0	0	0	0	0.2	0.1	0.2	Tr	40
606	**Pangasius**, raw	0	0	0	0	0	0	0	0	0	0.5	0.4	0.2	Tr	36

Inorganic constituents per 100g edible portion

No.	Food	mg										µg	
		Na	K	Ca	Mg	P	Fe	Cu	Zn	Cl	Mn	Se	I

White fish

No.	Food	Na	K	Ca	Mg	P	Fe	Cu	Zn	Cl	Mn	Se	I
591	**Cod**, raw	91	322	12	25	169	0.1	0.02	0.3	165	0.01	23	196
592	baked	91	367	18	30	189	0.2	0.02	0.6	130	0.01	44	161
593	microwaved	108	427	16	32	216	0.2	0.02	0.5	168	0.01	44	243
594	in batter, baked	424	230	32	21	158	0.5	0.04	0.4	530	0.14	17	99
595	in batter, fried in rapeseed oil	424	230	32	21	158	0.5	0.04	0.4	530	0.14	17	99
596	in batter, fried, takeaway	175	326	79	26	208	0.4	0.04	0.5	220	0.09	22	214
597	in breadcrumbs, baked	330	245	41	22	137	0.5	0.05	0.4	480	0.17	21	99
598	**Coley**, raw	68	303	7	32	171	0.3	0.04	0.4	130	0.01	33	111
599	baked	92	410	10	43	231	0.4	0.05	0.6	176	0.01	45	151
600	**Haddock**, raw	68	315	11	25	163	0.1	0.02	0.3	110	0.01	34	320
601	grilled	92	433	20	33	232	0.2	0.02	0.5	130	0.01	48	421
602	steamed	84	376	14	28	199	0.2	0.03	0.4	120	0.01	51	381
603	smoked, poached	464	265	24	25	164	0.2	0.02	0.4	640	0.01	42	217
604	**Lemon sole**, raw	115	177	17	26	124	0.1	Tr	0.3	178	0.01	50	23
605	grilled	151	260	28	26	163	0.5	0.01	0.4	160	0.01	83	31
606	**Pangasius**, raw	204	293	10	29	166	0.1	0.02	0.3	190	0.01	18	3

Fish and fish products

Vitamins per 100g edible portion

No.	Food	Retinol	Carotene	Vitamin D	Vitamin E	Thiamin	Ribo-flavin	Niacin	Trypt 60	Vitamin B_6	Vitamin B_{12}	Folate	Panto-thenate	Biotin	Vitamin C
		µg	µg	µg	mg	mg	mg	mg	mg	mg	µg	µg	mg	µg	mg
White fish															
591	**Cod**, raw	2	Tr	Tr	0.66	0.06	0.08	2.3	2.6	0.14	2	7	0.25	1	Tr
592	baked	2	Tr	Tr	0.95	0.10	0.09	2.0	4.1	0.12	2	8	0.30	1	Tr
593	microwaved	2	Tr	Tr	0.86	0.08	0.10	1.8	3.7	0.13	2	8	0.28	1	Tr
594	in batter, baked	Tr	N	Tr	2.38	0.07	0.07	0.9	2.7	0.20	2	12	0.09	1	Tr
595	in batter, fried in rapeseed oil	Tr	Tr	Tr	3.73	0.07	0.07	0.9	2.8	0.20	2	12	0.09	1	Tr
596	in batter, fried, takeaway	Tr	Tr	Tr	1.48	0.07	0.12	2.1	3.6	0.24	2	16	0.18	1	Tr
597	in breadcrumbs, baked	Tr	N	Tr	1.84	0.08	0.11	1.6	2.9	0.19	1	7	0.17	3	Tr
598	**Coley**, raw	4	Tr	Tr	0.57	0.23	0.17	2.6	3.7	0.27	3	5	0.33	4	Tr
599	baked	5	Tr	Tr	0.77	0.22	0.18	2.8	5.0	0.33	4	6	0.36	5	Tr
600	**Haddock**, raw	1	Tr	Tr	0.49	0.13	0.15	4.9	3.1	0.29	2	10	0.27	2	Tr
601	grilled	1	Tr	Tr	0.52	0.09	0.14	4.0	4.3	0.29	2	6	0.28	2	Tr
602	steamed	1	Tr	Tr	0.57	0.07	0.11	3.9	4.1	0.24	2	9	0.29	2	Tr
603	smoked, poached	2	Tr	N	0.77	0.11	0.14	6.3	5.1	0.22	2	8	0.28	2	Tr
604	**Lemon sole**, raw	Tr	Tr	Tr	0.73	0.15	0.08	4.3	2.5	0.15	1	13	0.30	4	Tr
605	grilled	Tr	Tr	Tr	0.85	0.12	0.10	3.7	3.9	0.13	1	10	0.29	5	Tr
606	**Pangasius**, raw	Tr	Tr	1.4	0.23	0.02	0.06	6.3	3.5	0.12	1	10	0.66	38	Tr

Composition of food per 100g edible portion

No.	Food	Description and main data sources	Main data reference	Water (g)	Total nitrogen (g)	Protein (g)	Fat (g)	Carbo-hydrate (g)	Energy value kcal	Energy value kJ
White fish *continued*										
607	**Pangasius**, baked	Flesh only, frozen and chilled. Calculated from raw using weight loss on cooking	73	76.1	3.50	21.8	2.3	0	109	458
608	**Plaice**, raw	Flesh only, frozen and chilled. Analytical data, 2010-2011	73	80.4	2.62	16.4	1.2	0	76	323
609	baked	Flesh only, frozen and chilled. Calculated from raw using weight loss on cooking	73	74.6	3.40	21.3	1.6	0	99	419
610	in breadcrumbs, baked	Frozen and chilled. Analytical data, 2010-2011	73	52.8	2.30	14.4	11.6	21.5	243	1018
611	**Pollock**, Alaskan, raw	Flesh only, frozen and chilled. Analytical data, 2010-2011	73	83.7	2.62	16.4	0.7	0	72	305
612	Alaskan, baked	Flesh only, frozen and chilled. Calculated from raw using weight loss on cooking	73	72.0	4.51	28.2	1.2	0	124	523
613	**Sea bass**, baked	Flesh only, frozen and chilled. Analytical data, 2010-2011	73	69.0	3.71	23.2	6.8	0	154	646
Fatty fish										
614	**Anchovies**, canned in oil, drained	FFP Supplement, 1993; and industry data, 2013	13	46.4	4.03	25.2	10.0	0	191	798
615	**Herring**, grilled	Samples gutted. FFP Supplement, 1993	13	63.9	3.22	20.1	11.2[a]	0	181	756
616	**Kippers**, grilled	Flesh only, frozen and chilled. Analytical data, 2010-2011	73	58.6	3.47	21.7	17.6	0	245	1020
617	boil in the bag, with butter, cooked	Flesh only, frozen and chilled. Analytical data, 2010-2011	73	63.6	2.98	18.6	13.2	Tr	193	805
618	**Mackerel**, raw	Flesh only, frozen and chilled. Analytical data, 2010-2011	73	61.9[b]	2.88	18.0	17.9[c]	0	233	968
619	grilled	Flesh only, frozen and chilled. Analytical data, 2010-2011	73	53.8	3.25	20.3	22.4	0	283	1174
620	smoked	Flesh only, frozen and chilled. Analytical data, 2010-2011	73	50.9	3.38	21.1	24.1	0	301	1250
621	**Salmon**, farmed, raw	Fresh fillets, flesh only. Analytical data, 2002-2003	65	65.5	3.26	20.4	15.0	0	217	902

[a] Herring lose much of their accumulated energy between winter and spring

[b] Levels range from 56g to 74g water per 100g

[c] Levels range from 6g to 23g fat per 100g

No.	Food	Starch	Total sugars	Gluc	Fruct	Sucr	Malt	Lact	Dietary fibre NSP	Dietary fibre AOAC	Satd	Mono-unsatd	Poly-unsatd	Trans	Cholesterol
		g	g	g	g	g	g	g	g	g	g	g	g	g	mg
White fish continued															
607	**Pangasius**, baked	0	0	0	0	0	0	0	0	0	0.7	0.7	0.3	Tr	53
608	**Plaice**, raw	0	0	0	0	0	0	0	0	0	0.2	0.3	0.3	Tr	66
609	baked	0	0	0	0	0	0	0	0	0	0.3	0.3	0.3	Tr	86
610	in breadcrumbs, baked	20.2	1.3	0.2	Tr	Tr	1.1	Tr	0.5	1.5	1.2	5.6	4.0	Tr	39
611	**Pollock**, Alaskan, raw	0	0	0	0	0	0	0	0	0	0.1	0.2	0.2	Tr	49
612	Alaskan, baked	0	0	0	0	0	0	0	0	0	0.2	0.3	0.3	Tr	85
613	**Sea bass**, baked	0	0	0	0	0	0	0	0	0	1.5	2.3	2.1		49
Fatty fish															
614	**Anchovies**, canned in oil, drained	0	0	0	0	0	0	0	0	0	1.6	5.3	1.8	Tr	63
615	**Herring**, grilled	0	0	0	0	0	0	0	0	0	2.8	4.7	2.3	Tr	43
616	**Kippers**, grilled	0	0	0	0	0	0	0	0	0	3.7	7.4	3.7	Tr	65
617	boil in the bag, with butter, cooked	0	Tr	0	0	0	0	Tr	0	0	3.0	5.8	2.4	Tr	71
618	**Mackerel**, raw	0	0	0	0	0	0	0	0	0	3.9	6.7	4.5	Tr	60
619	grilled	0	0	0	0	0	0	0	0	0	5.1	8.3	5.4	Tr	75
620	smoked	0	0	0	0	0	0	0	0	0	5.0	9.4	6.1	Tr	63
621	**Salmon**, farmed, raw	0	0	0	0	0	0	0	Tr	0.2	2.8	6.0	4.1	Tr	68

Inorganic constituents per 100g edible portion

No.	Food	mg										µg	
		Na	K	Ca	Mg	P	Fe	Cu	Zn	Cl	Mn	Se	I
White fish continued													
607	**Pangasius**, baked	299	430	14	42	243	0.1	0.03	0.5	279	0.01	27	2
608	**Plaice**, raw	147	226	17	21	157	0.1	0.01	0.4	180	Tr	35	31
609	baked	191	293	22	27	203	0.1	0.01	0.6	233	Tr	45	40
610	in breadcrumbs, baked	275	178	61	22	126	0.8	0.05	0.6	390	0.19	30	16
611	**Pollock**, Alaskan, raw	68	216	12	30	120	0.2	0.03	0.4	100	0.01	27	56
612	Alaskan, baked	117	371	21	51	207	0.3	0.05	0.7	172	0.02	46	97
613	**Sea bass**, baked	80	390	31	35	231	0.3	0.04	0.8	100	0.03	24	10
Fatty fish													
614	**Anchovies**, canned in oil, drained	5870	230	300	56	300	4.1	0.17	3.0	9100	0.18	N	N
615	**Herring**, grilled	160	430	79	42	310	1.6	0.19	1.2	220	0.05	46	38
616	**Kippers**, grilled	947	384	39	47	270	1.5	0.11	1.1	1360	0.02	57	24
617	boil in the bag, with butter, cooked	860	254	47	38	208	1.1	0.12	1.5	1220	0.03	40	13
618	**Mackerel**, raw	153	335	20	37	220	1.0	0.08	0.5	250	0.01	42	29
619	grilled	163	349	17	38	236	1.3	0.10	0.8	290	0.01	60	35
620	smoked	746	319	33	38	237	1.1	0.07	0.9	1010	0.02	59	28
621	**Salmon**, farmed, raw	43	357	10	26	226	0.3	0.05	0.4	59	0.09	18	12

Fish and fish products *continued*

Vitamins per 100g edible portion

No.	Food	Retinol µg	Carotene µg	Vitamin D µg	Vitamin E mg	Thiamin mg	Ribo-flavin mg	Niacin mg	Trypt 60 mg	Vitamin B6 mg	Vitamin B12 µg	Folate µg	Panto-thenate mg	Biotin µg	Vitamin C mg
White fish continued															
607	**Pangasius**, baked	Tr	Tr	2.0	0.34	0.02	0.07	7.4	5.1	0.16	1	12	0.77	50	Tr
608	**Plaice**, raw	Tr	Tr	Tr	0.57	0.33	0.14	2.5	3.0	0.23	1	12	0.77	36	Tr
609	baked	Tr	Tr	Tr	0.74	0.30	0.15	2.5	3.9	0.27	2	12	0.80	42	Tr
610	in breadcrumbs, baked	N	N	Tr	3.32	0.32	0.14	2.3	2.7	0.09	2	9	0.43	35	Tr
611	**Pollock**, Alaskan, raw	Tr	Tr	Tr	0.60	0.03	0.09	2.6	2.6	0.04	2	5	0.22	1	Tr
612	Alaskan, baked	Tr	Tr	Tr	1.03	0.04	0.12	3.6	4.5	0.06	4	7	0.30	2	Tr
613	**Sea bass**, baked	24	Tr	Tr	0.33	0.19	0.18	2.6	4.9	0.14	3	4	0.63	3	Tr
Fatty fish															
614	**Anchovies**, canned in oil, drained	57	Tr	N	N	Tr	0.10	3.8	4.7	N	11	18	N	N	Tr
615	**Herring**, grilled	34	Tr	16.1	0.64	Tr	0.27	4.0	3.8	0.35	15	10	0.78	7	Tr
616	**Kippers**, grilled	26	Tr	10.1	0.47	Tr	0.27	5.1	4.5	0.29	11	3	0.81	6	Tr
617	boil in the bag, with butter, cooked	30	15	11.1	0.23	0.01	0.24	4.2	4.3	0.22	10	3	0.57	6	Tr
618	**Mackerel**, raw	54	Tr	8.0	0.43	0.17	0.30	11.3	4.4	0.40	9	1	0.63	6	Tr
619	grilled	61	Tr	8.5	0.46	0.14	0.37	11.1	4.4	0.27	9	1	0.57	5	Tr
620	smoked	36	Tr	8.2	0.46	0.15	0.37	6.9	4.6	0.28	10	4	0.61	4	Tr
621	**Salmon**, farmed, raw	16	1	4.7	3.95	0.45	0.07	7.7	3.4	0.21	4	5	1.20	1	Tr

Composition of food per 100g edible portion

Fatty fish continued

No.	Food	Description and main data sources	Main data reference	Water g	Total nitrogen g	Protein g	Fat g	Carbo-hydrate g	Energy value kcal	kJ
622	**Salmon**, farmed, grilled	Fresh fillets, flesh only. Analytical data, 2002-2003	65	60.4	3.94	24.6	15.6	0	239	995
623	farmed, steamed	Fresh fillets, flesh only. Analytical data, 2002-2003	65	58.9	3.78	23.6	18.5	0	261	1086
624	farmed, baked	Fresh fillets, flesh only. Analytical data, 2002-2003	65	59.7	4.03	25.2	14.6	0	232	969
625	wild, raw	Fresh steaks, flesh only. Analytical data, 2003-2003	65	67.5	3.53	22.1	10.1	0	179	749
626	smoked (cold-smoked)	Cured using salt and smoked at a low temperature; most smoked salmon is cold-smoked. Chilled. Analytical data, 2010-2011	73	64.5	3.65	22.8	10.1	0.5	184	769
627	smoked (hot-smoked)	Smoked over heat, flesh only. Analytical data, 2010-2011	73	60.1	4.06	25.4	8.8	1.3	186	778
628	pink, canned in brine, drained	Includes skin and some bones, large bones removed. Analytical data, 2010-2011	73	71.4	3.78	23.6	4.8	0	138	579
629	red, canned in brine, drained	Includes skin and some bones, large bones removed. Analytical data, 2010-2011	73	66.5	3.76	23.5	7.3	0	160	670
630	red, skinless and boneless, canned in brine, drained	Analytical data, 2010-2011	73	68.5	3.71	23.2	6.7	0	153	642
631	**Sardines**, grilled	Flesh only, frozen and chilled. Calculated from raw (analytical data 2010-2011) using weight loss on cooking	73	67.2	4.06	25.4	7.8	0	172	720
632	canned in brine, drained	Analytical data, 2010-2011	73	66.1	3.54	22.1	9.1	0	170	712
633	canned in tomato sauce, whole contents	Analytical data, 2010-2011	73	67.3	2.96	18.5	10.8	0.9	175	729

Fatty fish continued

No.	Food	Starch g	Total sugars g	Gluc g	Fruct g	Sucr g	Malt g	Lact g	Dietary fibre NSP g	AOAC g	Satd g	Mono-unsatd g	Poly-unsatd g	Trans g	Cholesterol mg
622	**Salmon**, farmed, grilled	0	0	0	0	0	0	0	Tr	Tr	3.0	6.2	4.2	Tr	72
623	farmed, steamed	0	0	0	0	0	0	0	Tr	Tr	3.5	7.3	4.9	Tr	85
624	farmed, baked	0	0	0	0	0	0	0	Tr	Tr	2.8	5.8	3.9	Tr	67
625	wild, raw	0	0	0	0	0	0	0	0	0	2.1	4.1	2.5	Tr	51
626	smoked (cold-smoked)	0	0.5	Tr	Tr	Tr	0.5	0	0	0	2.1	3.1	2.8	Tr	45
627	smoked (hot-smoked)	0	1.3	Tr	Tr	0.8	0.4	0	0	0	1.9	2.6	2.9	Tr	72
628	pink, canned in brine, drained	0	0	0	0	0	0	0	0	0	0.9	1.7	1.4	Tr	61
629	red, canned in brine, drained	0	0	0	0	0	0	0	0	0	1.4	3.0	1.8	Tr	62
630	red, skinless and boneless, canned in brine, drained	0	0	0	0	0	0	0	0	0	1.3	2.8	1.7	Tr	61
631	**Sardines**, grilled	0	0	0	0	0	0	0	0	0	2.4	2.3	2.0	Tr	65
632	canned in brine, drained	0	0	0	0	0	0	0	0	0	2.6	2.3	2.7	Tr	66
633	canned in tomato sauce, whole contents	Tr	0.9	0.3	0.6	Tr	0	0	Tr	Tr	2.9	2.7	3.5	Tr	71

Inorganic constituents per 100g edible portion

Fatty fish continued

No.	Food	Na	K	Ca	Mg	P	Fe	Cu	Zn	Cl	Mn	Se	I
						mg						µg	
622	**Salmon**, farmed, grilled	49	412	11	30	262	0.5	0.05	0.6	86	0.05	20	14
623	farmed, steamed	51	425	11	31	269	0.4	0.06	0.5	70	0.11	21	14
624	farmed, baked	49	412	11	30	262	0.5	0.05	0.6	86	0.05	20	14
625	wild, raw	48	382	15	29	250	0.5	0.07	0.5	83	Tr	27	12
626	smoked (cold-smoked)	1180	442	8	31	266	0.2	0.02	0.4	1480	0.01	19	9
627	smoked (hot-smoked)	848	460	8	32	293	0.3	0.05	0.5	1200	0.01	24	9
628	pink, canned in brine, drained	352	326	109	25	234	0.8	0.07	0.7	500	0.01	34	18
629	red, canned in brine, drained	430	305	164	29	291	0.7	0.06	0.8	670	0.02	37	22
630	red, skinless and boneless, canned in brine, drained	379	304	6	27	214	0.6	0.07	0.5	580	0.01	38	24
631	**Sardines**, grilled	174	496	63	40	329	2.0	0.17	0.9	256	0.04	65	101
632	canned in brine, drained	368	287	679	42	545	2.7	0.13	2.2	560	0.18	41	26
633	canned in tomato sauce, whole contents	315	371	455	38	417	2.7	0.12	2.0	480	0.18	39	26

Fish and fish products *continued*

Vitamins per 100g edible portion

No.	Food	Retinol	Carotene	Vitamin D	Vitamin E	Thiamin	Ribo-flavin	Niacin	Trypt 60	Vitamin B_6	Vitamin B_{12}	Folate	Panto-thenate	Biotin	Vitamin C
		µg	µg	µg	mg	mg	mg	mg	mg	mg	µg	µg	mg	µg	mg
Fatty fish continued															
622	**Salmon**, farmed, grilled	18	Tr	7.8	3.94	0.21	0.10	8.6	4.2	0.16	3	9	1.50	2	Tr
623	farmed, steamed	21	Tr	9.3	4.70	0.21	0.08	7.7	4.5	0.17	2	6	1.30	2	Tr
624	farmed, baked	17	Tr	7.3	3.70	0.26	0.09	8.6	4.2	0.14	3	8	1.50	3	Tr
625	wild, raw	27	Tr	8.6	1.11	0.19	0.10	9.8	2.9	0.16	7	1	1.30	2	Tr
626	smoked (cold-smoked)	28	Tr	8.9	2.03	0.43	0.12	8.3	5.4	0.73	3	15	1.22	5	Tr
627	smoked (hot-smoked)	28	Tr	11.0	2.29	0.41	0.16	9.5	6.5	0.51	4	14	1.35	4	Tr
628	pink, canned in brine, drained	12	Tr	13.6	0.76	0.02	0.21	7.4	6.0	0.19	5	19	0.68	5	Tr
629	red, canned in brine, drained	7	Tr	10.9	1.65	0.03	0.21	7.6	6.1	0.20	5	14	0.88	4	Tr
630	red, skinless and boneless, canned in brine, drained	10	Tr	11.8	1.47	0.04	0.22	6.9	6.1	0.23	5	12	0.82	5	Tr
631	**Sardines**, grilled	13	Tr	5.1	0.40	Tr	0.39	11.6	6.8	0.36	11	9	0.84	12	Tr
632	canned in brine, drained	10	Tr	3.3	0.24	0.01	0.22	5.5	4.2	0.07	11	4	0.64	5	Tr
633	canned in tomato sauce, whole contents	10	276	3.3	1.84	0.03	0.22	5.5	5.2	0.25	9	4	0.63	6	Tr

Fatty fish continued

Composition of food per 100g edible portion

No.	Food	Description and main data sources	Main data reference	Water g	Total nitrogen g	Protein g	Fat g	Carbo-hydrate g	Energy value kcal	kJ
634	**Sardines**, canned in sunflower oil, drained	Calculated from sardines in brine and sunflower oil; and industry data, 2013	73	58.6	3.73	23.3	14.1[a]	0	220	918
635	canned in olive oil, drained	Calculated from sardines in brine and olive oil; and industry data, 2013	73	58.6	3.73	23.3	14.1[a]	0	220	918
636	**Trout**, rainbow, raw	Flesh only, frozen and chilled. Analytical data, 2010-2011	73	76.1	3.18	19.9	5.3	0	127	534
637	rainbow, baked	Flesh only, frozen and chilled. Analytical data, 2010-2011	73	70.1	3.81	23.8	6.1[b]	0	150	630
638	**Tuna**, baked	Flesh only, frozen and chilled. Analytical data, 2010-2011	73	68.2	5.17	32.3	0.8	0	136	579
639	canned in brine, drained	Analytical data, 2010-2011	73	74.3	3.98	24.9	1.0	0	109	460
640	canned in sunflower oil, drained	Analytical data, 2010-2011	73	67.1	4.06	25.4	6.4	0	159	669
Crustacea										
641	**Crab**, canned in brine, drained	FFP Supplement, 1993; and industry data, 2013	13	79.2	2.90	18.1	0.5	Tr	77	326
642	cooked	Frozen and chilled, purchased cooked. Average of brown and white crab meat. Analytical data, 2010-2011	73	72.1	3.14	19.7	4.1	Tr	115	484
643	**Prawns**, king, raw	Warm-water prawns, frozen and chilled. Analytical data, 2010-2011	73	81.9	2.82	17.6	0.7	0	77	325
644	king, grilled from raw	Warm-water prawns, frozen and chilled. Analytical data, 2010-2011	73	73.8	3.76	23.5	0.9	0	102	433
645	king, cooked	Warm-water prawns, frozen and chilled, purchased cooked. Analytical data, 2010-2011	73	82.4	2.59	16.2	0.4	0	68	290

[a] If not drained the fat content is approximately 24.4g per 100g

[b] Skin contains 17.3g fat per 100g

Fish and fish products *continued*

Composition of food per 100g edible portion

No.	Food	Starch g	Total sugars g	Gluc g	Fruct g	Sucr g	Malt g	Lact g	NSP g	AOAC g	Satd g	Mono- unsatd g	Poly- unsatd g	Trans g	Cholest- erol mg
					Individual sugars				Dietary fibre		Fatty acids				
Fatty fish *continued*															
634	**Sardines**, canned in sunflower oil, drained	0	0	0	0	0	0	0	0	0	3.2	3.3	5.9	Tr	66
635	canned in olive oil, drained	0	0	0	0	0	0	0	0	0	3.3	6.0	3.1	Tr	66
636	**Trout**, rainbow, raw	0	0	0	0	0	0	0	0	0	1.2	1.5	1.8	Tr	60
637	rainbow, baked	0	0	0	0	0	0	0	0	0	1.4	1.6	2.2	Tr	69[a]
638	**Tuna**, baked	0	0	0	0	0	0	0	0	0	0.3	0.2	0.2	Tr	40
639	canned in brine, drained	0	0	0	0	0	0	0	0	0	0.3	0.2	0.4	Tr	47
640	canned in sunflower oil, drained	0	0	0	0	0	0	0	0	0	0.8	1.6	3.6	Tr	47
Crustacea															
641	**Crab**, canned in brine, drained	Tr	Tr	0	0	0	0	0	0	0	0.1	0.1	0.1	Tr	72
642	cooked	Tr	Tr	0	0	0	0	0	0	0	0.7	0.9	0.8	Tr	169
643	**Prawns**, king, raw	0	0	0	0	0	0	0	0	0	0.2	0.1	0.2	Tr	150
644	king, grilled from raw	0	0	0	0	0	0	0	0	0	0.2	0.1	0.3	Tr	193
645	king, cooked	0	0	0	0	0	0	0	0	0	0.1	0.1	0.1	Tr	162

[a] Skin contains 230mg cholesterol per 100g

Fish and fish products *continued*

Inorganic constituents per 100g edible portion

No.	Food	Na	K	Ca	Mg	P	Fe	Cu	Zn	Cl	Mn	Se	I
		mg										µg	
Fatty fish continued													
634	**Sardines**, canned in sunflower oil, drained	400	410	500	46	520	2.3	0.11	2.2	550	0.19	49	23
635	canned in olive oil, drained	400	410	500	46	520	2.3	0.11	2.2	550	0.19	49	23
636	**Trout**, rainbow, raw	110	383	21	26	228	0.3	0.04	0.5	150	0.01	19	5
637	rainbow, baked	93	434	19[a]	29	254[a]	0.4	0.05	0.6[a]	160	0.01	23	8
638	**Tuna**, baked	63	450	11	41	290	0.9	0.03	0.5	130	0.01	92	23
639	canned in brine, drained	293	230	10	27	171	1.5	0.07	0.9	490	0.01	69	12
640	canned in sunflower oil, drained	368	267	11	35	204	1.2	0.05	0.8	610	0.01	87	12
Crustacea													
641	**Crab**, canned in brine, drained	550	100	120	32	140	2.8	0.42	5.7	830	N	N	N
642	cooked	337	204	226	42	318	1.5	1.72	6.6	515	0.19	156	218
643	**Prawns**, king, raw	215	126	44	28	155	0.7	0.21	1.2	260	0.04	34	5
644	king, grilled from raw	305	181	59	37	209	0.4	0.35	1.6	310	0.05	41	7
645	king, cooked	643	65	49	21	125	0.3	0.23	1.0	740	0.03	30	12

[a] Skin contains 890mg Ca, 750mg P and 4.1mg Zn per 100g

Fish and fish products *continued*

Vitamins per 100g edible portion

No.	Food	Retinol µg	Carotene µg	Vitamin D µg	Vitamin E mg	Thiamin mg	Ribo-flavin mg	Niacin mg	Trypt 60 mg	Vitamin B6 mg	Vitamin B12 µg	Folate µg	Panto-thenate mg	Biotin µg	Vitamin C mg
Fatty fish continued															
634	**Sardines,** canned in sunflower oil, drained	11	Tr	3.6	2.73	0.01	0.29	6.9	4.4	0.18	15	8	0.89	5	Tr
635	canned in olive oil, drained	11	N	3.6	0.52	0.01	0.29	6.9	4.4	0.18	15	8	0.89	5	Tr
636	**Trout,** rainbow, raw	25	Tr	7.9	0.44	0.16	0.12	7.3	4.2	0.31	3	9	1.23	3	Tr
637	rainbow, baked	44	Tr	8.2[a]	0.89[a]	0.13	0.13	6.4	5.3	0.19	3	11	1.11	4	Tr
638	**Tuna,** baked	78	Tr	3.1	0.13	0.12	0.07	17.4	7.5	0.23	2	5	0.21	3	Tr
639	canned in brine, drained	26	Tr	1.1	0.42	Tr	0.11	10.3	6.2	0.31	3	3	0.19	3	Tr
640	canned in sunflower oil, drained	26	Tr	1.1	2.84	Tr	0.11	10.3	6.2	0.31	3	3	0.19	3	Tr
Crustacea															
641	**Crab,** canned in brine, drained	Tr	Tr	Tr	N	Tr	N	1.1	3.4	N	N	N	N	N	Tr
642	cooked	3	Tr	Tr	4.73	0.05	0.88	0.7	5.5	0.16	13	13	1.61	9	Tr
643	**Prawns,** king, raw	Tr	Tr	Tr	1.80	Tr	0.05	0.1	3.6	0.11	1	11	0.16	4	Tr
644	king, grilled from raw	Tr	Tr	Tr	1.64	Tr	0.07	0.1	3.4	0.14	2	10	0.20	4	Tr
645	king, purchased cooked	Tr	Tr	Tr	1.64	Tr	0.05	0.1	3.4	0.05	1	10	0.20	4	Tr

[a] Skin contains 24µg vitamin D and 2.9mg vitamin E per 100g

267

Composition of food per 100g edible portion

No.	Food	Description and main data sources	Main data reference	Water g	Total nitrogen g	Protein g	Fat g	Carbo- hydrate g	Energy value kcal	kJ
Crustacea continued										
646	**Prawns**, standard, cooked	Cold-water/Atlantic prawns, frozen and chilled, purchased cooked. Analytical data, 2010-2011	73	84.0	2.46	15.4	0.9	0	70	295
647	**Scampi**, coated in breadcrumbs, baked	Frozen and chilled. Analytical data, 2010-2011	73	50.7	1.86	11.6	10.5	24.3	232	975
648	coated in breadcrumbs, fried in rapeseed oil[a]	Calculated from baked using analysed water and fat values	73	51.6	1.70	10.6	13.0	22.2	243	1016
649	coated in breadcrumbs, fried in sunflower oil	Calculated from baked using analysed water and fat values	73	51.6	1.70	10.6	13.0	22.2	243	1016
Molluscs										
650	**Calamari**, coated in batter, baked	Frozen. Analytical data, 2010-2011	73	42.1	1.36	8.5	17.5	25.9	288	1206
651	**Cockles**, boiled	Fresh and frozen. Analytical data, 1986-1987	29	83.0	1.92	12.0	0.6	Tr	53	226
652	**Mussels**, cooked	Frozen and chilled, purchased cooked. Analytical data, 2010-2011	73	75.5	2.83	17.7	2.2	3.5[b]	104	438
653	in white wine sauce, cooked	Frozen and chilled. Analytical data, 2010-2011	73	82.0	1.55	9.7	3.2	3.7	82	347
Fish products and dishes										
654	**Curry**, fish, Bangladeshi, homemade	Containing boal, rohu, spices, water and onion. Recipe		71.5	1.98	12.4	8.0	1.5[c]	125	520
655	fish, homemade	Containing white fish, onions, tomatoes and spices. Analytical data, 2007	69	73.5	1.81	11.3	9.6	1.9	139	578

[a] Most unspecified vegetable oils are made from rapeseed oil

[b] As glycogen

[c] Includes oligosaccharides

Composition of food per 100g edible portion

No.	Food	Starch g	Total sugars g	Gluc g	Fruct g	Sucr g	Malt g	Lact g	Dietary fibre		Fatty acids				Cholest-erol mg
									NSP g	AOAC g	Satd g	Mono-unsatd g	Poly-unsatd g	Trans g	
Crustacea continued															
646	**Prawns**, standard, cooked	0	0	0	0	0	0	0	0	0	0.2	0.2	0.2	Tr	143
647	**Scampi**, coated in breadcrumbs, baked	23.5	0.8	Tr	Tr	Tr	0.8	Tr	0.3	1.5	0.9	6.3	2.7	Tr	64
648	coated in breadcrumbs, fried in rapeseed oil	21.5	0.7	Tr	Tr	Tr	0.7	Tr	0.3	1.4	1.0	7.8	3.5	Tr	58
649	coated in breadcrumbs, fried in sunflower oil	21.5	0.7	Tr	Tr	Tr	0.7	Tr	0.3	1.4	1.2	6.8	4.3	Tr	58
Molluscs															
650	**Calamari**, coated in batter, baked	25.9	Tr	Tr	Tr	Tr	Tr	0	0.4	1.9	2.1	4.7	9.8	Tr	85
651	**Cockles**, boiled	Tr	Tr	0	0	0	0	0	0	0	0.2	0.1	0.2	Tr	53
652	**Mussels**, cooked	Tr	Tr	0	0	0	0	0	0	0	0.3	0.3	0.6	Tr	45
653	in white wine sauce, cooked	2.9	0.8	0	0	0	0	0.8	Tr	Tr	1.3	0.8	0.9	Tr	25
Fish products and dishes															
654	**Curry**, fish, Bangladeshi, homemade	Tr	1.2[a]	0.4	0.4	0.4	0	0	0.2	0.8	0.8	1.4	4.1	Tr	N
655	fish, homemade	Tr	1.9[b]	0.5	0.7	0.4	0	0	1.5	2.1	1.7	3.5	3.8	Tr	14

[a] Not including oligosaccharides

[b] Including galactose

Inorganic constituents per 100g edible portion

No.	Food	Na	K	Ca	Mg	P	Fe	Cu	Zn	Cl	Mn	Se	I
						mg						µg	
Crustacea *continued*													
646	**Prawns**, standard, cooked	588	74	65	36	127	1.0	0.28	1.0	770	0.02	30	13
647	**Scampi**, coated in breadcrumbs, baked	561	234	105	34	260	1.9	0.18	0.8	620	0.27	26	101
648	coated in breadcrumbs, fried in rapeseed oil	512	213	96	31	237	1.7	0.16	0.7	565	0.25	24	92
649	coated in breadcrumbs, fried in sunflower oil	512	213	96	31	237	1.7	0.16	0.7	565	0.25	24	92
Molluscs													
650	**Calamari**, coated in batter, baked	1180	88	41	33	259	0.5	0.12	0.8	1280	0.19	17	3
651	**Cockles**, boiled	490	110	91	46	140	28.0	0.38	2.1	750	0.84	43	160
652	**Mussels**, cooked	401	116	40	50	258	3.3	0.17	3.4	700	0.18	66	247
653	in white wine sauce, cooked	608	173	68	76	122	1.5	0.08	1.5	970	0.07	32	282
Fish products and dishes													
654	**Curry**, fish, Bangladeshi, homemade	N	257	N	N	261	1.1	0.09	N	N	N	N	N
655	fish, homemade	430	323	45	27	112	1.1	0.08	0.4	662	N	15	N

Fish and fish products *continued*

Vitamins per 100g edible portion

No.	Food	Retinol µg	Carotene µg	Vitamin D µg	Vitamin E mg	Thiamin mg	Ribo-flavin mg	Niacin mg	Trypt 60 mg	Vitamin B$_6$ mg	Vitamin B$_{12}$ µg	Folate µg	Panto-thenate mg	Biotin µg	Vitamin C mg
Crustacea continued															
646	**Prawns**, standard, cooked	Tr	Tr	Tr	3.63	Tr	0.05	Tr	3.6	0.03	2	10	0.14	4	Tr
647	**Scampi**, coated in breadcrumbs, baked	Tr	Tr	Tr	3.18	0.16	0.06	2.1	2.4	0.06	2	14	0.29	2	Tr
648	coated in breadcrumbs, fried in rapeseed oil	Tr	Tr	Tr	3.74	0.15	0.05	1.9	2.2	0.05	1	13	0.26	2	Tr
649	coated in breadcrumbs, fried in sunflower oil	Tr	Tr	Tr	4.41	0.15	0.05	1.9	2.2	0.05	1	13	0.26	2	Tr
Molluscs															
650	**Calamari**, coated in batter, baked	64	Tr	Tr	0.75	0.05	0.40	1.2	2.2	0.03	2	3	0.68	3	Tr
651	**Cockles**, boiled	40	Tr	Tr	N	0.05	0.11	1.2	2.6	0.04	47	N	0.27	9	Tr
652	**Mussels**, cooked	117	Tr	Tr	1.72	0.02	0.26	1.0	4.6	0.03	11	25	0.32	11	Tr
653	in white wine sauce, cooked	10	3	Tr	0.84	0.05	0.18	0.8	1.8	0.03	9	26	0.39	5	Tr
Fish products and dishes															
654	**Curry**, fish, Bangladeshi, homemade	N	78	N	N	N	N	0.7	N	N	4	N	N	N	Tr
655	fish, homemade	Tr	112	1.4	3.24	Tr	0.04	1.7	N	Tr	1	9	0.12	7	Tr

Fish and fish products *continued*

Composition of food per 100g edible portion

No.	Food	Description and main data sources	Main data reference	Water g	Total nitrogen g	Protein g	Fat g	Carbohydrate g	Energy value kcal	kJ
	Fish products and dishes continued									
656	**Curry**, prawn, takeaway	Including bhuna and madras. Analytical data, 1997	53	76.4	1.31	8.2	8.5	2.3	118	491
657	**Fishcakes**, white fish, coated in breadcrumbs, baked	Frozen and chilled. Analytical data, 2010-2011	73	56.9	1.49	9.3	9.4	22.6	206	867
658	salmon, coated in breadcrumbs, baked	Frozen and chilled. Analytical data, 2010-2011	73	54.7	1.82	11.4	13.7	20.4	245	1027
659	**Fish fingers**, cod, grilled/baked	Frozen. Analytical data, 2010-2011	73	54.5	2.29	14.3	9.2	22.0	223	936
660	cod, fried in rapeseed oil[a]	Calculated from grilled/baked using analysed water and fat values	73	54.5	2.08	13.0	12.6	19.9	240	1006
661	cod, fried in sunflower oil	Calculated using analysed water and fat values	73	54.5	2.08	13.0	12.6	19.9	240	1006
662	pollock, grilled	Frozen. Analytical data, 2010	72	54.6	2.22	13.9	9.2	20.0	213	897
663	salmon, grilled/baked	Frozen. Analytical data, 2010-2011	73	50.8	2.75	17.2	11.2	20.7	247	1038
664	**Fish paste**	Sardine, crab, lobster and salmon. FFP Supplement, 1993; and industry data, 2013	13	67.1	2.45	15.3	10.5	3.7	170	708
665	**Fish pie**, white fish	Frozen and chilled. Analytical data, 2010-2011	73	73.8	1.06	6.6	4.8	14.4	124	521
666	**Kedgeree**, homemade	Recipe		67.5	2.55	15.9	7.7	9.1	167	699
667	**Salmon en croute**	Calculated from manufacturers' proportions		49.3	1.93	11.8	19.1	18.0	288	1202
668	**Seafood selection**	Calculated from mussels, prawns, squid and cockles		75.3	2.50	15.6	1.5	2.9[b]	87	369
669	**Seafood sticks**	Frozen and chilled. Analytical data, 2010-2011	73	73.3	1.17	7.3	1.9	14.9	102	433
670	**Sesame prawn toast**, takeaway	Analytical data, 1997	53	35.8	2.06	12.9	29.8	16.7[c]	382	1589
671	**Sushi**, salmon nigiri	Analytical data, 2002-2003; and industry data, 2013	65	59.8	1.39	8.7	2.5	25.2[c]	152	644

[a] Most unspecified vegetable oils are made from rapeseed oil

[b] As glycogen

[c] Includes oligosaccharides

Composition of food per 100g edible portion

| No. | Food | Starch g | Total sugars g | Individual sugars | | | | | Dietary fibre | | Fatty acids | | | | Cholesterol mg |
				Gluc g	Fruct g	Sucr g	Malt g	Lact g	NSP g	AOAC g	Satd g	Mono-unsatd g	Poly-unsatd g	Trans g	erol mg
	Fish products and dishes continued														
656	**Curry**, prawn, takeaway	0.9	1.4	0.5	0.6	0.1	0.1	0.1	2.0	2.5	1.4	3.8	2.9	Tr	144
657	**Fishcakes**, white fish, coated in breadcrumbs, baked	20.8	1.8	0.2	0.2	0.1	1.3	Tr	0.4	1.7	1.0	5.5	2.3	Tr	30
658	salmon, coated in breadcrumbs, baked	18.8	1.6	0.1	0.2	Tr	1.3	Tr	0.4	1.7	2.0	7.0	3.7	Tr	25
659	**Fish fingers**, cod, grilled/baked	20.6	1.5	Tr	Tr	0.2	1.3	Tr	1.6	2.0	1.2	4.4	3.0	Tr	36
660	cod, fried in rapeseed oil	18.6	1.3	Tr	Tr	0.2	1.1	Tr	1.4	1.8	1.4	6.4	4.0	Tr	36
661	cod, fried in sunflower oil	18.6	1.3	Tr	Tr	0.2	1.1	Tr	1.4	1.8	1.6	5.1	5.2	Tr	33
662	pollock, grilled	18.7	1.3	0.4	0.1	Tr	0.8	Tr	1.6	2.0	1.2	4.3	3.2	Tr	44
663	salmon, grilled/baked	19.6	1.1	0.1	0.1	Tr	0.9	Tr	1.6	2.0	1.1	5.8	3.6	Tr	29
664	**Fish paste**	3.2	0.5	Tr	Tr	0.5	Tr	0	N	2.6	N	N	N	N	N
665	**Fish pie**, white fish	12.7	1.8	0.2	Tr	0.3	Tr	1.3	0.6	2.1	2.6	1.5	0.3	0.1	29
666	**Kedgeree**, homemade	9.1	Tr	Tr	Tr	Tr	0	Tr	Tr	0.2	2.4	3.2	1.3	Tr	129
667	**Salmon en croute**	17.1	0.9	0.1	Tr	0.1	0.5	0.2	N	N	N	N	N	N	31
668	**Seafood selection**	Tr	Tr	0	0	0	0	0	0	0	0.3	0.2	0.5	N	115
669	**Seafood sticks**	10.1	4.8	Tr	Tr	4.8	0	0	0	0	0.3	0.7	0.7	Tr	16
670	**Sesame prawn toast**, takeaway	13.9	0.8^a	Tr	Tr	Tr	0.8	Tr	1.8	3.6	3.8	15.1	9.5	Tr	48
671	**Sushi**, salmon nigiri	21.9	3.2^a	0.5	0.5	1.5	0.7	0	0.7	1.2	0.5	1.0	0.7	Tr	21

a Not including oligosaccharides

273

Inorganic constituents per 100g edible portion

No.	Food	Na	K	Ca	Mg	P	Fe	Cu	Zn	Cl	Mn	Se	I
		mg										µg	
Fish products and dishes *continued*													
656	**Curry**, prawn, takeaway	311	198	97	26	95	4.2	0.12	0.8	440	0.31	14	34
657	**Fishcakes**, white fish, coated in breadcrumbs, baked	356	233	51	19	102	0.8	0.06	0.4	520	0.17	13	58
658	salmon, coated in breadcrumbs, baked	322	269	42	21	150	0.8	0.05	0.4	470	0.15	13	6
659	**Fish fingers**, cod, grilled/baked	317	254	32	25	142	0.6	0.05	0.5	460	0.20	18	117
660	cod, fried in rapeseed oil	287	230	29	23	129	0.5	0.05	0.4	417	0.18	16	106
661	cod, fried in sunflower oil	287	230	29	23	129	0.5	0.05	0.4	417	0.18	16	106
662	pollock, grilled	401	263	23	26	143	0.5	0.08	0.5	580	0.21	15	47
663	salmon, grilled/baked	288	300	14	30	194	0.8	0.07	0.6	420	0.32	24	7
664	**Fish paste**	430	300	280	33	310	N	0.60	2.0	660	N	N	310[a]
665	**Fish pie**, white fish	254	300	86	21	119	0.4	0.04	0.5	380	0.08	7	33
666	**Kedgeree**, homemade	343	181	33	19	150	0.6	0.05	0.7	474	0.08	31	127
667	**Salmon en croute**	190	200	47	18	140	0.6	0.08	0.5	320	0.13	N	N
668	**Seafood selection**	620	160	52	32	170	5.6	0.36	2.4	940	0.20	N	N
669	**Seafood sticks**	714	21	50	8	61	0.2	0.01	0.3	940	0.02	19	21
670	**Sesame prawn toast**, takeaway	470	143	114	60	180	1.8	0.24	1.5	610	0.38	19	13
671	**Sushi**, salmon nigiri	360	132	10	13	90	0.2	0.07	0.4	564	0.18	8	4

[a] Crab paste contains 240µg I and salmon paste 370µg I per 100g

Vitamins per 100g edible portion

Fish products and dishes continued

No.	Food	Retinol µg	Carotene µg	Vitamin D µg	Vitamin E mg	Thiamin mg	Ribo- flavin mg	Niacin mg	Trypt 60 mg	Vitamin B6 mg	Vitamin B12 µg	Folate µg	Panto- thenate mg	Biotin µg	Vitamin C mg
656	**Curry**, prawn, takeaway	7	279	Tr	3.16	0.02	0.05	0.6	1.2	0.08	Tr	4	0.30	2	2
657	**Fishcakes**, white fish, coated in breadcrumbs, baked	1	Tr	Tr	1.98	0.25	0.07	1.7	1.9	0.09	1	6	0.31	2	Tr
658	salmon, coated in breadcrumbs, baked	2	Tr	5.7	2.79	0.38	0.10	4.7	2.8	0.22	2	14	0.74	2	Tr
659	**Fish fingers**, cod, grilled/baked	1	Tr	Tr	2.75	0.17	0.08	1.2	3.4	0.09	2	9	0.24	1	Tr
660	cod, fried in rapeseed oil	1	Tr	Tr	3.51	0.15	0.07	1.1	3.1	0.08	1	8	0.22	1	Tr
661	cod, fried in sunflower oil	1	Tr	Tr	4.42	0.15	0.07	1.1	3.1	0.08	1	8	0.22	1	Tr
662	pollock, grilled	Tr	Tr	Tr	2.70	0.09	0.12	0.8	3.3	0.18	Tr	32	0.16	Tr	Tr
663	salmon, grilled/baked	7	Tr	4.5	2.82	0.41	0.11	5.3	4.1	0.22	2	15	0.58	3	Tr
664	**Fish paste**	19[a]	Tr	N	0.87	0.02	0.20	4.1	2.9	N	N	N	N	N	Tr
665	**Fish pie**, white fish	83	6	2.8	0.51	0.11	0.13	0.8	1.6	0.02	1	9	0.40	3	2
666	**Kedgeree**, homemade	N	44	N	N	0.09	0.20	3.5	3.8	0.15	2	14	0.5	5	Tr
667	**Salmon en croute**	30	13	3.4	N	0.13	0.07	2.5	2.3	0.31	2	12	N	N	Tr
668	**Seafood selection**	6	Tr	Tr	0.56	0.03	0.20	1.2	3.3	0.14	15	N	0.30	N	Tr
669	**Seafood sticks**	Tr	Tr	Tr	0.47	0.01	0.06	1.2	2.0	0.03	1	12	0.30	3	Tr
670	**Sesame prawn toast**, takeaway	Tr	1	Tr	5.05	0.10	0.05	1.6	1.8	0.08	1	13	0.24	1	Tr
671	**Sushi**, salmon nigiri	2	Tr	2.5	0.17	0.04	0.05	2.7	1.2	0.15	1	6	0.46	Tr	Tr

[a] Salmon paste contains 49µg retinol per 100g

Composition of food per 100g edible portion

No.	Food	Description and main data sources	Main data reference	Water g	Total nitrogen g	Protein g	Fat g	Carbo-hydrate g	Energy value kcal	Energy value kJ

Fish products and dishes continued

No.	Food	Description and main data sources	Main data reference	Water g	Total nitrogen g	Protein g	Fat g	Carbo-hydrate g	kcal	kJ
672	**Sushi**, tuna nigiri	Analytical data, 2002-2003; and industry data, 2013	65	61.5	1.34	8.4	2.5	30.3[a]	170	720
673	**Szechuan prawns with vegetables**, takeaway	Analytical data, 1997	53	81.1	1.25	7.8	4.7	2.5[a]	83	347
674	**Taramasalata**	Greek dish based on cod roe. FFP Supplement, 1993; and industry data, 2013	13	35.9	0.51	3.2	52.9	7.4	517	2130
675	**Tuna pate**	Industry data, 2013		53.4	2.59	16.2	26.8	1.5	312	1291

[a] Includes oligosaccharides

276

Fish products and dishes continued

No.	Food	Starch g	Total sugars g	Individual sugars					Dietary fibre		Fatty acids				Cholest- erol mg
				Gluc g	Fruct g	Sucr g	Malt g	Lact g	NSP g	AOAC g	Satd g	Mono- unsatd g	Poly- unsatd g	Trans g	
672	**Sushi**, tuna nigiri	25.5	4.7[a]	1.0	0.5	2.2	0.9	0.1	0.7	1.2	0.7	0.8	0.7	Tr	8
673	**Szechuan prawns with vegetables**, takeaway	1.2	0.8[a]	0.4	0.4	Tr	Tr	Tr	1.4	1.2	0.7	2.4	1.4	Tr	56
674	**Taramasalata**	6.2	1.2	N	N	N	Tr	Tr	Tr	0.3	4.1	29.3	16.7	Tr	25
675	**Tuna pate**	1.1	0.4	0.1	0.1	0.2	0	0	N	0.7	3.9	12.1	9.0	N	N

[a] Not including oligosaccharides

Inorganic constituents per 100g edible portion

No.	Food	Na	K	Ca	Mg	P	Fe	Cu	Zn	Cl	Mn	Se	I
							mg					μg	

Fish products and dishes continued

No.	Food	Na	K	Ca	Mg	P	Fe	Cu	Zn	Cl	Mn	Se	I
672	**Sushi**, tuna nigiri	331	137	8	15	88	0.3	0.07	0.4	523	0.18	20	4
673	**Szechuan prawns with vegetables,** takeaway	536	102	40	15	65	1.1	0.11	0.4	827	Tr	N	N
674	**Taramasalata**	450	60	21	6	50	0.4	N	0.4	720	0.12	N	N
675	**Tuna pate**	390	170	12	21	130	0.8	0.05	0.5	640	Tr	N	17

Fish and fish products *continued*

Vitamins per 100g edible portion

No.	Food	Retinol µg	Carotene µg	Vitamin D µg	Vitamin E mg	Thiamin mg	Ribo-flavin mg	Niacin mg	Trypt 60 mg	Vitamin B$_6$ mg	Vitamin B$_{12}$ µg	Folate µg	Panto-thenate mg	Biotin µg	Vitamin C mg
Fish products and dishes continued															
672	**Sushi,** tuna nigiri	N	Tr	3.6	Tr	0.02	0.04	4.4	1.0	0.14	1	3	0.14	Tr	Tr
673	**Szechuan prawns with vegetables,** takeaway	Tr	569	N	1.99	0.02	N	0.4	N	0.06	N	12	N	N	2
674	**Taramasalata**	N	N	N	N	0.08	0.10	0.3	0.6	N	3	4	N	N	1
675	**Tuna pate**	N	N	N	N	0.02	0.09	10.1	3.2	0.34	3	4	0.22	1	1

Vegetables

Section 2.7

Vegetables

New analytical data (2012)[74] for a range of the most commonly consumed vegetables (including potatoes) and a few vegetable products have been incorporated into this section. There are also analytical data for a few vegetables that have not previously been analysed, including pak choi, baby spinach and rocket. For other vegetables, the values have largely been taken from the *Vegetables, Herbs and Spices* (1991)[9] and *Vegetable Dishes* (1992)[12] supplements, based on analytical data from the 1980s[24,25,26,31].

Because many of the vegetables and pulses eaten in the UK are imported, a larger number of literature values from sources outside the UK have been used in this food group than in many other food groups in the Tables.

For boiled vegetables, values are based on boiling in unsalted water. The amount of salt added to vegetables when boiled can vary considerably, but values for some vegetables boiled in water containing 0.5% salt are available in the CoFID. For fried foods, the type of oil used for frying has been included in the name and will determine the fatty acid profile of that particular food. Most values for cooked foods were obtained by analysis, but some were calculated from raw foods. Nutrient losses for these foods were estimated using the factors shown in Section 4.3. The changes in weight of beans, lentils and some other vegetables when soaked and cooked are shown in Section 4.3.

Samples of vegetables always vary somewhat in composition. Some nutrients differ in a consistent way between varieties of a vegetable and with season. There are also differences with the length of storage, the depth of peeling, the number of outer leaves removed and with cooking conditions (such as the extent to which a vegetable is cut up, the amount of water and the length of cooking).

Canned vegetables were analysed after draining liquid contents, therefore values are for the vegetable portion only, except where otherwise stated, e.g. tomatoes, canned, whole contents. Data from manufacturers has been used to review and update canned and processed vegetables, vegetable products and potato products to reflect reductions made in salt and sugar content.

Users should note that all values are expressed per 100g edible portion. Guidance for calculating nutrient content 'as purchased' or 'as served' (e.g. with or without pods, tough skin and outer leaves) is given in Section 4.2. Taxonomic names for foods in this part of the Tables can be found in Section 4.5.

Composition of food per 100g edible portion

No.	Food	Description and main data sources	Main data reference	Water g	Total nitrogen g	Protein g	Fat g	Carbo-hydrate g	Energy value kcal	kJ
Potatoes										
676	**New and salad potatoes**, boiled in, unsalted water, flesh and skin	Small potatoes with thin skins, including salad potatoes such as Charlotte, Anya and Exquisa boiled for 12-23 mins. Analytical data, 2011	74	81.5	0.29	1.8	0.1	14.9	64	272
677	**Old potatoes**, raw, flesh only	Autumn and winter, white and red varieties including Desiree, Maris Piper, King Edwards and Harmony. Analytical data, 2011-2012	74	78.1	0.31	1.9	0.1	19.6	82	349
678	boiled in unsalted water, flesh only	As raw, boiled for 10-25 mins. Analytical data, 2011-2012	74	78.9	0.28	1.8	0.1	17.5	74	315
679	baked, flesh and skin	As raw, baked for 40-60 mins. Analytical data, 2011-2012	74	71.0	0.40	2.5	0.2	22.6	97	413
680	microwaved, flesh and skin	As raw, cooked for 5-9 mins. Analytical data, 2012	74	73.2	0.41	2.6	0.1	21.5	92	392
681	mashed with butter	Calculated from 100g boiled potatoes, 5g salted butter, 7g semi-skimmed milk.		76.7	0.29	1.9	3.9	15.9	102	430
682	mashed with reduced fat spread	Calculated from 100g boiled potatoes, 5g polyunsaturated reduced fat spread (41-62%), 7g semi-skimmed milk.		77.8	0.28	1.8	2.8	15.9	93	391
683	roasted in rapeseed oil[a]	Calculated from raw, parboiled for 5-10 mins and roasted for 50 mins. Water and fat analysed, 2012	74	64.9	0.42	2.6	5.7	26.4	161	678
684	roasted in sunflower oil	Calculated from raw, parboiled for 5-10 mins and roasted for 50 mins. Water and fat analysed, 2012	74	64.9	0.42	2.6	5.7	26.4	161	678
685	wedges with skin, homemade, cooked in rapeseed oil[a]	Calculated from baked. Water and fat analysed, 2012	74	62.6	0.46	2.9	3.8	26.5	145	614

[a] Most unspecified vegetable oils are made from rapeseed oil

Composition of food per 100g edible portion

Potatoes

No.	Food	Starch g	Total sugars g	Individual sugars					Dietary fibre		Fatty acids				Cholesterol mg
				Gluc g	Fruct g	Sucr g	Malt g	Lact g	NSP g	AOAC g	Satd g	Mono-unsatd g	Poly-unsatd g	Trans g	
676	**New and salad potatoes**, boiled in unsalted water, flesh and skin	13.8	1.1	0.5	0.4	0.2	0	0	0.9	1.8	Tr	Tr	Tr	0	0
677	**Old potatoes**, raw, flesh only	18.7	0.9	0.5	0.4	Tr	0	0	0.8	2.0	Tr	Tr	Tr	0	0
678	boiled in unsalted water, flesh only	16.7	0.8	0.3	0.3	0.2	0	0	1.0	1.6	Tr	Tr	Tr	0	0
679	baked, flesh and skin	21.2	1.4	0.6	0.5	0.3	0	0	1.4	2.6	0.1	Tr	Tr	0	0
680	microwaved, flesh and skin	19.4	2.1	0.9	0.8	0.4	0	0	1.4	2.7	Tr	Tr	Tr	0	0
681	mashed with butter	14.9	1.0	0.3	0.3	0.2	0	0.3	0.9	1.4	2.4	1.0	0.1	0.1	10
682	mashed with reduced fat spread	14.9	1.0	0.3	0.3	0.2	Tr	0.3	0.9	1.4	0.7	0.8	1.1	Tr	Tr
683	roasted in rapeseed oil	25.2	1.2	0.7	0.5	Tr	0	0	1.1	2.7	0.4	3.3	1.7	Tr	0
684	roasted in sunflower oil	25.2	1.2	0.7	0.5	Tr	0	0	1.1	2.7	0.7	1.2	3.6	Tr	0
685	wedges with skin, homemade, cooked in rapeseed oil	24.8	1.7	0.7	0.6	0.4	0	0	1.6	3.0	0.3	2.2	1.1	Tr	0

Inorganic constituents per 100g edible portion

No.	Food	Na	K	Ca	Mg	P	Fe	Cu	Zn	Cl	Mn	Se	I
						mg						µg	
676	**New and salad potatoes**, boiled in unsalted water, flesh and skin	3	377	11	18	44	0.6	0.08	0.2	88	0.1	Tr	Tr
Potatoes													
677	**Old potatoes**, raw, flesh only	2	443	7	21	34	0.3	0.06	0.3	83	0.1	Tr	1
678	boiled in unsalted water, flesh only	1	365	6	18	31	0.3	0.06	0.2	74	0.1	Tr	1
679	baked, flesh and skin	2	600	11	27	45	0.6	0.09	0.4	114	0.2	Tr	1
680	microwaved, flesh and skin	2	585	13	27	43	0.8	0.09	0.4	121	0.2	Tr	1
681	mashed with butter	36	337	14	17	35	0.3	0.05	0.2	56	0.1	Tr	4
682	mashed with reduced fat spread	30	337	13	17	34	0.3	0.05	0.2	45	0.1	Tr	3
683	roasted in rapeseed oil	3	597	9	28	46	0.4	0.08	0.4	112	0.2	Tr	2
684	roasted in sunflower oil	3	597	9	28	46	0.4	0.08	0.4	112	0.2	Tr	1
685	wedges with skin, homemade, cooked in rapeseed oil	2	702	13	32	52	0.7	0.11	0.4	133	0.2	Tr	1

Vitamins per 100g edible portion

No.	Food	Retinol µg	Carotene µg	Vitamin D µg	Vitamin E mg	Thiamin mg	Ribo-flavin mg	Niacin mg	Trypt 60 mg	Vitamin B_6 mg	Vitamin B_{12} µg	Folate µg	Panto-thenate mg	Biotin µg	Vitamin C mg
676	**New and salad potatoes**, boiled in unsalted water, flesh and skin	0	Tr	0	0.11	0.13	0.01	0.7	0.4	0.13	0	21	0.51	0.3	7
Potatoes															
677	**Old potatoes**, raw, flesh only	0	Tr	0	0.01	0.20	0.01	0.3	0.4	0.14	0	13	0.44	0.3	14[a]
678	boiled in unsalted water, flesh only	0	Tr	0	0.01	0.21	Tr	0.5	0.4	0.06	0	18	0.43	0.3	9
679	baked, flesh and skin	0	Tr	0	0.05	0.20	0.02	0.9	0.4	0.11	0	18	0.46	0.3	6
680	microwaved, flesh and skin	0	Tr	0	0.13	0.23	0.01	0.8	0.4	0.14	0	33	0.48	0.3	5
681	mashed with butter	44	28	0	0.09	0.19	0.02	0.3	0.4	0.06	0.1	17	0.43	0.5	8
682	mashed with reduced fat spread	28	21	0.3	1.19	0.19	0.02	0.3	0.4	0.06	0.1	17	0.43	0.5	8
683	roasted in rapeseed oil	0	Tr	0	N	0.22	0.01	0.4	0.5	0.14	0	8	0.47	0.3	13
684	roasted in sunflower oil	0	Tr	0	2.77	0.22	0.01	0.4	0.5	0.14	0	8	0.47	0.3	13
685	wedges with skin, homemade, cooked in rapeseed oil	0	Tr	0	N	0.23	0.02	1.1	0.5	0.13	0	21	0.54	0.4	7

[a] It has been reported that freshly dug potatoes contain 21mg vitamin C per 100g which falls to 9mg per 100g after 3 months storage and to 7mg after 9 months

Composition of food per 100g edible portion

No.	Food	Description and main data sources	Main data reference	Water g	Total nitrogen g	Protein g	Fat g	Carbohydrate g	Energy value kcal	kJ
Potatoes continued										
686	**Old potatoes,** wedges with skin, homemade, cooked in sunflower oil	Calculated from baked. Water and fat analysed, 2012	74	62.6	0.46	2.9	3.8	26.5	145	614
Potato products										
687	**Chips,** fine cut, from fast food outlets	Including McDonald's, Burger King, Wimpy, KFC. Analytical data, 2011	72	38.5	0.55	3.5	14.2[a]	39.7	290	1219
688	fried in commercial oil, from takeaway fish and chip shops	Cooked in beef fat or commercial vegetable oil. Analytical data, 2011	72	51.0	0.56	3.5	8.4[a]	33.2	214	902
689	homemade, fried in rapeseed oil[b]	Calculated from raw and deep fried in corn oil	74, 9	55.9	0.57	3.6	6.7[a]	34.1	202	854
690	microwave, cooked	Cooked as packet directions. Analytical data, 1990; and industry data, 2013	31	50.4	0.58	3.6	9.6	32.1	221	930
691	oven ready, no batter, baked	Straight cut and crinkle cut. Analytical data, 2011	72	54.2	0.51	3.2	4.9	35.3	189	800
692	oven ready, with batter, baked	Including McCain Homefries and Crispy French Fries, Aunt Bessie's Homestyle Chips and own brands. Analytical data, 2011	72	51.9	0.54	3.4	6.1	35.6	202	852
693	**Instant potato powder,** made up with water	Calculated from ingredients, made up as packet directions. VHS Supplement, 1991; and industry data, 2013	9	83.3	0.24	1.5	0.1	13.5	57	245
694	**Potato products,** shaped, baked	Frozen, including waffles, smiley faces and letters. Analytical data, 2012	74	55.4	0.40	2.5	8.3	28.1	190	799

[a] The fat content of chips will be variable and dependent on a number of factors related to their preparation

[b] Most unspecified vegetable oils are made from rapeseed oil

Potatoes continued

Potato products

| No. | Food | Starch g | Total sugars g | Individual sugars | | | | | Dietary fibre | | Fatty acids | | | | Cholest-erol mg |
				Gluc g	Fruct g	Sucr g	Malt g	Lact g	NSP g	AOAC g	Satd g	Mono-unsatd g	Poly-unsatd g	Trans g	
686	**Old potatoes**, wedges with skin, homemade, cooked in sunflower oil	24.8	1.7	0.7	0.6	0.4	0	0	1.6	3.0	0.5	0.8	2.4	Tr	0
687	**Chips**, fine cut, from fast food outlets	39.4	0.3	Tr	Tr	0.3	Tr	Tr	3.2	3.8	2.5	7.8	3.2	Tr	Tr
688	fried in commercial oil, from takeaway fish and chip shops	32.7	0.6	0.1	0.1	0.3	Tr	Tr	3.7	3.2	4.3	3.2	0.5	0.2	1
689	homemade, fried in rapeseed oil	33.2	0.9	0.5	0.4	Tr	0	0	1.4	3.4	0.4	3.9	1.9	Tr	0
690	microwave, cooked	31.5	0.6	0.2	0.1	0.3	0	0	2.9	2.9	0.6	N	N	N	0
691	oven ready, no batter, baked	34.3	1.0	0.4	0.3	0.4	Tr	Tr	2.7	3.5	0.8	1.4	2.5	Tr	0
692	oven ready, with batter, baked	35.2	0.4	0.1	Tr	0.3	Tr	Tr	2.9	3.3	1.3	1.8	2.8	Tr	Tr
693	**Instant potato powder**, made up with water	12.7	0.7	0.1	0.1	Tr	0	0.6	1.0	1.2	Tr	Tr	0.1	Tr	0
694	**Potato products**, shaped, baked	27.7	0.4	0.2	Tr	0.2	0	0	2.8	2.7	0.9	3.3	3.7	Tr	0

Vegetables continued

Inorganic constituents per 100g edible portion

No.	Food	mg										µg	
		Na	K	Ca	Mg	P	Fe	Cu	Zn	Cl	Mn	Se	I
Potatoes continued													
686	**Old potatoes**, wedges with skin, homemade, cooked in sunflower oil	2	702	13	32	52	0.7	0.11	0.4	133	0.2	Tr	1
Potato products													
687	**Chips**, fine cut, from fast food outlets	193[a]	544	18	29	143	0.7	0.08	0.4	260	0.2	Tr	2
688	fried in commercial oil, from takeaway fish and chip shops	16[b]	804	16	32	63	0.7	0.14	0.4	120[b]	0.2	Tr	2
689	homemade, fried in rapeseed oil	3	812	15	39	57	0.6	0.11	0.6	151	0.3	Tr	2
690	microwave, cooked	40[c]	530	17	30	99	1.0	0.14	0.4	64	0.2	Tr	1
691	oven ready, no batter, baked	31	641	14	31	95	0.7	0.12	0.4	100	0.2	Tr	2
692	oven ready, with batter, baked	193	602	17	32	111	0.7	0.15	0.4	320	0.2	Tr	1
693	**Instant potato powder**, made up with water	100	260	13	12	41	0.4	0.04	0.2	150	0.1	N	N
694	**Potato products**, shaped, baked	254	423	29	22	55	0.7	0.13	0.4	423	0.2	Tr	N

[a] The composite sample included sub-samples with and without added salt, unsalted french fries contain approximately 35mg Na per 100g

[b] No salt added to purchased products

[c] Value is for unsalted products. Salted products contain 250mg Na per 100g

No.	Food	Retinol µg	Carotene µg	Vitamin D µg	Vitamin E mg	Thiamin mg	Ribo-flavin mg	Niacin mg	Trypt 60 mg	Vitamin B_6 mg	Vitamin B_{12} µg	Folate µg	Panto-thenate mg	Biotin µg	Vitamin C mg
	Potatoes continued														
686	**Old potatoes** wedges with skin, homemade, cooked in sunflower oil	0	Tr	0	N	0.23	0.02	1.1	0.5	0.13	0	21	0.54	0.4	7
	Potato products														
687	**Chips**, fine cut, from fast food outlets	0	Tr	0	3.28	0.07	0.09	0.6	0.4	0.04	0	38	0.49	0.2	2
688	fried in commercial oil, from takeaway fish and chip shops	Tr	Tr	0	0.32	0.10	0.10	0.6	0.5	0.05	0	46	0.51	0.3	2
689	homemade, fried in rapeseed oil	0	Tr	0	N	0.23	0.01	0.3	0.7	0.10	0	16	0.30	0.4	11
690	microwave, cooked	0	Tr	0	N	0.12	0.07	2.1	0.9	0.29	0	20	N	N	11
691	oven ready, no batter, baked	0	Tr	0	1.37	0.05	0.12	1.4	0.7	0.20	0	22	0.25	0.3	1
692	oven ready, with batter, baked	0	Tr	0	1.84	0.09	0.11	3.2	0.7	0.20	0	13	0.22	0.5	1
693	**Instant potato powder**, made up with water	0	3	0	0.05	0.01	0.03	1.2	0.4	0.15	0	2	N	N	23
694	**Potato products**, shaped, baked	0	Tr	0	2.70	0.19	0.02	0.8	0.5	0.10	0	17	0.29	0.8	44

No.	Food	Description and main data sources	Main data reference	Water g	Total nitrogen g	Protein g	Fat g	Carbo-hydrate g	Energy value kcal	kJ

Composition of food per 100g edible portion

Potato products continued

No.	Food	Description and main data sources	Main data reference	Water g	Total nitrogen g	Protein g	Fat g	Carbo-hydrate g	Energy value kcal	kJ
695	**Potato wedges**, retail, cooked	Frozen. Analytical data, 2002	65	61.5	0.45	2.8	5.5	30.6	176	741

Beans and lentils

No.	Food	Description and main data sources	Main data reference	Water g	Total nitrogen g	Protein g	Fat g	Carbo-hydrate g	Energy value kcal	kJ
696	**Baked beans**, canned in tomato sauce	Analytical data, 2013	74	72.8	0.81	5.0	0.5	15.0	81	343
697	canned in tomato sauce, reduced sugar, reduced salt	Analytical data, 2013; and industry data, 2013	74	72.8	0.81	5.0	0.5	13.5	75	320
698	**Beans**, green, raw	Autumn and winter. Analytical data, 2011	74	91.3	0.33	2.1	0.4	3.1	24	102
699	green, boiled in unsalted water	As raw, boiled for 3-6 minutes. Analytical data, 2011	74	89.6	0.33	2.1	0.3	4.0	26	108
700	**Beansprouts**, mung, raw	Analytical data, 1984-87	24	90.4	0.47	2.9	0.5	4.0	31	131
701	mung, stir-fried in rapeseed oil[a]	Stir-fried for 2 minutes. Analytical data, 1990	31	88.4	0.30	1.9	6.1	2.5	72	298
702	**Blackeye beans**, dried, boiled in unsalted water	Soaked and boiled. Analytical data, 1990	31	66.2	1.41	8.8	0.7	19.9[b]	116	494
703	**Broad beans**, boiled in unsalted water	Without pods, boiled for 20 minutes. Analytical data, 1984-87	24	82.8	0.82	5.1	0.8	5.6[b]	48	204
704	**Butter beans**, canned in water, re-heated, drained	No added salt. VHS Supplement, 1991; and industry data, 2013	9	74.0	0.95	5.9	0.5	13.0[b]	77	327
705	**Chick peas**, whole, dried, boiled in unsalted water	Soaked and boiled. Analytical data, 1990	31	65.8	1.35	8.4	2.1	18.2[b]	121	512

[a] Most unspecified vegetable oils are made from rapeseed oil

[b] Includes oligosaccharides

Composition of food per 100g edible portion

No.	Food	Starch g	Total sugars g	Gluc g	Fruct g	Sucr g	Malt g	Lact g	Dietary fibre NSP g	AOAC g	Fatty acids Satd g	Mono- unsatd g	Poly- unsatd g	Trans g	Cholest- erol mg
Potato products continued															
695	**Potato wedges**, retail, cooked	29.7	0.8	0.2	0.2	0.3	0.1	0	3.2	4.3	2.5	2.2	0.5	0.3	0
Beans and lentils															
696	**Baked beans**, canned in tomato sauce	10.2	4.8	0.6	0.8	3.4	0	0	3.8	4.9	0.1	0.1	0.3	Tr	0
697	canned in tomato sauce, reduced sugar, reduced salt	10.2	3.3	0.6	0.8	1.9	0	0	3.8	4.9	0.1	0.1	0.3	Tr	0
698	**Beans**, green, raw	1.0	2.2	0.8	1.4	Tr	0	0	2.5	3.4	0.1	Tr	0.2	0	0
699	green, boiled in unsalted water	0.9	3.0	1.3	1.2	0.5	0	0	2.5	4.1	0.1	Tr	0.2	0	0
700	**Beansprouts**, mung, raw	1.8	2.2	1.1	1.1	Tr	0	0	1.5	N	0.1	0.1	0.2	0	0
701	mung, stir-fried in rapeseed oil	1.1	1.4	0.6	0.8	Tr	0	0	0.9	N	0.5	3.4	1.8	Tr	0
702	**Blackeye beans**, dried, boiled in unsalted water	18.0	1.1[a]	0.1	Tr	0.9	Tr	0	3.5	N	0.2	0.1	0.3	0	0
703	**Broad beans**, boiled in unsalted water	4.3	0.9[a]	0.1	0.2	0.6	0	0	5.4	N	0.1	0.1	0.4	0	0
704	**Butter beans**, canned in water, re-heated, drained	10.9	1.1[a]	Tr	Tr	1.1	0	0	4.6	N	0.1	Tr	0.2	0	0
705	**Chick peas**, whole, dried, boiled in unsalted water	16.6	1.0[a]	Tr	0.1	0.9	0	0	4.3	N	0.2	0.4	1.0	Tr	0

[a] Not including oligosaccharides

No.	Food	Inorganic constituents per 100g edible portion											
		mg										µg	
		Na	K	Ca	Mg	P	Fe	Cu	Zn	Cl	Mn	Se	I
Potato products *continued*													
695	**Potato wedges**, retail, cooked	198	516	21	26	92	2.5	0.16	0.5	315	0.2	1	1
Beans and lentils													
696	**Baked beans**, canned in tomato sauce	261	272	42	30	88	1.4	0.24	0.6	471	0.3	3	Tr
697	canned in tomato sauce, reduced sugar, reduced salt	190	272	42	30	88	1.4	0.24	0.6	340	0.3	3	Tr
698	**Beans**, green, raw	Tr	286	52	25	38	1.0	0.06	0.4	69	0.3	1	2
699	green, boiled in unsalted water	Tr	304	61	28	44	1.1	0.07	0.4	54	0.4	1	2
700	**Beansprouts**, mung, raw	5	74	20	18	48	1.7	0.08	0.3	15	0.3	1	N
701	mung, stir-fried in rapeseed oil	3	45	12	11	29	1.0	0.05	0.2	9	0.2	1	N
702	**Blackeye beans**, dried, boiled in unsalted water	5	320	21	45	140	1.9	0.22	1.1	N	0.5	3	N
703	**Broad beans**, boiled in unsalted water	20	190	18	19	100	0.8	0.13	0.7	14	0.2	N	4
704	**Butter beans**, canned in water, re-heated, drained	Tr[a]	290	15	27	68	1.5	0.14	0.6	N[a]	0.3	3	N
705	**Chick peas**, whole, dried, boiled in unsalted water	5	270	46	37	83	2.1	0.28	1.2	7	0.7	1	N

[a] Butter beans canned in salted water contain 200mg Na and 310mg Cl per 100g

Vitamins per 100g edible portion

No.	Food	Retinol µg	Carotene µg	Vitamin D µg	Vitamin E mg	Thiamin mg	Ribo-flavin mg	Niacin mg	Trypt 60 mg	Vitamin B$_6$ mg	Vitamin B$_{12}$ µg	Folate µg	Panto-thenate mg	Biotin µg	Vitamin C mg
Potato products continued															
695	**Potato wedges**, retail, cooked	0	10	Tr	N	0.08	0.06	2.2	0.4	0.10	0	10	0.39	0.5	Tr
Beans and lentils															
696	**Baked beans**, canned in tomato sauce	0	23	0	0.35	0.21	0.03	0.7	1.0	0.13	0	29	0.11	2.5	Tr
697	canned in tomato sauce, reduced sugar, reduced salt	0	23	0	0.35	0.21	0.03	0.7	1.0	0.13	0	29	0.11	2.5	Tr
698	**Beans**, green, raw	0	253	0	0.44	0.12	0.09	0.8	0.4	0.06	0	58	0.11	1.0	8
699	green, boiled in unsalted water	0	143	0	0.26	0.08	0.08	0.7	0.4	0.02	0	58	0.12	0.7	6
700	**Beansprouts**, mung, raw	0	40	0	N	0.11	0.04	0.5	0.5	0.10	0	61	0.38	N	7
701	mung, stir-fried in rapeseed oil	0	24	0	N	0.06	0.02	0.3	0.3	0.07	0	43	0.23	N	7
702	**Blackeye beans**, dried, boiled in unsalted water	0	13	0	N	0.19	0.05	0.5	1.9	0.10	0	210	0.30	7.0	Tr
703	**Broad beans**, boiled in unsalted water	0	145	0	0.40	0.03	0.06	3.0	0.8	0.08	0	32	3.80	2.1	20
704	**Butter beans**, canned in water, re-heated, drained	0	Tr	0	0.33	0.05	0.03	0.2	0.9	0.05	0	12	N	N	Tr
705	**Chick peas**, whole, dried, boiled in unsalted water	0	23	0	1.10	0.10	0.07	0.7	1.1	0.14	0	66	0.29	N	Tr

Composition of food per 100g edible portion

No.	Food	Description and main data sources	Main data reference	Water (g)	Total nitrogen (g)	Protein (g)	Fat (g)	Carbohydrate (g)	Energy value kcal	Energy value kJ
	Beans and lentils continued									
706	**Chick peas**, canned in water, re-heated, drained	No added salt. VHS Supplement, 1991; and industry data, 2013	9	67.5	1.15	7.2	2.9	16.1[a]	115	487
707	**Gram flour**	Analytical data, 2003	68	9.0	3.62	22.7	5.4	57.0[a]	353	1498
708	**Houmous**	Industry data, 2013		51.7	1.09	6.8	26.7	10.5[a]	307	1272
709	**Lentils**, red, split, dried, raw	VHS Supplement, 1991	9	11.1	3.80	23.8	1.3	56.3[a]	318	1353
710	red, split, dried, boiled in unsalted water	Boiled for 20 minutes. VHS Supplement, 1991	9	72.1	1.22	7.6	0.4	17.5[a]	100	424
711	**Mung beans**, whole, dried, boiled in unsalted water	Literature sources	9	69.3	1.21	7.6	0.4	15.3[a]	91	389
712	**Red kidney beans**, dried, raw	Analytical data, 1990	31	11.2	3.54	22.1	1.4	44.1[a]	266	1133
713	dried, boiled in unsalted water	Soaked and boiled. Analytical data, 1990	31	66.0	1.35	8.4	0.5	17.4[a]	103	440
714	canned in water, re-heated, drained	VHS Supplement, 1991; and industry data, 2013	9	70.1	1.11	6.9	0.6	15.7[a]	92	391
715	**Runner beans**, raw	Ends and sides trimmed. Analytical data, 1984-87	24	91.2	0.26	1.6	0.4	3.2	22	93
716	boiled in unsalted water	Sliced and boiled for 20 minutes. Analytical data, 1984-87	24	92.8	0.19	1.2	0.5	2.3	18	76
717	**Soya beans**, dried, raw	Analytical data, 1990	31	8.5	5.74	35.9	18.6	15.8[a]	370	1551
718	dried, boiled in unsalted water	Analytical data, 1990	31	64.3	2.24	14.0	7.3	5.1[a]	141	590
719	**Tofu**, soya bean, steamed	Soya bean curd. VHS Supplement, 1991	9	85.0	1.29	8.1	4.2	0.7[a]	73	304
720	soya bean, steamed, fried	Calculated from steamed; and literature sources, 1986	135	51.0	3.76	23.5	17.7	2.0[a]	261	1086

[a] Includes oligosaccharides

Beans and lentils continued

No.	Food	Starch g	Total sugars g	Gluc g	Fruct g	Sucr g	Malt g	Lact g	NSP g	AOAC g	Satd g	Mono-unsatd g	Poly-unsatd g	Trans g	Cholesterol mg
				Individual sugars					Dietary fibre		Fatty acids				
706	Chick peas, canned in water, re-heated, drained	15.1	0.4[a]	Tr	Tr	0.4	0	0	4.1	N	0.3	0.7	1.3	Tr	0
707	Gram flour	51.5	2.3[a]	Tr	Tr	2.3	0	0	9.1	10.1	0.3	0.4	1.1	Tr	0
708	Houmous	9.3	0.6[a]	Tr	0.1	0.5	0	0	N	4.9	N	N	N	N	0
709	Lentils, red, split, dried, raw	50.8	2.4[a]	Tr	0.2	2.2	0	0	4.9	N	0.2	0.2	0.5	Tr	0
710	red, split, dried, boiled in unsalted water	16.2	0.8[a]	Tr	0.1	0.7	0	0	1.9	N	Tr	0.1	0.2	Tr	0
711	Mung beans, whole, dried, boiled in unsalted water	14.1	0.5[a]	0.1	0.1	0.3	0	0	3.0	N	0.1	Tr	0.2	Tr	0
712	Red kidney beans, dried, raw	38.0	2.5[a]	0.2	0.1	2.2	0	0	15.7	N	0.2	0.1	0.8	Tr	0
713	dried, boiled in unsalted water	14.5	1.0[a]	0.1	Tr	0.8	0	0	6.7	N	0.1	Tr	0.3	Tr	0
714	canned in water, re-heated, drained	13.7	0.6[a]	0.1	Tr	0.5	0	0	6.2	N	0.1	0.1	0.3	Tr	0
715	Runner beans, raw	0.4	2.8	0.9	1.3	0.6	0	0	2.0	N	0.1	Tr	0.2	0	0
716	boiled in unsalted water	0.3	2.0	0.6	0.9	0.5	0	0	1.9	N	0.1	Tr	0.3	0	0
717	Soya beans, dried, raw	4.8	5.5[a]	0.2	0.5	4.8	0	0	15.7	N	2.3	3.5	9.1	Tr	0
718	dried, boiled in unsalted water	1.9	2.1[a]	0.1	0.2	1.9	0	0	6.1	N	0.9	1.4	3.5	Tr	0
719	Tofu, soya bean, steamed	0.3	0.3[a]	Tr	Tr	0.2	0	0	N	N	0.5	0.8	2.0	Tr	0
720	soya bean, steamed, fried	0.9	0.9[a]	0.1	0.1	0.6	0	0	N	N	N	N	N	Tr	0

[a] Not including oligosaccharides

Inorganic constituents per 100g edible portion

Beans and lentils continued

No.	Food	mg										µg	
		Na	K	Ca	Mg	P	Fe	Cu	Zn	Cl	Mn	Se	I
706	**Chick peas**, canned in water, re-heated, drained	Tr[a]	110	43	24	81	1.5	0.05	0.8	N[a]	0.8	1	N
707	**Gram flour**	2	297	58	62	220	2.6	0.27	1.5	71	1.6	4	Tr
708	**Houmous**	410	190	41	62	160	1.9	0.30	1.4	N	0.5	4	N
709	**Lentils**, red, split, dried, raw	36	710	51	83	320	7.6	0.58	3.1	64	N	6	N
710	red, split, dried, boiled in unsalted water	12	220	16	26	100	2.4	0.19	1.0	20	N	2	N
711	**Mung beans**, whole, dried, boiled in unsalted water	2	270	24	43	81	1.4	0.19	0.9	4	0.3	5	N
712	**Red kidney beans**, dried, raw	18	1370	100	150	410	6.4	0.68	3.0	2	1.2	16	N
713	dried, boiled in unsalted water	2	420	37	45	130	2.5	0.23	1.0	1	0.5	6	N
714	canned in water, re-heated, drained	Tr	280	71	30	130	2.0	Tr	0.7	N	0.3	6	N
715	**Runner beans**, raw	Tr	220	33	19	34	1.2	0.02	0.2	21	0.2	N	2
716	boiled in unsalted water	1	130	22	14	21	1.0	0.01	0.2	5	0.2	N	Tr
717	**Soya beans**, dried, raw	5	1730	240	250	660	9.7	1.55	4.3	7	2.6	14	6
718	dried, boiled in unsalted water	1	510	83	63	250	3.0	0.32	0.9	3	0.7	5	2
719	**Tofu**, soya bean, steamed	4	63	N[b]	23[b]	95	1.2	0.20	0.7	N	0.4	N	N
720	soya bean, steamed, fried	12	180	N	67	270	3.5	0.58	2.0	N	1.2	N	N

[a] Chick peas canned in salted water contain 220mg Na and 280mg Cl per 100g

[b] If nigari is used as a coagulant Ca and Mg are 150mg and 59mg per 100g respectively

Vegetables continued

Vitamins per 100g edible portion

No.	Food	Retinol µg	Carotene µg	Vitamin D µg	Vitamin E mg	Thiamin mg	Ribo-flavin mg	Niacin mg	Trypt 60 mg	Vitamin B_6 mg	Vitamin B_{12} µg	Folate µg	Panto-thenate mg	Biotin µg	Vitamin C mg
	Beans and lentils continued														
706	**Chick peas**, canned in water, re-heated, drained	0	21	0	1.55	0.05	0.03	0.2	1.0	0.04	0	11	N	N	Tr
707	**Gram flour**	0	32	0	2.54	0.45	0.17	1.9	4.2	0.45	0	193	1.24	8.4	Tr
708	**Houmous**	0	N	0	N	0.16	0.05	1.1	1.0	0.15	0	42	0.39	N	1
709	**Lentils**, red, split, dried, raw	0	60	0	N	0.50	0.20	2.0	3.2	0.60	0	35	1.36	N	Tr
710	red, split, dried, boiled in unsalted water	0	20	0	N	0.11	0.04	0.4	1.0	0.11	0	33	0.31	N	Tr
711	**Mung beans**, whole, dried, boiled in unsalted water	0	12	0	N	0.09	0.07	0.5	1.2	0.07	0	35	0.41	N	Tr
712	**Red kidney beans**, dried, raw	0	11	0	0.52	0.65	0.19	2.1	3.5	0.40	0	130	0.78	N	4
713	dried, boiled in unsalted water	0	4	0	0.20	0.17	0.05	0.6	1.3	0.12	0	42	0.22	N	1
714	canned in water, re-heated, drained	0	4	0	0.19	0.21	0.06	0.6	1.1	0.11	0	15	0.15	N	Tr
715	**Runner beans**, raw	0	145	0	0.23	0.06	0.03	Tr	0.4	0.08	0	60	0.05	0.7	18
716	boiled in unsalted water	0	120	0	0.23	0.05	0.02	Tr	0.3	0.04	0	42	0.04	0.5	10
717	**Soya beans**, dried, raw	0	12	0	2.90	0.61	0.27	2.2	5.7	0.38	0	370	0.79	65.0	Tr
718	dried, boiled in unsalted water	0	6	0	1.13	0.12	0.09	0.5	2.2	0.23	0	54	0.18	25.0	Tr
719	**Tofu**, soya bean, steamed	0	2	0	0.95	0.06	0.02	0.1	1.3	0.07	0	15	0.05	N	0
720	soya bean, steamed, fried	0	2	0	N	0.09	0.02	0.1	3.8	0.10	0	27	0.14	N	0

Composition of food per 100g edible portion

No.	Food	Description and main data sources	Main data reference	Water g	Total nitrogen g	Protein g	Fat g	Carbo-hydrate g	Energy value kcal	Energy value kJ
Peas										
721	**Mange-tout peas**, raw	Whole pods, ends trimmed. Analytical data, 1990	31	88.7	0.58	3.6	0.2	4.2	32	136
722	boiled in unsalted water	As raw, boiled for 3 minutes. Analytical data, 1990; and calculated from raw	31	89.2	0.51	3.2	0.1	3.3	26	111
723	stir-fried in rapeseed oil[a]	As raw, stir-fried for 5 minutes. Analytical data, 1990; and calculated from raw	31	83.6	0.61	3.8	4.8	3.5	71	298
724	**Marrowfat peas**, canned, re-heated, drained	Analytical data, 1985; and industry data, 2013	25	69.0	1.10	6.9	0.8	13.8[b]	87	368
725	**Mushy peas**, canned, re-heated	Analytical data, 1985; and industry data, 2013	25	76.5	0.92	5.8	0.7	13.8[b]	81	345
726	**Peas**, raw	Whole peas, no pods. Analytical data, 1984-87	24	74.6	1.10	6.9	1.5	11.3[b]	83	354
727	boiled in unsalted water	As raw, boiled for 20 minutes. Analytical data, 1984-87	24	75.6	1.07	6.7	1.6	10.0[b]	79	329
728	canned in water, re-heated, drained	No added salt. VHS Supplement, 1991; and industry data, 2013	9	77.9	0.85	5.3	0.9	8.0	59	251
729	frozen, raw	Garden peas and petit pois. Analytical data, 2012	74	78.9	0.85	5.3	0.7	10.7	68	288
730	frozen, boiled in unsalted water	Calculated from raw using a weight loss of 3.8%	74	76.6	0.88	5.5	0.7	11.2	70	299
731	frozen, microwaved	As raw, cooked for 2-4.5 minutes. Analytical data, 2012	74	77.6	0.91	5.7	0.9	10.8	71	303
Vegetables, general										
732	**Asparagus**, raw	Tough base of stems removed. Analytical data, 1984-87	24	91.4	0.47	2.9	0.6	2.0	25	103
733	boiled in unsalted water	Soft tips only, boiled for 15 minutes. Analytical data, 1984-87	24	91.5	0.55	3.4	0.8	1.4	26	110

[a] Most unspecified vegetable oils are made from rapeseed oil

[b] Includes oligosaccharides

No.	Food	Starch	Total sugars	Individual sugars					Dietary fibre		Fatty acids				Cholest-erol
				Gluc	Fruct	Sucr	Malt	Lact	NSP	AOAC	Satd	Mono-unsatd	Poly-unsatd	Trans	
		g	g	g	g	g	g	g	g	g	g	g	g	g	mg
Peas															
721	**Mange-tout peas**, raw	0.8	3.4	2.6	0.3	0.5	0	0	2.3	N	N	N	N	Tr	0
722	boiled in unsalted water	0.5	2.8	2.1	0.1	0.6	0	0	2.2	2.4	Tr	Tr	Tr	Tr	0
723	stir-fried in rapeseed oil	0.2	3.3	2.4	0.2	0.7	0	0	2.4	2.4	0.3	2.9	1.4	Tr	0
724	**Marrowfat peas**, canned, re-heated, drained	11.3	0.9[a]	Tr	Tr	0.9	0	0	4.1	5.0	0.1	0.2	0.3	Tr	0
725	**Mushy peas**, canned, re-heated	10.7	1.7[a]	Tr	Tr	1.6	0	0	1.8	3.1	0.1	0.1	0.3	Tr	0
726	**Peas**, raw	7.0	2.3[a]	0.1	0.1	2.1	0	0	4.7	5.3	0.6	0.5	0.2	Tr	0
727	boiled in unsalted water	7.6	1.2[a]	Tr	Tr	1.2	0	0	4.5	5.6	0.3	0.2	0.8	Tr	0
728	canned in water, re-heated, drained	6.3	1.7	Tr	Tr	1.7	0	0	5.1	5.3	0.2	0.1	0.4	Tr	0
729	frozen, raw	5.1	5.7	Tr	Tr	5.7	0	0	3.9	5.3	0.1	0.1	0.4	Tr	0
730	frozen, boiled in unsalted water	5.3	5.9	Tr	Tr	5.9	0	0	4.0	5.5	0.1	0.1	0.4	Tr	0
731	frozen, microwaved	4.2	6.6	Tr	Tr	6.6	0	0	4.5	5.6	0.2	0.1	0.5	Tr	0
Vegetables, general															
732	**Asparagus**, raw	0.1	1.9	0.7	1.1	0.1	0	0	1.7	N	0.1	0.1	0.2	0	0
733	boiled in unsalted water	Tr	1.4	0.5	0.7	0.2	0	0	1.4	N	0.1	0.2	0.3	0	0

[a] Not including oligosaccharides

Vegetables *continued*

Inorganic constituents per 100g edible portion

No.	Food	Na	K	Ca	Mg	P	Fe	Cu	Zn	Cl	Mn	Se	I
		mg										µg	
Peas													
721	**Mange-tout peas**, raw	2	200	44	28	62	0.8	0.06	0.5	28	0.3	Tr	N
722	boiled in unsalted water	2	170	35	22	55	0.8	0.06	0.4	28	0.3	Tr	N
723	stir-fried in rapeseed oil	2	210	46	29	65	0.8	0.06	0.5	29	0.3	Tr	N
724	**Marrowfat peas**, canned, re-heated, drained	160	160	26	22	100	1.5	0.04	0.7	230	0.2	N	N
725	**Mushy peas**, canned, re-heated	220	170	14	22	100	1.3	0.11	0.7	320	0.2	N	N
726	**Peas**, raw	1	330	21	34	130	2.8	0.05	1.1	39	0.4	Tr	2
727	boiled in unsalted water	Tr	230	19	29	130	1.5	0.03	1.0	8	0.4	Tr	2
728	canned in water, re-heated, drained	Tr	130	30	20	81	1.9	0.02	0.6	N	0.2	Tr	N
729	frozen, raw	4	171	36	26	86	1.8	0.13	0.8	59	0.4	Tr	2
730	frozen, boiled in unsalted water	4	177	37	27	90	1.8	0.13	0.8	59	0.4	Tr	2
731	frozen, microwaved	4	179	36	27	91	1.8	0.14	0.8	73	0.4	Tr	2
Vegetables, general													
732	**Asparagus**, raw	1	260	27	13	72	0.7	0.08	0.7	60	0.2	1	Tr
733	boiled in unsalted water	1	220	25	13	50	0.6	0.08	0.7	60	0.2	1	Tr

No.	Food	Retinol µg	Carotene µg	Vitamin D µg	Vitamin E mg	Thiamin mg	Ribo-flavin mg	Niacin mg	Trypt 60 mg	Vitamin B$_6$ mg	Vitamin B$_{12}$ µg	Folate µg	Panto-thenate mg	Biotin µg	Vitamin C mg
Peas															
721	**Mange-tout peas**, raw	0	695	0	0.39	0.22	0.15	0.6	0.6	0.18	0	10	0.72	5.3	54
722	boiled in unsalted water	0	665	0	0.37	0.14	0.16	0.4	0.5	0.14	0	8	0.67	3.7	28
723	stir-fried in rapeseed oil	0	725	0	N	0.17	0.14	0.6	0.6	0.17	0	9	0.68	5.0	51
724	**Marrowfat peas**, canned, re-heated, drained	0	60	0	0.30	0.10	0.04	0.4	1.1	0.10	0	11	0.04	Tr	Tr
725	**Mushy peas**, canned, re-heated	0	Tr	0	0.30	N	N	N	0.9	N	0	N	N	Tr	Tr
726	**Peas**, raw	0	300	0	0.21	0.74	0.02	2.5	1.1	0.12	0	62	0.15	0.5	24
727	boiled in unsalted water	0	250	0	0.21	0.70	0.03	1.8	1.1	0.09	0	27	0.15	0.4	16
728	canned in water, re-heated, drained	0	534	0	0.22	0.09	0.07	1.2	0.9	0.06	0	25	0.04	Tr	1
729	frozen, raw	0	266	0	0.11	0.60	0.08	2.3	0.8	0.12	0	50	0.11	0.5	22
730	frozen, boiled in unsalted water	0	276	0	0.12	0.40	0.07	1.7	0.8	0.07	0	31	0.09	0.4	12
731	frozen, microwaved	0	285	0	0.14	0.59	0.08	2.2	0.8	0.11	0	60	0.10	0.4	17
Vegetables, general															
732	**Asparagus**, raw	0	315	0	1.16	0.16	0.06	1.0	0.5	0.09	0	175	0.17	0.4	12
733	boiled in unsalted water	0	389	0	1.16	0.12	0.06	0.8	0.6	0.07	0	173	0.16	0.4	10

Composition of food per 100g edible portion

No.	Food	Description and main data sources	Main data reference	Water g	Total nitrogen g	Protein g	Fat g	Carbohydrate g	Energy value kcal	Energy value kJ
	Vegetables, general, continued									
734	**Aubergine**, raw	Ends trimmed. Analytical data, 1984-87	24	92.9	0.14	0.9	0.4	2.2	15	64
735	fried in corn oil	Sliced, shallow fried for 10 minutes. Analytical data, 1984-87	24	59.5	0.19	1.2	31.9	2.8	302	1246
736	**Beetroot**, boiled in unsalted water	Top and root trimmed, peeled, boiled for 45 minutes. Analytical data, 1984-87	24	82.4	0.37	2.3	0.1	9.5	46	195
737	pickled, drained	Whole and sliced. Analytical data, 1990	31	88.6	0.19	1.2	0.2	5.6	28[a]	117[a]
738	**Broccoli**, green, raw	Autumn and winter. Analytical data, 2011	74	88.2	0.69	4.3	0.6	3.2[b]	34	146
739	green, boiled in unsalted water	As raw, boiled for 3-8 minutes. Analytical data, 2011	74	90.8	0.52	3.3	0.5	2.8[b]	28	120
740	green, steamed	As raw, steamed for 3-9 minutes. Analytical data, 2011	74	88.4	0.66	4.1	0.5	3.5[b]	34	142
741	**Brussels sprouts**, raw	Base trimmed, outer leaves removed. Analytical data, 1984-87	24	84.3	0.56	3.5	1.4	4.1[b]	42	177
742	boiled in unsalted water	As raw, boiled for 15 minutes. Analytical data, 1984-87	24	86.9	0.46	2.9	1.3	3.5[b]	35	153
743	**Cabbage**, green, raw	Autumn and winter. Analytical data, 2011-2012	74	88.4	0.38	2.4	0.2	4.1	27	114
744	green, boiled in unsalted water	As raw, boiled for 4-8 minutes. Analytical data, 2011-2012	74	91.9	0.24	1.5	0.2	2.3	17	70
745	red, boiled in unsalted water	Outer leaves and stem removed, shredded and boiled for 19 minutes. Analytical data, 1984-87	24	92.6	0.12	0.8	0.3	2.3[b]	15	61
746	white, raw	Autumn and winter. Analytical data, 2011-2012	74	90.1	0.19	1.2	0.1	4.8	24	101
747	**Carrots**, old, raw	Autumn and winter. Analytical data, 2011-2012	74	89.0	0.07	0.5	0.4	7.7[b]	34	146
748	old, boiled in unsalted water	As raw, boiled for 5-10 minutes. Analytical data, 2011-2012	74	90.0	0.08	0.5	0.5	6.0[b]	29	123
749	old, microwaved	As raw, cooked for 3-8 minutes. Analytical data, 2011-2012	74	87.5	0.09	0.6	0.2	7.5[b]	32	138

[a] Acetic acid from vinegar will contribute to the energy value

[b] Includes oligosaccharides

Composition of food per 100g edible portion

Vegetables, general, continued

No.	Food	Starch g	Total sugars g	Gluc g	Fruct g	Sucr g	Malt g	Lact g	NSP g	AOAC g	Satd g	Mono- unsatd g	Poly- unsatd g	Trans g	Cholest- erol mg
						Individual sugars			Dietary fibre		Fatty acids				
734	Aubergine, raw	0.2	2.0	1.1	0.8	0.1	0	0	2.0	N	0.1	Tr	0.2	0	0
735	fried in corn oil	0.2	2.6	1.4	1.1	0.1	0	0	2.3	N	4.1	7.9	18.5	N	0
736	**Beetroot**, boiled in unsalted water	0.7	8.8	0.2	0.1	8.5	0	0	1.9	N	Tr	Tr	0.1	0	0
737	pickled, drained	Tr	5.6	0.6	0.6	4.4	0	0	1.7	N	Tr	Tr	0.1	0	0
738	**Broccoli**, green, raw	0.6	1.9[a]	0.7	1.2	Tr	0	0	2.5	4.0	0.2	0.1	0.3	Tr	0
739	green, boiled in unsalted water	0.7	1.6[a]	0.8	0.8	Tr	0	0	2.3	2.8	0.1	0.1	0.2	Tr	0
740	green, steamed	0.8	2.0[a]	0.8	0.9	0.3	0	0	2.6	3.8	0.1	0.1	0.2	Tr	0
741	**Brussels sprouts**, raw	0.8	3.1[a]	1.1	1.3	0.7	0	0	4.1	N	0.3	0.1	0.7	0	0
742	boiled in unsalted water	0.3	3.0[a]	1.3	1.1	0.6	0	0	3.1	N	0.3	0.1	0.7	0	0
743	**Cabbage**, green, raw	0	4.1	2.0	1.8	0.3	0	0	2.7	4.1	Tr	Tr	0.1	0	0
744	green, boiled in unsalted water	0	2.3	1.0	0.9	0.4	0	0	2.6	2.2	Tr	Tr	0.1	0	0
745	red, boiled in unsalted water	0.1	2.0[a]	0.9	0.9	0.2	0	0	2.0	2.3	Tr	Tr	0.2	0	0
746	white, raw	0	4.8	2.4	2.1	0.3	0	0	2.0	3.0	Tr	Tr	0.1	0	0
747	**Carrots**, old, raw	0.1	7.2[a]	1.1	1.1	5.0	0	0	2.1	3.9	0.1	0.1	0.1	Tr	0
748	old, boiled in unsalted water	0.3	5.5[a]	0.9	0.7	3.9	0	0	2.1	2.8	0.2	0.2	0.1	Tr	0
749	old, microwaved	Tr	7.2[a]	1.1	1.1	5.0	0	0	2.2	2.8	0.1	0.1	Tr	Tr	0

[a] Not including oligosaccharides

Inorganic constituents per 100g edible portion

No.	Food	mg										µg	
		Na	K	Ca	Mg	P	Fe	Cu	Zn	Cl	Mn	Se	I
Vegetables, general, *continued*													
734	**Aubergine**, raw	2	210	10	11	16	0.3	0.01	0.2	14	0.1	1	1
735	fried in corn oil	2	170	8	8	25	0.5	0.03	0.1	16	0.2	1	1
736	**Beetroot**, boiled in unsalted water	90	510	29	16	87	0.8	0.03	0.5	80	0.9	Tr	N
737	pickled, drained	120	190	19	13	17	0.5	0.04	0.3	210	0.2	Tr	N
738	**Broccoli**, green, raw	9	397	48	22	81	1.1	0.08	0.7	73	0.3	1	2
739	green, boiled in unsalted water	6	212	35	14	59	0.6	0.05	0.4	50	0.2	1	2
740	green, steamed	7	373	44	21	74	0.8	0.08	0.6	70	0.3	1	2
741	**Brussels sprouts**, raw	6	450	26	8	77	0.7	0.02	0.5	38	0.2	N	1
742	boiled in unsalted water	2	310	20	13	61	0.5	0.03	0.3	16	0.2	N	1
743	**Cabbage**, green, raw	7	288	56	14	37	0.5	0.04	0.3	75	0.2	1	1
744	green, boiled in unsalted water	5	187	54	9	29	0.4	0.03	0.2	79	0.1	1	1
745	red, boiled in unsalted water	6	130	44	6	34	0.3	0.01	0.1	36	0.2	2	2
746	white, raw	7	227	56	12	26	0.4	0.03	0.2	94	0.1	1	2
747	**Carrots**, old, raw	27	178	26	7	16	0.2	0.03	0.1	122	0.1	Tr	Tr
748	old, boiled in unsalted water	29	166	31	8	17	0.3	0.04	0.1	84	0.1	Tr	Tr
749	old, microwaved	44	267	36	11	23	0.3	0.05	0.2	130	0.1	Tr	Tr

Vitamins per 100g edible portion

No.	Food	Retinol µg	Carotene µg	Vitamin D µg	Vitamin E mg	Thiamin mg	Ribo-flavin mg	Niacin mg	Trypt 60 mg	Vitamin B6 mg	Vitamin B12 µg	Folate µg	Panto-thenate mg	Biotin µg	Vitamin C mg
	Vegetables, general, continued														
734	**Aubergine**, raw	0	70	0	0.03	0.02	0.01	0.1	0.2	0.08	0	18	0.08	N	4
735	fried in corn oil	0	125	0	5.50	Tr	Tr	Tr	0.2	0.07	0	5	0.07	N	1
736	**Beetroot**, boiled in unsalted water	0	27	0	Tr	0.01	0.01	0.1	0.3	0.04	0	110	0.10	Tr	5
737	pickled, drained	0	Tr	0	Tr	0.02	0.03	0.1	0.2	0.04	0	2	0.10	Tr	N
738	**Broccoli**, green, raw	0	581	0	1.72	0.15	0.12	0.8	0.9	0.13	0	95	0.61	4.1	79
739	green, boiled in unsalted water	0	598	0	1.67	0.04	0.06	0.5	0.9	0.11	0	34	0.28	3.5	44
740	green, steamed	0	364	0	1.84	0.29	0.15	0.8	0.8	0.13	0	72	0.58	3.8	60
741	**Brussels sprouts**, raw	0	215	0	1.00	0.15	0.11	0.2	0.7	0.37	0	135	1.00	0.4	115
742	boiled in unsalted water	0	320	0	0.90	0.07	0.09	Tr	0.5	0.19	0	110	0.28	0.3	60
743	**Cabbage**, green, raw	0	454[a]	0	0.08	0.33	0.04	0.6	0.3	0.14	0	45	0.36	0.1	48
744	green, boiled in unsalted water	0	317[a]	0	0.27	0.15	0.05	0.3	0.3	0.07	0	40	0.21	Tr	45
745	red, boiled in unsalted water	0	12	0	0.20	0.02	0.01	0.2	0.1	0.04	0	31	0.22	0.1	32
746	white, raw	0	Tr	0	0.05	0.23	0.02	0.3	0.1	0.12	0	84	0.21	0.1	47
747	**Carrots**, old, raw	0	11800	0	0.09	0.13	0.01	0.2	0.2	0.06	0	8	0.27	0.3	2
748	old, boiled in unsalted water	0	11100	0	0.09	0.09	0.02	0.2	0.2	0.04	0	8	0.23	0.3	3
749	old, microwaved	0	11300	0	0.09	0.14	0.02	0.3	0.1	0.06	0	17	0.37	0.3	3

[a] Average figures. The amount of carotene in leafy vegetables depends on the amount of chlorophyll, and the outer green leaves may contain 50 times as much as inner white ones

Composition of food per 100g edible portion

No.	Food	Description and main data sources	Main data reference	Water g	Total nitrogen g	Protein g	Fat g	Carbohydrate g	Energy value kcal	kJ
	Vegetables, general, continued									
750	**Carrots**, young, raw	Ends trimmed, scrubbed. Analytical data, 1984-87	24	88.8	0.11	0.7	0.5	6.0[a]	30	125
751	young, boiled in unsalted water	As raw, boiled for 15 minutes. Analytical data, 1984-87	24	90.7	0.09	0.6	0.4	4.4[a]	22	93
752	canned in water, re-heated, drained	No added salt. Analytical data, 1985; and industry data, 2013	25	91.9	0.09	0.5	0.3	4.2[a]	20	87
753	**Cauliflower**, raw	Autumn and winter. Analytical data, 2011-2012	74	91.1	0.40	2.5	0.4	4.4[a]	30	128
754	boiled in unsalted water	As raw, boiled for 4-8 minutes. Analytical data, 2011-2012	74	92.3	0.31	1.9	0.9	3.5[a]	29	122
755	**Celery**, raw	Stem only. Analytical data, 1984-87	24	95.1	0.08	0.5	0.2	0.9	7	30
756	boiled in unsalted water	As raw, boiled for 20 minutes. Analytical data, 1984-87	24	95.2	0.08	0.5	0.3	0.8	8	34
757	**Chicory**, raw	Stem and inner leaves, pale variety. Analytical data, 1984-87	24	94.3	0.09	0.5	0.6	2.8[b]	11[b]	45[b]
758	**Courgette**, raw	Ends trimmed. Analytical data, 1984-87	24	93.7	0.29	1.8	0.4	1.8	18	74
759	boiled in unsalted water	Analysis and calculation from raw. Analytical data, 1984-87	24	93.0	0.32	2.0	0.4	2.0	19	81
760	fried in corn oil	As raw, sliced and shallow fried for 5 minutes. Analytical data, 1984-87	24	86.8	0.41	2.6	4.8	2.6	63	265
761	**Cucumber**, raw, flesh and skin	Autumn and winter. Analytical data, 2011	74	96.5	0.16	1.0	0.6	1.2	14	60
762	**Curly kale**, raw	Main ribs and stalks removed. Analytical data, 1984-87	24	88.4	0.55	3.4	1.6	1.4	33	140
763	boiled in unsalted water	As raw, shredded and boiled for 7 minutes. Analytical data, 1984-87	24	90.9	0.39	2.4	1.1	1.0	24	100
764	**Fennel**, Florence, raw	Inner leaves and bulb only. Analytical data, 1984-87	24	94.2	0.15	0.9	0.2	1.8	12	50

[a] Includes oligosaccharides

[b] Contains inulin; 32 per cent total carbohydrate taken to be available for energy purposes

Composition of food per 100g edible portion

No.	Food	Starch g	Total sugars g	Individual sugars					Dietary fibre		Fatty acids				Cholest-erol mg
				Gluc g	Fruct g	Sucr g	Malt g	Lact g	NSP g	AOAC g	Satd g	Mono-unsatd g	Poly-unsatd g	Trans g	
Vegetables, general, continued															
750	**Carrots**, young, raw	0.2	5.6ᵃ	1.7	1.5	2.4	0	0	2.4	N	0.1	Tr	0.3	0	0
751	young, boiled in unsalted water	0.2	4.2ᵃ	1.3	1.1	1.8	0	0	2.3	N	0.1	Tr	0.2	0	0
752	canned, re-heated, drained	0.4	3.7ᵃ	0.8	0.7	2.2	0	0	1.9	2.6	0.1	Tr	0.2	0	0
753	**Cauliflower**, raw	0.2	2.9ᵃ	1.2	1.3	0.4	0	0	1.8	1.8	0.1	Tr	0.2	0	0
754	boiled in unsalted water	Tr	2.4ᵃ	0.9	1.0	0.5	0	0	1.6	1.9	0.2	0.1	0.5	0	0
755	**Celery**, raw	Tr	0.9	0.4	0.3	0.2	0	0	1.1	N	Tr	Tr	0.1	0	0
756	boiled in unsalted water	Tr	0.8	0.3	0.3	0.2	0	0	1.2	N	0.1	0.1	0.1	0	0
757	**Chicory**, raw	0.2	0.7	0.3	0.4	Tr	0	0	0.9	N	0.2	Tr	0.3	0	0
758	**Courgette**, raw	0.1	1.7	0.7	0.8	0.2	0	0	0.9	N	0.1	Tr	0.2	0	0
759	boiled in unsalted water	0.1	1.9	0.8	0.9	0.2	0	0	1.2	N	0.1	Tr	0.2	0	0
760	fried in corn oil	0.1	2.5	1.0	1.2	0.3	0	0	1.2	N	0.6	1.2	2.8	N	0
761	**Cucumber**, raw, flesh and skin	Tr	1.2ᵇ	0.5	0.7	0	0	0	0.7	0.7	N	N	N	0	0
762	**Curly kale**, raw	0.1	1.3	0.6	0.6	0.1	0	0	3.1	N	0.2	0.1	0.9	0	0
763	boiled in unsalted water	0.1	0.9	0.4	0.4	0.1	0	0	2.8	N	0.2	0.1	0.6	0	0
764	**Fennel**, Florence, raw	0.1	1.7	0.9	0.7	0.1	0	0	2.4	N	Tr	Tr	Tr	0	0

ᵃ Not including oligosaccharides

ᵇ Peeled cucumbers contain approximately 2.0g total sugars per 100g as equal quantities of glucose and fructose

Vegetables, general, continued

Inorganic constituents per 100g edible portion

No.	Food	Na	K	Ca	Mg	P	Fe	Cu	Zn	Cl	Mn	Se	I
		mg										µg	
750	Carrots, young, raw	40	240	34	9	25	0.4	0.02	0.2	39	0.1	1	2
751	young, boiled in unsalted water	23	160	30	6	15	0.4	0.02	0.2	28	0.1	1	2
752	canned in water, re-heated, drained	Tr[a]	110	25	5	14	0.6	0.04	0.1	N[a]	0.1	1	N
753	Cauliflower, raw	7	252	17	12	37	0.4	0.03	0.3	73	0.1	1	N
754	boiled in unsalted water	7	215	19	12	45	0.5	0.03	0.2	54	0.1	1	N
755	Celery, raw	60	320	41	5	21	0.4	0.01	0.1	130	0.1	3	N
756	boiled in unsalted water	60	230	45	4	20	0.3	0.01	0.1	130	0.1	3	N
757	Chicory, raw	1	170	21	6	27	0.4	0.05	0.2	25	0.3	N	N
758	Courgette, raw	1	360	25	22	45	0.8	0.02	0.3	45	0.1	1	N
759	boiled in unsalted water	1	210	19	17	36	0.6	0.01	0.2	26	0.1	1	N
760	fried in corn oil	1	490	38	32	61	1.4	0.05	0.5	65	0.1	1	N
761	Cucumber, raw, flesh and skin	4	156	21	10	23	0.3	0.03	0.1	67	0.1	Tr	3
762	Curly kale, raw	43	450	130	34	61	1.7	0.03	0.4	68	0.8	2	N
763	boiled in unsalted water	34	160	150	8	39	2.0	0.02	0.2	53	0.4	2	N
764	Fennel, Florence, raw	11	440	24	8	26	0.3	0.02	0.5	27	N	N	N

[a] Carrots canned in salted water contain approximately 370mg Na and 490mg Cl per 100g

Vitamins per 100g edible portion

Vegetables, general, continued

No.	Food	Retinol µg	Carotene µg	Vitamin D µg	Vitamin E mg	Thiamin mg	Ribo-flavin mg	Niacin mg	Trypt 60 mg	Vitamin B_6 mg	Vitamin B_{12} µg	Folate µg	Panto-thenate mg	Biotin µg	Vitamin C mg
750	**Carrots**, young, raw	0	7810	0	0.56	0.04	0.02	0.2	0.1	0.07	0	28	0.25	0.6	4
751	young, boiled in unsalted water	0	7700	0	0.56	0.05	0.01	0.1	0.1	0.05	0	17	0.18	0.4	2
752	canned in water, re-heated, drained	0	2070	0	0.64	0.01	0.02	0.2	0.1	0.07	0	8	0.10	0.4	1
753	**Cauliflower**, raw	0	Tr	0	0.09	0.06	0.09	0.6	0.4	0.14	0	55	1.04	1.7	56
754	boiled in unsalted water	0	Tr	0	0.11	0.09	0.03	0.4	0.5	0.15	0	48	0.47	1.2	30
755	**Celery**, raw	0	50	0	0.20	0.06	0.01	0.3	0.1	0.03	0	16	0.40	0.1	8
756	boiled in unsalted water	0	50	0	0.20	0.06	0.01	Tr	0.1	0.03	0	10	0.28	Tr	4
757	**Chicory**, raw	0	120	0	N	0.14	Tr	0.1	0.2	0.01	0	14	N	N	5
758	**Courgette**, raw	0	610	0	N	0.12	0.02	0.3	0.3	0.15	0	52	0.08	N	21
759	boiled in unsalted water	0	440	0	N	0.08	0.02	0.2	0.3	0.09	0	31	0.11	N	11
760	fried in corn oil	0	500	0	0.83	0.10	0.01	0.4	0.4	0.09	0	42	N	N	15
761	**Cucumber**, raw, flesh and skin	0	74[a]	0	0.04	0.03	0.02	0.2	0.1	0.01	0	14	0.32	0.8	2
762	**Curly kale**, raw	0	3150	0	1.70	0.08	0.09	1.0	0.7	0.26	0	120	0.09	0.5	110
763	boiled in unsalted water	0	3380	0	1.33	0.02	0.06	0.8	0.5	0.13	0	86	0.05	0.4	71
764	**Fennel**, Florence, raw	0	140	0	N	0.06	0.01	0.6	N	0.06	0	42	N	N	5

[a] Carotene can be as high as 260µg per 100g. In peeled cucumbers the carotene ranges from 0µg to 35µg per 100g

Composition of food per 100g edible portion

No.	Food	Description and main data sources	Main data reference	Water g	Total nitrogen g	Protein g	Fat g	Carbo-hydrate g	Energy value kcal	Energy value kJ
	Vegetables, general, continued									
765	**Fennel**, Florence, boiled in unsalted water	As raw, boiled for 14 minutes. Analytical data, 1984-87	24	94.4	0.14	0.9	0.2	1.5	11	47
766	**Garlic**, raw	Peeled cloves. Analytical data, 1984-87	24	64.3	1.27	7.9	0.6	16.3	98	411
767	**Gherkins**, pickled, drained	VHS Supplement, 1991	9	92.8	0.14	0.9	0.1	2.6	14[a]	61[a]
768	**Leeks**, raw	Trimmed and outer leaves removed. Analytical data, 1984-87	24	90.8	0.26	1.6	0.5	2.9[b]	22	93
769	boiled in unsalted water	As raw, chopped and boiled for 22 minutes. Analytical data, 1984-87	24	92.2	0.20	1.2	0.7	2.6[b]	21	87
770	**Lettuce**, average, raw	Autumn and winter, including shredded, Iceberg, Romaine and Little Gem. Analytical data, 2011	74	96.1	0.19	1.2	0.1	1.4	11	48
771	**Mixed vegetables**, frozen, boiled in unsalted water	Assorted varieties, boiled for 3-7 minutes. Analytical data, 1989-90; and industry data, 2013	31	85.8	0.53	3.3	0.5	6.6	42	180
772	**Mushrooms**, white, raw	Closed cap and button. Analytical data, 2011	74	92.9	0.40[c]	1.0[d]	0.2	0.3	7	29
773	white, stewed in water	As raw, stewed for 5-10 minutes. Analytical data, 2011	74	93.1	0.58[c]	1.4[d]	0.3	0.1	9	37
774	white, fried in rapeseed oil[e]	Calculated from raw, cooked for 6-10 minutes. Water and fat analysed, 2011	74	79.1	0.56[c]	1.4[d]	11.0	0.4	106	437
775	**Mustard and cress**, raw	Leaves and cut stems. Analytical data, 1984-87	24	95.3	0.26	1.6	0.6	0.4	13	56
776	**Okra**, raw	Ends trimmed. Literature sources; and analytical data, 1984-87	24	86.6	0.40	2.8	1.0	3.0	31	130
777	boiled in unsalted water	Calculated from raw	24	87.9	0.40	2.5	0.9	2.7	28	119

[a] Not including contribution of acetic acid from vinegar

[b] Includes oligosaccharides

[c] 60 per cent of this nitrogen is non-protein nitrogen

[d] (Total N - non-protein N) x 6.25

[e] Most unspecified vegetable oils are made from rapeseed oil

Vegetables, general, continued

No.	Food	Starch g	Total sugars g	Gluc g	Fruct g	Sucr g	Malt g	Lact g	NSP g	AOAC g	Satd g	Mono- unsatd g	Poly- unsatd g	Trans g	Cholest- erol mg
					Individual sugars				Dietary fibre		Fatty acids				
765	**Fennel**, Florence, boiled in unsalted water	0.1	1.4	0.7	0.6	0.1	0	0	2.3	N	Tr	Tr	Tr	0	0
766	**Garlic**, raw	14.7	1.6	0.4	0.6	0.6	0	0	4.1	N	0.1	Tr	0.3	0	0
767	**Gherkins**, pickled, drained	0.2	2.4	0.5	0.8	1.1	0	0	1.2	1.5	Tr	Tr	Tr	0	0
768	**Leeks**, raw	0.3	2.2[a]	0.8	0.9	0.5	0	0	2.2	N	0.1	Tr	0.3	0	0
769	boiled in unsalted water	0.2	2.0[a]	0.7	0.8	0.5	0	0	1.7	2.0	0.1	Tr	0.4	0	0
770	**Lettuce**, average, raw	Tr	1.4	0.6	0.8	Tr	0	0	1.3	1.5	Tr	Tr	0.1	0	0
771	**Mixed vegetables**, frozen, boiled in unsalted water	3.0	3.6	0.4	0.4	2.8	0	0	N	N	N	N	N	0	0
772	**Mushrooms**, white, raw	Tr	0.3	Tr	0.3	Tr	0	0	1.2	0.7	Tr	Tr	0.1	0	0
773	white, stewed in water	0.1	Tr	Tr	Tr	Tr	0	0	2.0	2.6	0.1	Tr	0.2	0	0
774	white, fried in rapeseed oil	Tr	0.4	Tr	0.4	Tr	0	0	1.7	1.0	0.8	6.4	3.3	Tr	0
775	**Mustard and cress**, raw	Tr	0.4	N	N	N	0	0	1.1	N	Tr	0.2	0.2	0	0
776	**Okra**, raw	0.5	2.5	0.6	0.9	0.9	0	0	4.0	N	0.3	0.1	0.3	0	0
777	boiled in unsalted water	0.5	2.3	0.6	0.8	0.9	0	0	3.6	N	0.3	0.1	0.3	0	0

[a] Not including oligosaccharides

311

Inorganic constituents per 100g edible portion

Vegetables, general, continued

No.	Food	Na	K	Ca	Mg	P	Fe	Cu	Zn	Cl	Mn	Se	I
		mg										µg	
765	Fennel, Florence, boiled in unsalted water	11	300	20	7	21	0.2	0.01	0.4	27	N	N	N
766	Garlic, raw	4	620	19	25	170	1.9	0.06	1.0	73	0.5	2	3
767	Gherkins, pickled, drained	690	110	20	11	22	0.7	0.10	0.3	1060	0.1	N	N
768	Leeks, raw	2	260	24	3	44	1.1	0.02	0.2	59	0.2	1	N
769	boiled in unsalted water	6	150	20	2	32	0.7	0.02	0.2	43	0.2	1	N
770	Lettuce, average, raw	9	222	24	9	22	0.1	0.03	0.2	78	0.1	Tr	1
771	Mixed vegetables, frozen, boiled in unsalted water	15	130	35	16	57	0.8	0.02	0.4	30	0.2	N	N
772	Mushrooms, white, raw	4	378	3	10	94	0.2	0.28	0.6	125	0.1	17	2
773	white, stewed in water	3	216	3	8	75	0.3	0.35	0.9	93	0.1	16	2
774	white, fried in rapeseed oil	6	542	4	14	135	0.3	0.40	0.9	179	0.1	24	3
775	Mustard and cress, raw	19	110	50	22	33	1.0	0.01	0.3	39	N	N	N
776	Okra, raw	8	330	160	71	59	1.1	0.13	0.6	41	N	1	N
777	boiled in unsalted water	5	310	120	57	54	0.6	0.09	0.5	N	N	1	N

Vegetables *continued*

Vitamins per 100g edible portion

No.	Food	Retinol µg	Carotene µg	Vitamin D µg	Vitamin E mg	Thiamin mg	Ribo- flavin mg	Niacin mg	Trypt 60 mg	Vitamin B$_6$ mg	Vitamin B$_{12}$ µg	Folate µg	Panto- thenate mg	Biotin µg	Vitamin C mg
	Vegetables, general, continued														
765	**Fennel**, Florence, boiled in unsalted water	0	60	0	N	0.05	0.01	0.4	N	0.08	0	26	N	N	2
766	**Garlic**, raw	0	Tr	0	0.01	0.13	0.03	0.3	1.9	0.38	0	5	N	N	17
767	**Gherkins**, pickled, drained	0	2	0	N	Tr	0.02	0.1	0.1	N	0	6	N	N	1
768	**Leeks**, raw	0	177	0	0.92	0.29	0.05	0.4	0.2	0.48	0	56	0.12	1.4	17
769	boiled in unsalted water	0	150	0	0.78	0.02	0.02	0.4	0.2	0.05	0	40	0.10	1.0	7
770	**Lettuce**, average, raw	0	60[a]	0	0.64	0.14	0.05	0.5	0.1	0.02	0	60	0.19	0.7	1
771	**Mixed vegetables**, frozen, boiled in unsalted water	0	2520	0	N	0.12	0.09	0.8	0.5	0.11	0	52	N	N	13
772	**Mushrooms**, white, raw	0	0	0	0.01	0.13	0.27	2.5	0.5	0.10	0	40	2.38	11.7	1
773	white, stewed in water	0	0	0	0.01	0.09	0.26	1.8	0.8	0.06	0	15	1.29	10.9	Tr
774	white, fried in rapeseed oil	0	Tr	0	2.41	0.15	0.39	3.6	0.7	0.11	0	26	2.73	13.4	1
775	**Mustard and cress**, raw	0	1280	0	0.70	0.04	0.04	1.0	0.3	0.15	0	60	N	N	33
776	**Okra**, raw	0	515	0	N	0.20	0.06	1.0	0.4	0.21	0	88	0.25	N	21
777	boiled in unsalted water	0	465	0	N	0.13	0.05	0.9	0.3	0.19	0	46	0.21	N	16

[a] Average figures. The outer green leaves may contain 50 times as much as the inner white ones

Composition of food per 100g edible portion

No.	Food	Description and main data sources	Main data reference	Water g	Total nitrogen g	Protein g	Fat g	Carbo-hydrate g	Energy value kcal	Energy value kJ
778	**Okra**, stir-fried in corn oil	As raw, sliced and stir-fried for 5 minutes. Literature sources; and analytical data, 1984-87	24	54.5	0.69	4.3	26.1	4.4	269	1109
	Vegetables, general, continued									
779	**Onions**, raw	Brown, autumn and winter. Analytical data, 2011-2012	74	89.1	0.16	1.0	0.1	8.0[a]	35	150
780	boiled in unsalted water	As raw, boiled for 5-10 minutes. Analytical data, 2011-2012	74	92.5	0.11	0.7	0.3	5.4[a]	25	108
781	fried in sunflower oil	Calculated from raw, fried for 5-10 minutes. Nitrogen, fat and water analysed, 2011	74	79.9	0.19	1.2	5.3	11.2[a]	95	396
782	pickled, drained	Analytical data, 1990	31	90.6	0.14	0.9	0.2	4.9[a]	24[b]	101[b]
783	**Pak choi**, steamed	Autumn and winter, steamed for 2-5 minutes. Analytical data, 2011-2012	74	94.8	0.24	1.5	0.1	1.9	14	58
784	**Parsnip**, raw	Ends trimmed and peeled. Analytical data, 1984-87	24	79.3	0.29	1.8	1.1	12.5[a]	64	271
785	boiled in unsalted water	As raw, sliced and boiled for 12 minutes. Analytical data, 1984-87	24	78.7	0.26	1.6	1.2	12.9[a]	66	278
786	**Peppers, capsicum**, chilli, green, raw	Literature sources, 1980/89	91, 131	85.7	0.46	2.9	0.6	0.7	20	83
787	green, raw	Stalk and seeds removed. Analytical data, 1984-87	24	93.3	0.13	0.8	0.3	2.6[a]	15	65
788	green, boiled in unsalted water	As raw, sliced and boiled for 15 minutes. Analytical data, 1984-87	24	92.6	0.16	1.0	0.5	2.6[a]	18	76
789	red, raw	Autumn and winter. Analytical data, 2011	74	92.9	0.13	0.8	0.2	4.3[a]	21	89
790	red, boiled in unsalted water	As raw, boiled for 5-10 minutes. Analytical data, 2011	74	93.3	0.13	0.8	0.1	3.4[a]	17	72
791	yellow, raw	Autumn and winter. Analytical data, 2011	74	92.8	0.13	0.8	0.2	4.6[a]	23	96

[a] Includes oligosaccharides

[b] Acetic acid from vinegar will contribute to the energy value

Composition of food per 100g edible portion

No.	Food	Starch g	Total sugars g	Gluc g	Fruct g	Sucr g	Malt g	Lact g	Dietary fibre NSP g	AOAC g	Satd g	Mono- unsatd g	Poly- unsatd g	Trans g	Cholest- erol mg
Vegetables, general, continued															
778	**Okra**, stir-fried in corn oil	0.8	3.6	0.9	1.3	1.4	0	0	6.3	N	3.3	6.5	15.1	N	0
779	**Onions**, raw	Tr	6.2[a]	2.3	1.8	2.1	0	0	1.1	2.2	Tr	Tr	0.1	0	0
780	boiled in unsalted water	Tr	4.2[a]	1.6	1.2	1.4	0	0	1.3	2.3	Tr	Tr	0.1	0	0
781	fried in sunflower oil	0.1	8.6[a]	3.2	2.5	2.9	0	0	1.5	3.0	0.6	1.1	3.4	Tr	0
782	pickled, drained	Tr	3.5[a]	0.9	1.4	1.2	0	0	1.2	1.6	Tr	Tr	0.1	0	0
783	**Pak choi**, steamed	0.4	1.5	0.8	0.6	0.1	0	0	N	2.0	Tr	Tr	Tr	0	0
784	**Parsnip**, raw	6.2	5.7[a]	0.8	0.5	4.3	0	0	4.6	4.7	0.2	0.5	0.2	0	0
785	boiled in unsalted water	6.4	5.9[a]	0.8	0.5	4.5	0	0	4.7	N	0.2	0.5	0.2	0	0
786	**Peppers, capsicum**, chilli, green, raw	Tr	0.7	0.4	0.2	0.1	0	0	N	N	N	N	N	0	0
787	green, raw	0.1	2.4[a]	1.0	1.4	Tr	0	0	1.6	N	0.1	Tr	0.2	0	0
788	green, boiled in unsalted water	0.2	2.3[a]	0.9	1.4	Tr	0	0	1.8	N	0.1	Tr	0.3	0	0
789	red, raw	Tr	4.2[a]	2.0	2.2	Tr	0	0	1.0	2.2	0.1	Tr	0.1	0	0
790	red, boiled in unsalted water	Tr	3.3[a]	1.2	1.9	0.2	0	0	0.8	2.4	Tr	Tr	0.1	0	0
791	yellow, raw	Tr	4.4[a]	1.8	2.6	Tr	0	0	1.0	2.2	Tr	Tr	0.1	0	0

[a] Not including oligosaccharides

Vegetables *continued*

Inorganic constituents per 100g edible portion

No.	Food	Na	K	Ca	Mg	P	Fe	Cu	Zn	Cl	Mn	Se	I
		mg										µg	
Vegetables, general, continued													
778	**Okra**, stir-fried in corn oil	13	480	220	110	89	1.5	0.19	1.0	64	N	2	N
779	**Onions**, raw	3	138	30	8	23	0.3	0.04	0.1	54	0.1	Tr	2
780	boiled in unsalted water	2	105	25	7	23	0.3	0.05	0.2	49	0.1	Tr	2
781	fried in sunflower oil	4	189	41	11	31	0.4	0.06	0.2	73	0.1	Tr	2
782	pickled, drained	450	93	22	5	23	0.2	0.04	0.1	730	0.1	1	3
783	**Pak choi**, steamed	39	287	73	16	47	1.0	0.06	0.4	129	0.3	Tr	1
784	**Parsnip**, raw	10	450	41	23	74	0.6	0.05	0.3	49	0.5	2	N
785	boiled in unsalted water	4	350	50	23	76	0.6	0.04	0.3	33	0.3	N	N
786	**Peppers, capsicum**, chilli, green, raw	7	220	30	24	80	1.2	N	0.4	15	N	N	N
787	green, raw	4	120	8	10	19	0.4	0.02	0.1	19	0.1	Tr	1
788	green, boiled in unsalted water	4	140	9	10	23	0.4	0.03	0.2	21	0.1	Tr	1
789	red, raw	1	216	7	11	23	0.4	0.05	0.2	48	0.1	Tr	3
790	red, boiled in unsalted water	Tr	159	7	10	20	0.4	0.05	0.2	29	0.1	Tr	3
791	yellow, raw	1	189	7	10	21	0.5	0.05	0.2	64	0.1	Tr	3

Vitamins per 100g edible portion

No.	Food	Retinol (µg)	Carotene (µg)	Vitamin D (µg)	Vitamin E (mg)	Thiamin (mg)	Ribo-flavin (mg)	Niacin (mg)	Trypt 60 (mg)	Vitamin B_6 (mg)	Vitamin B_{12} (µg)	Folate (µg)	Panto-thenate (mg)	Biotin (µg)	Vitamin C (mg)
	Vegetables, general, continued														
778	**Okra**, stir-fried in corn oil	0	560	0	4.50	0.17	0.06	0.9	0.6	0.20	0	83	0.23	N	21
779	**Onions**, raw	0	10	0	0.29	0.11	0.02	0.3	0.3	0.10	0	11	0.04	1.0	3
780	boiled in unsalted water	0	5	0	0.31	0.03	Tr	0.3	0.2	0.07	0	8	0.06	0.7	4
781	fried in sunflower oil	0	14	0	2.85	0.12	0.03	0.4	0.4	0.10	0	7	0.04	1.1	3
782	pickled, drained	0	10	0	0.31	0.02	Tr	0.1	0.2	0.10	0	14	N	N	Tr
783	**Pak choi**, steamed	0	328	0	0.40	0.07	0.04	0.5	0.3	0.04	0	80	0.14	1.0	15
784	**Parsnip**, raw	0	30	0	1.00	0.23	0.01	1.0	0.5	0.11	0	87	0.50	0.1	17
785	boiled in unsalted water	0	30	0	1.00	0.07	0.01	0.7	0.4	0.09	0	41	0.35	Tr	10
786	**Peppers, capsicum**, chilli, green, raw	0	175	0	N	0.07	0.08	1.1	0.5	N	0	29	N	N	120
787	green, raw	0	265	0	0.80	0.01	0.01	0.1	0.1	0.30	0	36	0.08	N	120
788	green, boiled in unsalted water	0	240	0	0.80	0.01	0.02	Tr	0.2	0.26	0	19	0.06	N	69
789	red, raw	0	580	0	0.95	0.07	0.06	0.5	0.1	0.23	0	75	0.27	3.3	126
790	red, boiled in unsalted water	0	617	0	1.03	0.05	0.05	0.5	0.1	0.20	0	26	0.16	1.5	89
791	yellow, raw	0	134	0	0.64	0.11	0.02	0.4	0.1	0.16	0	30	0.35	3.9	121

Composition of food per 100g edible portion

No.	Food	Description and main data sources	Main data reference	Water g	Total nitrogen g	Protein g	Fat g	Carbo-hydrate g	Energy value kcal	Energy value kJ
	Vegetables, general, continued									
792	**Peppers, capsicum**, yellow, boiled in unsalted water	Calculated from raw using 13.1% weight loss		91.7	0.14	0.9	0.3	5.3[a]	26	111
793	**Plantain**, boiled in unsalted water, flesh only	Boiled for 30 minutes. VHS Supplement, 1991; and literature sources	9	68.5	0.13	0.8	0.2	28.5	112	477
794	ripe, fried in rapeseed oil[b]	VHS Supplement, 1991	9	34.7	0.24	1.5	9.2	47.5	267	1126
795	**Pumpkin**, boiled in unsalted water	Peeled thickly, seeds removed, boiled for 15 minutes. Analytical data, 1984-87	24	94.9	0.10	0.6	0.3	1.9	12	52
796	**Quorn**, pieces, as purchased	Industry data, 2013		75.2	2.24[c]	14	1.4	1.1	73	307
797	**Radish**, red, raw, flesh and skin	Ends trimmed. Analytical data, 1984-87	24	95.4	0.11	0.7	0.2	1.9	12	49
798	**Rocket**, raw	Autumn and winter. Analytical data, 2011	74	93.1	0.57	3.6	0.4	Tr	18	74
799	**Spinach**, mature, raw	Ribs and stems removed. Analytical data, 1984-87	24	89.7	0.45	2.8	0.8	1.6	25	103
800	mature, boiled in unsalted water	As raw, shredded. Analytical data, 1984-87	24	91.8	0.35	2.2	0.8	0.8	19	79
801	frozen, boiled in unsalted water	Boiled for 2-10 minutes. Analytical data, 1985	26	91.6	0.50	3.1	0.8	0.5	21	90
802	baby, raw	Autumn and winter. Analytical data, 2011	74	93.5	0.42	2.6	0.6	0.2	16	69
803	baby, boiled in unsalted water	Calculated from raw	74	91.9	0.52	3.2	0.7	0.2	20	86
804	**Spring onions**, bulbs and tops, raw	Peeled bulb and leaves. Analytical data, 1984-87	24	92.2	0.32	2.0	0.5	3.0	23	98
805	**Squash**, butternut, baked	VHS Supplement, 1991	9	87.8	0.14	0.9	0.1	7.4[a]	32	137
806	**Swede**, boiled in unsalted water, flesh only	Peeled thinly, diced and boiled for 22 minutes. Analytical data, 1984-87	24	95.8	0.05	0.3	0.1	2.3	11	46
807	**Sweet potato**, raw, flesh only	Yellow variety. Analytical data 1984-87 and 1990	24, 31	73.7	0.19	1.2	0.3	21.3	87	372

[a] Includes oligosaccharides

[b] Most unspecified vegetable oils are made from rapeseed oil

[c] Additional non-protein nitrogen from chitin is present in variable amounts

No.	Food	Starch g	Total sugars g	Gluc g	Fruct g	Sucr g	Malt g	Lact g	Dietary fibre NSP g	Dietary fibre AOAC g	Satd g	Mono- unsatd g	Poly- unsatd g	Trans g	Cholesterol mg
792	**Peppers, capsicum**, yellow, boiled in unsalted water	Tr	5.1[a]	2.1	3.0	Tr	0	0	0.8	2.4	Tr	Tr	0.1	0	0
	Vegetables, general, continued														
793	**Plantain**, boiled in unsalted water, flesh only	23.0	5.5	0.8	0.9	3.9	0	0	1.2	N	0.1	Tr	0.1	0	0
794	ripe, fried in rapeseed oil	36.0	11.5	2.3	2.3	6.9	0	0	2.3	N	0.7	5.3	2.7	Tr	0
795	**Pumpkin**, boiled in unsalted water	0.1	1.8	0.7	0.6	0.4	0	0	1.1	N	0.1	Tr	Tr	0	0
796	**Quorn**, pieces, as purchased	0.7	0.4	0.4	Tr	Tr	Tr	Tr	N	8.3	0.4	N	N	Tr	0
797	**Radish**, red, raw, flesh and skin	Tr	1.9	1.2	0.7	Tr	0	0	0.9	N	0.1	Tr	0.1	0	0
798	**Rocket**, raw	Tr	Tr	Tr	Tr	Tr	0	0	1.3	1.7	0.1	Tr	0.2	0	0
799	**Spinach**, mature, raw	0.1	1.5	0.5	0.5	0.5	0	0	2.1	N	0.1	0.1	0.5	0	0
800	mature, boiled in unsalted water	Tr	0.8	0.3	0.3	0.3	0	0	2.1	N	0.1	0.1	0.5	0	0
801	frozen, boiled in unsalted water	0.2	0.3	0.1	Tr	0.1	0	0	2.1	N	0.1	0.1	0.5	0	0
802	baby, raw	0.2	Tr	Tr	Tr	Tr	0	0	1.2	1.0	0.1	0.1	0.4	0	0
803	baby, boiled in unsalted water	0.2	Tr	Tr	Tr	Tr	0	0	1.5	1.2	0.2	0.1	0.3	0	0
804	**Spring onions**, bulbs and tops, raw	0.2	2.8	1.2	1.4	0.2	0	0	1.5	N	0.1	0.1	0.2	0	0
805	**Squash**, butternut, baked	3.0	3.9[a]	1.3	1.3	1.3	0	0	1.4	N	Tr	Tr	Tr	0	0
806	**Swede**, boiled in unsalted water, flesh only	0.1	2.2	1.2	0.9	0.1	0	0	0.7	N	Tr	Tr	0.1	0	0
807	**Sweet potato**, raw, flesh only	15.6	5.7	0.7	0.6	4.4	Tr	0	2.4	N	0.1	Tr	0.1	0	0

[a] Not including oligosaccharides

Inorganic constituents per 100g edible portion

Vegetables, general, continued

No.	Food	mg										µg	
		Na	K	Ca	Mg	P	Fe	Cu	Zn	Cl	Mn	Se	I
792	**Peppers, capsicum**, yellow, boiled in unsalted water	1	218	8	11	24	0.6	0.06	0.2	73	0.1	Tr	3
793	**Plantain**, boiled in unsalted water, flesh only	4	400	5	33	31	0.5	0.08	0.2	50	N	2	N
794	ripe, fried in rapeseed oil	3	610	6	54	66	0.8	0.20	0.4	110	N	3	N
795	**Pumpkin**, boiled in unsalted water	Tr	84	23	7	15	0.1	0.02	0.2	37	0.1	N	N
796	**Quorn**, pieces, as purchased	300	120	N	37	237	0.6	0.10	7.0	N	2.8	N	N
797	**Radish**, red, raw, flesh and skin	11	240	19	5	20	0.6	0.01	0.2	37	0.1	2	1
798	**Rocket**, raw	30	326	216	28	44	1.3	0.19	0.4	93	0.4	2	5
799	**Spinach**, mature, raw	140	500	170	54	45	2.1	0.04	0.7	98	0.6	1	2
800	mature, boiled in unsalted water	120	230	160	34	28	1.6	0.01	0.5	56	0.5	1	2
801	frozen, boiled in unsalted water	16	340	150	31	48	1.7	0.09	0.6	31	0.2	1	2
802	baby, raw	30	682	119	80	44	1.9	0.16	0.9	112	0.9	5	4
803	baby, boiled in unsalted water	42	950	166	112	61	2.6	0.22	1.3	156	1.2	7	5
804	**Spring onions**, bulbs and tops, raw	7	260	39	12	29	1.9	0.06	0.4	31	0.2	N	N
805	**Squash**, butternut, baked	4	280	41	29	27	0.6	0.07	0.1	37	0.1	N	N
806	**Swede**, boiled in unsalted water, flesh only	14	86	26	4	11	0.1	Tr	0.1	9	0.1	1	N
807	**Sweet potato**, raw, flesh only	40	370	24	18	50	0.7	0.14	0.3	65	0.4	1	2

Vegetables continued

Vitamins per 100g edible portion

No.	Food	Retinol µg	Carotene µg	Vitamin D µg	Vitamin E mg	Thiamin mg	Ribo- flavin mg	Niacin mg	Trypt 60 mg	Vitamin B6 mg	Vitamin B12 µg	Folate µg	Panto- thenate mg	Biotin µg	Vitamin C mg
792	**Peppers, capsicum**, yellow, boiled in unsalted water	0	154	0	0.74	0.08	0.02	0.3	0.1	0.11	0	21	0.32	3.6	77
	Vegetables, general, continued														
793	**Plantain**, boiled in unsalted water, flesh only	0	350	0	0.20	0.03	0.04	0.5	0.1	0.24	0	22	0.25	N	9
794	ripe, fried in rapeseed oil	0	N	0	N	0.11	0.02	0.6	0.2	1.00	0	37	0.73	N	12
795	**Pumpkin**, boiled in unsalted water	0	955	0	1.06	0.14	Tr	0.1	0.1	0.03	0	10	0.30	0.4	7
796	**Quorn**, pieces, as purchased	0	0	0	0	0.10	0.39	0.3	2.7	0.08	0.3	21	0.36	5.9	0
797	**Radish**, red, raw, flesh and skin	0	Tr	0	0	0.03	Tr	0.4	0.1	0.07	0	38	0.18	N	17
798	**Rocket**, raw	0	1140	0	0.22	0.19	0.18	0.7	0.9	0.08	0	88	0.29	1.3	20
799	**Spinach**, mature, raw	0	3540	0	1.71	0.07	0.09	1.2	0.7	0.17	0	114	0.27	0.1	26
800	mature, boiled in unsalted water	0	3840	0	1.71	0.06	0.05	0.9	0.6	0.09	0	81	0.21	0.1	8
801	frozen, boiled in unsalted water	0	6600	0	1.71	0.06	0.05	0.9	0.8	0.09	0	52	0.21	0.1	6
802	baby, raw	0	1560	0	0.48	0.09	0.18	1.0	0.7	0.12	0	161	0.28	0.1	29
803	baby, boiled in unsalted water	0	2170	0	0.67	0.08	0.20	0.9	1.0	0.10	0	135	0.31	0.1	22
804	**Spring onions**, bulbs and tops, raw	0	620	0	N	0.05	0.03	0.5	0.5	0.13	0	54	0.07	N	26
805	**Squash**, butternut, baked	0	3260	0	1.83	0.07	0.02	0.6	0.2	0.12	0	19	0.36	0.4	15
806	**Swede**, boiled in unsalted water, flesh only	0	165	0	Tr	0.13	0.01	1.0	0.1	0.04	0	18	0.07	Tr	15
807	**Sweet potato**, raw, flesh only	0	3930[a]	0	0.28	0.17	Tr	0.5	0.3	0.09	0	17	0.59	N	23

[a] Value for orange fleshed varieties. Carotene can range from 1820µg to 16000µg per 100g. White fleshed varieties contain approximately 69µg per 100g

Composition of food per 100g edible portion

No.	Food	Description and main data sources	Main data reference	Water g	Total nitrogen g	Protein g	Fat g	Carbo-hydrate g	Energy value kcal	kJ

Vegetables, general, continued

808	**Sweet potato**, boiled in unsalted water, flesh only	As raw, boiled for 27 minutes. Analytical data, 1984-87	24	74.7	0.18	1.1	0.3	20.5	84	358
809	**Sweetcorn**, baby, fresh and frozen, boiled in unsalted water	Boiled for 5 minutes. Analytical data, 1990	31	89.8	0.40	2.5	0.4	2.7	24	101
810	kernels, canned in water, drained	No added salt. Analytical data, 2012	74	78.7	0.41	2.6	1.7	13.9[a]	78	330
811	kernels, boiled 'on the cob' in unsalted water	Autumn and winter, boiled for 4-10 minutes. Analytical data, 2011	74	76.0	0.58	3.6	1.9	9.5[a]	67	284
812	**Tomatoes**, standard, raw	Autumn and winter, 'on the vine' and loose. Analytical data, 2011	74	94.6	0.08	0.5	0.1	3.0	14	61
813	standard, grilled, flesh and seeds only	As raw, grilled for 6-9 minutes. Analytical data, 2011	74	93.3	0.09	0.6	0.2	3.4	17	72
814	cherry, raw	Autumn and winter, 'on the vine' and loose. Analytical data, 2011	74	91.4	0.17	1.1	0.5	3.6	22	94
815	canned, whole contents	Whole and chopped, not containing added salt. Analytical data, 2012	74	92.9	0.18	1.1	0.1	3.8	19	80
816	**Turnip**, boiled in unsalted water	Peeled thinly, diced and boiled for 19 minutes. Analytical data, 1984-87	24	93.1	0.10	0.6	0.2	2.0	12	51
817	**Watercress**, raw	Large stalks removed. Analytical data, 1984-87	24	92.5	0.48	3.0	1.0	0.4	22	94
818	**Yam**, boiled in unsalted water, flesh only	Boiled for 25 minutes. Analytical data, 1984-87	24	64.4	0.27	1.7	0.3	33.0	133	568

[a] Includes oligosaccharides

Vegetables, general, continued

No.	Food	Starch g	Total sugars g	Individual sugars					Dietary fibre		Fatty acids				Cholest-erol mg
				Gluc g	Fruct g	Sucr g	Malt g	Lact g	NSP g	AOAC g	Satd g	Mono-unsatd g	Poly-unsatd g	Trans g	
808	**Sweet potato**, boiled in unsalted water, flesh only	8.9	11.6	N	N	N	N	0	2.3	N	0.1	Tr	0.1	0	0
809	**Sweetcorn**, baby, fresh and frozen, boiled in unsalted water	0.8	1.9	1.4	0.5	Tr	0	0	2.0	N	N	N	N	0	0
810	kernels, canned in water, drained	6.2	7.5[a]	0.3	0.1	7.1	Tr	0	2.5	3.1	0.3	0.4	0.7	0	0
811	kernels, boiled 'on the cob' in unsalted water	6.8	2.5[a]	2.4	0.1	Tr	Tr	0	2.6	5.1	0.3	0.5	0.8	0	0
812	**Tomatoes**, standard, raw	Tr	3.0	1.4	1.6	Tr	0	0	1.0	1.0	Tr	Tr	0.1	0	0
813	standard, grilled, flesh and seeds only	Tr	3.4	1.6	1.8	Tr	0	0	1.0	Tr	Tr	Tr	0.1	0	0
814	cherry, raw	Tr	3.6	1.6	2.0	Tr	0	0	1.2	1.3	0.1	0.1	0.2	0	0
815	canned, whole contents	Tr	3.8	1.9	1.9	Tr	0	0	0.7	0.8	Tr	Tr	Tr	0	0
816	**Turnip**, boiled in unsalted water	0.1	1.9	0.9	0.7	0.3	0	0	1.9	N	Tr	Tr	0.1	0	0
817	**Watercress**, raw	Tr	0.4	0.2	0.1	0.1	0	0	1.5	N	0.3	0.1	0.4	0	0
818	**Yam**, boiled in unsalted water, flesh only	32.3	0.7	0.2	0.1	0.4	0	0	1.4	N	0.1	Tr	0.1	0	0

[a] Not including oligosaccharides

Inorganic constituents per 100g edible portion

Vegetables, general, continued

No.	Food	mg										µg	
		Na	K	Ca	Mg	P	Fe	Cu	Zn	Cl	Mn	Se	I
808	Sweet potato, boiled in unsalted water, flesh only	40	300	23	45	50	0.7	0.14	0.3	65	0.4	1	2
809	Sweetcorn, baby, fresh and frozen, boiled in unsalted water	Tr	170	16	21	57	0.5	0.04	0.6	N	0.4	N	N
810	kernels, canned in water, drained	1[a]	158	3	16	52	0.3	0.04	0.4	84[a]	0.1	Tr	Tr
811	kernels, boiled 'on the cob' in unsalted water	Tr	333	4	42	107	0.7	0.09	0.9	63	0.3	1	Tr
812	Tomatoes, standard, raw	2	223	8	8	22	0.2	0.03	0.1	84	0.1	Tr	2
813	standard, grilled, flesh and seeds only	2	209	10	9	21	0.3	0.04	0.1	93	0.1	Tr	2
814	cherry, raw	4	274	10	12	31	0.3	0.05	0.2	95	0.1	Tr	2
815	canned, whole contents	5	212	11	10	17	0.6	0.07	0.1	74	0.1	Tr	3
816	Turnip, boiled in unsalted water	28	200	45	6	31	0.2	0.01	0.1	31	0.1	1	N
817	Watercress, raw	49	230	170	15	52	2.2	0.01	0.7	170	0.6	N	N
818	Yam, boiled in unsalted water, flesh only	17	260	12	12	21	0.4	0.03	0.4	40	Tr	N	N

[a] Products with added salt contain 270mg Na and 390mg Cl per 100g

Vitamins per 100g edible portion

No.	Food	Retinol (µg)	Carotene (µg)	Vitamin D (µg)	Vitamin E (mg)	Thiamin (mg)	Riboflavin (mg)	Niacin (mg)	Trypt 60 (mg)	Vitamin B$_6$ (mg)	Vitamin B$_{12}$ (µg)	Folate (µg)	Pantothenate (mg)	Biotin (µg)	Vitamin C (mg)
	Vegetables, general, continued														
808	**Sweet potato**, boiled in unsalted water, flesh only	0	3960[a]	0	0.28	0.07	0.01	0.5	0.3	0.05	0	8	0.53	N	17
809	**Sweetcorn**, baby, fresh and frozen, boiled in unsalted water	0	140	0	N	0.07	0.17	0.6	0.3	0.21	0	N	N	N	39
810	kernels, canned in water, drained	0	41	0	0.63	0.26	0.06	1.9	0.4	0.13	0	45	0.12	1.1	24
811	kernels, boiled 'on the cob' in unsalted water	0	28	0	0.42	0.25	0.08	2.2	0.7	0.02	0	24	0.40	1.0	4
812	**Tomatoes**, standard, raw	0	349	0	0.52	0.04	0.01	0.6	0.1	0.06	0	23	0.29	1.4	22
813	standard, grilled, flesh and seeds only	0	355	0	0.89	0.05	0.01	0.6	0.1	0.15	0	14	0.19	1.3	30
814	cherry, raw	0	479	0	0.89	0.05	0.02	0.4	0.1	0.06	0	24	0.19	1.8	15
815	canned, whole contents	0	328	0	1.36	0.13	0.04	1.0	0.1	0.12	0	11	0.11	1.4	11
816	**Turnip**, boiled in unsalted water	0	20	0	Tr	0.05	0.02	0.2	0.1	0.04	0	8	0.14	Tr	10
817	**Watercress**, raw	0	2520	0	1.46	0.16	0.06	0.3	0.5	0.23	0	45	0.10	0.4	62
818	**Yam**, boiled in unsalted water, flesh only	0	Tr	0	N	0.14	0.01	0.2	0.4	0.12	0	6	0.31	N	4

[a] Carotene can range from 1820µg to 16000µg per 100g. White fleshed varieties contain approximately 66µg per 100g

Composition of food per 100g edible portion

Vegetable Dishes

No.	Food	Description and main data sources	Main data reference	Water g	Total nitrogen g	Protein g	Fat g	Carbo-hydrate g	Energy value kcal	Energy value kJ
819	**Bhindi subji**, homemade	Containing okra and tomatoes. Analytical data, 2007	69	74.3	0.46	2.9	4.6	4.9	71	298
820	**Casserole**, vegetable, homemade	Recipe		84.1	0.34	2.1	0.4	10.6[a]	52	220
821	**Cauliflower cheese**	Retail. Industry data, 2013; and calculated		78.4	0.67	4.2	5.8	5.0	88	366
822	homemade with semi-skimmed milk	Recipe		81.1	0.84	5.3	5.9	6.2[a]	97	407
823	**Chilli**, vegetable, homemade	Recipe		84.0	0.41	2.5	0.8	8.6[a]	49	210
824	**Coleslaw**, not low calorie	Analytical data, 2010	72	73.0	0.13	0.8	16.3	6.0	173	714
825	with reduced calorie dressing	Including economy products. Analytical data, 2010	72	80.8	0.14	0.9	9.1	6.5	110	456
826	**Curry**, chick pea dhal, homemade	Punjabi dish containing split chick peas and tomato. Recipe		64.1	1.26	7.9	6.1	17.8[a]	152	639
827	Thai, stir-fry vegetable, takeaway and restaurant	Analytical data, 1997	53	77.9	0.61	3.8	8.2	3.3	101	421
828	vegetable, ready meal, cooked	Frozen and chilled, including generic vegetable curry, korma, dhansak and jalfrezi, no added rice. Analytical data, 2002-2003; and industry data, 2013	65	79.8	0.33	2.1	6.0	8.4	94	392
829	**Garlic mushrooms**, not coated, homemade	Recipe		77.8	0.45	1.2	14.1	0.5	134	552
830	**Lasagne**, vegetable	Retail, cooked in microwave and conventional ovens. Analytical data, 1990; and industry data, 2013	31	72.6	0.77	4.8	5.3	13.4	117	492
831	**Mixed dhal**, homemade	Mixed lentils in spices. Analytical data, 2007	69	78.2	0.78	4.9	0.7	9.1[b]	60	254

[a] Includes oligosaccharides

[b] Not including oligosaccharides

Vegetable Dishes

No.	Food	Starch g	Total sugars g	Gluc g	Fruct g	Sucr g	Malt g	Lact g	Dietary fibre		Fatty acids			Trans g	Cholest- erol mg
									NSP g	AOAC g	Satd g	Mono- unsatd g	Poly- unsatd g		
819	**Bhindi subji**, homemade	0.6	4.4	1.8	1.5	1.1	0	0	3.4	7.2	0.4	2.2	1.8	Tr	4
820	**Casserole**, vegetable, homemade	5.3	5.1ᵃ	1.6	1.4	2.1	Tr	0	1.9	2.4	0.1	0.1	0.2	Tr	0
821	**Cauliflower cheese**	3.1	1.9	0.6	0.5	0.1	Tr	0.7	N	1.6	N	N	N	N	N
822	homemade with semi-skimmed milk	2.1	3.2ᵃ	0.8	0.9	0.3	0	1.2	1.3	1.3	3.1	1.9	0.6	0.2	11
823	**Chilli**, vegetable, homemade	4.2	3.8ᵃ	0.8	0.8	2.2	Tr	0	2.6	N	0.1	0.2	0.3	Tr	Tr
824	**Coleslaw**, not low calorie	Tr	6.0	1.4	1.2	3.5	Tr	Tr	1.7	1.2	1.7	10.1	3.7	Tr	11
825	with reduced calorie dressing	Tr	6.5	1.6	1.3	3.7	Tr	Tr	1.8	1.6	0.7	5.5	2.4	Tr	12
826	**Curry**, chick pea dhal, homemade	14.6	1.9ᵃ	0.4	0.5	1.0	0	0	N	N	0.7	1.2	3.6	Tr	0
827	Thai, stir-fry vegetable, takeaway and restaurant	1.7	1.6	0.8	0.8	Tr	Tr	Tr	2.6	3.1	4.0	2.3	1.6	Tr	20
828	vegetable, ready meal, cooked	5.0	3.4	0.9	0.9	1.1	Tr	0.6	1.5	1.8	1.9	2.3	1.5	0.2	4
829	**Garlic mushrooms**, not coated, homemade	0.1	0.4	0	0.3	0	0	0.1	1.3	N	8.9	3.5	0.6	0.5	36
830	**Lasagne**, vegetable	9.0	4.4	0.7	0.7	0.2	1.6	1.2	N	N	N	N	N	N	N
831	**Mixed dhal**, homemade	8.5	0.5ᵃ	Tr	0.2	0.3	0	0	2.4	3.1	0.1	0.3	0.3	Tr	3

ᵃ Not including oligosaccharides

Inorganic constituents per 100g edible portion

Vegetable Dishes

No.	Food	Na	K	Ca	Mg	P	Fe	Cu	Zn	Cl	Mn	Se	I
		mg										µg	
819	Bhindi subji, homemade	437	372	108	56	78	0.8	0.13	0.6	673	N	3	N
820	Casserole, vegetable, homemade	36	311	24	17	46	0.6	0.07	0.3	127	0.2	1	3
821	Cauliflower cheese	200	309	119	18	119	0.6	0.03	0.8	316	0.2	1	9
822	homemade with semi-skimmed milk	104	223	116	14	101	0.4	0.03	0.7	202	0.1	2	10
823	Chilli, vegetable, homemade	127	235	29	17	53	0.8	0.04	0.3	N	0.2	2	N
824	Coleslaw, not low calorie	296	156	36	8	21	0.3	Tr	0.1	450	0.1	1	3
825	with reduced calorie dressing	197	175	40	8	20	0.2	0.02	0.1	320	0.1	1	3
826	Curry, chick pea dhal, homemade	32	390	24	40	118	2.0	0.36	1.3	48	0.6	1	N
827	Thai, stir-fry vegetable, takeaway and restaurant	570	207	28	21	54	1.7	0.10	0.4	690	0.4	4	15
828	vegetable, ready meal, cooked	200	259	41	19	47	0.8	0.12	0.3	330	0.3	2	3
829	Garlic mushrooms, not coated, homemade	128	409	6	11	105	0.2	0.30	0.6	322	0.1	18	9
830	Lasagne, vegetable	210	190	73	18	87	0.8	0.02	0.4	330	0.2	N	N
831	Mixed dhal, homemade	237	234	21	28	72	0.7	0.16	0.6	365	N	N	N

Vegetable Dishes

No.	Food	Retinol µg	Carotene µg	Vitamin D µg	Vitamin E mg	Thiamin mg	Ribo-flavin mg	Niacin mg	Trypt 60 mg	Vitamin B6 mg	Vitamin B12 µg	Folate µg	Panto-thenate mg	Biotin µg	Vitamin C mg
819	**Bhindi subji**, homemade	0	275	0	4.10	0.67	0.14	0.4	N	Tr	0	25	N	N	Tr
820	**Casserole**, vegetable, homemade	0	1350	0	0.78	0.20	0.11	1.3	0.4	0.12	0	33	0.24	0.7	8
821	**Cauliflower cheese**	N	N	N	N	0.11	0.11	0.4	1.5	0.18	N	N	0.48	1.9	N
822	homemade with semi-skimmed milk	N	33	N	N	0.05	0.13	0.4	1.1	0.10	0.5	22	0.74	2.1	20
823	**Chilli**, vegetable, homemade	0	1470	0	0.54	0.13	0.03	0.5	0.4	0.09	0	14	0.13	N	8
824	**Coleslaw**, not low calorie	37	694	Tr	3.93	0.02	0.42	0.2	0.3	0.13	0.1	56	0.12	0.6	1
825	with reduced calorie dressing	N	N	N	1.41	0.02	0.42	0.2	0.3	0.13	N	56	0.12	0.6	1
826	**Curry**, chick pea dhal, homemade	0	140	0	3.10	0.12	0.07	0.7	1.0	0.17	0	32	0.46	N	2
827	Thai, stir-fry vegetable, takeaway and restaurant	3	514	0	1.48	0.02	N	0.7	0.7	0.09	0	3	0.38	2.4	3
828	vegetable, ready meal, cooked	15	580	Tr	1.97	0.06	0.05	0.8	0.2	0.08	Tr	56	0.36	2.5	Tr
829	**Garlic mushrooms**, not coated, homemade	162	103	0.2	0.32	0.11	0.24	2.1	0.6	0.09	0.1	21	2.02	9.9	1
830	**Lasagne**, vegetable	N	N	N	N	0.25	0.29	2.0	1.1	0.44	N	6	N	N	N
831	**Mixed dhal**, homemade	0	69	0	1.36	0.09	0.07	0.3	N	N	0	62	N	N	Tr

Composition of food per 100g edible portion

No.	Food	Description and main data sources	Main data reference	Water g	Total nitrogen g	Protein g	Fat g	Carbohydrate g	Energy value kcal	Energy value kJ
	Vegetable Dishes continued									
832	**Mixed vegetables** cooked with onion, spice and tomatoes, homemade	South Asian style, including spices, salt, ginger and vegetable oil. Analytical data, 2007	69	80.3	0.38	2.4	5.3	6.6	82	342
833	**Moussaka**, vegetable	Retail, cooked in microwave and conventional ovens Analytical data, 1990; and industry data, 2013	31	75.4	0.94	5.9	4.9	8.0	98	410
834	**Nut roast**, homemade	Recipe		38.7	2.41	13.2	23.5	18.8[a]	335	1395
835	**Pakora/bhajia**, vegetable	Recipe from manufacturer; and industry data, 2013		50.5	1.04	6.4	14.7	21.4[a]	238	995
836	**Pancakes**, stuffed with vegetables, homemade	Tomato, mushroom and onion stuffing. Recipe		74.4	0.69	4.1	4.2	15.8[a]	113	474
837	**Pasty**, vegetable, homemade	Recipe		44.6	0.73	4.2	19.1	30.0	301	1259
838	**Pilau**, vegetable, homemade	Analytical data, 2007	69	69.2	0.53	3.3	1.5	22.6	112	474
839	**Quiche**, vegetable	Retail, including broccoli, tomato, spinach, roasted vegetables, asparagus and vegetable and cheese Analytical data, 2002; and industry data, 2013	65	49.9	1.30	8.1	19.7	21.2[a]	289	1205
840	**Ratatouille**, homemade	Recipe		84.7	0.20	1.2	7.0	3.8[a]	82	339
841	**Salad**, green	Lettuce, cucumber, pepper and celery. Recipe		95.4	0.16	1.0	0.4	1.6	13	57
842	potato, with mayonnaise	Recipe from manufacturers; and industry data, 2013		73.2	0.25	1.5	11.8	12.3	158	658
843	rice, homemade	Rice, vegetables, nut and raisin. Recipe		65.6	0.54	3.1	7.0	24.5	168	706
844	**Samosas**, vegetable	Mixed vegetable filling. Analytical data, 1990	31	51.3	0.82	5.1	9.3	30.0	217	911

[a] Includes oligosaccharides

Vegetables *continued*

Composition of food per 100g edible portion

No.	Food	Starch	Total sugars	Individual sugars					Dietary fibre		Fatty acids				Cholest- erol
				Gluc	Fruct	Sucr	Malt	Lact	NSP	AOAC	Satd	Mono- unsatd	Poly- unsatd	Trans	
		g	g	g	g	g	g	g	g	g	g	g	g	g	mg
Vegetable Dishes *continued*															
832	**Mixed vegetables** cooked with onion, spice and tomatoes, homemade	3.1	3.4	1.4	1.4	0.6	0	0	2.2	3.3	0.7	2.3	2.0	Tr	2
833	**Moussaka**, vegetable	3.5	4.5	1.0	1.0	0.5	0.9	1.1	N	N	N	N	N	N	N
834	**Nut roast**, homemade	14.4	4.1[a]	0.4	0.4	2.8	0.5	0	4.0	N	3.6	12.1	6.5	Tr	0
835	**Pakora/bhajia**, vegetable	17.5	2.4[a]	0.7	0.6	1.1	Tr	0	3.6	N	1.0	7.6	4.8	N	0
836	**Pancakes**, stuffed with vegetables, homemade	11.0	4.4[a]	1.1	1.0	0.4	0	1.9	1.0	1.2	1.0	1.0	1.9	Tr	24
837	**Pasty**, vegetable, homemade	28.1	1.8	0.5	0.3	0.7	0.3	Tr	2.0	2.8	7.1	8.0	3.0	Tr	1
838	**Pilau**, vegetable, homemade	22.3	0.3	Tr	0.3	Tr	0	0	N	2.2	0.3	0.6	0.5	Tr	4
839	**Quiche**, vegetable	17.5	3.5[a]	0.6	0.4	0.2	0.5	1.8	1.8	2.8	8.3	7.8	2.4	0.8	83
840	**Ratatouille**, homemade	0.2	3.3[a]	1.5	1.4	0.4	0	0	1.7	N	0.9	1.4	4.4	Tr	0
841	**Salad**, green	0	1.6	0.7	0.9	0	0	0	1.1	N	Tr	Tr	0.1	0	0
842	potato, with mayonnaise	10.4	1.9	0.4	0.2	1.3	0	0	0.8	1.2	N	N	N	N	N
843	rice, homemade	19.6	4.9	2.0	1.9	1.0	Tr	0	0.8	N	1.0	2.3	3.4	Tr	0
844	**Samosas**, vegetable	27.3	2.7	0.3	0.2	1.1	1.1	0	2.5	3.5	1.1	4.7	3.2	0.3	1

[a] Not including oligosaccharides

Inorganic constituents per 100g edible portion

Vegetable Dishes continued

No.	Food	mg										µg	
		Na	K	Ca	Mg	P	Fe	Cu	Zn	Cl	Mn	Se	I
832	**Mixed vegetables** cooked with onion, spice and tomatoes, homemade	374	377	40	24	58	0.9	0.13	0.3	576	N	N	N
833	**Moussaka**, vegetable	210	330	76	25	100	1.0	0.06	0.5	320	0.2	N	N
834	**Nut roast**, homemade	154	419	76	114	260	2.1	0.54	2.0	260	1.4	4	8
835	**Pakora/bhajia**, vegetable	430	490	99	47	130	3.7	0.21	1.1	N	0.7	1	N
836	**Pancakes**, stuffed with vegetables, homemade	29	235	74	14	82	0.8	0.09	0.4	113	0.2	4	16
837	**Pasty**, vegetable, homemade	138	169	62	12	47	0.8	0.02	0.3	218	0.3	2	Tr
838	**Pilau**, vegetable, homemade	170	88	16	10	36	0.5	0.07	0.4	262	0.4	N	4
839	**Quiche**, vegetable	200	183	170	19	151	0.9	0.04	0.9	370	0.2	4	18
840	**Ratatouille**, homemade	3	273	18	15	30	0.5	0.03	0.2	50	0.1	1	N
841	**Salad**, green	8	172	19	9	22	0.3	0.03	0.1	60	0.1	Tr	2
842	potato, with mayonnaise	160	180	6	9	29	0.4	0.05	0.2	290	0.1	N	14
843	rice, homemade	171	156	22	22	60	0.9	0.17	0.6	303	0.3	5	N
844	**Samosas**, vegetable	390	150	65	19	65	1.5	0.11	0.5	590	0.3	N	N

Vitamins per 100g edible portion

No.	Food	Retinol	Carotene	Vitamin D	Vitamin E	Thiamin	Ribo-flavin	Niacin	Trypt 60	Vitamin B_6	Vitamin B_{12}	Folate	Panto-thenate	Biotin	Vitamin C
		μg	μg	μg	mg	mg	mg	mg	mg	mg	μg	μg	mg	μg	mg
832	**Mixed vegetables** cooked with onion, spice and tomatoes, homemade	0	792	0	N	0.08	0.09	0.3	N	N	0	6	N	N	6
	Vegetable Dishes continued														
833	**Moussaka**, vegetable	N	N	N	N	0.06	0.07	0.7	1.3	0.18	Tr	12	N	N	N
834	**Nut roast**, homemade	0	17	0	6.56	0.51	0.31	6.2	2.9	0.28	Tr	89	1.00	29.3	0
835	**Pakora/bhajia**, vegetable	0	965	0	3.66	0.17	0.10	1.2	1.0	0.23	0	30	0.53	N	7
836	**Pancakes**, stuffed with vegetables, homemade	15	144	0.2	1.34	0.12	0.14	0.9	0.9	0.11	0.5	12	0.54	4.1	4
837	**Pasty**, vegetable, homemade	0	720	0	2.09	0.11	0.01	0.7	0.8	0.06	0	13	0.36	1.3	5
838	**Pilau**, vegetable, homemade	N	311	0.1	0.83	0.01	0.06	Tr	0.5	0.09	Tr	8	0.19	3.3	Tr
839	**Quiche**, vegetable	121	202	Tr	0.62	0.09	0.17	0.7	1.0	0.06	0.2	15	0.41	4.0	Tr
840	**Ratatouille**, homemade	0	301	0	1.77	0.05	0.01	0.3	0.3	0.11	0	16	0.12	N	15
841	**Salad**, green	0	123	0	0.42	0.05	0.02	0.3	0.1	0.10	0	32	0.22	N	35
842	potato, with mayonnaise	N	N	0.1	N	0.12	0.03	0.3	0.4	0.21	N	18	N	N	4
843	rice, homemade	0	129	0	2.32	0.09	0.02	0.8	0.7	0.10	0	22	0.13	0.9	13
844	**Samosas**, vegetable	0	N	0	N	0.12	0.08	1.1	0.7	0.15	0	44	N	N	N

Vegetables *continued*

845 to 854

Composition of food per 100g edible portion

Vegetable Dishes continued

No.	Food	Description and main data sources	Main data reference	Water g	Total nitrogen g	Protein g	Fat g	Carbo-hydrate g	Energy value kcal	kJ
845	**Sauerkraut**	Bottled and canned, drained. Analytical data, 1985	25	91.0	0.17	1.1	Tr	1.1	9	36
846	**Shepherd's pie**, vegetable	Vegetable, lentil and barley base with potato topping. Recipe from manufacturer, 1992; and industry data, 2013	12	77.5	0.30	1.9	4.9	13.3[a]	101	425
847	**Sushi**, vegetable	Analytical data, 2002-2003	65	61.0	0.54	3.4	1.3	32.8[a]	148	630
848	**Vegeburger**, grilled	Soya protein based, grilled for 6-10 minutes. Analytical data, 1990; and industry data, 2013	31	63.7	2.91	16.6	7.2	8.0	161	677
849	**Vegetable and cheese grill/burger**, in crumbs, baked/grilled	Including cheese grills and cheese and onion crispbakes. Analytical data, 1995; and industry data, 2013	57	53.6	1.12	7.0	14.0	23.0[a]	240	1005
850	**Vegetable bake**, homemade	Recipe		74.5	0.68	4.3	5.9	13.7[a]	121	509
851	**Vegetable pie**, homemade	Recipe		68.4	0.51	2.9	9.4	17.1[a]	160	668
852	**Vegetable stir-fry mix**, fried in rapeseed oil[b]	Frozen, assorted, stir-fried for 4-7 minutes. Analytical data, 1990	31	83.8	0.32	2.0	3.6	6.4	64	270
853	**Vegetables, stir-fried**, takeaway	Analytical data, 1997	53	88.1	0.29	1.8	4.1	2.1[a]	52	216
854	**Vegetarian sausages**, baked/grilled	Soya and wheat based. Analytical data, 1995; and industry data, 2013	57	57.8	2.38	14.9	9.4	9.2[a]	179	748

[a] Includes oligosaccharides

[b] Most unspecified vegetable oils are made from rapeseed oil

Composition of food per 100g edible portion

No.	Food	Starch	Total sugars	Individual sugars					Dietary fibre		Fatty acids				Cholest-
				Gluc	Fruct	Sucr	Malt	Lact	NSP	AOAC	Satd	Mono-unsatd	Poly-unsatd	Trans	erol
		g	g	g	g	g	g	g	g	g	g	g	g	g	mg

Vegetable Dishes continued

No.	Food	Starch	Total sugars	Gluc	Fruct	Sucr	Malt	Lact	NSP	AOAC	Satd	Mono-unsatd	Poly-unsatd	Trans	Cholesterol
845	**Sauerkraut**	Tr	1.1	0.7	0.3	0.1	0	0	2.2	N	Tr	Tr	Tr	Tr	0
846	**Shepherd's pie**, vegetable	11.4	1.7[a]	0.6	0.5	0.5	Tr	0.1	1.2	N	2.0	1.2	1.4	Tr	7
847	**Sushi**, vegetable	25.6	7.0[a]	2.5	2.4	0.5	1.4	0.1	1.2	1.6	N	N	N	0	0
848	**Vegeburger**, grilled	4.4	3.6	0.5	0.4	1.8	0.9	0	4.2	4.5	N	N	N	N	N
849	**Vegetable and cheese grill/burger,** in crumbs, baked/grilled	18.6	1.3[a]	0.2	0.2	0.2	0.3	0.4	1.6	N	4.6	4.4	3.0	0.8	N
850	**Vegetable bake**, homemade	8.9	4.6[a]	0.6	0.6	1.2	0.2	1.9	0.9	1.2	2.7	2.1	0.6	0.1	8
851	**Vegetable pie**, homemade	15.9	2.8[a]	1.0	1.0	0.6	0.1	Tr	1.5	N	2.6	3.1	2.2	Tr	1
852	**Vegetable stir-fry mix**, fried in rapeseed oil	2.5	3.9	1.4	0	1.2	1.1	0.2	N	N	0.2	2.1	1.1	Tr	0
853	**Vegetables, stir-fried**, takeaway	1.6	0.2[a]	Tr	0.2	Tr	Tr	0	1.8	2.1	0.8	2.2	0.6	Tr	1
854	**Vegetarian sausages**, baked/grilled	2.9	1.3[a]	0.5	0.5	0.2	0.1	0	2.6	N	2.3	4.1	1.9	N	0

[a] Not including oligosaccharides

Vegetable Dishes continued

Inorganic constituents per 100g edible portion

No.	Food	mg										µg	
		Na	K	Ca	Mg	P	Fe	Cu	Zn	Cl	Mn	Se	I
845	**Sauerkraut**	590	180	50	10	23	1.2	0.05	0.3	860	0.2	Tr	1
846	**Shepherd's pie**, vegetable	210	240	12	14	36	0.6	0.07	0.3	350	0.1	7	N
847	**Sushi**, vegetable	521	88	23	14	48	0.5	0.11	0.5	665	0.3	4	20
848	**Vegeburger**, grilled	490	610	100	80	240	4.5	0.40	1.6	660	1.1	8	N
849	**Vegetable and cheese grill/burger**, in crumbs, baked/grilled	290	260	154	20	147	0.9	0.10	0.8	460	0.2	4	32
850	**Vegetable bake**, homemade	107	257	109	17	92	0.4	0.04	0.6	216	0.1	1	15
851	**Vegetable pie**, homemade	107	253	39	14	46	0.7	0.05	0.3	290	0.2	1	N
852	**Vegetable stir-fry mix**, fried in rapeseed oil	11	230	30	16	46	0.5	0.11	0.3	27	0.1	Tr	N
853	**Vegetables, stir-fried**, takeaway	399	119	13	9	32	1.0	0.05	0.2	616	0.1	Tr	N
854	**Vegetarian sausages**, baked/grilled	550	351	136	54	193	3.1	0.24	1.0	830	0.8	4	Tr

Vitamins per 100g edible portion

No.	Food	Retinol µg	Carotene µg	Vitamin D µg	Vitamin E mg	Thiamin mg	Ribo-flavin mg	Niacin mg	Trypt 60 mg	Vitamin B6 mg	Vitamin B12 µg	Folate µg	Panto-thenate mg	Biotin µg	Vitamin C mg
Vegetable Dishes continued															
845	**Sauerkraut**	0	18	0	N	0.04	0.01	0.2	0.2	0.15	0	16	0.23	N	10
846	**Shepherd's pie**, vegetable	29	585	Tr	0.75	0.11	0.01	0.4	0.4	0.18	Tr	10	0.24	0.5	4
847	**Sushi**, vegetable	0	163	0	0.55	0.03	0.06	0.5	0.7	0.04	0	6	0.13	1.6	4
848	**Vegeburger**, grilled	N	Tr	N	N	N	N	N	3.9	N	N	95	N	N	N
849	**Vegetable and cheese grill/burger**, in crumbs, baked/grilled	17	265	N	1.12	0.07	0.11	1.0	1.2	0.05	0.4	8	0.30	2.0	2
850	**Vegetable bake**, homemade	N	2390	N	N	0.11	0.12	0.3	0.9	0.08	0.4	9	0.35	1.6	4
851	**Vegetable pie**, homemade	0	1330	0	1.94	0.15	0.13	1.2	0.5	0.15	Tr	35	0.24	1.0	9
852	**Vegetable stir-fry mix**, fried in rapeseed oil	0	N	0	N	0.07	0.13	1.0	0.3	0.25	0	16	N	N	8
853	**Vegetables, stir-fried**, takeaway	Tr	575	0	1.26	0.03	0.13	0.3	0.3	0.05	0	3	0.30	3.3	2
854	**Vegetarian sausages**, baked/grilled	0	N	0	N	1.72	0.14	1.1	2.5	0.05	N	34	0.30	5.5	Tr

Section 2.8

Herbs and spices

The foods in this section of the Tables have been taken from the *Vegetables, Herbs, and Spices* (1991)[9] supplement. The majority of values are derived from literature sources, including values from food composition tables published in other countries, e.g. the United States Department of Agriculture National Nutrient Database for Standard Reference[169].

Starch and sugars have not been analysed for many herbs and spices and reliable values are not available. Total carbohydrate, energy, starch and sugars for some herbs and spices have therefore been given as 'unknown', i.e. as 'N'. Variation in the nutrient content of spices may arise due to the processing methods used, e.g. contamination from processing machinery can result in variation of the iron content of ground spices.

Taxonomic names for foods in this part of the Tables can be found in Section 4.5.

Composition of food per 100g edible portion

No.	Food	Description and main data sources	Main data reference	Water (g)	Total nitrogen (g)	Protein (g)	Fat (g)	Carbo-hydrate (g)	Energy value kcal	Energy value kJ
855	Basil, fresh	Analytical data, 1990; literature sources 1982 and 1972	31, 159 176	88.0	0.50	3.1	0.8	5.1	40	169
Herbs and spices										
856	**Chilli powder**	Data from USDA SR26, 2013[a]	169	10.8	2.16	13.5	14.3	N	N	N
857	**Chinese 5 spice**	Recipe from VHS Supplement, 1991	9	9.1	1.53	9.5	8.7	N	N	N
858	**Chives**, fresh	Data from USDA SR26, 2013	169	90.7	0.53	3.3	0.7	1.9	27	112
859	**Cinnamon**, ground	Data from USDA SR26, 2013	169	10.6	0.64	4.0	1.2	N	N	N
860	**Coriander** leaves, fresh	Data from USDA SR26, 2013	169	92.2	0.34	2.1	0.5	1.2	18	74
861	seeds	Data from USDA SR26, 2013	169	8.9	1.98	12.4	17.8	N	N	N
862	**Cumin** seeds	Data from USDA SR26, 2013	169	8.1	2.85	17.8	22.3	N	N	N
863	**Curry powder**	VHS Supplement, 1991[b]	9	8.5	1.52	9.5	10.8	26.1	233	979
864	**Garam masala**	Literature sources, 1983	172	10.1	2.50	15.6	15.1	45.2	379	1592
865	**Ginger**, ground	VHS Supplement, 1991	9	9.4	1.19	7.4	3.3	60.0	284	1208
866	fresh	Data from USDA SR26, 2013	169	78.9	0.29	1.8	0.8	8.1	44	188
867	**Mint**, fresh	Literature sources, 1972-1982. VHS Supplement, 1991	9	86.4	0.61	3.8	0.7	5.3	43	181
868	**Mixed herbs**, dried	Calculated from 25g marjoram, 25g parsley, 25g sage and 25g thyme		8.1	1.93	12.1	8.5	36.3	261	1092
869	**Mustard powder**	MSF Supplement, 1994	14	5.0	4.62	28.9	28.7	20.7	452	1884
870	**Nutmeg**, ground	Data from USDA SR26, 2013	169	6.2	1.10	5.8	36.3	N	N	N
871	**Oregano**, dried, ground	Data from USDA SR26, 2013	169	9.9	1.44	9.0	4.3	N	N	N
872	**Paprika**	Data from USDA SR26, 2013	169	11.2	2.26	14.1	12.9	N	N	N

[a] Mix of chilli pepper, other spices and salt

[b] Composition will vary according to variety

Composition of food per 100g edible portion

No.	Food	Starch g	Total sugars g	Individual sugars					Dietary fibre		Fatty acids				Cholesterol mg
				Gluc g	Fruct g	Sucr g	Malt g	Lact g	NSP g	AOAC g	Satd g	Mono-unsatd g	Poly-unsatd g	Trans g	
	Herbs and spices														
855	**Basil**, fresh	Tr	N	N	N	N	0	0	N	N	N	N	N	0	0
856	**Chilli powder**	N	7.2	2.1	4.3	0.8	0	0	N	34.8	2.5	3.2	8.0	0	0
857	**Chinese 5 spice**	N	N	N	N	N	0	0	N	N	N	N	N	0	0
858	**Chives**, fresh	Tr	1.9	0.9	1.0	Tr	0	0	1.9	2.5	0.2	0.1	0.3	0	0
859	**Cinnamon**, ground	N	2.2	1.0	1.1	Tr	0	0	N	53.1	0.4	0.3	0.1	0	0
860	**Coriander** leaves, fresh	0.3	0.9	0.5	0.4	Tr	0	0	N	2.8	N	N	N	0	0
861	seeds	N	N	N	N	N	0	0	N	41.9	1.0	13.6	1.8	0	0
862	**Cumin** seeds	N	2.3	N	N	N	0	0	N	10.5	1.5	14.0	3.3	0	0
863	**Curry powder**	N	N	N	N	N	0	0	23.0	N	N	N	N	0	0
864	**Garam masala**	N	N	N	N	N	0	0	N	N	N	N	N	0	0
865	**Ginger**, ground	40.2	19.8	9.6	10.2	0	0	0	N	14.1	1.6	1.0	0.1	0	0
866	fresh	6.4	1.7	0.8	0.9	0	0	0	N	2.0	0.2	0.2	0.2	0	0
867	**Mint**, fresh	N	N	N	N	N	0	0	N	N	N	N	N	0	0
868	**Mixed herbs**, dried	N	N	N	N	N	0	0	N	N	N	N	N	0	0
869	**Mustard powder**	N	N	N	N	N	0	0	N	N	1.5	19.8	5.4	0	0
870	**Nutmeg**, ground	N	28.5	N	N	N	0	0	N	20.8	25.9	3.2	0.3	0	0
871	**Oregano**, dried, ground	N	4.1[a]	1.9	1.1	0.9	0	0	N	42.5	1.6	0.7	1.4	0	0
872	**Paprika**	N	10.3[a]	2.6	6.7	0.8	0	0	N	34.9	2.1	1.7	7.8	0	0

[a] Contains galactose

Inorganic constituents per 100g edible portion

No.	Food	Na	K	Ca	Mg	P	Fe	Cu	Zn	Cl	Mn	Se	I
		mg										µg	
Herbs and spices													
855	**Basil**, fresh	9	300	250	11	37	5.5	N	0.7	N	N	N	N
856	**Chilli powder**	4000[a]	1950	330	149	300	17.3	1.00	4.3	5980[a]	1.7	N	N
857	**Chinese 5 spice**	63	1070	1040	210	260	25.6	0.74	2.9	N	8.4	N	N
858	**Chives**, fresh	3	296	92	42	58	1.6	0.16	0.6	N	0.4	Tr	N
859	**Cinnamon**, ground	10	431	1000	60	64	8.3[b]	0.34	1.8	N	17.5	3	N
860	**Coriander** leaves, fresh	46	521	67	26	48	1.8	0.23	0.5	N	0.4	N	N
861	seeds	35	1270	709	330	409	16.3	0.97	4.7	N	1.9	26	N
862	**Cumin** seeds	168	1790	931	366	499	66.4	0.87	4.8	N	3.3	N	N
863	**Curry powder**	450	1830	640	280	270	58.3	1.04	4.1	470	4.7	N	N
864	**Garam masala**	97	1450	760	330	390	32.6	1.62	3.8	N	6.0	N	N
865	**Ginger**, ground	34	910	97	130	140	46.8	0.45	4.7	40	28.0	N	N
866	fresh	13	415	16	43	34	0.6	0.23	0.3	N	0.2	N	N
867	**Mint**, fresh	15	260	210	N	75	9.5	N	N	34	1.4	N	N
868	**Mixed herbs**, dried	81	1870	1650	280	235	69.0	0.73	4.6	N	9.8	N	N
869	**Mustard powder**	5	940	330	260	180	9.5	0.20	6.5	62	1.7	N	N
870	**Nutmeg**, ground	16	350	180	180	210	3.0	1.03	2.2	N	2.9	2	N
871	**Oregano**, dried, ground	25	1260	1600	270	148	36.8	0.63	2.7	N	5.0	5	N
872	**Paprika**	68	2280	229	178	314	21.1	0.71	4.3	N	1.6	6	N

[a] Contains added salt

[b] Whole unground cinnamon contains 4mg Fe per 100g

Vitamins per 100g edible portion

No.	Food	Retinol µg	Carotene µg	Vitamin D µg	Vitamin E mg	Thiamin mg	Ribo-flavin mg	Niacin mg	Trypt 60 mg	Vitamin B$_6$ mg	Vitamin B$_{12}$ µg	Folate µg	Panto-thenate mg	Biotin µg	Vitamin C mg
	Herbs and spices														
855	**Basil**, fresh	0	3950	0	N	0.08	0.31	1.1	N	N	0	N	N	N	26
856	**Chilli powder**	0	17800	0	N	0.25	0.94	11.6	N	2.10	0	28	0.89	N	1
857	**Chinese 5 spice**	0	138	0	N	0.21	0.24	5.3	N	N	0	0	N	N	0
858	**Chives**, fresh	0	2610	0	0.21	0.08	0.12	0.7	0.7	0.14	0	105	0.33	N	58
859	**Cinnamon**, ground	0	177	0	N	0.02	0.04	1.3	N	0.16	0	6	0.36	N	4
860	**Coriander leaves**, fresh	0	4050	0	2.50	0.07	0.12	1.1	0.4	0.15	0	62	0.57	N	27
861	seeds	0	Tr	0	N	0.24	0.29	2.1	N	N	0	0	N	N	21
862	**Cumin seeds**	0	762	0	3.33	0.63	0.33	4.6	N	0.44	0	10	N	N	8
863	**Curry powder**	0	100	0	N	0.25	0.28	3.5	N	1.11	0	56	N	N	1
864	**Garam masala**	0	340	0	N	0.35	0.33	2.5	N	N	0	0	N	N	0
865	**Ginger**, ground	0	220	0	N	0.05	0.19	5.1	0.9	1.01	0	0	1.27	N	0
866	fresh	0	0	0	0.26	0.02	0.03	0.8	0.2	0.16	0	11	0.20	N	5
867	**Mint**, fresh	0	740	0	5.00	0.12	0.33	1.1	N	N	0	110	N	N	31
868	**Mixed herbs, dried**	0	8100	0	N	N	0.34	5.0	N	N	N	N	N	N	43
869	**Mustard powder**	0	N	0	N	N	N	N	8.5	N	0	0	N	N	0
870	**Nutmeg**, ground	0	60	0	N	0.35	0.06	1.3	N	0.16	0	76	N	N	3
871	**Oregano**, dried, ground	0	1021	0	N	0.18	0.53	4.6	N	1.04	0	237	0.92	N	2
872	**Paprika**	0	29600	0	N	0.33	1.23	10.1	N	2.14	0	49	2.51	N	1

Composition of food per 100g edible portion

No.	Food	Description and main data sources	Main data reference	Water g	Total nitrogen g	Protein g	Fat g	Carbo-hydrate g	Energy value kcal	Energy value kJ

Herbs and spices continued

No.	Food	Description and main data sources	Main data reference	Water g	Total nitrogen g	Protein g	Fat g	Carbo-hydrate g	kcal	kJ
873	**Parsley**, fresh	Tough stalks removed. Analytical data, 1984-87	24	83.1	0.47	3.0	1.3	2.7	34	141
874	**Pepper**, black	Data from USDA SR26, 2013	169	12.5	1.66	10.4	3.3	N	N	N
875	white	Data from USDA SR26, 2013	169	11.4	1.95	10.4	2.1	N	N	N
876	**Rosemary**, dried	Literature sources, 1977; and data from USDA SR26, 2013	144, 169	9.3	0.78	4.9	15.2	46.4	331	1387
877	**Thyme**, dried, ground	Literature sources, 1977; and data from USDA SR26, 2013	144, 169	7.8	1.46	9.1	7.4	45.3	276	1156

344

Composition of food per 100g edible portion

No.	Food	Starch g	Total sugars g	Gluc g	Fruct g	Sucr g	Malt g	Lact g	Dietary fibre NSP g	Dietary fibre AOAC g	Satd g	Mono- unsatd g	Poly- unsatd g	Trans g	Cholest- erol mg
						Individual sugars							Fatty acids		
Herbs and spices continued															
873	**Parsley,** fresh	0.4	2.3[a]	1.4	0.9	Tr	0	0	5.0	N	N	N	N	0	0
874	**Pepper,** black	Tr	0.6[a]	0.2	0.2	Tr	0	0	N	25.3	1.4	0.7	1.0	0	0
875	white	Tr	N	N	N	N	0	0	N	26.2	0.6	0.8	0.6	0	0
876	**Rosemary,** dried	N	N	N	N	N	0	0	N	42.6	7.4	3.0	2.3	0	0
877	**Thyme,** dried, ground	N	1.7	N	N	N	0	0	N	37.0	2.7	0.5	1.2	0	0

[a] Includes galactose

345

Inorganic constituents per 100g edible portion

No.	Food	Na	K	Ca	Mg	P	Fe	Cu	Zn	Cl	Mn	Se	I
						mg						μg	
Herbs and spices continued													
873	**Parsley**, fresh	33	760	200	23	64	7.7	0.03	0.7	160	0.2	1	N
874	**Pepper**, black	20	1330	443	171	158	9.7	1.33	1.2	30	12.8	5	N
875	white	5	73	270	90	180	14.3	0.91	1.1	60	4.3	3	N
876	**Rosemary**, dried	50	950	1280	220	70	29.3	0.55	3.2	N	1.9	5	N
877	**Thyme**, dried, ground	55	810	1890	220	200	123.6	0.86	6.2	N	7.9	5	N

Vitamins per 100g edible portion

No.	Food	Retinol µg	Carotene µg	Vitamin D µg	Vitamin E mg	Thiamin mg	Ribo-flavin mg	Niacin mg	Trypt 60 mg	Vitamin B₆ mg	Vitamin B₁₂ µg	Folate µg	Panto-thenate mg	Biotin µg	Vitamin C mg
	Herbs and spices continued														
873	**Parsley**, fresh	0	4040	0	1.70	0.23	0.06	1.0	0.5	0.09	0	170	0.30	0.4	190
874	**Pepper**, black	0	329	0	N	0.11	0.18	1.1	N	0.29	0	17	1.40	N	0
875	white	0	Tr	0	N	0.02	0.13	0.2	N	0.10	0	10	N	N	21
876	**Rosemary**, dried	0	1880	0	N	0.51	0.43	1.0	N	1.74	0	307	N	N	61
877	**Thyme**, dried, ground	0	2280	0	N	0.51	0.40	4.9	3.1	0.55	0	274	N	N	50

Fruit

Section 2.9

Fruit

New analytical data (2012)[74] for a range of the most commonly consumed fruit have been incorporated into this section. For other fruit, the data have been taken from the *Fruit and Nuts* (1992)[11] supplement, based on analysis in the 1980s[27,28,31]. Data from manufacturers has been used to review and update sugar content of canned and processed fruit products.

The nutrient content of fruit samples can vary widely, often being greater within the same fruit type than between different varieties of fruit. Factors affecting the nutrient content include the degree of ripening, cultivar, length and conditions of storage, depth of peeling and cooking conditions.

During the process of stewing fruit, sucrose becomes inverted into glucose and fructose, the extent depending on the length of cooking time and level of acidity. A factor of 10% hydrolysis of sucrose has been applied to all stewed fruit. The nutrient values for stewed fruits have been derived from both analyses and calculation. The proportions of sugar used for cooking and the method of calculation of the data have been included in the description of the food. For fruit cooked with a different proportion of sugar, the values for fruit 'stewed without sugar' can be used, with the appropriate quantity of sugar added. Corrections have been made for both vitamin losses (see Section 4.3 for the factors used) and evaporative losses of 10% during stewing.

Values for canned fruit include either syrup or juice, unless it is stated that the contents have been drained. It has been found by analysis that sugar diffuses between the syrup or juice and the fruit until it reaches an equilibrium, so that there are no significant differences between the levels of sugars in the fruit and the syrup or juice.

Users should note that all values are expressed per 100g edible portion. Guidance for calculating nutrient content 'as purchased' or 'as served' (e.g. including citrus rind and inedible stones) is given in Section 4.2. Taxonomic names for foods included in this part of the Tables can be found in Section 4.5.

Composition of food per 100g edible portion

Fruit, general

No.	Food	Description and main data sources	Main data reference	Water g	Total nitrogen g	Protein g	Fat g	Carbo-hydrate g	Energy value kcal	Energy value kJ
878	**Apples,** cooking, stewed with sugar, flesh only	Calculated from stewed without sugar	74	77.5	0.03	0.2	0.3	20.8	81	346
879	cooking, stewed without sugar, flesh only	Autumn and winter, UK grown pre-packed and loose, including Bramley and unspecified varieties, stewed with 1 tbsp water/100g for 5-10 minutes. Analytical data, 2011-2012	74	87.3	0.02	0.2	0.3	9.7	40	169
880	eating, raw, flesh and skin	Autumn and winter, UK grown and imported, pre-packed and loose, including Gala, Braeburn, Golden Delicious, Pink Lady, Cox and Granny Smith. Analytical data, 2011-2012	74	86.2	0.10	0.6	0.5	11.6	51	215
881	**Apricots,** raw, flesh and skin	Analytical data, 1990	31	87.2	0.14	0.9	0.1	7.2	31	134
882	ready-to-eat	No stones, semi-dried. Analytical data, 1990	31	29.7	0.63	4.0	0.6	36.5	158	674
883	**Avocado,** average	Fuede and Hass varieties. Analytical data, 1990	31	72.5[a]	0.30	1.9	19.5[b]	1.9[c]	190	784
884	**Bananas,** flesh only	Including Fairtrade and organic, pre-packed and loose. Analytical data, 2011	74	75.0	0.18	1.2	0.1	20.3	81	348
885	**Blackberries,** raw	Cultivated and wild berries. whole fruit. Analytical data, 1985-86	28	85.0	0.14	0.9	0.2	5.1	25	104
886	stewed without sugar	Calculated from 700g fruit, 210g water		87.2	0.12	0.8	0.2	4.4	21	88
887	**Blackcurrants,** raw	Whole fruit, stalks removed. MW1, 1940	1	77.4	0.15	0.9	Tr	6.6	28	121
888	stewed without sugar	Calculated from 700g fruit, 210g water		80.7	0.13	0.8	Tr	5.6	24	103

[a] Water can range from 50g to 80g per 100g
[b] Fat can range from 10g to 40g per 100g
[c] Including mannoheptulose

Fruit, general

No.	Food	Starch g	Total sugars g	Gluc g	Fruct g	Sucr g	Malt g	Lact g	Dietary fibre NSP g	AOAC g	Fatty acids Satd g	Mono-unsatd g	Poly-unsatd g	Trans g	Cholest-erol mg
878	**Apples**, cooking, stewed with sugar, flesh only	Tr	20.8	3.1	6.7	11.0	0	0	1.0	1.4	0.1	Tr	0.1	0	0
879	cooking, stewed without sugar, flesh only	Tr	9.7	2.1	5.9	1.7	0	0	1.3	1.7	0.1	Tr	0.1	0	0
880	eating, raw, flesh and skin	Tr	11.6	2.1	6.7	2.8	0	0	1.3	1.2	0.1	Tr	0.2	0	0
881	**Apricots**, raw, flesh and skin	0	7.2	1.6	0.9	4.6	0	0	1.7	N	Tr	Tr	Tr	0	0
882	ready-to-eat	0	36.5	17.5	8.4	10.6	0	0	6.3	N	N	N	N	0	0
883	**Avocado**, average	Tr	0.5[a]	0.3	0.1	0.1	0	0	3.4	N	4.1	12.1	2.2	0	0
884	**Bananas**, flesh only	2.2[b]	18.1[b]	7.9	7.5	2.7	0	0	0.8	1.4	Tr	Tr	Tr	0	0
885	**Blackberries**, raw	0	5.1	2.5	2.6	Tr	0	0	3.1	N	Tr	0.1	0.1	0	0
886	stewed without sugar	0	4.4	2.1	2.2	Tr	0	0	2.6	N	Tr	0.1	0.1	0	0
887	**Blackcurrants**, raw	0	6.6	3.0	3.4	0.3	0	0	3.6	N	Tr	Tr	Tr	0	0
888	stewed without sugar	0	5.6	2.5	2.9	0.2	0	0	3.1	N	Tr	Tr	Tr	0	0

[a] Not including mannoheptulose

[b] Including a range of ripeness. The starch content falls and the sugar content rises on ripening

Inorganic constituents per 100g edible portion

Fruit, general

No.	Food	mg										µg	
		Na	K	Ca	Mg	P	Fe	Cu	Zn	Cl	Mn	Se	I
878	**Apples**, cooking, stewed with sugar, flesh only	1	81	3	3	6	0.1	0.03	Tr	73	Tr	Tr	4
879	cooking, stewed without sugar, flesh only	1	87	3	3	7	0.1	0.03	Tr	73	Tr	Tr	4
880	eating, raw, flesh and skin	1	100	5	4	8	0.1	0.03	Tr	44	Tr	Tr	4
881	**Apricots**, raw, flesh and skin	2	270	15	11	20	0.5	0.06	0.1	3	0.1	1	N
882	ready-to-eat	14	1380	73	43	82	3.4	0.35	0.5	29	0.3	5	N
883	**Avocado**, average	6	450	11	25	39	0.4	0.19	0.4	6	0.2	Tr	2
884	**Bananas**, flesh only	Tr	330	6	27	23	0.3	0.10	0.2	109	0.4	Tr	3
885	**Blackberries**, raw	2	160	41	23	31	0.7	0.11	0.2	22	1.4	Tr	N
886	stewed without sugar	1	140	35	19	26	0.6	0.09	0.2	18	1.2	Tr	N
887	**Blackcurrants**, raw	3	370	60	17	43	1.3	0.14	0.3	15	0.3	N	N
888	stewed without sugar	2	320	51	14	36	1.1	0.12	0.3	12	0.3	N	N

Vitamins per 100g edible portion

No.	Food	Retinol µg	Carotene µg	Vitamin D µg	Vitamin E mg	Thiamin mg	Ribo-flavin mg	Niacin mg	Trypt 60 mg	Vitamin B$_6$ mg	Vitamin B$_{12}$ µg	Folate µg	Panto-thenate mg	Biotin µg	Vitamin C mg
Fruit, general															
878	**Apples**, cooking, stewed with sugar, flesh only	0	Tr	0	0.10	0.02	0.03	0.2	0.1	0.05	0	Tr	0.11	0.9	11[a]
879	cooking, stewed without sugar, flesh only	0	Tr	0	0.11	0.02	0.03	0.2	0.1	0.05	0	Tr	0.11	1.0	12
880	eating, raw, flesh and skin	0	14	0	0.09	0.04	0.04	0.1	Tr	0.07	0	Tr	0.10	1.1	6
881	**Apricots**, raw, flesh and skin	0	405[b]	0	N	0.04	0.05	0.5	0.1	0.08	0	5	0.24	N	6
882	ready-to-eat	0	545	0	N	Tr	0.16	2.3	0.5	0.14	0	11	0.58	N	1
883	**Avocado**, average	0	16	0	3.20	0.10	0.18	1.1	0.3	0.36	0	11	1.10	3.6	6
884	**Bananas**, flesh only	0	26	0	0.16	0.15	0.04	0.7	0.2	0.31	0	14	0.35	2.5	9
885	**Blackberries**, raw	0	80	0	2.37	0.02	0.05	0.5	0.1	0.05	0	34	0.25	0.4	15
886	stewed without sugar	0	68	0	2.03	0.01	0.03	0.3	0.1	0.03	0	5	0.16	0.3	10
887	**Blackcurrants**, raw	0	100	0	1.00	0.03	0.06	0.3	0.1	0.08	0	N	0.40	2.4	200[c]
888	stewed without sugar	0	85	0	0.83	0.02	0.04	0.2	0.1	0.05	0	N	0.26	1.5	130

[a] Frozen apple slices, stewed with sugar, contain 12mg vitamin C per 100g

[b] Levels ranged from 200µg to 3370µg carotene per 100g

[c] Levels ranged from 150mg to 230mg per 100g

Composition of food per 100g edible portion

Fruit, general continued

No.	Food	Description and main data sources	Main data reference	Water g	Total nitrogen g	Protein g	Fat g	Carbo-hydrate g	Energy value kcal	Energy value kJ
889	**Blueberries**	Summer and winter, UK grown and imported. Analytical data, 2011	74	85.7	0.14	0.9	0.2	9.1	40	169
890	**Cherries**, raw, flesh and skin	Black and red cherries. Analytical data, 1985-86	28	82.8	0.14	0.9	0.1	11.5	48	203
891	glacé	Red and multicoloured. Analytical data, 1985-86; and industry data, 2013	27	23.6	0.07	0.4	Tr	78.1[a]	294	1256
892	**Citrus fruit**, soft/easy peelers, flesh only	Early and late winter, including clementines, mandarins, satsumas and tangerines. Analytical data, 2011-2012	74	85.8	0.12	0.7	0.2	9.6	41	173
893	**Dates**, dried, flesh and skin	FAN Supplement, 1992	11	14.6	0.53	3.3	0.2	68.0	270	1151
894	**Dried mixed fruit**	Calculated as sultanas 49%, currants 24%, raisins 18% and peel 9%		15.5	0.37	2.3	0.4	68.1	268	1144
895	**Figs**, ready-to-eat	Semi-dried. Analytical data, 1990	31	23.6	0.52	3.3	1.5	48.6	209	889
896	**Fruit cocktail**, canned in juice	Analytical data, 1985-86; and industry data, 2013	27	86.9	0.07	0.4	Tr	11.7	45	194
897	canned in syrup	Analytical data, 1990; and calculation from recipe proportions[b]	31	81.8	0.06	0.4	Tr	14.8	57	244
898	**Fruit salad**, homemade	Recipe, including eating apples, oranges, bananas, kiwi fruit, grapes and strawberries		82.6	0.11	0.7	0.3	14.3	59	252
899	**Gooseberries**, cooking, stewed with sugar	1000g fruit, 150g water, 120g sugar. Analytical data, 1985-86	28	82.1	0.11	0.7	0.3	12.9	54	229
900	**Grapefruit**, raw, flesh only	Analytical data, 1985-86	28	89.0	0.13	0.8	0.1	6.8	30	126
901	canned in juice	Analytical data, 1985-86	27	88.6	0.09	0.6	Tr	7.3	30	120

[a] Includes oligosaccharides

[b] Calculated as pears 42%, peaches 41%, pineapple 8%, grapes 5% and cherries 4%

Composition of food per 100g edible portion

Fruit, general continued

No.	Food	Starch g	Total sugars g	Gluc g	Fruct g	Sucr g	Malt g	Lact g	Dietary fibre NSP g	AOAC g	Satd g	Mono- unsatd g	Poly- unsatd g	Trans g	Cholest- erol mg
889	**Blueberries**	Tr	9.1	3.9	5.2	Tr	0	0	1.5	1.5	Tr	Tr	0.1	0	0
890	**Cherries**, raw, flesh and skin	0	11.5	5.9	5.3	0.2	0	0	0.9	N	Tr	Tr	Tr	0	0
891	glace	Tr	N	N	N	N	N	0	0.9	N	Tr	Tr	Tr	0	0
892	**Citrus fruit**, soft/easy peelers, flesh only	0	9.6	1.6	1.9	6.1	0	0	1.2	1.5	Tr	0.1	0.1	0	0
893	**Dates**, dried, flesh and skin	0	68.0	35.4	32.6	Tr	0	0	4.0	N	0.1	0.1	Tr	0	0
894	**Dried mixed fruit**	0	68.1	33.3	31.6	0.8	2.3	0	2.2	N	N	N	N	0	0
895	**Figs**, ready-to-eat	0	48.6	26.2	20.8	1.5	0	0	6.9	N	N	N	N	0	0
896	**Fruit cocktail**, canned in juice	0	11.7	5.2	5.7	0.8	0	0	1.0	N	Tr	Tr	Tr	0	0
897	canned in syrup	0	14.8	6.1	6.4	1.9	0.3	0	1.0	N	Tr	Tr	Tr	0	0
898	**Fruit salad**, homemade	0.3	14.0	3.3	4.6	6.2	0	0	1.1	N	N	N	N	0	0
899	**Gooseberries**, cooking, stewed with sugar	0	12.9	2.4	2.6	7.8	0	0	1.9	N	N	N	N	0	0
900	**Grapefruit**, raw, flesh only	0	6.8	2.1	2.3	2.4	0	0	1.3	N	Tr	Tr	Tr	0	0
901	canned in juice	0	7.3	3.6	3.4	0.3	0	0	0.4	N	Tr	Tr	Tr	0	0

Fruit, general continued

No.	Food	Na	K	Ca	Mg	P	Fe	Cu	Zn	Cl	Mn	Se	I
		mg										µg	
889	**Blueberries**	2	66	10	5	16	0.6	0.06	0.1	53	0.7	Tr	2
890	**Cherries**, raw, flesh and skin	1	210	13	10	21	0.2	0.07	0.1	Tr	0.1	1	Tr
891	glacé	27	24	56	5	9	0.9	0.08	0.1	N	Tr	Tr	N[a]
892	**Citrus fruit**, soft/easy peelers, flesh only	1	128	25	9	15	0.1	0.04	Tr	55	Tr	Tr	1
893	**Dates**, dried, flesh and skin	10	700	45	41	60	1.3	0.26	0.4	370	0.3	3	N
894	**Dried mixed fruit**	48	880	73	29	73	2.2	0.47	0.4	13	0.4	N	N
895	**Figs**, ready-to-eat	57	890	230	73	82	3.9	0.27	0.6	160	0.5	Tr	N
896	**Fruit cocktail**, canned in juice	3	95	9	7	14	0.4	0.04	0.1	2	0.1	Tr	N[a]
897	canned in syrup	3	95	5	5	9	0.3	0.02	0.1	3	0.1	Tr	N[a]
898	**Fruit salad**, homemade	1	155	12	9	15	0.2	0.05	Tr	55	0.1	Tr	N
899	**Gooseberries**, cooking, stewed with sugar	7	140	19	6	22	0.3	0.07	0.1	5	0.3	Tr	Tr
900	**Grapefruit**, raw, flesh only	3	200	23	9	20	0.1	0.02	Tr	3	Tr	1	N
901	canned in juice	10	72	22	8	16	0.3	0.01	Tr	5	Tr	Tr	N

[a] Iodine from erythrosine is present but largely unavailable

356

Vitamins per 100g edible portion

Fruit, general continued

No.	Food	Retinol μg	Carotene μg	Vitamin D μg	Vitamin E mg	Thiamin mg	Ribo-flavin mg	Niacin mg	Trypt 60 mg	Vitamin B$_6$ mg	Vitamin B$_{12}$ μg	Folate μg	Panto-thenate mg	Biotin μg	Vitamin C mg
889	**Blueberries**	0	14	0	0.94	0.04	0.04	0.3	0.2	0.01	0	8	0.20	1.5	6
890	**Cherries**, raw, flesh and skin	0	25	0	0.13	0.03	0.03	0.2	0.1	0.05	0	5	0.26	0.4	11
891	glace	0	7	0	Tr	Tr	Tr	Tr	Tr	Tr	0	Tr	Tr	Tr	Tr
892	**Citrus fruit**, soft/easy peelers, flesh only	0	105	0	0.21	0.17	0.03	0.4	0.1	0.06	0	19	0.15	1.4	42
893	**Dates**, dried, flesh and skin	0	40	0	N	0.07	0.09	1.8	1.5	0.19	0	13	0.78	N	Tr
894	**Dried mixed fruit**	0	9	0	N	0.10	0.05	0.7	0.2	0.22	0	15	0.09	3.9	Tr
895	**Figs**, ready-to-eat	0	59	0	N	0.07	0.09	0.7	0.4	0.24	0	8	0.47	N	1
896	**Fruit cocktail**, canned in juice	0	54	0	N	0.01	0.01	0.3	0.1	0.04	0	6	0.05	0.3	14
897	canned in syrup	0	54	0	N	0.02	0.01	0.4	0.1	0.03	0	5	0.05	0.1	4
898	**Fruit salad**, homemade	0	23	0	N	0.09	0.03	0.3	0.1	0.09	0	N	N	N	24
899	**Gooseberries**, cooking, stewed with sugar	0	41	0	0.29	0.01	0.02	0.2	0.1	0.01	0	6	0.17	0.3	11
900	**Grapefruit**, raw, flesh only	0	17[a]	0	0.19	0.05	0.02	0.3	0.1	0.03	0	26	0.28	1.0	36
901	canned in juice	0	Tr	0	0.10	0.04	0.01	0.3	0.1	0.02	0	6	0.12	1.0	33

[a] Pink varieties contain approximately 770μg carotene per 100g

Composition of food per 100g edible portion

No.	Food	Description and main data sources	Main data reference	Water g	Total nitrogen g	Protein g	Fat g	Carbo-hydrate g	Energy value kcal	Energy value kJ
	Fruit, general continued									
902	**Grapes**, green	Seedless, autumn and winter, including Sugarone, Thompson and Prime. Analytical data, 2011-2012	74	82.7	0.11	0.7	0.2	15.2	62	263
903	red	Seedless, autumn and winter, including Crimson and Flame. Analytical data, 2011-2012	74	81.1	0.09	0.6	0.1	17.0	67	286
904	**Kiwi fruit**, flesh and seeds	FAN Supplement, 1992	11	84.0	0.18	1.1	0.5	10.6	49	207
905	**Lemon peel**	Literature sources, 1982; and USDA SR26, 2013	129, 169	81.6	0.24	1.5	0.3	N	N	N
906	**Lemons**, whole, without pips	Includes peel but no pips. FAN Supplement, 1992	11	86.3	0.16	1.0	0.3	3.2	19	79
907	**Lychees**, raw, flesh only	FAN Supplement, 1992	11	81.1	0.14	0.9	0.1	14.3	58	248
908	**Mandarin oranges**, canned in juice	Analytical data, 1985-86	27	89.6	0.11	0.7	Tr	7.7	32	135
909	**Mangoes**, ripe, raw, flesh only	Literature sources. FAN Supplement, 1992	11	82.4	0.11	0.7	0.2	14.1	57	245
910	**Melon**, Canteloupe-type, flesh only	Canteloupe, Charantais and Rock. Analytical data, 1985-86	28	92.1	0.10	0.6	0.1	4.2	19	81
911	Galia, flesh only	Analytical data, 1990	31	91.7	0.08	0.5	0.1	5.6	24	102
912	yellow flesh, flesh only	Honeydew, autumn and winter, whole and pre-prepared slices. Analytical data, 2011	74	91.0	0.08	0.5	0.1	6.8	29	122
913	watermelon, flesh only	Literature sources. FAN Supplement, 1992	11	92.3	0.07	0.5	0.3	7.1	31	133
914	**Mixed peel**	Analytical data, 1985-86; and industry data, 2013	27	20.9	0.05	0.3	0.9	74.1	287	1224
915	**Nectarines**, flesh and skin	Analytical data, 1985-86	28	88.9	0.22	1.4	0.1	9.0	40	171
916	**Olives**, in brine	Bottled, drained, flesh and skin, green. MW1, 1940; and industry data, 2013	1	76.5	0.14	0.9	11.0	Tr	103	422

Composition of food per 100g edible portion

Fruit, general continued

No.	Food	Starch g	Total sugars g	Individual sugars					Dietary fibre		Fatty acids				Cholest-erol mg
				Gluc g	Fruct g	Sucr g	Malt g	Lact g	NSP g	AOAC g	Satd g	Mono-unsatd g	Poly-unsatd g	Trans g	
902	**Grapes**, green	0	15.2	7.3	7.9	Tr	0	0	0.7	1.2	0.1	Tr	0.1	0	0
903	red	0	17.0	7.7	9.3	Tr	0	0	0.6	1.3	Tr	Tr	Tr	0	0
904	**Kiwi fruit**, flesh and seeds	0.3	10.3	4.6	4.3	1.3	0	0	1.9	N	N	N	N	0	0
905	**Lemon peel**	0	N	N	N	N	0	0	N	10.6	0.1	Tr	0.1	0	0
906	**Lemons**, whole, without pips	0	3.2	1.4	1.4	0.4	0	0	N	N	0.1	Tr	0.1	0	0
907	**Lychees**, raw, flesh only	0	14.3	7.0	7.3	Tr	0	0	0.7	N	Tr	Tr	Tr	0	0
908	**Mandarin oranges**, canned in juice	0	7.7	2.8	3.1	1.8	0	0	0.3	N	Tr	Tr	Tr	0	0
909	**Mangoes**, ripe, raw, flesh only	0.3	13.8	0.7	3.0	10.1	0	0	2.6	N	0.1	Tr	Tr	0	0
910	**Melon**, Canteloupe-type, flesh only	0	4.2	1.8	2.2	0.1	0	0	1.0	1.8	Tr	Tr	Tr	0	0
911	Galia, flesh only	0	5.6	1.6	2.0	2.0	0	0	0.4	N	Tr	Tr	Tr	0	0
912	yellow flesh, flesh only	0	6.8	1.7	2.5	2.6	0	0	0.4	0.7	Tr	Tr	0.1	0	0
913	watermelon, flesh only	0	7.1	1.3	2.3	3.4	0	0	0.1	N	0.1	0.1	0.1	0	0
914	**Mixed peel**	22.9	51.2	16.7	3.8	8.1	22.6	0	4.8	4.5	N	N	N	0	0
915	**Nectarines**, flesh and skin	0	9.0	1.3	1.3	6.3	0	0	1.2	N	Tr	Tr	Tr	0	0
916	**Olives**, in brine	0	Tr	Tr	Tr	Tr	0	0	2.9	N	1.7	5.7	1.3	0	0

Inorganic constituents per 100g edible portion

No.	Food	mg										µg	
		Na	K	Ca	Mg	P	Fe	Cu	Zn	Cl	Mn	Se	I
Fruit, general continued													
902	**Grapes,** green	1	217	8	6	19	0.2	0.07	Tr	44	0.1	Tr	1
903	red	1	213	11	7	18	0.2	0.10	Tr	63	0.1	Tr	1
904	**Kiwi fruit,** flesh and seeds	4	290	25	15	32	0.4	0.13	0.1	39	0.1	N	N
905	**Lemon peel**	6	160	130	15	12	0.8	N	0.3	N	N	N	N
906	**Lemons,** whole, without pips	5	150	85	12	18	0.5	0.26	0.1	5	N	1	N
907	**Lychees,** raw, flesh only	1	160	6	9	30	0.5	0.15	0.3	3	0.1	N	N
908	**Mandarin oranges,** canned in juice	6	85	17	9	13	0.5	Tr	0.1	2	Tr	Tr	Tr
909	**Mangoes,** ripe, raw, flesh only	2	180	12	13	16	0.7	0.12	0.1	N	0.3	N	N
910	**Melon,** Canteloupe-type, flesh only	8	210	20	11	13	0.3	Tr	0.1	44	Tr	Tr	4
911	Galia, flesh only	31	150	13	12	10	0.2	Tr	0.1	75	Tr	Tr	N
912	yellow flesh, flesh only	11	180	6	6	6	0.2	0.02	0.1	97	Tr	Tr	Tr
913	watermelon, flesh only	2	100	7	8	9	0.3	0.03	0.2	N	Tr	Tr	Tr
914	**Mixed peel**	280	21	130	12	6	1.3	0.15	0.2	N	0.1	N	N
915	**Nectarines,** flesh and skin	1	170	7	10	22	0.4	0.06	0.1	5	0.1	1	3
916	**Olives,** in brine	1330	91	61	22	17	1.0	0.23	N	2220	N	N	N

Fruit, general continued

Vitamins per 100g edible portion

No.	Food	Retinol µg	Carotene µg	Vitamin D µg	Vitamin E mg	Thiamin mg	Ribo-flavin mg	Niacin mg	Trypt 60 mg	Vitamin B6 mg	Vitamin B12 µg	Folate µg	Panto-thenate mg	Biotin µg	Vitamin C mg
902	**Grapes**, green	0	Tr	0	0.18	0.04	0.01	0.2	0.1	0.04	0	6	0.14	0.2	2
903	red	0	14	0	0.20	0.09	0.01	0.2	0.1	0.04	0	6	0.12	0.2	3
904	**Kiwi fruit**, flesh and seeds	0	40	0	N	0.01	0.03	0.3	0.3	0.15	0	N	N	N	59
905	**Lemon peel**	0	30	0	0.25	0.06	0.08	0.4	0.2	0.17	0	11	0.19	N	130
906	**Lemons**, whole, without pips	0	18	0	N	0.05	0.04	0.2	0.1	0.11	0	N	0.23	0.5	58
907	**Lychees**, raw, flesh only	0	0	0	N	0.04	0.06	0.5	0.1	N	0	N	N	N	45
908	**Mandarin oranges**, canned in juice	0	95	0	Tr	0.08	0.01	0.2	0.1	0.03	0	12	0.15	0.8	20
909	**Mangoes**, ripe, raw, flesh only	0	696	0	1.05	0.04	0.05	0.5	1.3	0.13	0	N	0.16	N	37
910	**Melon**, Canteloupe-type, flesh only	0	1770	0	0.10	0.04	0.02	0.6	Tr	0.11	0	5	0.13	N	26
911	Galia, flesh only	0	N	0	0.10	0.03	0.01	0.4	Tr	0.09	0	3	0.17	N	15
912	yellow flesh, flesh only	0	7	0	0.07	0.07	0.01	0.4	0.1	0.07	0	13	0.24	2.6	8
913	watermelon, flesh only	0	116	0	0.10	0.05	0.01	0.1	Tr	0.14	0	2	0.21	1	8
914	**Mixed peel**	0	Tr	0	N	N	N	N	0.1	N	0	N	N	N	Tr
915	**Nectarines**, flesh and skin	0	114	0	N	0.02	0.04	0.6	0.3	0.03	0	Tr	0.16	0.2	37
916	**Olives**, in brine	0	180[a]	0	1.99	Tr	Tr	Tr	0.1	0.02	0	Tr	0.02	Tr	0

[a] Value is for green olives. Ripe black olives contain 40µg carotene per 100g

Fruit *continued*

Composition of food per 100g edible portion

Fruit, general continued

No.	Food	Description and main data sources	Main data reference	Water g	Total nitrogen g	Protein g	Fat g	Carbo-hydrate g	Energy value kcal	Energy value kJ
917	**Oranges**, flesh only	Early and late winter, including Navel and Valencia. Analytical data, 2011-2012	74	87.0	0.13	0.8	0.2	8.2	36	152
918	**Passion fruit**, flesh and pips	FAN Supplement, 1992	11	74.9	0.45	2.6	0.4	5.8	36	152
919	**Papaya**, raw, flesh only	FAN Supplement, 1992	11	88.5	0.08	0.5	0.1	8.8	36	153
920	**Peaches**, raw, flesh and skin	Analytical data, 1985-86	28	88.9	0.16	1.0	0.1	7.6	33	142
921	canned in juice	Halves and slices. Analytical data, 1985-86	27	86.7	0.09	0.6	Tr	9.7	39	165
922	canned in syrup	Halves and slices. Analytical data, 1985-86	27	81.1	0.08	0.5	Tr	14.0	55	233
923	**Pears**, raw, flesh and skin	Autumn and winter, UK grown and imported, pre-packed and loose, including Conference, Comice, Concorde, Rocha, Green Williams. Analytical data, 2011-2012	74	85.2	0.05	0.3	0.1	10.9	43	182
924	canned in juice	Analytical data, 1985-86	27	86.8	0.04	0.3	Tr	8.5	33	141
925	**Pineapple**, raw, flesh only	Analytical data, 1985-86	28	86.5	0.06	0.4	0.2	10.1	41	176
926	canned in juice	Cubes and slices. Analytical data, 1985-86	27	86.8	0.05	0.3	Tr	12.2	47	200
927	canned in syrup	Cubes and slices. Analytical data, 1985-86	27	82.2	0.08	0.5	Tr	16.5	64	273
928	**Plums**, average, raw, flesh and skin	Assorted varieties. FAN Supplement, 1992	11	83.9	0.09	0.6	0.1	8.8	36	155
929	average, stewed with sugar	Calculated from 1350g fruit, 100g water, 162g sugar; stones removed.		76.5	0.08	0.5	0.1	17.9	70	299
930	**Pomegranate**, flesh and pips	FAN Supplement, 1992	11	80.0	0.21	1.3	0.2	11.8	51	218
931	**Prunes**, canned in juice	Stones removed. Analytical data, 1985-86	27	74.1	0.12	0.7	0.2	19.7	79	335
932	ready-to-eat	Semi-dried. Analytical data, 1990	31	31.1	0.40	2.5	0.4	34.0	141	601

Fruit *continued*

Fruit, general continued

No.	Food	Starch	Total sugars	Individual sugars					Dietary fibre		Fatty acids				Cholesterol
				Gluc	Fruct	Sucr	Malt	Lact	NSP	AOAC	Satd	Mono-unsatd	Poly-unsatd	Trans	erol
		g	g	g	g	g	g	g	g	g	g	g	g	g	mg
917	**Oranges**, flesh only	0	8.2	2.0	2.2	4.0	0	0	1.7	1.2	0.1	0.1	0.1	0	0
918	**Passion fruit**, flesh and pips	0	5.8	2.2	1.9	1.7	0	0	3.3	N	0.1	0.1	0.1	0	0
919	**Papaya**, raw, flesh only	0	8.8	2.8	2.8	3.1	0	0	2.2	N	Tr	Tr	Tr	0	0
920	**Peaches**, raw, flesh and skin	0	7.6	1.1	1.1	5.2	0	0	1.5	N	Tr	Tr	Tr	0	0
921	canned in juice	0	9.7	2.4	3.7	3.6	0	0	0.8	N	Tr	Tr	Tr	0	0
922	canned in syrup	0	14.0	3.7	3.6	6.7	0	0	0.9	N	Tr	Tr	Tr	0	0
923	**Pears**, raw, flesh and skin	0	10.9	3.1	6.6	1.2	0	0	1.6	2.7	Tr	Tr	Tr	0	0
924	canned in juice	0	8.5	2.3	5.7	0.6	0	0	1.4	N	Tr	Tr	Tr	0	0
925	**Pineapple**, raw, flesh only	0	10.1	2.0	2.5	5.5	0	0	1.2	N	Tr	0.1	0.1	0	0
926	canned in juice	0	12.2	4.0	4.0	4.2	0	0	0.5	N	Tr	Tr	Tr	0	0
927	canned in syrup	0	16.5	6.0	4.8	5.8	0	0	0.7	N	Tr	Tr	Tr	0	0
928	**Plums**, average, raw, flesh and skin	0	8.8	4.3	2.0	2.5	0	0	1.6	N	Tr	Tr	Tr	0	0
929	average, stewed with sugar	0	17.9	3.6	1.7	12.6	0	0	1.3	N	Tr	Tr	Tr	0	0
930	**Pomegranate**, flesh and pips	0	11.8	6.4	5.2	0.2	0	0	3.4	N	Tr	0.1	0.1	0	0
931	**Prunes**, canned in juice	0	19.7	10.2	8.4	1.1	0	0	2.4	N	Tr	0.1	0.1	0	0
932	ready-to-eat	0	34.0	17.9	12.1	4.1	0	0	5.7	N	N	N	N	0	0

Inorganic constituents per 100g edible portion

No.	Food	Na	K	Ca	Mg	P	Fe	Cu	Zn	Cl	Mn	Se	I
					mg							µg	

Fruit, general continued

No.	Food	Na	K	Ca	Mg	P	Fe	Cu	Zn	Cl	Mn	Se	I
917	**Oranges**, flesh only	1	122	24	8	16	0.1	0.03	Tr	73	Tr	Tr	1
918	**Passion fruit**, flesh and pips	19	200	11	29	64	1.3	N	0.8	N	N	N	N
919	**Papaya**, raw, flesh only	5	200	23	11	13	0.5	0.08	0.2	11	0.1	N	N
920	**Peaches**, raw, flesh and skin	1	160	7	9	22	0.4	0.06	0.1	Tr	0.1	1	3
921	canned in juice	12	170	4	7	19	0.4	0.04	0.1	4	0.1	Tr	N
922	canned in syrup	4	110	3	5	11	0.2	Tr	Tr	4	Tr	Tr	N
923	**Pears**, raw, flesh and skin	1	105	7	5	9	0.1	0.05	0.1	64	0.1	Tr	1
924	canned in juice	3	81	6	5	10	0.2	Tr	0.1	3	Tr	Tr	Tr
925	**Pineapple**, raw, flesh only	2	160	18	16	10	0.2	0.11	0.1	29	0.5	Tr	Tr
926	canned in juice	1	71	8	13	5	0.5	0.08	0.1	4	0.9	Tr	Tr
927	canned in syrup	2	79	6	11	5	0.2	0.02	0.1	4	0.9	Tr	Tr
928	**Plums**, average, raw, flesh and skin	2	240	13	8	23	0.4	0.10	0.1	Tr	0.1	Tr	Tr
929	average, stewed with sugar	2	201	12	7	19	0.4	0.10	0.1	Tr	0.1	Tr	Tr
930	**Pomegranate**, flesh and pips	2	240	12	11	29	0.7	0.17	0.4	2	N	N	N
931	**Prunes**, canned in juice	18	340	26	15	30	2.2	0.09	1.0	N	0.1	Tr	N
932	ready-to-eat	11	760	34	24	73	2.6	0.14	0.4	3	0.3	3	N

Vitamins per 100g edible portion

No.	Food	Retinol µg	Carotene µg	Vitamin D µg	Vitamin E mg	Thiamin mg	Ribo-flavin mg	Niacin mg	Trypt 60 mg	Vitamin B₆ mg	Vitamin B₁₂ µg	Folate µg	Panto-thenate mg	Biotin µg	Vitamin C mg
	Fruit, general continued														
917	**Oranges**, flesh only	0	55[a]	0	0.35	0.22	0.03	0.5	0.1	0.05	0	33	0.27	1.0	52
918	**Passion fruit**, flesh and pips	0	750	0	N	0.03	0.12	1.5	0.4	N	0	N	N	N	23
919	**Papaya**, raw, flesh only	0	810	0	N	0.03	0.04	0.3	0.1	0.03	0	1	0.22	N	60
920	**Peaches**, raw, flesh and skin	0	114	0	N	0.02	0.04	0.6	0.2	0.02	0	3	0.17	0.2	31
921	canned in juice	0	67	0	N	0.01	0.01	0.6	0.1	0.02	0	2	0.06	0.2	6
922	canned in syrup	0	75	0	N	0.01	0.01	0.6	0.1	0.02	0	7	0.05	0.1	5
923	**Pears**, raw, flesh and skin	0	14	0	0.12	0.03	0.04	0.2	0.1	0.04	0	6	0.08	0.3	3
924	canned in juice	0	Tr	0	Tr	0.01	0.01	0.2	Tr	0.03	0	4	0.04	0.2	3
925	**Pineapple**, raw, flesh only	0	18	0	0.10	0.08	0.03	0.3	0.1	0.09	0	5	0.16	0.3	12
926	canned in juice	0	12	0	0.05	0.09	0.01	0.2	0.1	0.09	0	1	0.11	0.1	11
927	canned in syrup	0	11	0	0.06	0.07	0.01	0.2	0.1	0.07	0	1	0.07	0.1	13
928	**Plums**, average, raw, flesh and skin	0	376	0	0.61	0.05	0.03	1.1	0.1	0.05	0	3	0.15	Tr	4
929	average, stewed with sugar	0	315	0	0.51	0.03	0.02	0.7	0.1	0.03	0	1	0.09	Tr	3
930	**Pomegranate**, flesh and pips	0	33	0	N	0.05	0.04	0.3	0.2	0.31	0	N	0.57	N	13
931	**Prunes**, canned in juice	0	140	0	N	0.02	0.02	0.5	0.1	0.06	0	5	0.07	Tr	Tr
932	ready-to-eat	0	140	0	N	0.09	0.18	1.3	0.4	0.21	0	3	0.41	Tr	Tr

[a] Blood oranges have been found to contain 155µg carotene per 100g

Composition of food per 100g edible portion

No.	Food	Description and main data sources	Main data reference	Water g	Total nitrogen g	Protein g	Fat g	Carbo-hydrate g	Energy value kcal	kJ
Fruit, general *continued*										
933	**Raisins**	Large stoned variety. Analytical data, 1985-86	27	13.2	0.34	2.1	0.4	69.3	272	1159
934	**Raspberries**, raw	Whole fruit. Analytical data, 1985-86	28	87.0	0.22	1.4	0.3	4.6	25	109
935	**Rhubarb**, stewed with sugar	1000g fruit, 100g water, 120g sugar. Analytical data, 1985-86	28	84.6	0.14	0.9	0.1	11.5	48	203
936	**Strawberries**, raw	Summer and autumn, UK grown and imported, including Elsanta, Sonata, Ava, Portola and unspecified varieties. Analytical data, 2011	74	91.6	0.09	0.6	0.5	6.1	30	126
937	**Sultanas**	Whole fruit. Analytical data, 1985-86	27	15.2	0.43	2.7	0.4	69.4	275	1171

Composition of food per 100g edible portion

Fruit, general continued

No.	Food	Starch (g)	Total sugars (g)	Individual sugars					Dietary fibre		Fatty acids				Cholesterol (mg)
				Gluc (g)	Fruct (g)	Sucr (g)	Malt (g)	Lact (g)	NSP (g)	AOAC (g)	Satd (g)	Mono-unsatd (g)	Poly-unsatd (g)	Trans (g)	erol (mg)
933	**Raisins**	0	69.3	34.5	34.8	Tr	0	0	2.0	N	N	N	N	0	0
934	**Raspberries**, raw	0	4.6	1.9	2.4	0.2	0	0	2.5	N	0.1	0.1	0.1	0	0
935	**Rhubarb**, stewed with sugar	0	11.5	1.2	1.2	9.1	0	0	1.2	N	Tr	Tr	Tr	0	0
936	**Strawberries**, raw	0	6.1	3.0	3.1	Tr	0	0	1.0	3.8	Tr	0.1	0.3	0	0
937	**Sultanas**	0	69.4	34.8	34.6	Tr	0	0	2.0	N	N	N	N	0	0

Inorganic constituents per 100g edible portion

No.	Food	Na	K	Ca	Mg	P	Fe	Cu	Zn	Cl	Mn	Se	I
		mg										µg	
Fruit, general continued													
933	**Raisins**	60	1020	46	35	76	3.8	0.39	0.7	9	0.3	8	N
934	**Raspberries**, raw	3	170	25	19	31	0.7	0.10	0.3	22	0.4	N	N
935	**Rhubarb**, stewed with sugar	1	210	33	6	18	0.1	0.02	Tr	75	0.3	Tr	N
936	**Strawberries**, raw	1	170	17	12	26	0.3	0.03	0.1	62	0.3	Tr	1
937	**Sultanas**	19	1060	64	31	86	2.2	0.40	0.3	16	0.3	N	N

Vitamins per 100g edible portion

Fruit, general continued

No.	Food	Retinol µg	Carotene µg	Vitamin D µg	Vitamin E mg	Thiamin mg	Ribo-flavin mg	Niacin mg	Trypt 60 mg	Vitamin B_6 mg	Vitamin B_{12} µg	Folate µg	Panto-thenate mg	Biotin µg	Vitamin C mg
933	**Raisins**	0	12	0	N	0.12	0.05	0.6	0.2	0.25	0	10	0.15	2.0	1
934	**Raspberries**, raw	0	6	0	0.48	0.03	0.05	0.5	0.3	0.06	0	33	0.24	1.9	32
935	**Rhubarb**, stewed with sugar	0	28	0	0.17	0.03	0.02	0.2	0.1	0.02	0	4	0.08	N	5
936	**Strawberries**, raw	0	Tr	0	0.39	0.02	0.02	0.6	0.1	0.03	0	61	0.37	1.2	57
937	**Sultanas**	0	12	0	0.70	0.09	0.05	0.8	0.2	0.25	0	27	0.09	4.8	Tr

Nuts and seeds

Section 2.10

Nuts and seeds

Most of the data in this section of the Tables have been taken from the *Fruit and Nuts* (1992)[11] supplement, based on analysis in the 1980s[31,39]. However, values for processed nuts and nut products have been reviewed, using data from manufacturers, and updated where necessary, in particular for sodium.

Users should note that all values are expressed per 100g edible portion. Guidance for calculating nutrient content 'as purchased' or 'as served' (e.g. including shells) is given in Section 4.2. Cooked foods including nuts are not included in this section. Taxonomic names for foods in this part of the Tables can be found in Section 4.5.

Composition of food per 100g edible portion

No.	Food	Description and main data sources	Main data reference	Water g	Total nitrogen g	Protein g	Fat g	Carbo-hydrate g	Energy value kcal	kJ
Nuts and seeds										
938	**Almonds**	Flaked and ground. Analytical data, 1990/91	39	4.2	4.07	21.1	55.8	6.9	612	2534
939	**Brazil nuts**	Kernel only. Analytical data, 1990/91	39	2.8	2.61	14.3	68.2	3.1	683	2816
940	**Cashew nuts**, roasted and salted	Analytical data, 1990/91	39	2.4	3.87	20.5	50.9	18.8	611	2533
941	**Chestnuts**, raw	MW1, 1940, literature sources	1	51.7	0.37	2.0	2.7	36.6	170	719
942	**Coconut**, creamed block	Block of dried kernel. Analytical data, 1990	31	2.5	1.14	6.0	68.8	7.0	669	2760
943	desiccated	MW1, 1940	1	2.3	1.05	5.6	62.0	6.4	604	2492
944	**Coconut milk**	Retail. Industry data, 2013		78.3	0.21	1.1	16.9	3.3	169	697
945	reduced fat	Retail. Industry data, 2013		89.5	0.13	0.7	7.7	2.0	79	328
946	**Hazelnuts**	Kernel only. Analytical data, 1990; and industry data, 2013	31	4.6	2.66	14.1	63.5	6.0	650	2685
947	**Macadamia nuts**, salted	Analytical data, 1990/91; and industry data, 2013	39	1.3	1.49	7.9	77.6	4.8	748	3082
948	**Marzipan**	Analytical data, 1990; and industry data, 2013	31	8.1	1.02	5.3	12.7	67.6	389	1642
949	**Mixed nuts**	Calculated as plain peanuts 68%, almonds 17%, cashews 8% and hazelnuts 7%		5.7	4.36	23.8	49.1	11.6	581	2407
950	**Peanut butter**, smooth	MW4, 1978; and industry data, 2013	4	1.1	4.17	22.8	51.8	13.1	607	2514
951	**Peanuts and raisins**	Calculated as peanuts 56% and raisins 44%		9.3	2.80	15.4	25.9	37.5	436	1821
952	**Peanuts**, plain	Kernel only, unsalted. Analytical data, 1990/91	39	6.3	4.73	25.8	46.0	12.5	564	2341
953	dry roasted	Analytical data, 1990/91; and industry data, 2013	39	1.8	4.71	25.7	49.8	10.3	590	2444
954	roasted and salted	Analytical data, 1990/91; and industry data, 2013	39	1.9	4.53	24.7	53.0	7.1	602	2495
955	**Pecan nuts**	Analytical data, 1990/91	39	3.7	1.74	9.2	70.1	5.8	689	2843

Nuts and seeds

No.	Food	Starch g	Total sugars g	Gluc g	Fruct g	Sucr g	Malt g	Lact g	Dietary fibre NSP g	Dietary fibre AOAC g	Satd g	Mono-unsatd g	Poly-unsatd g	Trans g	Cholesterol mg
938	**Almonds**	2.7	4.2	Tr	Tr	4.2	0	0	7.4	N	4.4	38.2	10.5	0	0
939	**Brazil nuts**	0.7	2.4	0	0	2.4	0	0	4.3	N	17.4	22.4	25.4	0	0
940	**Cashew nuts**, roasted and salted	13.2	5.6	0	0	5.6	0	0	3.2	4.3	10.1	29.4	9.1	Tr	0
941	**Chestnuts**, raw	29.6	7.0	Tr	Tr	7.0	0	0	4.1	N	0.5	1.0	1.1	0	0
942	**Coconut**, creamed block	0	7.0	Tr	0.1	6.9	0	0	N	N	59.3	3.9	1.6	0	0
943	desiccated	0	6.4	Tr	0.8	5.6	0	0	13.7	N	53.4	3.5	1.5	0	0
944	**Coconut milk**	1.3	2.0	N	N	N	0	0	N	0.4	14.6	N	N	0	0
945	reduced fat	0.9	1.1	N	N	N	0	0	N	0.1	6.4	N	N	0	0
946	**Hazelnuts**	2.0	4.0	0.2	0.1	3.7	0	0	6.5	6.9	4.6	49.2	6.6	0	0
947	**Macadamia nuts**, salted	0.8	4.0	0.1	0.1	3.8	0	0	5.3	N	11.2	60.8	1.6	0	0
948	**Marzipan**	0	67.6	2.7	1.1	62.2	1.6	0	1.9	2.4	1.0	8.0	3.1	0	0
949	**Mixed nuts**	6.0	5.6	0	0	5.6	0	0	6.2	N	7.7	27.3	11.8	0	0
950	**Peanut butter**, smooth	6.4	6.7	0	0	6.7	0	0	5.4	6.6	12.8	19.9	16.8	Tr	0
951	**Peanuts and raisins**	3.5	34.0	15.2	15.3	3.5	0	0	4.4	N	4.9	12.3	7.3	0	0
952	**Peanuts**, plain	6.3	6.2	0	0	6.2	0	0	6.2	N	8.7	22.0	13.1	0	0
953	dry roasted	6.5	3.8	0	0	3.8	0	0	6.4	7.6	8.9	22.8	15.5	0	0
954	roasted and salted	3.3	3.8	0	0	3.8	0	0	6.0	8.0	9.5	24.2	16.5	0	0
955	**Pecan nuts**	1.5	4.3	0.3	0.3	3.7	0	0	4.7	N	5.7	42.5	18.7	0	0

Inorganic constituents per 100g edible portion

No.	Food	mg										µg	
		Na	K	Ca	Mg	P	Fe	Cu	Zn	Cl	Mn	Se	I
	Nuts and seeds												
938	**Almonds**	14	780	240	270	550	3.0	1.00	3.2	18	1.7	2	2
939	**Brazil nuts**	3	660	170	410	590	2.5	1.76	4.2	57	1.2	254[a]	20
940	Cashew nuts, roasted and salted	290	730	35	250	510	6.2	2.04	5.7	490	1.8	34	11
941	**Chestnuts**, raw	11	500	46	33	74	0.9	0.23	0.5	15	0.5	Tr	N
942	**Coconut**, creamed block	30	650	23	73	170	3.7	0.56	0.9	190	1.8	12	2
943	desiccated	28	660	23	90	160	3.6	0.55	0.9	200	1.8	12	3
944	**Coconut milk**	Tr	N	N	N	N	N	N	N	N	N	N	N
945	reduced fat	Tr	N	N	N	N	N	N	N	N	N	N	N
946	**Hazelnuts**	6	730	140	160	300	3.2	1.23	2.1	18	4.9	2	17
947	**Macadamia nuts**, salted	400	300	47	100	200	1.6	0.43	1.1	560	5.5	7	N
948	**Marzipan**	20	160	66	68	130	0.9	0.24	0.8	23	0.4	1	Tr
949	**Mixed nuts**	5	696	94	222	452	2.9	1.12	3.5	10	2.2	5	16
950	**Peanut butter**, smooth	350	700	37	180	330	2.1	0.70	3.0	500	1.7	3	N
951	**Peanuts and raisins**	28	824	54	133	274	3.1	0.74	2.3	8	1.3	5	N
952	**Peanuts**, plain	2	670	60	210	430	2.5	1.02	3.5	7	2.1	3	20
953	dry roasted	790	730	52	190	420	2.1	0.64	3.3	1140	2.2	3	19
954	roasted and salted	400	810	37	180	410	1.3	0.54	2.9	660	1.9	4	19
955	**Pecan nuts**	1	520	61	130	310	2.2	1.07	5.3	15	4.6	12	N

[a] Selenium can range from 85µg to 690µg per 100g

Vitamins per 100g edible portion

No.	Food	Retinol µg	Carotene µg	Vitamin D µg	Vitamin E mg	Thiamin mg	Ribo-flavin mg	Niacin mg	Trypt 60 mg	Vitamin B$_6$ mg	Vitamin B$_{12}$ µg	Folate µg	Panto-thenate mg	Biotin µg	Vitamin C mg
Nuts and seeds															
938	**Almonds**	0	0	0	23.96	0.21	0.75	3.1	3.4	0.15	0	48	0.44	64.0	0
939	**Brazil nuts**	0	0	0	7.18	0.67	0.03	0.3	3.0	0.31	0	21	0.41	11.0	0
940	**Cashew nuts**, roasted and salted	0	6	0	1.30	0.41	0.16	1.3	5.2	0.43	0	68	1.08	13.0	0
941	**Chestnuts**, raw	0	0	0	1.20	0.14	0.02	0.5	0.4	0.34	0	N	0.49	1.4	Tr
942	**Coconut**, creamed block	0	0	0	1.40	0.03	0.05	0.9	1.2	N	0	9	0.50	N	N
943	desiccated	0	0	0	1.26	0.03	0.05	0.9	1.1	0.09	0	9	0.50	N	0
944	**Coconut milk**	0	0	0	N	N	N	N	N	N	0	N	N	N	N
945	reduced fat	0	0	0	N	N	N	N	N	N	0	N	N	N	N
946	**Hazelnuts**	0	0	0	24.98	0.43	0.16	1.1	4.0	0.59	0	72	1.51	76.0	0
947	**Macadamia nuts**, salted	0	0	0	1.49	0.28	0.06	1.6	1.7	0.28	0	N	0.61	6.0	0
948	**Marzipan**	0	0	0	6.18	0.05	0.19	0.7	0.9	0.04	0	12	0.11	16.0	0
949	**Mixed nuts**	0	0	0	12.78	0.89	0.22	10.0	5.0	0.51	0	93	2.07	66.1	0
950	**Peanut butter**, smooth	0	0	0	4.99	0.17	0.09	12.5	4.9	0.58	0	53	1.56	94.0	0
951	**Peanuts and raisins**	0	5	0	5.65	0.69	0.08	8.0	3.2	0.44	0	66	1.56	41.2	0
952	**Peanuts**, plain	0	0	0	10.09	1.14	0.10	13.8	5.5	0.59	0	110	2.66	72.0	0
953	dry roasted	0	0	0	1.11	0.18	0.13	13.1	5.5	0.54	0	44	1.59	130.0	0
954	roasted and salted	0	0	0	0.66	0.18	0.10	13.6	5.3	0.63	0	52	1.70	102.0	0
955	**Pecan nuts**	0	50	0	4.34	0.71	0.15	1.4	4.1	0.19	0	39	1.71	N	0

Composition of food per 100g edible portion

Nuts and seeds continued

No.	Food	Description and main data sources	Main data reference	Water g	Total nitrogen g	Protein g	Fat g	Carbo-hydrate g	Energy value kcal	kJ
956	**Pine nuts**	Pine kernels. Analytical data, 1990/91	39	2.7	2.64	14.0	68.6	4.0	688	2840
957	**Pistachio nuts**, roasted and salted	Analytical data, 1990/91	39	2.1	3.38	17.9	55.4	8.2	601	2485
958	**Pumpkin seeds**	FAN Supplement, 1992	11	5.6	4.61	24.4	45.6	15.2	565	2345
959	**Sesame seeds**	With and without hulls. Analytical data, 1990/91	39	4.6	3.44	18.2	58.0	0.9	598	2470
960	**Sunflower seeds**	FAN Supplement, 1992	11	4.4	3.74	19.8	47.5	18.6[a]	576	2392
961	**Tahini paste**	Literature sources, 1982	147	3.1	3.49	18.5	58.9	0.9	607	2508
962	**Trail mix**	Mix of nuts and dried fruit. Analytical data, 1987; and industry data, 2013	27	8.9	1.45	9.1	28.5	37.2	432	1804
963	**Walnuts**	Kernel only. Analytical data, 1990/91	39	2.8	2.77	14.7	68.5	3.3	688	2837

[a] Includes oligosaccharides

Nuts and seeds *continued*

Composition of food per 100g edible portion

Nuts and seeds continued

No.	Food	Starch g	Total sugars g	Individual sugars					Dietary fibre		Fatty acids				Cholest-erol mg
				Gluc g	Fruct g	Sucr g	Malt g	Lact g	NSP g	AOAC g	Satd g	Mono-unsatd g	Poly-unsatd g	Trans g	
956	Pine nuts	0.1	3.9	0.1	0.1	3.7	0	0	1.9	N	4.6	19.9	41.1	0	0
957	Pistachio nuts, roasted and salted	2.5	5.7	Tr	Tr	5.7	0	0	6.1	7.4	7.4	27.6	17.9	0	0
958	Pumpkin seeds	14.1	1.1	0	0	1.1	0	0	5.3	N	7.0	11.2	18.3	0	0
959	Sesame seeds	0.5	0.4	0.1	0.1	0.2	0	0	7.9	N	10.5	22.1	25.5	0	0
960	Sunflower seeds	16.3	1.7[a]	0	0	1.7	0	0	6.0	N	6.6	10.7	28.2	0	0
961	Tahini paste	0.5	0.4	0.1	0.1	0.2	0	0	8.0	N	8.4	22.0	25.8	N	0
962	Trail mix	0.1	37.1	17.3	16.1	3.4	0.4	0	4.3	5.1	N	N	N	N	0
963	Walnuts	0.7	2.6	0.2	0.2	2.2	0	0	3.5	N	7.5	10.7	46.8	0	0

[a] Not including oligosaccharides

377

Inorganic constituents per 100g edible portion

Nuts and seeds continued

No.	Food	Na	K	Ca	Mg	P	Fe	Cu	Zn	Cl	Mn	Se	I
						mg						µg	
956	Pine nuts	1	780	11	270	650	5.6	1.32	6.5	41	7.9	N	N
957	Pistachio nuts, roasted and salted	530	1040	110	130	420	3.0	0.83	2.2	810	0.9	6	N
958	Pumpkin seeds	18	820	39	270	850	10.0	1.57	6.6	N	N	6	N
959	Sesame seeds	20	570	670	370	720	10.4	1.46	5.3	10	1.5	N	N
960	Sunflower seeds	3	710	110	390	640	6.4	2.27	5.1	N	2.2	49	N
961	Tahini paste	20	580	680	380	730	10.6	1.48	5.4	10	1.5	N	N
962	Trail mix	27	620	69	110	210	3.7	0.55	1.5	N	1.6	N	N
963	Walnuts	7	450	94	160	380	2.9	1.34	2.7	24	3.4	3	9

Nuts and seeds continued

Vitamins per 100g edible portion

No.	Food	Retinol µg	Carotene µg	Vitamin D µg	Vitamin E mg	Thiamin mg	Ribo-flavin mg	Niacin mg	Trypt 60 mg	Vitamin B$_6$ mg	Vitamin B$_{12}$ µg	Folate µg	Panto-thenate mg	Biotin µg	Vitamin C mg
956	Pine nuts	0	10	0	13.65	0.73	0.19	3.8	3.1	N	0	N	N	N	Tr
957	Pistachio nuts, roasted and salted	0	130	0	4.16	0.70	0.23	1.7	3.9	N	0	58	N	N	0
958	Pumpkin seeds	0	230	0	N	0.23	0.32	1.7	7.1	N	0	N	N	N	0
959	Sesame seeds	0	6	0	2.53	0.93	0.17	5.0	5.4	0.75	0	97	2.14	11.0	0
960	Sunflower seeds	0	15	0	37.77	1.60	0.19	4.1	5.0	N	0	N	N	N	0
961	Tahini paste	0	6	0	2.57	0.94	0.17	5.1	4.1	0.76	0	99	2.17	11.0	0
962	Trail mix	0	47	0	4.53	0.23	0.09	2.0	1.5	N	0	25	N	N	Tr
963	Walnuts	0	0	0	3.85	0.40	0.14	1.2	2.8	0.67	0	66	1.60	19.0	0[a]

[a] Value for ripe dried walnuts. Unripe walnuts contain 1300mg to 3000mg vitamin C per 100g

Sugar, preserves and snacks

Section 2.11

Sugars, preserves and snacks

New analytical data have been incorporated into this section for a range of the most commonly consumed chocolate[72] and sugar confectionery items[72]. Where new analytical data are not available, values have generally been taken from the *Miscellaneous Foods* (1994)[14] supplement, updated using data from manufacturers to reflect the reformulation of some confectionery products to reduce the saturated fat and/or sugar content.

New analytical data have also been incorporated into this section for a range of the most commonly consumed crisp and savoury snack products[72]. Where new analytical data are not available, values have generally been taken from the *Miscellaneous Foods* (1994)[14] supplement, updated using data from manufacturers to reflect the reformulation of some products to reduce the saturated fat and/or salt content.

Values for sugars, syrups and preserves have generally been taken from the *Miscellaneous Foods* (1994)[14] supplement. Values have been reviewed, using data from manufacturers, and updated where necessary to reflect the reformulation of some products to reduce the saturated fat and/or sugar content.

Composition of food per 100g edible portion

No.	Food	Description and main data sources	Main data reference	Water (g)	Total nitrogen (g)	Protein (g)	Fat (g)	Carbohydrate (g)	Energy value kcal	Energy value kJ
	Sugars, syrups and preserves									
964	**Chocolate spread**	Analytical data, 2011	72	1.0	0.52	3.3	37.7	59.4	575	2402
965	**Chocolate nut spread**	Analytical data, 1992; and industry data, 2013	35	Tr	0.99	6.2	33.0	60.5	549	2294
966	**Honey**	Assorted types. Analytical data, 1992	35	17.5	0.06	0.4	0	76.4	288	1229
967	**Ice cream sauce**, topping[a]	Analytical data, 1992; and industry data, 2013	35	26.7	0.06	0.4	0.2	72.7[b]	276	1177
968	**Jam**, fruit with edible seeds	Analytical data,1994	43	29.8	0.10	0.6	0	69.0	261	1114
969	reduced sugar	Assorted flavours. Analytical data, 1992	35	65.3	0.08	0.5	0.1	31.9	123	523
970	stone fruit	Analytical data, 1994; and industry data, 2013	43	29.6	0.06	0.4	0	69.3	261	1116
971	**Lemon curd**	MW4, 1978; and industry data, 2013	4	35.9	0.09	0.6	4.9	58.4	266	1126
972	**Marmalade**	Analytical data, 1994	43	28.0	0.01	0.1	0	69.5[c]	261	1114
973	**Mincemeat**	MSF Supplement, 1994	14	27.5	0.10	0.6	4.3	62.1	274	1163
974	**Sugar**, brown	Analytical data, 1994	43	Tr	0.02	0.1	0	101.3	380[d]	1623[d]
975	Demerara	Analytical data, 1994	43	Tr	0.08	0.5	0	104.5	394	1681
976	white	Granulated and caster sugar. Analytical data, 1994	43	Tr	Tr	Tr	0	105.0	394	1680
977	**Syrup**, golden	Analytical data, 1994	43	20.0	0.05	0.3	0	79.0	298	1269
978	**Treacle**, black	Analytical data, 1994; and industry data, 2013	43	28.5	0.19	1.2	0	67.2[b]	257	1096
	Chocolate confectionery									
979	**Bounty bar** and own brand equivalents	Industry data, 2013		8.6	0.59	3.7	26.3	61.0	480	2012

[a] Fruit and chocolate flavours

[b] Oligosaccharides may be present

[c] Reduced sugar marmalade contains about 40.0g carbohydrate per 100g

[d] Light muscovado sugar provides 376kcal, 1705kJ per 100g. Dark muscovado sugar provides 355 kcal, 1607kJ per 100g

Composition of food per 100g edible portion

No.	Food	Starch	Total sugars	Gluc	Fruct	Sucr	Malt	Lact	Dietary fibre NSP	Dietary fibre AOAC	Satd	Mono-unsatd	Poly-unsatd	Trans	Cholesterol
		g	g	g	g	g	g	g	g	g	g	g	g	g	mg
Sugars, syrups and preserves															
964	**Chocolate spread**	Tr	59.4	Tr	Tr	49.5	Tr	10.0	1.0	2.0	8.1	19.9	7.6	Tr	9
965	**Chocolate nut spread**	0.8	59.7	Tr	Tr	56.7	0	3.0	0.8	3.0	9.3	16.8	5.4	Tr	2
966	**Honey**	0	76.4	34.6	41.8	Tr	Tr	0	0	0	0	0	0	0	0
967	**Ice cream sauce**, topping	N	62.3	28.0	28.0	6.2	0	0	N	N	Tr	Tr	Tr	Tr	0
968	**Jam**, fruit with edible seeds	0	69.0	27.4	14.9	18.7	8.0	0	N	N	0	0	0	0	0
969	reduced sugar	0	31.9	10.4	15.0	6.5	0	0	0.8	1.7	Tr	Tr	Tr	Tr	0
970	stone fruit	0	69.3	27.5	14.9	18.8	8.0	0	N	1.0	0	0	0	0	0
971	**Lemon curd**	5.9	52.5	21.4	9.9	15.6	5.6	0	0.2	N	1.5	2.0	1.2	Tr	21
972	**Marmalade**	0	69.5	27.6	15.0	18.8	8.0	0	0.3	0.5	0	0	0	0	0
973	**Mincemeat**	Tr	62.1	30.7	30.8	0.6	Tr	0	1.3	N	N	N	N	N	Tr
974	**Sugar**, brown	0	101.3	0	0	101.3	0	0	0	0	0	0	0	0	0
975	Demerara	0	104.5	0	0	104.5	0	0	0	0	0	0	0	0	0
976	white	0	105.0	0	0	105.0	0	0	0	0	0	0	0	0	0
977	**Syrup**, golden	0	79.0	23.1	23.0	32.8	0	0	0	0	0	0	0	0	0
978	**Treacle**, black	0	66.8	17.4	16.7	32.7	0	0	Tr	Tr	0	0	0	0	0
Chocolate confectionery															
979	**Bounty bar** and own brand equivalents	10.6	50.4	3.2	0.1	41.7	3.0	2.4	3.2	3.2	20.5	4.8	0.8	0.1	4

Inorganic constituents per 100g edible portion

No.	Food	Na	K	Ca	Mg	P	Fe	Cu	Zn	Cl	Mn	Se	I
		mg										µg	

Sugars, syrups and preserves

No.	Food	Na	K	Ca	Mg	P	Fe	Cu	Zn	Cl	Mn	Se	I
964	**Chocolate spread**	58	362	91	51	128	4.9	0.32	0.7	160	0.39	1	15
965	**Chocolate nut spread**	50	390	130	65	180	2.2	0.48	1.0	60	1.10	N	N
966	**Honey**	11	51	5	2	17	0.4	0.05	0.9	18	0.30	1	Tr
967	**Ice cream sauce**, topping	Tr	68	9	15	26	0.8	0.09	0.1	N	0.14	N	N
968	**Jam**, fruit with edible seeds	29	43	12	5	10	0.2	0.01	0.1	9	0.13	Tr	7
969	reduced sugar	20	123	19	7	15	0.4	0.05	Tr	Tr	0.10	0	2
970	stone fruit	46	67	10	3	6	0.2	0.02	Tr	4	0.02	Tr	7
971	**Lemon curd**	65	11	9	2	15	0.2	0.30	1.3	150	N	N	N
972	**Marmalade**	64	35	26	3	6	0.2	0.03	0.1	7	0.01	1	7
973	**Mincemeat**	18	44	35	4	13	0.6	0.12	0.2	7	N	1	7
974	**Sugar**, brown	31	140	56	17	4	1.7	0.06	0.1	N	Tr	Tr	Tr
975	Demerara	5	48	29	9	3	0.9	0.11	0.1	35	Tr	Tr	Tr
976	white	5	5	10	2	1	0.2	0.12	0.1	Tr	Tr	Tr	Tr
977	**Syrup**, golden	270	58	16	3	1	0.4	0.06	0.1	42	0.01	Tr	Tr
978	**Treacle**, black	180	1760	550	180	29	14.0	0.78	0.8	820	2.67	N	N

Chocolate confectionery

No.	Food	Na	K	Ca	Mg	P	Fe	Cu	Zn	Cl	Mn	Se	I
979	**Bounty bar** and own brand equivalents	180	320	57	39	102	1.5	0.47	0.6	400	N	N	N

Vitamins per 100g edible portion

No.	Food	Retinol	Carotene	Vitamin D	Vitamin E	Thiamin	Ribo-flavin	Niacin	Trypt 60	Vitamin B_6	Vitamin B_{12}	Folate	Panto-thenate	Biotin	Vitamin C
		µg	µg	µg	mg	mg	mg	mg	mg	mg	µg	µg	mg	µg	mg
Sugars, syrups and preserves															
964	**Chocolate spread**	Tr	Tr	Tr	7.70	0.17	Tr	0.3	0.6	0.19	Tr	10	0.26	1	0
965	**Chocolate nut spread**	Tr	Tr	Tr	N	0.03	0.10	0.5	1.5	0.10	Tr	N	N	N	Tr
966	**Honey**	0	0	0	0	Tr	0.05	0.2	Tr	N	0	N	N	N	0
967	**Ice cream sauce**, topping	0	Tr	0	N	Tr	Tr	Tr	Tr	Tr	0	Tr	Tr	Tr	0
968	**Jam**, fruit with edible seeds	0	Tr	0	0	Tr	Tr	Tr	Tr	Tr	0	Tr	Tr	Tr	10[a]
969	reduced sugar	0	26	0	0.14	Tr	Tr	Tr	Tr	Tr	0	Tr	Tr	Tr	26
970	stone fruit	0	Tr	0	0	Tr	Tr	Tr	Tr	Tr	0	Tr	Tr	Tr	N
971	**Lemon curd**	10	Tr	0.1	N	Tr	0.02	Tr	0.1	Tr	Tr	Tr	0.10	1	Tr
972	**Marmalade**	0	50	0	Tr	Tr	Tr	Tr	Tr	Tr	0	5	Tr	Tr	10
973	**Mincemeat**	0	9	Tr	N	0.04	0.02	0.4	0.1	0.10	Tr	8	0.03	Tr	Tr
974	**Sugar**, brown	0	0	0	0	Tr	Tr	Tr	Tr	Tr	0	Tr	Tr	Tr	0
975	Demerara	0	0	0	0	Tr	Tr	Tr	Tr	Tr	0	Tr	Tr	Tr	0
976	white	0	0	0	0	0	0	0	0	0	0	0	0	0	0
977	**Syrup**, golden	0	0	0	0	Tr	Tr	Tr	Tr	Tr	0	Tr	Tr	Tr	0
978	**Treacle**, black	0	0	0	0	Tr	Tr	Tr	Tr	Tr	0	Tr	Tr	Tr	0
Chocolate confectionery															
979	**Bounty bar** and own brand equivalents	15	40	0.3	0.32	0.04	0.13	0.3	0.8	0.03	Tr	4	0.25	1	0

[a] Blackcurrant jam contains 24mg vitamin C per 100g

Composition of food per 100g edible portion

No.	Food	Description and main data sources	Main data reference	Water g	Total nitrogen g	Protein g	Fat g	Carbohydrate g	Energy value kcal	kJ
	Chocolate confectionery continued									
980	**Caramel bars and sweets**, chocolate covered	Including Cadbury's Caramel, Curly Wurly, Rolo, Galaxy Caramel, Toffee Poppets and own brands. Analytical data, 2010; and industry data, 2013	72	4.8	0.66	4.2	23.6	70.2[a]	493	2068
981	**Chocolate covered bar with caramel and cereal**	Including Balisto, Lion Bar, Picnic and Crispy Caramel. Analytical data, 2010[b]	72	5.0	0.81	5.2	25.8	66.2[a]	501	2102
982	**Chocolate covered wafer biscuit**	Including Kit Kat, Blue Riband, Time Out, Taxi. Analytical data, 2008	70	2.6	0.96	5.5	28.6	61.1	509	2130
983	**Chocolate covered caramel and biscuit fingers**	Including Twix and own brands. Analytical data, 2010	72	3.6	0.79	5.0	23.6	70.0[a]	495	2079
984	**Chocolate**, fancy and filled	Analytical data, 1992	34	6.1	0.78	4.9	21.3	62.9[a]	447	1878
985	milk	Analytical data, 2010	72	1.6	1.15	7.3	31.1	56.0	519	2171
986	plain	36-50% cocoa solids. Analytical data, 1992	34	0.6	0.80	5.0	28.0	63.5	510	2137
987	white	Buttons and bars. Analytical data, 1992	33	0.6	1.28	8.0	30.9	58.3	529	2212
988	**Creme egg**	Analytical data, 1989; and industry data, 2013	30	6.7	0.64	4.0	15.9	71.0[a]	425	1792
989	**Dark chocolate with crème or mint fondant centres**	Including After Eights and similar products. Analytical data, 2010	72	5.4	0.58	3.7	16.3	71.9[a]	431	1816
990	**Maltesers** and similar products	Analytical data, 2010	72	1.8	1.19	7.6	23.3	63.0	476	1998
991	**Mars bar** and own brand equivalents	Including standard, snack and fun size. Analytical data, 2012	72	7.1	0.65	4.1	15.3	66.6	404	1703

[a] Includes oligosaccharides

[b] Some products may include fortified cereals

Sugars, preserves and snacks *continued*

Composition of food per 100g edible portion

Chocolate confectionery *continued*

No.	Food	Starch g	Total sugars g	Gluc g	Fruct g	Sucr g	Malt g	Lact g	Dietary fibre NSP g	AOAC g	Fatty acids Satd g	Mono-unsatd g	Poly-unsatd g	Trans g	Cholesterol mg
980	Caramel bars and sweets, chocolate covered	Tr	56.0ᵃ	4.7	Tr	39.6	4.2	7.5	0.3	0.7	13.8	7.5	1.1	0.1	13
981	Chocolate covered bar with caramel and cereal	11.6	46.4ᵃ	2.1	Tr	32.9	2.0	9.4	0.8	1.9	16.3	7.1	1.1	0.1	9
982	Chocolate covered wafer biscuit	16.1	45.1	Tr	Tr	38.2	Tr	6.9	1.4	2.7	17.5	7.8	1.2	0.6	16
983	Chocolate covered caramel and biscuit fingers	12.2	45.4ᵃ	4.5	Tr	31.6	3.5	5.8	1.5	2.5	13.5	7.5	1.3	0.1	10
984	Chocolate, fancy and filled	0.2	60.0ᵃ	5.4	3.1	45.7	2.2	3.6	1.3	N	11.3	8.0	1.0	0.1	11
985	milk	Tr	56.0	Tr	Tr	46.8	Tr	9.2	1.3	2.3	18.7	9.6	1.1	0.2	22
986	plain	0.9	62.6	Tr	Tr	62.4	Tr	0.2	2.5	N	16.8	9.0	1.0	0.1	6
987	white	Tr	58.3	Tr	Tr	47.6	Tr	10.7	N	N	18.4	10.0	1.1	N	N
988	Creme egg	Tr	58.0ᵃ	3.6	1.8	45.7	2.0	4.9	0.5	N	9.7	N	N	N	10
989	Dark chocolate with crème or mint fondant centres	Tr	62.9ᵃ	4.0	2.4	56.5	Tr	Tr	1.9	4.7	9.8	5.1	0.5	Tr	3
990	Maltesers and similar products	7.5	55.5	2.3	Tr	36.9	2.1	14.2	0.4	1.7	14.2	7.0	1.0	0.1	12
991	Mars bar and own brand equivalents	3.3	63.3	7.8	0.3	38.7	7.8	8.7	0.8	1.5	7.3	6.4	0.8	0.1	10

ᵃ Not including oligosaccharides

Inorganic constituents per 100g edible portion

Chocolate confectionery continued

No.	Food	Na	K	Ca	Mg	P	Fe	Cu	Zn	Cl	Mn	Se	I
		mg										µg	
980	**Caramel bars and sweets**, chocolate covered	160	297	154	37	156	1.3	0.17	0.8	280	0.20	2	40
981	**Chocolate covered bar with caramel and cereal**	161	329	140	40	158	4.6	0.24	0.8	230	0.40	4	N
982	**Chocolate covered wafer biscuit**	90	340	167	41	151	2.4	0.27	0.8	130	0.35	4	22
983	**Chocolate covered caramel and biscuit fingers**	191	242	100	30	118	1.6	0.13	0.6	310	0.30	1	16
984	**Chocolate**, fancy and filled	88	270	110	48	150	1.2	0.30	0.8	140	0.39	2	N
985	milk	89	451	226	57	224	2.1	0.31	1.1	190	0.30	3	51
986	plain	6	300	33	89	140	2.3	0.71	1.3	9	0.63	4	3
987	white	110	350	270	26	230	0.2	Tr	0.9	250	0.02	N	N
988	**Creme egg**	63	145	85	27	130	0.8	0.10	0.6	110	0.10	Tr	N
989	**Dark chocolate with crème or mint fondant centres**	6	389	49	13	104	0.7	0.06	0.6	30	0.10	3	8
990	**Maltesers** and similar products	156	565	266	50	269	2.0	0.20	1.0	270	0.20	5	53
991	**Mars bar** and own brand equivalents	174	269	118	35	125	1.7	0.18	0.6	346	0.22	1	N

Vitamins per 100g edible portion

Chocolate confectionery continued

No.	Food	Retinol µg	Carotene µg	Vitamin D µg	Vitamin E mg	Thiamin mg	Ribo-flavin mg	Niacin mg	Trypt 60 mg	Vitamin B$_6$ mg	Vitamin B$_{12}$ µg	Folate µg	Panto-thenate mg	Biotin µg	Vitamin C mg
980	**Caramel bars and sweets,** chocolate covered	90	15	Tr	1.46	0.02	0.30	0.2	1.1	Tr	Tr	4	0.55	2	0
981	**Chocolate covered bar with caramel and cereal**	15	7	N	0.94	N	N	N	0.9	N	N	N	N	2	0
982	**Chocolate covered wafer biscuit**	28	Tr	Tr	0.83	0.07	0.20	0.8	1.2	0.05	0	11	0.83	14	0
983	**Chocolate covered caramel and biscuit fingers**	33	12	0.3	1.28	0.03	0.23	0.2	1.0	Tr	0.5	4	0.40	2	0
984	**Chocolate,** fancy and filled	81	120	Tr	1.65	0.05	0.20	0.4	0.9	0.03	Tr	17	0.73	3	0
985	milk	66	22	Tr	1.60	0.12	0.53	0.3	2.4	0.21	2.1	9	0.73	2	0
986	plain	15	15	0	1.44	0.04	0.06	0.4	0.7	0.03	0	12	0.30	3	0
987	white	13	75	Tr	1.14	0.08	0.49	0.2	2.6	0.07	Tr	10	0.59	3	0
988	**Creme egg**	47	55	0.6	1.07	0.06	0.34	0.2	1.3	0.03	1.0	12	0.59	3	0
989	**Dark chocolate with crème or mint fondant centres**	74	15	Tr	1.52	0.16	0.01	0.5	0.6	0.35	Tr	1	0.04	2	0
990	**Maltesers** and similar products	48	Tr	Tr	0.84	0.04	0.47	0.6	1.4	0.02	1.3	14	0.78	5	0
991	**Mars bar** and own brand equivalents	33	15	0.1	2.00	0.17	0.20	0.4	1.0	0.03	Tr	5	0.54	2	0

Composition of food per 100g edible portion

No.	Food	Description and main data sources	Main data reference	Water g	Total nitrogen g	Protein g	Fat g	Carbo-hydrate g	Energy value kcal	Energy value kJ
Chocolate confectionery continued										
992	**Milky Way** and own brand equivalents	Including standard and fun size. Analytical data, 2012	72	5.8	0.60	3.8	15.7	76.6	444	1872
993	**Smartie-type sweets**	Including Smarties and M&M's. Analytical data, 1992	33	1.5	0.86	5.4	17.5	73.9	456	1922
994	**Topic/Snickers** and own brand equivalents	Including standard, snack and fun size. Analytical data, 2012	72	5.4	1.39	7.5	28.2	52.1	479	2005
Non-chocolate confectionery										
995	**Boiled sweets**	MW3, 1960	3	16.6	Tr	Tr	Tr	87.1[a]	327	1394
996	**Chew sweets**	Including Starburst, Chewits, Blackjacks. Analytical data, 2010	72	3.8	0.15	0.9	6.0	85.1[b]	377	1599
997	**Fruit gums/jellies**	Assorted flavours. Analytical data, 1992	34	14.0	1.04	6.5	0	79.5[b]	324	1383
998	**Fruit pastilles**	Assorted flavours. Analytical data, 1992	34	9.1	0.45	2.8	0	84.2[b]	327	1395
999	**Fudge**, homemade	Recipe		5.8	0.54	3.4	13.1	80.8	435	1836
1000	**Liquorice allsorts**	Analytical data, 1992	34	8.4	0.59	3.7	5.2	76.7[b]	349	1483
1001	**Marshmallows**	Analytical data, 1992	34	17.4	0.62	3.9	0	83.1[b]	327	1396
1002	**Peppermints**	MW3, 1960	3	0.2	0.08	0.5	0.7	102.7	393	1678
1003	**Sherbet sweets**	Including Refreshers, Parma Violets, Fizzers and Love Hearts. Analytical data, 1992	34	0.2	0.10	0.6	0	93.9	355	1513
1004	**Toffees**, mixed	Including liquorice and mint. Analytical data, 2010; and industry data, 2013	72	4.0	0.34	2.1	15.9	62.9[b]	387	1630

[a] Oligosaccharides may be present

[b] Includes oligosaccharides

Sugars, preserves and snacks *continued*

Composition of food per 100g edible portion

No.	Food	Starch	Total sugars	Individual sugars					Dietary fibre		Fatty acids				Cholest-erol
				Gluc	Fruct	Sucr	Malt	Lact	NSP	AOAC	Satd	Mono-unsatd	Poly-unsatd	Trans	
		g	g	g	g	g	g	g	g	g	g	g	g	g	mg
Chocolate confectionery continued															
992	**Milky Way** and own brand equivalents	6.9	69.7	6.5	0.3	47.1	7.5	8.3	0.6	1.0	7.7	6.4	0.7	0.1	9
993	**Smartie-type sweets**	3.1	70.8	0.3	Tr	65.6	0.1	4.8	N	N	10.4	5.7	0.6	N	17
994	**Topic/Snickers** and own brand equivalents	6.1	46.1	4.8	0.1	31.0	4.4	5.8	2.4	2.8	9.2	15.6	2.1	Tr	5
Non-chocolate confectionery															
995	**Boiled sweets**	0.4	86.7	8.5	1.4	67.5	9.3	0	0	0	0	0	0	0	0
996	**Chew sweets**	Tr	54.5[a]	6.3	Tr	40.5	7.7	Tr	Tr	Tr	3.6	1.7	0.4	Tr	0
997	**Fruit gums/jellies**	1.9	58.7[a]	6.3	Tr	46.4	6.0	Tr	N	N	0	0	0	0	0
998	**Fruit pastilles**	3.4	59.3[a]	6.5	2.1	45.4	5.3	Tr	N	N	0	0	0	0	0
999	**Fudge**, homemade	0	80.8	0	0	75.7	0	5.0	0	0	8.3	3.4	0.4	N	37
1000	**Liquorice allsorts**	9.4	62.4[a]	5.9	2.5	51.1	2.9	Tr	2.0	N	3.6	1.2	0.2	Tr	0
1001	**Marshmallows**	4.5	64.5[a]	12.1	0.7	41.5	10.2	Tr	0	0	N	N	0	N	0
1002	**Peppermints**	0	102.7	1.0	0	101.7	0	0	0	0	N	N	N	N	0
1003	**Sherbet sweets**	Tr	93.9	0.2	Tr	93.7	Tr	Tr	Tr	Tr	0	0	0	0	0
1004	**Toffees**, mixed	Tr	39.1[a]	5.9	Tr	29.9	3.3	Tr	Tr	Tr	8.6	5.3	1.1	0.1	17

[a] Not including oligosaccharides

Inorganic constituents per 100g edible portion

No.	Food	Na	K	Ca	Mg	P	Fe	Cu	Zn	Cl	Mn	Se	I
						mg						µg	
Chocolate confectionery continued													
992	**Milky Way** and own brand equivalents	220	240	117	25	114	2.0	0.13	0.5	354	0.13	1	N
993	**Smartie-type sweets**	58	280	150	48	160	1.5	0.25	0.9	120	0.25	N	N
994	**Topic/Snickers** and own brand equivalents	187	388	101	80	210	1.9	0.35	1.4	385	0.60	6	N
	Non-chocolate confectionery												
995	**Boiled sweets**	25	8	5	2	12	0.4	0.09	N	68	N	Tr	N
996	**Chew sweets**	30	10	3	2	4	0.1	Tr	Tr	30	Tr	Tr	N
997	**Fruit gums/jellies**	30	8	5	1	4	0.1	0.02	Tr	N	Tr	Tr	N
998	**Fruit pastilles**	33	28	28	6	4	0.4	0.04	Tr	29	0.02	Tr	N
999	**Fudge**, homemade	156	153	126	13	105	0.2	0.09	0.5	231	Tr	1	15
1000	**Liquorice allsorts**	57	600	170	76	44	7.3	0.34	0.5	N	1.14	N	N
1001	**Marshmallows**	29	2	4	2	4	0.3	Tr	Tr	36	Tr	N	N
1002	**Peppermints**	9	Tr	7	3	Tr	0.2	0.04	N	22	N	Tr	N
1003	**Sherbet sweets**	N	15	42	69	Tr	0.2	0.04	Tr	6	0.02	N	N
1004	**Toffees**, mixed	312	132	85	11	65	0.3	0.04	0.3	460	0.03	1	20

Vitamins per 100g edible portion

No.	Food	Retinol µg	Carotene µg	Vitamin D µg	Vitamin E mg	Thiamin mg	Ribo-flavin mg	Niacin mg	Trypt 60 mg	Vitamin B$_6$ mg	Vitamin B$_{12}$ µg	Folate µg	Panto-thenate mg	Biotin µg	Vitamin C mg
Chocolate confectionery continued															
992	**Milky Way** and own brand equivalents	24	Tr	0.2	1.96	0.18	0.21	0.4	1.0	0.03	Tr	5	0.56	2	0
993	**Smartie-type sweets**	5	28	Tr	0.80	0.08	0.79	0.3	1.7	0.03	Tr	4	0.67	2	0
994	**Topic/Snickers** and own brand equivalents	10	7	N	4.28	0.12	0.16	2.1	1.7	0.04	Tr	11	0.69	2	0
Non-chocolate confectionery															
995	**Boiled sweets**	0	0	0	0	0	0	0	0	0	0	0	0	0	0
996	**Chew sweets**	0	152	0	1.20	Tr	Tr	N	N	Tr	0	Tr	Tr	Tr	N
997	**Fruit gums/jellies**	0	N	0	0	0	0	0	0	0	0	0	0	0	0
998	**Fruit pastilles**	0	N	0	0	0	0	0	0	0	0	0	0	0	0
999	**Fudge**, homemade	151	105	0.9	0.28	0.02	0.17	0.1	0.7	0.03	0.3	4	0.35	2	0
1000	**Liquorice allsorts**	0	0	0	0	0	0	0	0.2	0	0	0	0	0	0
1001	**Marshmallows**	0	0	0	0	0	0	Tr	Tr	0	0	0	0	0	0
1002	**Peppermints**	0	0	0	0	0	0	0	0	0	0	0	0	0	0
1003	**Sherbet sweets**	0	0	0	0	0	0	Tr	Tr	0	0	0	0	0	0
1004	**Toffees**, mixed	0	0	N	Tr	0	Tr	0	0.7	0	0.2	1	0.21	Tr	0

Composition of food per 100g edible portion

No.	Food	Description and main data sources	Main data reference	Water g	Total nitrogen g	Protein g	Fat g	Carbo-hydrate g	Energy value kcal	kJ
	Non-chocolate confectionery continued									
1005	**Turkish delight**, without nuts	MW5, 1991	10	16.1	0.10	0.6	0	77.9	295	1257
	Savoury snacks									
1006	**Bombay mix**	Savoury mix of gram flour, assorted peas, lentils, nuts and seeds. Analytical data, 1990/91; and industry data, 2013	39	3.5	3.01	18.8	32.9	35.1	503	2099
1007	**Corn snacks**	Including Wotsits and Monster Munch. Analytical data, 2010	72	1.3	0.95	6.0	30.4	60.8	526	2199
1008	**Popcorn**, candied	Industry data, 2013		4.2	1.10	6.9	23.8	60.7	469	1969
1009	salted	Industry data, 2013		4.3	1.44	9.0	23.5	59.3	470	1971
1010	**Pork scratchings**	Analytical data, 1990/91	39	2.1	7.66	47.9	46.0	0.2	606	2520
1011	**Potato crisps**, fried in sunflower oil	Assorted flavours, fried in high oleic sunflower oil, including Walkers and own brands. Analytical data, 2010	72	4.3	1.00	6.2	28.8	55.8	493	2064
1012	low fat	Plain and flavoured, not baked. Analytical data, 1990/91	39	1.1	1.06	6.6	21.5	63.5	458	1924
1013	**Potato rings**	Including Hula Hoops and own brands. Analytical data, 2010	72	2.0	0.57	3.6	22.4	70.5	480	2018
1014	**Potato snacks**, pringle type, fried in vegetable oil	Including Pringles and own brands. Analytical data, 2010	72	1.9	0.69	4.3	31.8	57.4	519	2168
1015	**Rice cakes**	Plain, salted. Analytical data, 2002-2003	65	3.6	1.24	7.4	3.4	79.3	358	1521
1016	**Tortilla chips**, fried in sunflower oil	Assorted flavours, fried in high oleic sunflower oil, including Doritos and own brands. Analytical data, 2010	72	1.3	1.16	7.2	27.4	60.8	504	2110

Composition of food per 100g edible portion

No.	Food	Starch g	Total sugars g	Individual sugars					Dietary fibre		Fatty acids				Cholest-erol mg
				Gluc g	Fruct g	Sucr g	Malt g	Lact g	NSP g	AOAC g	Satd g	Mono-unsatd g	Poly-unsatd g	Trans g	
Non-chocolate confectionery continued															
1005	**Turkish delight**, without nuts	9.3	68.6	N	N	N	N	0	0	0	0	0	0	0	0
Savoury snacks															
1006	**Bombay mix**	32.8	2.3	0.1	0.1	2.2	0	0	6.2	8.8	4.0	16.3	11.1	Tr	0
1007	**Corn snacks**	55.3	5.5	Tr	Tr	0.6	Tr	4.9	1.4	1.3	2.8	18.4	7.5	Tr	0
1008	**Popcorn**, candied	45.7	15.0	Tr	Tr	15.0	0	0	N	9.5	N	N	N	N	0
1009	salted	58.7	0.6	Tr	Tr	0.6	0	0	N	9.3	N	N	N	N	0
1010	**Pork scratchings**	Tr	0.2	0.2	Tr	Tr	0	0	0.3	N	16.6	23.9	3.7	0.2	129
1011	**Potato crisps**, fried in sunflower oil	54.9	0.9	Tr	Tr	0.9	Tr	Tr	4.6	4.4	2.5	22.4	2.5	Tr	0
1012	low fat	62.0	1.5	0.2	Tr	0.8	0	0.5	5.9	N	1.9	16.8	1.9	Tr	0
1013	**Potato rings**	70.2	0.3	Tr	Tr	0.3	Tr	Tr	1.7	2.6	1.9	17.1	2.3	Tr	0
1014	**Potato snacks**, pringle type, fried in vegetable oil	55.9	1.5	0.3	0.2	1.1	Tr	Tr	2.4	2.9	8.4	19.8	2.9	0.1	0
1015	**Rice cakes**	78.3	0.9	Tr	0.1	0.6	0.1	0	4.3	5.0	0.6	1.0	1.2	0	0
1016	**Tortilla chips**, fried in sunflower oil	58.3	2.5	0.2	0.2	1.1	Tr	1.0	5.7	5.9	2.9	20.1	3.1	0.1	0

Inorganic constituents per 100g edible portion

No.	Food	mg										µg	
		Na	K	Ca	Mg	P	Fe	Cu	Zn	Cl	Mn	Se	I
	Non-chocolate confectionery continued												
1005	**Turkish delight**, without nuts	31	4	10	2	7	0.2	0.12	0.7	110	Tr	Tr	Tr
	Savoury snacks												
1006	**Bombay mix**	640	770	58	100	290	3.8	0.62	2.5	1170	1.40	N	N
1007	**Corn snacks**	909	329	71	20	96	0.3	0.05	0.4	1120	0.20	9	N
1008	**Popcorn**, candied	Tr	N	N	N	N	N	N	N	N	N	N	Tr
1009	salted	730	N	N	N	N	N	N	N	1120	N	N	N
1010	**Pork scratchings**	1320	300	32	18	180	2.4	0.20	1.6	2090	0.09	N	N
1011	**Potato crisps**, fried in sunflower oil	604	1328	48	63	135	1.5	0.20	0.9	1000	0.40	1	2
1012	low fat	730	1020	36	48	130	1.8	0.38	0.9	1200	0.37	1	N
1013	**Potato rings**	845	781	26	34	108	0.8	0.16	0.6	1490	0.20	1	2
1014	**Potato snacks**, pringle type, fried in vegetable oil	599	706	35	40	103	1.1	0.17	0.7	850	0.30	Tr	2
1015	**Rice cakes**	87[a]	276	14	112	308	1.1	0.25	1.6	142	2.70	4	1
1016	**Tortilla chips**, fried in sunflower oil	636	285	103	78	234	1.5	0.10	1.2	900	0.40	5	N

[a] Unsalted rice cakes contain 10mg Na per 100g

Vitamins per 100g edible portion

No.	Food	Retinol	Carotene	Vitamin D	Vitamin E	Thiamin	Ribo-flavin	Niacin	Trypt 60	Vitamin B6	Vitamin B12	Folate	Panto-thenate	Biotin	Vitamin C
		µg	µg	µg	mg	mg	mg	mg	mg	mg	µg	µg	mg	µg	mg
Non-chocolate confectionery continued															
1005	**Turkish delight**, without nuts	0	0	0	0	0.13	N	N	N	N	N	N	N	N	0
Savoury snacks															
1006	**Bombay mix**	0	Tr	0	4.71	0.38	0.10	4.3	3.5	0.54	0	N	1.19	24	Tr
1007	**Corn snacks**	0	232	0	8.43	0.23	0.31	0.3	0.5	Tr	0	5	0.30	1	Tr
1008	**Popcorn**, candied	0	N	0	N	N	N	N	N	N	0	N	N	N	0
1009	salted	0	N	0	N	N	N	N	N	N	0	N	N	N	0
1010	**Pork scratchings**	0	0	Tr	N	0.56	0.20	4.2	2.5	0.05	N	N	N	N	0
1011	**Potato crisps**, fried in sunflower oil	0	29	0	9.05	0.09	0.16	3.9	0.9	0.31	0	62	0.78	1	17
1012	low fat	0	2	0	3.47	0.19	0.14	5.0	1.6	0.46	0	48	N	N	14
1013	**Potato rings**	0	29	0	7.64	0.05	0.27	1.1	0.8	0.40	0	5	0.28	Tr	3
1014	**Potato snacks**, pringle type, fried in vegetable oil	0	29	0	10.80	0.09	0.16	3.9	0.9	0.31	0	62	0.78	1	N
1015	**Rice cakes**	0	0	0	1.16	0.02	0.03	5.9	1.1	0.07	0	17	0.86	4	0
1016	**Tortilla chips**, fried in sunflower oil	0	208	0	7.11	0.11	0.18	0.5	0.9	0.15	0	10	0.28	1	Tr

1017

Composition of food per 100g edible portion

No.	Food	Description and main data sources	Main data reference	Water g	Total nitrogen g	Protein g	Fat g	Carbo-hydrate g	Energy value kcal	Energy value kJ

Savoury snacks continued

| 1017 | **Twiglets** | Savoury wholewheat sticks. Industry data, 2013; and analytical data, 1990/91 | 39 | 3.2 | 2.16 | 12.3 | 11.8 | 63.3 | 393 | 1659 |

No.	Food	Starch	Total sugars	Gluc	Fruct	Sucr	Malt	Lact	Dietary fibre NSP	Dietary fibre AOAC	Satd	Mono- unsatd	Poly- unsatd	Trans	Cholest- erol
		g	g	g	g	g	g	g	g	g	g	g	g	g	mg
Savoury snacks continued															
1017	**Twiglets**	62.7	0.6	Tr	Tr	0.6	0	Tr	10.3	12.4	1.6	N	N	N	0

Inorganic constituents per 100g edible portion

No.	Food	Na	K	Ca	Mg	P	Fe	Cu	Zn	Cl	Mn	Se	I
						mg						µg	
	Savoury snacks continued												
1017	**Twiglets**	800	460	45	81	370	2.9	0.32	2.0	1500	1.61	N	N

Vitamins per 100g edible portion

No.	Food	Retinol	Carotene	Vitamin D	Vitamin E	Thiamin	Ribo-flavin	Niacin	Trypt 60	Vitamin B$_6$	Vitamin B$_{12}$	Folate	Panto-thenate	Biotin	Vitamin C
		µg	µg	µg	mg	mg	mg	mg	mg	mg	µg	µg	mg	µg	mg
Savoury snacks continued															
1017	**Twiglets**	0	Tr	0	2.47	0.37	0.48	7.8	2.3	0.38	0	78	1.54	15	Tr

Beverages

Section 2.12

Beverages

Most of the values in this section of the Tables have been taken from the *Miscellaneous Foods* (1994)[14] supplement. However, new analytical data have been incorporated for a few beverages, e.g. cappuccino/latte coffee[65], orange juice[74] and apple juice[74]. Values for powdered beverages and soft drinks have been reviewed using data from manufacturers, with soft drink categories updated and expanded to reflect products currently available.

This section includes beverages that are made up with milk and distilled water (e.g. tea and coffee) as well as carbonated drinks, squash, cordials and fruit juices. Values for drinking chocolate have been given made-up with semi-skimmed milk. Examples of the amounts of powder and liquid that are recommended by manufacturers and that have been used to calculate the made-up or diluted form (available in CoFID) are given below. As it is difficult to cover the range of strengths in which instant coffee, squash and cordials are made up only one entry, for the undiluted form, is given in the main tables, although a few ready to drink products have been included.

Drink	Made-up/diluted form
Build-up powder, shake	38g powder with 200 ml milk
Cocoa powder	4g cocoa powder with 200 ml milk
Complan powder, savoury	57g powder with 200 ml water
Complan powder, original and sweet	60g powder with 200 ml water
Horlicks powder	25g powder with 200 ml milk
Milkshake powder	15g powder with 200 ml milk
Ovaltine powder	25g powder with 200 ml milk

Losses of labile vitamins assigned to made-up powdered drinks have been estimated from figures in Section 4.3.

The vitamin composition of beverages may be different from that quoted in these Tables if manufacturers have added to or changed the fortification of products. Concentrations of vitamin C in many fruit-based drinks can vary widely depending on fortification practices. Users requiring details of possible recent changes in fortification practices and brand-specific information should contact manufacturers directly.

Beverages *continued*

As many beverages may be sold or measured by volume, typical specific gravities (densities) of some of these products are given below. To convert values from per 100g to per 100ml, the values should be multiplied by the specific gravity.

Specific gravities of beverages	
Carbonated beverages	
Cola	1.040
Fruit juice drinks	1.040
Lemonade	1.020
Lucozade	1.070
Fruit juice drinks and cordials	
Blackcurrant juice drink/squash, undiluted	1.280
Fruit juice drinks/squash, undiluted	1.090 - 1.120
Fruit juice drinks/squash, ready to drink	1.030 - 1.040
Fruit juice drink, no added sugar, undiluted	1.010 - 1.030
Fruit juice drink, no added sugar, ready to drink	1.010
High juice drinks, undiluted	1.150
High juice drinks, ready to drink	1.040
Lime juice cordial, undiluted	1.102

Composition of food per 100g edible portion

No.	Food	Description and main data sources	Main data reference	Water g	Total nitrogen g	Protein g	Fat g	Carbo-hydrate g	Energy value kcal	kJ
Powdered drinks and infusions										
1018	**Build-up**, powder, shake	Average of chocolate, strawberry, banana and vanilla flavours. Industry data, 2013		4.2	3.28	20.5	0.7	63.0[a]	325	1383
1019	powder, soup	Average of chicken, vegetable, tomato and potato & leek flavours. Industry data, 2013		3.0	2.30	14.4	14.9	57.3[a]	407	1713
1020	**Cocoa**, powder	MW4, 1978	4	3.4	3.70[b]	18.5[c]	21.7	11.5	312	1301
1021	**Coffee**, infusion, average	As consumed. Average of strong and weak infusions. Analytical data, 1984	21	98.3	0.03	0.2	Tr	0.3	2	8
1022	cappuccino, latte	As consumed. Analytical data, 2002	65	93.2	0.32	2.0	0.8	3.2	27	114
1023	powder, instant	Analytical data, 1984	21	3.4	3.26[d]	14.6[c]	Tr	4.5	75	320
1024	**Coffeemate**, whitener powder	Industry data, 1989 and 2013		3.0	0.33	2.1	34.5	57.3[a]	534	2202
1025	**Complan**, powder, original and sweet	Including original, chocolate and vanilla. Industry data, 2013		3.5	2.45	15.6	14.7	64.8[a]	438	1846
1026	powder, savoury	Industry data, 2013		3.5	2.53	16.1	15.6	62.5[a]	439	1852
1027	**Drinking chocolate**, powder	Analytical data, 1993-1994	50	2.1	1.02	6.4	5.8	79.7[a]	377	1598
1028	powder, made up with semi-skimmed milk	Calculated from 18g powder to 200ml milk		82.3	0.58	3.6	2.0	10.9[a]	73	310
1029	powder, reduced fat	Analytical data, 1993-1994	50	2.0	1.02	6.4	2.3	82.1	354	1507
1030	**Horlicks**, powder	Industry data, 2013		2.5	1.50	9.4	3.1	83.7	379	1614

[a] Includes oligosaccharides

[b] Includes 0.74g purine nitrogen

[c] (Total N - purine N) x 6.25

[d] Includes 0.93g purine nitrogen

Powdered drinks and infusions

No.	Food	Starch g	Total sugars g	Individual sugars					Dietary fibre		Satd g	Fatty acids			Cholest-erol mg
				Gluc g	Fruct g	Sucr g	Malt g	Lact g	NSP g	AOAC g		Mono-unsatd g	Poly-unsatd g	Trans g	
1018	**Build-up**, powder, shake	Tr	62.0[a]	N	N	N	N	N	N	8.2	0.4	N	N	Tr	12
1019	powder, soup	26.4	14.3[a]	N	N	N	N	N	N	6.5	4.6	N	N	Tr	N
1020	**Cocoa**, powder	11.5	Tr	0	0	0	0	0	12.1	N	12.8	7.2	0.6	N	0
1021	**Coffee**, infusion, average	0	0.3	N	N	N	0	0	0	0	Tr	Tr	Tr	Tr	0
1022	cappuccino, latte	0.8	2.4	0	0	0	0	2.4	0	0	0.5	0.2	Tr	Tr	3
1023	powder, instant	4.5	0	0	0	0	0	0	0	0	Tr	Tr	Tr	Tr	0
1024	**Coffeemate**, whitener powder	Tr	9.4[a]	5.0	0	0	4.4	Tr	0	0	26.0	N	N	Tr	2
1025	**Complan**, powder, original and sweet	Tr	42.8[a,b]	0.4	0	4.9	2.6	34.9	Tr	Tr	6.5	6.3	1.6	Tr	N
1026	powder, savoury	6.8	6.2[a]	1.6	0.1	0.2	3.3	1.1	0.3	0.2	6.6	6.3	1.7	Tr	N
1027	**Drinking chocolate**, powder	Tr	77.7[a]	0	0	77.7	0	0	N	N	3.4	1.8	0.3	0	0
1028	powder, made up with semi-skimmed milk	Tr	10.7[a]	0	0	6.4	0	4.3	Tr	Tr	1.3	0.5	0.1	0.1	5
1029	powder, reduced fat	Tr	82.1	Tr	0.9	81.2	Tr	Tr	N	N	1.4	0.7	0.1	0	Tr
1030	**Horlicks**, powder	44.8	38.9	N	N	N	N	N	4.0	3.4	1.3	N	N	Tr	N

[a] Not including oligosaccharides

[b] Dependent on variety

Inorganic constituents per 100g edible portion

No.	Food	mg										µg	
		Na	K	Ca	Mg	P	Fe	Cu	Zn	Cl	Mn	Se	I

Powdered drinks and infusions

No.	Food	Na	K	Ca	Mg	P	Fe	Cu	Zn	Cl	Mn	Se	I
1018	**Build-up**, powder, shake	250	1070	725	263	600	13.4	4.90	14.0	N	2.60	N	150
1019	powder, soup	980	767	763	232	541	10.5	N	10.7	N	N	N	102
1020	**Cocoa**, powder	N	1500	130	520	660	10.5	3.90	6.9	N	N	N	N
1021	**Coffee**, infusion, average	Tr	92	3	8	7	0.1	Tr	Tr	3	0.05	Tr	Tr
1022	cappuccino, latte	25	129	65	10	50	0.1	0.02	0.2	60	0.04	1	9
1023	powder, instant	81	3780	140	330	310	4.6	0.62	1.1	65	2.10	9	Tr
1024	**Coffeemate**, whitener powder	400	900	4	N	350	N	N	N	N	N	N	N
1025	**Complan**, powder, original and sweet	190	660	540	96	440	7.4	0.53	5.3	450	0.53	19	79
1026	powder, savoury	900	730	420	96	490	7.4	0.53	5.3	1400	0.61	19	79
1027	**Drinking chocolate**, powder	228	495	39	132	193	3.5	3.69	5.6	107	1.00	N	165
1028	powder, made up with semi-skimmed milk	58	184	114	21	102	0.3	0.30	0.9	89	0.08	1	42
1029	powder, reduced fat	228	495	39	132	193	3.5	3.69	5.6	107	1.00	N	165
1030	**Horlicks**, powder	500	686	1910	39	300	10.5	0.20	N	N	N	N	N

Powdered drinks and infusions

No.	Food	Retinol µg	Carotene µg	Vitamin D µg	Vitamin E mg	Thiamin mg	Ribo-flavin mg	Niacin mg	Trypt 60 mg	Vitamin B₆ mg	Vitamin B₁₂ µg	Folate µg	Panto-thenate mg	Biotin µg	Vitamin C mg
1018	**Build-up**, powder, shake	900	Tr	4.5	10.00	1.60	2.60	16.0	5.8	2.20	2.3	180	9.00	130	65
1019	powder, soup	583	N	3.6	6.40	1.70	1.10	12.9	N	1.50	1.6	146	4.58	140	60
1020	**Cocoa**, powder	0	40	0	0.68	0.16	0.06	1.7	3.9	0.07	0	38	N	N	0
1021	**Coffee**, infusion, average	0	0	0	Tr	Tr	0.01	0.7	0	Tr	0	Tr	Tr	3	0
1022	cappuccino, latte	12	5	0.7	Tr	0.02	0.11	0.8	0.3	0.01	Tr	4	0.39	2	Tr
1023	powder, instant	0	N	0	Tr	0.04	0.21	24.8[a]	2.9	0.02	0	11	Tr	67	0
1024	**Coffeemate**, whitener powder	0	200	0	N	0	1.00	0	0.6	0	0	0	0	0	0
1025	**Complan**, powder, original and sweet	440	Tr	4.4	11.00	0.96	1.20	14.0	3.5	1.20	2.3	180	5.30	44	70
1026	powder, savoury	440	Tr	4.4	11.00	0.96	1.20	14.0	3.5	1.20	2.3	180	5.30	44	70
1027	**Drinking chocolate**, powder	0	N	0	0.41	0.02	0.06	0.6	1.2	0.01	0	7	0.30	9	0
1028	powder, made up with semi-skimmed milk	17	8	Tr	0.06	0.03	0.20	0.1	0.8	0.05	0.3	5	0.29	3	1
1029	powder, reduced fat	0	N	0	0.16	0.02	0.06	0.6	1.2	0.01	0	7	0.30	9	0
1030	**Horlicks**, powder	978	Tr	18.5	12.20	1.70	2.00	22.0	3.0	2.40	1.2	160	7.30	184	73

[a] Can be as high as 39mg per 100g. Decaffeinated instant coffee contains about the same

Composition of food per 100g edible portion

No.	Food	Description and main data sources	Main data reference	Water g	Total nitrogen g	Protein g	Fat g	Carbo-hydrate g	Energy value kcal	Energy value kJ
Powdered drinks and infusions *continued*										
1031	**Instant drinks powder**, chocolate, low calorie	Assorted flavours, including Ovaltine Options, Cadbury Highlights and own brands. Analytical data, 1993-1994; and industry data, 2013	50	4.5	2.56	16.0	11.1	52.0[a]	359	1515
1032	malted, unfortified	Own brands. Industry data, 2013; and analytical data, 1993-1994	50	3.4	0.91	5.7	6.2	82.5[a]	388	1646
1033	**Milk shake**, powder	MPE Supplement, 1989; and industry data, 2013	8	0.5	0.21	1.3	1.6	98.3[b]	388	1654
1034	**Ovaltine**, powder	Industry data, 2013		2.0	1.14	7.3	1.9	83.1	358	1524
1035	**Tea**, black, infusion, average	15g leaves per litre water, strained after 5 minutes. Analytical data, 1984	21	99.5	Tr	0.1	Tr	Tr	Tr	2
1036	green, infusion	Sencha Fukujyu and Banch type. Literature sources	14	99.7	0.02	0.1	0	Tr	Tr	Tr
1037	herbal, infusion	Literature sources, 1986	96	99.7	0	0	Tr	0.2	1	3
Carbonated drinks										
1038	**Cola**	Analytical data, 1993	38	89.7	Tr	Tr	0	10.9	41	174
1039	diet	Calculated from Cola		99.8	Tr	Tr	0	Tr	1	2
1040	**Energy drink**, carbonated	Including Red Bull, Monster, EQ8, Kx, Relentless and own brands. Industry data, 2013		88.9	Tr	Tr	0	11.1[b]	42	178
1041	**Fruit juice drink**, carbonated, ready to drink	Bottles and cans; orange, lemon, apple and tropical fruit flavours e.g. Citrus Spring, Fanta, Orangina and Tango. Industry data, 1999 and 2013		92.8	Tr	Tr	Tr	7.2[c]	27	116

[a] Contains oligosaccharides

[b] May contain oligosaccharides

[c] Carbohydrate typically varies from 2.2g to 13.5g per 100g

Composition of food per 100g edible portion

No.	Food	Starch g	Total sugars g	Individual sugars					Dietary fibre		Fatty acids				Cholest- erol mg
				Gluc g	Fruct g	Sucr g	Malt g	Lact g	NSP g	AOAC g	Satd g	Mono- unsatd g	Poly- unsatd g	Trans g	
Powdered drinks and infusions continued															
1031	**Instant drinks powder**, chocolate, low calorie	Tr	33.6[a]	0.7	Tr	Tr	Tr	32.9	N	N	8.1	1.7	0.9	0.1	3
1032	malted, unfortified	Tr	54.8[a]	3.7	0	10.7	14.3	26.1	N	2.1	3.8	N	N	Tr	4
1033	**Milk shake**, powder	Tr	98.3	0.1	0	95.2	2.8	0.2	N	0	N	N	N	N	Tr
1034	**Ovaltine**, powder	34.8	48.3	N	N	N	N	N	2.5	4.3	1.4	N	N	N	N
1035	**Tea**, black, infusion, average	0	Tr	0	0	0	0	0	0	0	Tr	Tr	Tr	Tr	0
1036	green, infusion	0	Tr	0	0	0	0	0	0	0	0	0	0	0	0
1037	herbal, infusion	0	0	0	0	0	0	0	0	0	Tr	Tr	Tr	0	0
Carbonated drinks															
1038	**Cola**	Tr	10.9	3.5	3.4	4.0	0	0	0	0	0	0	0	0	0
1039	diet	0	Tr	Tr	Tr	Tr	0	0	0	0	0	0	0	0	0
1040	**Energy drink**, carbonated	Tr	11.1	N	N	N	N	0	0	0	0	0	0	0	0
1041	**Fruit juice drink**, carbonated, ready to drink	0	7.2	N	N	N	N	0	Tr	Tr	Tr	Tr	Tr	0	0

[a] Not including oligosaccharides

Inorganic constituents per 100g edible portion

No.	Food	mg										µg	
		Na	K	Ca	Mg	P	Fe	Cu	Zn	Cl	Mn	Se	I
Powdered drinks and infusions continued													
1031	**Instant drinks**, powder, chocolate, low calorie	1170	1802	411	186	618	7.5	2.20	3.2	1860	1.10	N	178
1032	powder, malted, unfortified	400	1191	349	67	470	0.6	7.57	5.1	620	0.10	N	N
1033	**Milk shake**, powder	20	150	8	N	N	N	0.10	0.4	27	0.20	N	32
1034	**Ovaltine**, powder	120	156	800	375	N	14.0	N	10.0	125	N	N	N
1035	**Tea**, black, infusion, average	Tr	27	Tr	2	2	Tr	0.01	Tr	1	0.15	Tr	Tr
1036	green, infusion	1	20	2	Tr	1	0.1	Tr	Tr	Tr	Tr	Tr	Tr
1037	herbal, infusion	Tr	9	2	1	Tr	0.1	0.02	Tr	Tr	0.04	Tr	Tr
Carbonated drinks													
1038	**Cola**	5	1	6	1	30	Tr	Tr	Tr	Tr	Tr	Tr	Tr
1039	diet	5	1	6	1	30	Tr	Tr	Tr	Tr	Tr	Tr	Tr
1040	**Energy drink**, carbonated	60	N	N	N	N	N	N	N	N	N	N	N
1041	**Fruit juice drink**, carbonated, ready to drink	8	27	7	7	2	Tr	Tr	Tr	3	Tr	Tr	Tr

Vitamins per 100g edible portion

No.	Food	Retinol	Carotene	Vitamin D	Vitamin E	Thiamin	Ribo-flavin	Niacin	Trypt 60	Vitamin B_6	Vitamin B_{12}	Folate	Panto-thenate	Biotin	Vitamin C
		µg	µg	µg	mg	mg	mg	mg	mg	mg	µg	µg	mg	µg	mg

Powdered drinks and infusions continued

No.	Food	Retinol	Carotene	Vitamin D	Vitamin E	Thiamin	Ribo-flavin	Niacin	Trypt 60	Vitamin B_6	Vitamin B_{12}	Folate	Panto-thenate	Biotin	Vitamin C
1031	**Instant drinks**, powder, chocolate, low calorie	Tr	16	0.8	0.74	0.10	0.80	1.1	3.3	0.04	0.2	13	1.70	21	0
1032	powder, malted, unfortified	0	4	Tr	N	0.36	0.91	4.9	2.6	0.17	Tr	18	1.50	16	Tr
1033	**Milk shake**, powder	N	Tr	7.1	0.15	1.20	N	25.0	0.3	1.80	0	200	N	N	67
1034	**Ovaltine**, powder	800	Tr	N	12.00	1.10	1.40	16.0	N	1.40	2.5	200	6.00	50	80
1035	**Tea**, black, infusion, average	0	0	0	N	Tr	0.02	0	0	Tr	0	3	0.04	1	0
1036	green, infusion	0	0	0	N	0	0.02	0.1	0	Tr	0	Tr	Tr	Tr	3
1037	herbal, infusion	0	0	0	Tr	0.01	Tr	0	0	0	0	1	0.01	0	0
	Carbonated drinks														
1038	**Cola**	0	0	0	0	0	0	0	0	0	0	0	0	0	0
1039	diet	0	0	0	0	0	0	0	0	0	0	0	0	0	0
1040	**Energy drink**, carbonated	0	N	0	0	N	N	N[a]	N	N[b]	N[c]	N	N[d]	Tr	N
1041	**Fruit juice drink**, carbonated, ready to drink	0	94	0	Tr	Tr	Tr	Tr	Tr	Tr	Tr	1	Tr	Tr	1

[a] Fortified products contain between 3.2mg and 8.5mg per 100g

[b] Fortified products contain between 0.28mg and 2.00mg per 100g

[c] Fortified products contain between 0.5µg and 2.5µg per 100g

[d] Fortified products contain between 1.20mg and 2.00mg per 100g

No.	Food	Description and main data sources	Main data reference	Water g	Total nitrogen g	Protein g	Fat g	Carbo-hydrate g	Energy value kcal	kJ
Carbonated drinks continued										
1042	**Fruit juice drink**, carbonated, no added sugar, ready to drink	Estimated from fruit juice drink, carbonated and industry data, 2013		99.4	Tr	Tr	Tr	0.6	2	10
1043	**Lemonade**	Analytical data, 1993	38	93.8	Tr	Tr	0	5.8[a]	22	93
1044	**Lucozade**	Including lemon, orange and tropical flavours. MSF Supplement, 1994; and industry data, 2013	14	81.1	Tr	Tr	0	16.0[b]	60	256
1045	**Tonic water**	Industry data, 2013		94.1	0	0	0	5.9	22	94
Squashes and cordials										
1046	**Barley water**, undiluted	Orange and lemon flavours. MSF Supplement, 1994; and industry data, 2013	14	75.2	0.05	0.3	Tr	23.7	90	384
1047	**Blackcurrant juice drink/squash**, undiluted	Including Ribena. Analytical data, 1993; and industry data, 2013	38	47.5	0.02	0.1	0	54.2	204	869
1048	**Fruit juice drink/squash**, undiluted	Lemon, orange, apple and mixed fruit flavours. Analytical data, 1993; and industry data, 2013[c]	38	91.0	0.02	0.1	Tr	8.9	34	144
1049	ready to drink	Lemon, orange, apple and mixed fruit flavours, as purchased. Analytical data, 1993	38	89.5	0.02	0.1	Tr	9.8	37	159
1050	**Fruit juice drink**, no added sugar, undiluted	Lemon, orange and mixed fruit flavours, typically less than 3% sugar. Analytical data, 1993; and industry data, 2013	38	97.3	0.02	0.1	Tr	1.4	6	25
1051	no added sugar, ready to drink	Typically less than 3% sugar, as purchased. Analytical data, 1993; and industry data, 2013	38	96.6	0.03	0.2	Tr	0.9	4	18

[a] Carbohydrate typically varies from 2.4g to 12.8g per 100g

[b] Includes oligosaccharides

[c] Undiluted double concentrated fruit squash drinks contain approximately twice the carbohydrate, total sugars and energy

Beverages *continued*

Composition of food per 100g edible portion

No.	Food	Starch g	Total sugars g	Individual sugars					Dietary fibre		Fatty acids				Cholest-erol mg
				Gluc g	Fruct g	Sucr g	Malt g	Lact g	NSP g	AOAC g	Satd g	Mono-unsatd g	Poly-unsatd g	Trans g	
Carbonated drinks continued															
1042	**Fruit juice drink**, carbonated, no added sugar, ready to drink	0	0.6	0.1	0.2	0.3	0	0	Tr	Tr	Tr	Tr	Tr	0	0
1043	**Lemonade**	0	5.8[a]	1.5	1.4	2.8	0.1	0	0	0	0	0	0	0	0
1044	**Lucozade**	Tr	11.1[b]	N	N	N	N	0	0	0	0	0	0	0	0
1045	**Tonic water**	0	5.9	N	N	N	N	0	0	0	0	0	0	0	0
Squashes and cordials															
1046	**Barley water**, undiluted	2.2	21.5	N	N	N	N	0	Tr	Tr	Tr	Tr	Tr	0	0
1047	**Blackcurrant juice drink/squash**, undiluted	Tr	54.2	8.8	7.8	36.3	1.3	0	0	0	Tr	0	0	0	0
1048	**Fruit juice drink/squash**, undiluted	0	8.9	3.7	3.7	1.2	0.3	0	Tr	Tr	Tr	Tr	Tr	Tr	0
1049	ready to drink	0	9.8	2.7	3.7	3.4	Tr	0	Tr	Tr	Tr	Tr	Tr	Tr	0
1050	**Fruit juice drink**, no added sugar, undiluted	0	1.4	0.5	0.7	0.2	Tr	0	Tr	Tr	Tr	Tr	Tr	Tr	0
1051	no added sugar, ready to drink	0	0.9	0.3	0.3	0.3	Tr	0	Tr	Tr	Tr	Tr	Tr	Tr	0

[a] Total sugar typically varies from 2.4g to 12.8g per 100g

[b] Not including oligosaccharides

Inorganic constituents per 100g edible portion

No.	Food	Na	K	Ca	Mg	P	Fe	Cu	Zn	Cl	Mn	Se	I
						mg						µg	
Carbonated drinks continued													
1042	**Fruit juice drink**, carbonated, no added sugar, ready to drink	Tr	27	7	7	2	Tr	Tr	Tr	Tr	Tr	Tr	Tr
1043	**Lemonade**	7	15	5	1	Tr	Tr	Tr	Tr	2	Tr	Tr	Tr
1044	**Lucozade**	26	7	3	1	1	Tr	Tr	Tr	14	Tr	Tr	Tr
1045	**Tonic water**	4	0	1	0	0	Tr	Tr	Tr	Tr	Tr	Tr	Tr
Squashes and cordials													
1046	**Barley water**, undiluted	15	27	5	2	4	Tr	Tr	Tr	3	Tr	Tr	Tr
1047	**Blackcurrant juice drink/squash**, undiluted	16	92	8	2	3	0.2	0.01	0.1	2	Tr	Tr	Tr
1048	**Fruit juice drink/squash**, undiluted	40	27	6	1	2	Tr	Tr	Tr	4	Tr	Tr	Tr
1049	ready to drink	5	44	6	3	2	Tr	Tr	Tr	3	Tr	Tr	Tr
1050	**Fruit juice drink**, no added sugar, undiluted	110	31	5	1	2	Tr	Tr	Tr	3	Tr	Tr	Tr
1051	no added sugar, ready to drink	5	48	5	3	3	Tr	Tr	Tr	2	0.03	Tr	Tr

Vitamins per 100g edible portion

No.	Food	Retinol µg	Carotene µg	Vitamin D µg	Vitamin E mg	Thiamin mg	Ribo- flavin mg	Niacin mg	Trypt 60 mg	Vitamin B6 mg	Vitamin B12 µg	Folate µg	Panto- thenate mg	Biotin µg	Vitamin C mg
Carbonated drinks continued															
1042	**Fruit juice drink,** carbonated, no added sugar, ready to drink	0	94	0	Tr	Tr	Tr	Tr	Tr	Tr	0	1	Tr	Tr	1
1043	**Lemonade**	0	Tr	0	Tr	Tr	Tr	Tr	Tr	Tr	0	Tr	Tr	Tr	Tr
1044	**Lucozade**	0	835	0	0	Tr	Tr	Tr	Tr	Tr	0	1	Tr	Tr	8
1045	**Tonic water**	0	0	0	0	0	0	0	0	0	0	0	0	0	0
Squashes and cordials															
1046	**Barley water,** undiluted	0	630	0	N	Tr	Tr	0.1	Tr	0.01	0	5	Tr	Tr	10
1047	**Blackcurrant juice drink/squash,** undiluted	0	N	0	N	Tr	Tr	N	Tr	N	0	Tr	Tr	Tr	N[a]
1048	**Fruit juice drink/squash,** undiluted	0	690	0	N	Tr	Tr	0.1	Tr	0.01	0	2	Tr	Tr	N[b]
1049	ready to drink	0	N	0	N	Tr	Tr	0.1	Tr	0.01	0	2	Tr	Tr	N
1050	**Fruit juice drink,** no added sugar, undiluted	0	N	0	Tr	Tr	Tr	0.1	Tr	0.01	0	2	0.05	Tr	N
1051	no added sugar, ready to drink	0	Tr	0	Tr	0.02	Tr	0.1	Tr	0.01	0	2	0.06	Tr	5

[a] Vitamin C is added to some products and typically varies from 20mg to 120mg per 100g

[b] Unfortified and fortified products contain 7mg and 30-40mg vitamin C per 100g respectively

415

Composition of food per 100g edible portion

No.	Food	Description and main data sources	Main data reference	Water g	Total nitrogen g	Protein g	Fat g	Carbo-hydrate g	Energy value kcal	kJ
Squashes and cordials continued										
1052	**High juice drink**, undiluted	Typically 50% juice with 35-45% sugar. Analytical data, 1993; and industry data, 2013	38	57.1	0.04	0.3	Tr	42.6	161	687
1053	no added sugar, undiluted	Typically 50% juice. Estimated from high juice drink, undiluted and industry data, 2013		95.1	0.04	0.3	Tr	4.6	18	78
1054	**Lime juice cordial**, undiluted	MW3, 1960	3	70.5	0.01	0.1	0	29.8	112	479
Juices										
1055	**Apple juice**, clear, ambient and chilled	From concentrate. Analytical data, 2012	74	86.6	0.02	0.1	Tr	9.7	37	157
1056	**Cranberry fruit juice drink**	Industry data, 2013		87.9	Tr	Tr	0	12.1	45	194
1057	**Grape juice**, unsweetened	100% red juice. Analytical data, 1990; and industry data, 2013	31	83.6	0.05	0.3	0.1	16.0	62	265
1058	**Grapefruit juice**, unsweetened	Cartons, canned, bottled and frozen. Analytical data, 1990[a]	31	89.4	0.07	0.4	0.1	8.3	33	140
1059	**Lemon juice**, fresh	Analysis and literature sources. FAN Supplement, 1992	11	91.4	0.05	0.3	Tr	1.6	7	31
1060	**Mixed fruit juice**	Estimated from apple and orange juice and industry data, 2013		88.5	0.06	0.4	Tr	10.3	40	172
1061	**Orange juice**, chilled	Premium and from concentrate, including 'smooth' and 'with bits'. Analytical data, 2012	74	87.7	0.14	0.9	Tr	8.6	36	153
1062	ambient, UHT	From concentrate, including 'smooth' and 'with bits'. Analytical data, 2012	74	89.4	0.09	0.6	Tr	8.5	34	146

[a] Frozen samples were diluted as per manufacturers' instructions prior to analysis

Beverages *continued*

Composition of food per 100g edible portion

No.	Food	Starch g	Total sugars g	Gluc g	Fruct g	Sucr g	Malt g	Lact g	Dietary fibre NSP g	AOAC g	Satd g	Mono-unsatd g	Poly-unsatd g	Trans g	Cholest-erol mg
Squashes and cordials *continued*															
1052	**High juice drink**, undiluted	0	42.6	16.6	16.2	9.8	Tr	0	Tr	Tr	Tr	Tr	Tr	Tr	0
1053	no added sugar, undiluted	0	4.6	1.1	1.3	2.2	0	0	Tr	Tr	Tr	Tr	Tr	Tr	0
1054	**Lime juice cordial**, undiluted	Tr	29.8	11.5	11.0	5.9	1.4	0	0	0	0	0	0	0	0
Juices															
1055	**Apple juice**, clear, ambient and chilled	0	9.7	2.4	5.5	1.8	0	0	Tr	Tr	Tr	Tr	Tr	Tr	0
1056	**Cranberry fruit juice drink**	0	12.1	N	N	N	N	0	Tr	Tr	0	0	0	0	0
1057	**Grape juice**, unsweetened	0	16.0	7.5	8.5	Tr	0	0	0	0	Tr	Tr	Tr	Tr	0
1058	**Grapefruit juice**, unsweetened	0	8.3	3.0	3.3	2.0	0	0	Tr	Tr	Tr	Tr	Tr	Tr	0
1059	**Lemon juice**, fresh	0	1.6	0.5	0.9	0.2	0	0	0.1	N	Tr	Tr	Tr	Tr	0
1060	**Mixed fruit juice**	0	10.3	N	N	N	Tr	0	N	0.8	Tr	Tr	Tr	0	0
1061	**Orange juice**, chilled	0	8.6	2.0	2.4	4.2	0	0	0.2	Tr	Tr	Tr	Tr	Tr	0
1062	ambient, UHT	0	8.5	2.0	2.4	4.1	0	0	0.2	Tr	Tr	Tr	Tr	Tr	0

Inorganic constituents per 100g edible portion

No.	Food	Na	K	Ca	Mg	P	Fe	Cu	Zn	Cl	Mn	Se	I
						mg						µg	

Squashes and cordials continued

No.	Food	Na	K	Ca	Mg	P	Fe	Cu	Zn	Cl	Mn	Se	I
1052	**High juice drink**, undiluted	11	110	14	4	5	Tr	Tr	Tr	6	Tr	Tr	Tr
1053	no added sugar, undiluted	100	110	14	4	5	Tr	Tr	Tr	N	Tr	Tr	Tr
1054	**Lime juice cordial**, undiluted	8	49	9	4	5	0.3	0.07	N	4	Tr	Tr	Tr

Juices

No.	Food	Na	K	Ca	Mg	P	Fe	Cu	Zn	Cl	Mn	Se	I
1055	**Apple juice**, clear, ambient and chilled	3	89	6	4	6	0.1	0.01	Tr	64	0.03	Tr	Tr
1056	**Cranberry fruit juice drink**	Tr	N	N	N	N	N	N	N	N	N	0	N
1057	**Grape juice**, unsweetened	7	55	19	7	14	0.9	Tr	0.1	6	0.10	1	N
1058	**Grapefruit juice**, unsweetened	7	100	14	8	11	0.2	0.01	Tr	4	0.20	1	N
1059	**Lemon juice**, fresh	1	130	7	7	8	0.1	0.03	Tr	3	Tr	1	N
1060	**Mixed fruit juice**	2	123	7	7	11	0.1	0.02	Tr	65	0.03	Tr	Tr
1061	**Orange juice**, chilled	1	158	8	9	15	0.1	0.03	Tr	65	0.02	Tr	1
1062	ambient, UHT	3	164	12	10	16	0.1	0.03	0.1	70	0.03	Tr	1

Squashes and cordials continued

Juices

No.	Food	Retinol µg	Carotene µg	Vitamin D µg	Vitamin E mg	Thiamin mg	Ribo-flavin mg	Niacin mg	Trypt 60 mg	Vitamin B6 mg	Vitamin B12 µg	Folate µg	Panto-thenate mg	Biotin µg	Vitamin C mg
1052	**High juice drink**, undiluted	0	N	0	N	0.01	0.01	0.1	Tr	0.03	0	4	Tr	Tr	N
1053	no added sugar, undiluted	0	N	0	N	0.01	0.01	0.1	Tr	0.03	0	4	Tr	Tr	N[a]
1054	**Lime juice cordial**, undiluted	0	Tr	0	Tr	Tr	Tr	Tr	Tr	Tr	0	Tr	Tr	Tr	Tr
1055	**Apple juice**, clear, ambient and chilled	0	Tr	0	Tr	0.05	0.02	0.2	Tr	0.05	0	1	0.05	1	26
1056	**Cranberry fruit juice drink**	0	0	0	0	Tr	Tr	Tr	Tr	Tr	0	Tr	Tr	Tr	30
1057	**Grape juice**, unsweetened	0	Tr	0	Tr	Tr	0.01	0.1	Tr	0.04	0	1	0.03	1	Tr
1058	**Grapefruit juice**, unsweetened	0	1	0	0.19	0.04	0.01	0.2	Tr	0.02	0	6	0.08	1	31
1059	**Lemon juice**, fresh	0	12	0	N	0.03	0.01	0.1	Tr	0.05	0	13	0.10	0	36
1060	**Mixed fruit juice**	0	N	0	Tr	0.17	0.02	0.3	Tr	0.06	0	11	0.12	1	33
1061	**Orange juice**, chilled	0	40	0	0.15	0.28	0.02	0.4	Tr	0.06	0	22	0.15	1	40
1062	ambient, UHT	0	40	0	0.15	0.33	0.02	0.4	Tr	0.04	0	32	0.19	1	31

[a] Fortified products contain between 21mg and 80mg per 100g

Composition of food per 100g edible portion

No.	Food	Description and main data sources	Main data reference	Water g	Total nitrogen g	Protein g	Fat g	Carbo-hydrate g	Energy value kcal	Energy value kJ

Juices continued

No.	Food	Description and main data sources	Main data reference	Water g	Total nitrogen g	Protein g	Fat g	Carbo-hydrate g	kcal	kJ
1063	**Pineapple juice**, unsweetened	Cartons only. Analytical data, 1984	23	87.8	0.05	0.3	0.1	10.5	41	177
1064	**Pomegranate juice drink**	With added sugar. Industry data, 2013; and MW1, 1940	1	85.4	0.03	0.2	Tr	11.6	44	189
1065	**Smoothies**	Retail, chilled, yellow and red fruit smoothies. Not made with milk. Industry data, 2013		86.2	0.08	0.5	0.1	12.2	49	207
1066	**Tomato juice**	Analytical data, 1985	25	93.8	0.13	0.8	Tr	3.0	14	62

No.	Food	Starch	Total sugars	Gluc	Fruct	Sucr	Malt	Lact	Dietary fibre NSP	Dietary fibre AOAC	Fatty acids Satd	Mono-unsatd	Poly-unsatd	Trans	Cholest-erol
		g	g	g	g	g	g	g	g	g	g	g	g	g	mg
Juices *continued*															
1063	**Pineapple juice**, unsweetened	0	10.5	2.9	2.9	4.7	0	0	Tr	Tr	Tr	Tr	Tr	Tr	0
1064	**Pomegranate juice**, fresh	0	11.6	6.3	5.1	0.2	0	0	Tr	Tr	Tr	Tr	Tr	Tr	0
1065	**Smoothies**	0.6	11.6	N	N	N	Tr	0	N	1.0	Tr	Tr	Tr	0	0
1066	**Tomato juice**	Tr	3.0	1.4	1.6	Tr	0	0	0.6	N	Tr	Tr	Tr	Tr	0

Inorganic constituents per 100g edible portion

No.	Food	Na	K	Ca	Mg	P	Fe	Cu	Zn	Cl	Mn	Se	I
						mg						µg	
Juices continued													
1063	**Pineapple juice**, unsweetened	8	53	8	6	1	0.2	0.02	0.1	15	0.70	Tr	Tr
1064	**Pomegranate juice**, fresh	1	200	3	3	8	0.2	0.07	N	53	N	N	N
1065	**Smoothies**	Tr	N	N	N	N	N	N	N			N	Tr
1066	**Tomato juice**	230	230	10	10	19	0.4	0.06	0.1	400	0.10	Tr	2

Vitamins per 100g edible portion

No.	Food	Retinol	Carotene	Vitamin D	Vitamin E	Thiamin	Ribo-flavin	Niacin	Trypt 60	Vitamin B_6	Vitamin B_{12}	Folate	Panto-thenate	Biotin	Vitamin C
		µg	µg	µg	mg	mg	mg	mg	mg	mg	µg	µg	mg	µg	mg

Juices continued

No.	Food	Retinol	Carotene	Vitamin D	Vitamin E	Thiamin	Ribo-flavin	Niacin	Trypt 60	Vitamin B_6	Vitamin B_{12}	Folate	Panto-thenate	Biotin	Vitamin C
1063	Pineapple juice, unsweetened	0	8	0	0.03	0.06	0.01	0.1	0.1	0.05	0	8	0.07	Tr	11
1064	Pomegranate juice, fresh	0	33	0	N	0.02	0.03	0.2	Tr	0.31	0	N	0.57	N	30
1065	Smoothies	0	N	0	N	N	N	N	N	N	0	N	N	N	N
1066	Tomato juice	0	200	0	1.01	0.02	0.02	0.7	0.1	0.06	0	10	0.20	2	8

Alcoholic beverages

Section 2.13

Alcoholic beverages

Most of the data in this section of the Tables have been taken from the *Miscellaneous Foods* (1994)[14] supplement. However, values have been reviewed, using data from manufacturers, and updated where necessary. In addition, the categories have been updated and expanded to reflect products currently available.

The values for wines were selected to be typical values based on an extensive review of a range of products. However because of the range of alcohol content in wine, these values should be used only as a guide.

Alcoholic beverages are normally measured by volume; the data in this section (in contrast to all other sections of the book) are presented as amounts per 100ml. The strength of alcoholic beverages is shown on labels as percentage alcohol by volume (ABV). To convert from ABV to g/100ml, multiply by the specific gravity of ethyl alcohol 0.789, so 10 per cent alcohol by volume contains 7.9 grams of alcohol per 100ml.

	Alcohol contents of various strengths 'by volume'
% Alcohol by volume	*Alcohol (g/100ml)*
5	4.0
10	7.9
15	11.9
20	15.8
25	19.8
30	23.7
35	27.7
40	31.6

The specific gravities (densities) of alcoholic beverages are given below so that calculations can be made if the beverages are measured by weight. To convert from g/100ml to g/100g, the values are divided by the specific gravity (density). For example, if white wine, sweet has a specific gravity of 1.016 and ABV of 10%, in order to convert ABV to g/100g:

$$\text{Alcohol g/100g} = 10\% \text{ alcohol} \times 0.789 \div 1.016$$
$$= 7.76 \text{ g/100g}$$

Alcoholic beverages *continued*

The specific gravity varies with the composition of the drink and typical values are given below. In general, it increases with the amount of solids (mainly sugars) and decreases with the amount of alcohol because the specific gravity of ethyl alcohol itself is only 0.79.

Specific gravities of alcoholic beverages			
Beers		**Wines**	
Beer, bitter, average	1.004	**Red wine**	0.998
canned	1.008	**Rose wine**, medium	1.003
keg	1.001	**White wine**, dry	0.995
Brown ale, bottled	1.008	medium	1.005
Lager, bottled	1.005	sparkling	0.995
low alcohol	1.002	sweet	1.016
Stout, bottled	1.014		
		Fortified wines	
Ciders			
		Port	1.026
Cider, dry	1.007	**Sherry**, dry	0.988
low alcohol	1.020	medium	0.988
sweet	1.012	sweet	1.009
vintage	1.017	**Vermouth**, dry	1.005
		Liqueurs	
		cream liqueurs	1.070
		high strength, 35-40% ABV	1.035
		low-medium strength, 20-28% ABV	1.090
		Spirits	
		40% volume	0.950

Composition of food per 100ml

No.	Food	Description and main data sources	Main data reference	Water g	Alcohol g	Total nitrogen g	Protein g	Fat g	Carbohydrate g	Energy value kcal	kJ
Beers											
1067	**Beer, bitter**, average	<4% ABV, canned, draught and bottled, including Boddingtons, John Smith, Greene King IPA, Tetley's and Caffrey's. Analytical data, 1984	21	93.9	2.9	0.05	0.3	Tr	2.2	30	124
1068	best, premium	4-5% ABV, including Fuller's London Pride, Spitfire, Greene King Abbot. Analytical data, 1984	21	93.0	3.4	0.05	0.3	Tr	2.2	33	139
1069	strong	>5% ABV, including Old Speckled Hen, Hobgoblin, Old Peculier, Leffe and Marston's Old Empire. Estimated from beer, bitter, best, premium		93.0	4.7	0.05	0.3	Tr	2.2	42	175
1070	**Lager**, standard	<4.5% ABV, canned and draught, including Skol, Hofmeister, Tennent's, Carling Black Label, Stella Artois and Foster's. Analytical data, 1984; and industry data, 2013	21	93.0	3.2	0.05	0.3	Tr	Tr	24	98
1071	alcohol-free	Kaliber, Beck's Blue, Equator, Bitburger Drive, Cobra Zero and Holsten Pils Alcohol Free. Analytical data, 1993	38	96.3	Tr	0.06	0.4	Tr	1.5[a]	7	31
1072	low alcohol	2-3% ABV, including Bavaria Premium, Carling Zest, Carling C2, Beck's Premier Light and own brand. Estimated from standard lager and industry data, 2013		97.0	1.9	0.05	0.3	Tr	0.5	16	67

[a] Includes oligosaccharides

No.	Food	Starch	Total sugars	Gluc	Fruct	Sucr	Malt	Lact	Dietary fibre		Fatty acids			Trans	Cholest- erol
						Individual sugars			NSP	AOAC	Satd	Mono- unsatd	Poly- unsatd		
		g	g	g	g	g	g	g	g	g	g	g	g	g	mg
Beers															
1067	**Beer, bitter**, average	0	2.2	0	0	0	2.2	0	Tr	Tr	Tr	Tr	Tr	0	0
1068	best, premium	0	2.2	0.3	0	0	1.9	0	Tr	Tr	Tr	Tr	Tr	0	0
1069	strong	0	2.2	0.3	0	0	1.9	0	Tr	Tr	Tr	Tr	Tr	0	0
1070	**Lager**, standard	0	Tr	Tr	0	0	0	0	Tr	Tr	Tr	Tr	Tr	0	0
1071	alcohol-free	0	1.2[a]	0.6	0.4	Tr	0.2	0	Tr	Tr	Tr	Tr	Tr	0	0
1072	low alcohol	0	0.5	0.3	0.1	0	0.1	0	Tr	Tr	Tr	Tr	Tr	0	0

[a] Not including oligosaccharides

427

Inorganic constituents per 100ml

No.	Food	Na	K	Ca	Mg	P	Fe	Cu	Zn	Cl	Mn	Se	I
						mg						µg	
Beers													
1067	**Beer, bitter**, average	6	32	8	7	14	0.1	0.01	0.1	24	0.03	Tr	N
1068	best, premium	8	46	9	8	16	Tr	0.03	0.1	36	0.01	Tr	N
1069	strong	8	46	9	8	16	Tr	0.03	0.1	36	0.01	Tr	N
1070	**Lager**, standard	7	39	5	7	19	Tr	Tr	Tr	20	0.01	Tr	N
1071	alcohol-free	2	44	3	7	19	Tr	Tr	Tr	Tr	0.01	Tr	N
1072	low alcohol	10	48	7	14	15	Tr	Tr	Tr	N	0.01	Tr	N

Vitamins per 100ml

Beers

No.	Food	Retinol µg	Carotene µg	Vitamin D µg	Vitamin E mg	Thiamin mg	Ribo-flavin mg	Niacin mg	Trypt 60 mg	Vitamin B6 mg	Vitamin B12 µg	Folate µg	Panto-thenate mg	Biotin µg	Vitamin C mg
1067	**Beer, bitter**, average	0	Tr	0	N	Tr	0.03	0.2	0.2	0.07	Tr	5	0.05	1	0
1068	best, premium	0	Tr	0	N	Tr	0.04	0.8	0.2	0.09	Tr	8	0.07	1	0
1069	strong	0	Tr	0	N	Tr	0.04	0.8	0.2	0.09	Tr	8	0.07	1	0
1070	**Lager**, standard	0	Tr	0	N	Tr	0.04	0.7	0.3	0.06	Tr	12	0.03	1	0
1071	alcohol-free	0	Tr	0	N	Tr	0.02	0.6	0.4	0.03	Tr	5	0.09	Tr	0
1072	low alcohol	0	Tr	0	N	Tr	0.03	0.6	0.3	0.05	Tr	9	0.19	Tr	0

Composition of food per 100ml

No.	Food	Description and main data sources	Main data reference	Water g	Alcohol g	Total nitrogen g	Protein g	Fat g	Carbo-hydrate g	Energy value kcal	kJ
Beers continued											
1073	**Lager**, premium	Approx. 5% ABV, including Bitburger Pils, San Miguel, Stella Artois, Bud, Kronenbourg, Grolsch, Beck's and Carlsberg Export. Estimated from standard lager and industry data, 2013		93.0	3.9	0.05	0.3	Tr	Tr	29	118
1074	extra strong	Approx. 9% ABV, including Carlsberg Special Brew, Skol Super, Tennent's Super and Kestrel Super. Estimated from previous values for premium lager (analytical data, 1984) and industry data, 2013	21	88.7	7.1	0.05	0.3	Tr	2.4	60	249
1075	**Shandy**, bottled or canned	<1% ABV, typically 10-12% beer or lager. Analytical data, 1984	21	94.0	0.7	Tr	Tr	Tr	5.0	24	100
1076	50% lager	Calculated from standard lager and standard lemonade		93.4	1.6	0.03	0.2	Tr	2.9	23	96
1077	**Stout**, Guinness	Approx. 4% ABV, canned, bottled and draught. Analytical data, 1984; and industry data, 2013	21	90.2	3.3	0.06	0.4	Tr	3.2	37	153
Ciders											
1078	**Cider**, dry	4.7-5.5% ABV, including Strongbow, Blackthorn dry, Thatchers medium-dry and Savanna dry. MW3, 1960	3	92.5	3.8	Tr	Tr	0	2.6	36	152

No.	Food	Starch	Total sugars	Gluc	Fruct	Sucr	Malt	Lact	NSP	AOAC	Satd	Mono- unsatd	Poly- unsatd	Trans	Cholest- erol
		g	g	g	g	g	g	g	g	g	g	g	g	g	mg

Beers continued

No.	Food	Starch	Total sugars	Gluc	Fruct	Sucr	Malt	Lact	NSP	AOAC	Satd	Mono-unsatd	Poly-unsatd	Trans	Cholesterol
1073	**Lager**, premium	0	Tr	Tr	0	0	0	0	Tr	Tr	Tr	Tr	Tr	0	0
1074	extra strong	0	2.4	1.0	0	0	1.4	0	Tr	Tr	Tr	Tr	Tr	0	0
1075	**Shandy**, bottled or canned	0	5.0	1.6	1.7	1.7	0	0	Tr	Tr	Tr	Tr	Tr	0	0
1076	50% lager	0	2.9	0.8	0.7	1.4	0.1	0	Tr	Tr	Tr	Tr	Tr	0	0
1077	**Stout**, Guinness	0	3.2	Tr	Tr	0	3.2	Tr	Tr	Tr	Tr	Tr	Tr	0	0

Ciders

No.	Food	Starch	Total sugars	Gluc	Fruct	Sucr	Malt	Lact	NSP	AOAC	Satd	Mono-unsatd	Poly-unsatd	Trans	Cholesterol
1078	**Cider**, dry	0	2.6	0.6	0.5	0.7	0.8	0	0	0	0	0	0	0	0

431

Inorganic constituents per 100ml

No.	Food	Na	K	Ca	Mg	P	Fe	Cu	Zn	Cl	Mn	Se	I
						mg						µg	

Beers continued

No.	Food	Na	K	Ca	Mg	P	Fe	Cu	Zn	Cl	Mn	Se	I
1073	**Lager**, premium	7	39	5	7	19	Tr	Tr	Tr	20	0.01	Tr	N
1074	extra strong	7	39	5	7	19	Tr	Tr	Tr	20	0.01	Tr	N
1075	**Shandy**, bottled or canned	7	6	8	1	5	Tr	Tr	Tr	8	Tr	Tr	N
1076	50% lager	7	27	5	4	10	Tr	Tr	Tr	11	Tr	Tr	N
1077	**Stout**, Guinness	6	48	4	8	26	0.2	Tr	Tr	17	0.01	Tr	N

Ciders

No.	Food	Na	K	Ca	Mg	P	Fe	Cu	Zn	Cl	Mn	Se	I
1078	**Cider**, dry	7	72	8	3	3	0.5	0.04	Tr	6	Tr	Tr	N

Vitamins per 100ml

No.	Food	Retinol µg	Carotene µg	Vitamin D µg	Vitamin E mg	Thiamin mg	Ribo-flavin mg	Niacin mg	Trypt 60 mg	Vitamin B$_6$ mg	Vitamin B$_{12}$ µg	Folate µg	Panto-thenate mg	Biotin µg	Vitamin C mg
Beers continued															
1073	**Lager**, premium	0	Tr	0	N	Tr	0.04	0.7	0.3	0.06	Tr	12	0.03	1	0
1074	extra strong	0	Tr	0	N	Tr	0.04	0.7	0.3	0.06	Tr	12	0.03	1	0
1075	**Shandy**, bottled or canned	0	Tr	0	N	Tr	Tr	0.1	Tr	0.01	Tr	1	0.02	Tr	N
1076	50% lager	0	Tr	0	N	Tr	0.02	0.3	0.2	0.03	Tr	6	0.01	1	Tr
1077	**Stout**, Guinness	0	Tr	0	N	Tr	0.03	0.8	0.2	0.08	Tr	6	0.04	1	0
Ciders															
1078	**Cider**, dry	0	Tr	0	N	Tr	Tr	0	Tr	0.01	Tr	N	0.04	1	0

Ciders, continued

No.	Food	Description and main data sources	Main data reference	Water g	Alcohol g	Total nitrogen g	Protein g	Fat g	Carbo- hydrate g	Energy value kcal	kJ
1079	**Cider,** low alcohol	<1% ABV, including Kopparberg Pear non-alcoholic and own brands. Analytical data, 1993	38	94.9	0.6	Tr	Tr	0	3.6	17	74
1080	sweet	3.5-5.0% ABV, including Woodpecker, Magners, Bulmers, Kopparberg, Stella Artois Pear Cidre, Jacques fruit cider and Thatchers rose cider. MW3, 1960[a]	3	91.2	3.7	Tr	Tr	0	4.3	42	176
1081	strong	6-8.5% ABV, including vintage varieties, Aspall Premier Cru, K Cider, Scrumpy Strong and Diamond White. MW3, 1960	3	86.9	5.8	Tr	Tr	0	7.3	68	285
	Wines										
1082	**Red wine**	Typically 11-15% ABV, mixed sample from different countries. Industry data, 2010, 2013; and calculated from analytical data, 1984 and MW4	21, 4	88.4	10.7	0.03	0.1	0	0.2	76	315
1083	**Rose wine**, medium	9.5-13.5% ABV, mixed sample from different countries. MW4, 1978; and industry data, 2010, 2013	4	87.3	9.9	0.01	0.1	0	2.5	79	329
1084	**White wine**, dry	11-14% ABV, mixed sample from different countries. MW4, 1978; and industry data, 2010, 2013	4	89.1	10.3	0.02	0.1	0	0.6	75	309
1085	medium	8-13.5% ABV, mixed sample from different countries. Industry data, 2010, 2013; and calculated from analytical data, 1984 and MW4	21, 4	86.3	9.1	0.02	0.1	0	3.0	75	313

[a] Pear and other fruit ciders are similar in composition to sweet apple ciders

Composition of food per 100ml

No.	Food	Starch g	Total sugars g	Individual sugars Gluc g	Fruct g	Sucr g	Malt g	Lact g	Dietary fibre NSP g	AOAC g	Fatty acids Satd g	Mono- unsatd g	Poly- unsatd g	Trans g	Cholest- erol mg
Ciders continued															
1079	**Cider**, low alcohol	0	3.6	0.7	1.4	1.4	0.1	0	0	0	0	0	0	0	0
1080	sweet	0	4.3	1.0	0.7	1.2	1.3	0	0	0	0	0	0	0	0
1081	strong	0	7.3	1.8	1.3	2.0	2.3	0	0	0	0	0	0	0	0
Wines															
1082	**Red wine**	0	0.2	0.1	0.1	Tr	0	0	0	0	0	0	0	0	0
1083	**Rose wine**, medium	0	2.5	0.8	1.7	0	0	0	0	0	0	0	0	0	0
1084	**White wine**, dry	0	0.6	0.3	0.3	0	0	0	0	0	0	0	0	0	0
1085	medium	0	3.0	1.2	1.4	N	0	0	0	0	0	0	0	0	0

Inorganic constituents per 100ml

No.	Food	mg										µg	
		Na	K	Ca	Mg	P	Fe	Cu	Zn	Cl	Mn	Se	I
Ciders continued													
1079	**Cider**, low alcohol	3	81	7	2	4	0.1	0.03	Tr	2	0.01	Tr	Tr
1080	sweet	7	72	8	3	3	0.5	0.04	Tr	6	Tr	Tr	N
1081	strong	2	97	5	4	9	0.3	0.02	Tr	5	Tr	Tr	N
Wines													
1082	**Red wine**	7	110	7	11	13	0.9	0.06	0.1	11	0.10	Tr	N
1083	**Rose wine**, medium	4	75	12	7	6	1.0	0.02	Tr	7	0.10	Tr	N
1084	**White wine**, dry	4	61	9	8	6	0.5	0.01	Tr	10	0.10	Tr	N
1085	medium	11	81	12	8	8	0.8	Tr	Tr	3	0.10	Tr	N

Alcoholic beverages *continued*

Vitamins per 100ml

No.	Food	Retinol µg	Carotene µg	Vitamin D µg	Vitamin E mg	Thiamin mg	Ribo-flavin mg	Niacin mg	Trypt 60 mg	Vitamin B_6 mg	Vitamin B_{12} µg	Folate µg	Panto-thenate mg	Biotin µg	Vitamin C mg
	Ciders continued														
1079	**Cider,** low alcohol	0	Tr	0	N	Tr	Tr	0.1	Tr	Tr	Tr	2	0.07	Tr	0
1080	sweet	0	Tr	0	N	Tr	Tr	0	Tr	0.01	Tr	N	0.03	1	0
1081	strong	0	Tr	0	N	Tr	Tr	0	Tr	0.01	Tr	N	0.03	1	0
	Wines														
1082	**Red wine**	0	Tr	0	N	Tr	0.02	0.1	Tr	0.03	Tr	1	0.04	2	0
1083	**Rose wine,** medium	0	Tr	0	N	Tr	0.01	0.1	Tr	0.02	Tr	Tr	0.04	N	0
1084	**White wine,** dry	0	Tr	0	N	Tr	0.01	0.1	Tr	0.02	Tr	Tr	0.03	N	0
1085	medium	0	Tr	0	N	Tr	Tr	0.1	Tr	0.01	Tr	Tr	0.06	1	0

No.	Food	Description and main data sources	Main data reference	Water g	Alcohol g	Total nitrogen g	Protein g	Fat g	Carbo-hydrate g	Energy value kcal	kJ
Wines *continued*											
1086	**White wine**, sparkling	Approx. 11.5% ABV, mixed sample from different countries. Analytical data, 1984 and industry data, 2010, 2013[a]	21	85.8	9.1	0.04	0.3	0	5.1	84	351
1087	sweet	10-15% ABV, mixed sample from different countries. MW4, 1978	4	80.6	10.2	0.03	0.2	0	5.9	94	394
Fortified wines											
1088	**Port**	19-21% ABV. MW4, 1978	4	71.1	15.9	0.02	0.1	0	12.0	157	655
1089	**Sherry**, medium	15-19.5% ABV. Analytical data, 1984	21	78.8	13.3	0.02	0.1	0	5.9	116	482
1090	**Vermouth**, dry	15-19% ABV. MSF Supplement, 1994	14	82.1	13.9	0.01	0.1	0	3.0	109	453
Liqueurs											
1091	**Cream liqueurs**	17% ABV, Baileys Original Irish Cream. Analytical data, 1984; and industry data, 2013	21	48.7	13.5[b]	0.47	3.0	13.0	21.8	305	1272
1092	**Liqueurs**, high strength	35-40% ABV, including Pernod, Drambuie, Cointreau, Grand Marnier and Southern Comfort. Analytical data, 1984	21	28.0	31.8	Tr	Tr	0	24.4	314	1313
1093	low-medium strength	20-28% ABV, including cherry brandy, Tia Maria and Creme de Menthe. Analytical data, 1984	21	47.4	19.8	Tr	Tr	0	32.8	262	1099

[a] Not including champagne

[b] Other cream liqueurs contain 11.5g to 15.8g alcohol per 100ml

No.	Food	Starch g	Total sugars g	Gluc g	Fruct g	Sucr g	Malt g	Lact g	Dietary fibre NSP g	AOAC g	Fatty acids Satd g	Mono- unsatd g	Poly- unsatd g	Trans g	Cholest- erol mg
Wines continued
1086	**White wine**, sparkling	0	5.1	2.2	2.8	0.1	0	0	0	0	0	0	0	0	0
1087	sweet	0	5.9	2.6	3.3	0.1	0	0	0	0	0	0	0	0	0
Fortified wines
1088	**Port**	0	12.0	4.6	4.6	2.8	0	0	0	0	0	0	0	0	0
1089	**Sherry**, medium	0	5.9	3.0	2.9	0	0	0	0	0	0	0	0	0	0
1090	**Vermouth**, dry	0	3.0	1.1	1.2	0.7	0	0	0	0	0	0	0	0	0
Liqueurs
1091	**Cream liqueurs**	Tr	21.8	0	0	21.0	0	0.8	0	0	8.2	3.0	0.5	0.4	N
1092	**Liqueurs**, high strength	0	24.4	2.6	2.3	17.1	2.4	0	0	0	0	0	0	0	0
1093	low-medium strength	0	32.8	6.3	6.1	20.4	0	0	0	0	0	0	0	0	0

Inorganic constituents per 100ml

No.	Food	Na	K	Ca	Mg	P	Fe	Cu	Zn	Cl	Mn	Se	I
						mg						µg	

Wines continued

| 1086 | **White wine**, sparkling | 5 | 58 | 9 | 7 | 9 | 0.5 | 0.01 | Tr | 6 | 0.04 | Tr | N |
| 1087 | sweet | 13 | 110 | 14 | 11 | 13 | 0.6 | 0.05 | Tr | 7 | 0.10 | Tr | N |

Fortified wines

1088	**Port**	4	97	4	11	12	0.4	0.10	N	8	Tr	Tr	N
1089	**Sherry**, medium	27	55	8	5	24	0.4	0.04	Tr	10	0.01	Tr	N
1090	**Vermouth**, dry	11	34	7	6	6	0.3	0.03	Tr	7	Tr	Tr	N

Liqueurs

1091	**Cream liqueurs**	89	19	18	2	38	0.1	Tr	0.2	25	Tr	Tr	N
1092	**Liqueurs**, high strength	6	3	Tr	Tr	Tr	Tr	Tr	Tr	4	0.02	Tr	Tr
1093	low-medium strength	12	34	5	2	7	0.1	0.02	Tr	20	0.02	N	N

Alcoholic beverages *continued*

Vitamins per 100ml

No.	Food	Retinol	Carotene	Vitamin D	Vitamin E	Thiamin	Ribo-flavin	Niacin	Trypt 60	Vitamin B_6	Vitamin B_{12}	Folate	Panto-thenate	Biotin	Vitamin C
		µg	µg	µg	mg	mg	mg	mg	mg	mg	µg	µg	mg	µg	mg
Wines continued															
1086	**White wine**, sparkling	0	Tr	0	N	Tr	0.01	0.1	Tr	0.02	Tr	Tr	0.04	1	0
1087	sweet	0	Tr	0	N	Tr	0.01	0.1	Tr	0.01	Tr	Tr	0.03	N	0
Fortified wines															
1088	**Port**	0	Tr	0	0	Tr	0.01	0.1	Tr	0.01	Tr	Tr	N	N	0
1089	**Sherry**, medium	0	Tr	0	0	Tr	0.01	0.1	Tr	0.02	Tr	Tr	0.02	1	0
1090	**Vermouth**, dry	0	Tr	0	0	Tr	Tr	0	Tr	0.01	Tr	Tr	N	N	0
Liqueurs															
1091	**Cream liqueurs**	190	91	Tr	0.57	N	N	N	N	N	Tr	Tr	N	N	0
1092	**Liqueurs**, high strength	0	Tr	0	0	Tr	Tr	Tr	Tr	Tr	Tr	Tr	Tr	Tr	0
1093	low-medium strength	0	Tr	0	0	Tr	Tr	Tr	Tr	Tr	Tr	Tr	Tr	Tr	0

Composition of food per 100ml

No.	Food	Description and main data sources	Main data reference	Water g	Alcohol g	Total nitrogen g	Protein g	Fat g	Carbo-hydrate g	Energy value kcal	Energy value kJ
Spirits											
1094	**Spirits**, 40% volume	Mean of brandy, gin, rum, whisky and vodka. MW5, 1991	10	68.3	31.7	Tr	Tr	0	Tr	222	919
1095	**Pre-mixed spirit based drinks**	Approx. 4% ABV, including WKD, Bacardi Breezer, Smirnoff Ice and Caribbean Twist. Industry data, 2013		88.8	3.2	Tr	Tr	0	8.0	52	221

Composition of food per 100ml

No.	Food	Starch g	Total sugars g	Gluc g	Fruct g	Sucr g	Malt g	Lact g	Dietary fibre NSP g	AOAC g	Fatty acids Satd g	Mono-unsatd g	Poly-unsatd g	Trans g	Cholesterol mg
						Individual sugars									

Spirits

No.	Food	Starch g	Total sugars g	Gluc g	Fruct g	Sucr g	Malt g	Lact g	NSP g	AOAC g	Satd g	Mono-unsatd g	Poly-unsatd g	Trans g	Cholesterol mg
1094	**Spirits, 40% volume**	0	Tr	0	0	Tr	0	0	0	0	0	0	0	0	0
1095	**Pre-mixed spirit based drinks**	0	8.0	N	N	N	N	0	0	0	0	0	0	0	0

Inorganic constituents per 100ml

No.	Food	Na	K	Ca	Mg	P	Fe	Cu	Zn	Cl	Mn	Se	I
						mg						μg	

Spirits

| 1094 | **Spirits**, 40% volume | Tr | Tr | Tr | Tr | Tr | Tr | Tr | Tr | Tr | Tr | Tr | Tr |
| 1095 | **Pre-mixed spirit based drinks** | N | N | N | N | N | N | Tr | Tr | N | Tr | Tr | N |

No.	Food	Retinol	Carotene	Vitamin D	Vitamin E	Thiamin	Ribo-flavin	Niacin	Trypt 60	Vitamin B6	Vitamin B12	Folate	Panto-thenate	Biotin	Vitamin C
		µg	µg	µg	mg	mg	mg	mg	mg	mg	µg	µg	mg	µg	mg

Spirits

| 1094 | **Spirits**, 40% volume | 0 | 0 | 0 | 0 | 0 | 0 | 0 | 0 | 0 | 0 | 0 | 0 | 0 | 0 |
| 1095 | **Pre-mixed spirit based drinks** | 0 | Tr | 0 | N | Tr | Tr | N | N | N | 0 | N | N | N | N |

Soups, sauces and miscellaneous foods

Section 2.14

Soups, sauces and miscellaneous foods

New analytical data for a range of soups[65,72], pasta and cooking sauces[65,66] have been incorporated into this section, with the categories expanded to reflect products currently available. However, most of the values for other foods have been taken from the *Miscellaneous Foods* (1994)[14] supplement, updated using data from manufacturers to reflect reductions made in salt, sugar, and/or fat content. For some foods in this section, the range of nutrient composition varies considerably between brands, e.g. for stocks and table sauces, and the values given typically reflect brand leader products. Users requiring more detailed brand-specific information should contact manufacturers directly.

The foods in this group cover soups; dairy sauces; salad sauces; dressings and pickles; table sauces; cooking sauces and a selection of miscellaneous food items.

Condensed and dried soups have been made up according to the manufacturer's instructions using distilled water.

An entry for distilled water has been included in the miscellaneous foods section, mainly for use in recipe calculations. There is considerable variation in the composition of tap water both by area of the country and source of supply. The local water company will be able to provide information on the composition of tap water from a specific area.

Losses of labile vitamins assigned to recipes were estimated from figures in Section 4.3.

Soups, sauces and miscellaneous foods

Composition of food per 100g edible portion

No.	Food	Description and main data sources	Main data reference	Water g	Total nitrogen g	Protein g	Fat g	Carbohydrate g	Energy value kcal	kJ
Soups										
1096	**Broccoli and stilton soup**, carton, chilled	Analytical data, 2002-2003; and industry data, 2013	65	88.8	0.37	2.3	3.1	3.8[a]	51	215
1097	**Carrot and coriander soup**, carton, chilled	Analytical data, 2002-2003; and industry data, 2013	65	90.6	0.14	0.9	2.6	4.7	45	187
1098	**Chicken noodle soup**, dried, as served	Calculated from 35g soup powder to 570ml water. Analytical data, 1992	35	94.5	0.16	1.0	0.3	3.2[a]	19	79
1099	**Chicken soup**, cream of, canned	MW5, 1991; and industry data, 2013	10	87.9	0.27	1.7	3.8	4.5	58	242
1100	cream of, canned, condensed	MW5, 1991; and industry data, 2013	10	82.2	0.41	2.6	5.8	6.0	85	355
1101	cream of, canned, condensed, as served	Diluted with an equal volume of water. MW5, 1991; and industry data, 2013	10	91.1	0.20	1.3	2.9	3.0	43	177
1102	**Instant soup**, dried, as served	Calculated from instant soup powder, 24g powder made up with 225g water; assorted flavours. Analytical data, 2010	72	90.8	0.09	0.6	1.3	6.2[a]	37	156
1103	**Lentil soup**, canned	Analytical data, 1992; and industry data, 2013	35	88.2	0.50	3.1	0.2	8.5	46	196
1104	**Low calorie soup**, canned	Tomato, vegetable and minestrone varieties. Analytical data, 1992; and industry data, 2013	35	91.3	0.14	0.9	0.7	6.2	33	140
1105	**Minestrone soup**, canned	Industry data, 2013		91.2	0.18	1.1	0.2	6.6	31	132
1106	**Mushroom soup**, carton, chilled	Analytical data, 2002-2003	65	89.8	0.24	1.5	2.7	4.9[a]	48	203
1107	cream of, canned	MW4, 1978; and industry data, 2013	4	90.4	0.20	1.1	3.0	3.9	46	192
1108	**Oxtail soup**, canned	MW4, 1978; and industry data, 2013	4	88.5	0.38	2.4	1.7	5.1	44	185
1109	**Tomato soup**, carton, chilled	Analytical data, 2002-2003	65	90.3	0.15	0.9	1.9	4.3	37	154

[a] Includes oligosaccharides

Composition of food per 100g edible portion

No.	Food	Starch g	Total sugars g	Individual sugars					Dietary fibre		Fatty acids				Cholesterol
				Gluc g	Fruct g	Sucr g	Malt g	Lact g	NSP g	AOAC g	Satd g	Mono-unsatd g	Poly-unsatd g	Trans g	erol mg

Soups

No.	Food	Starch	Total sugars	Gluc	Fruct	Sucr	Malt	Lact	NSP	AOAC	Satd	Mono-unsatd	Poly-unsatd	Trans	Cholesterol
1096	**Broccoli and stilton soup**, carton, chilled	2.3	1.5[a]	0.2	0.3	0.2	0	0.6	N	N	1.7	1.0	0.2	0.1	48
1097	**Carrot and coriander soup**, carton, chilled	1.7	3.0	0.6	0.6	1.6	Tr	0.3	0.5	1.0	1.4	0.9	0.2	0.1	Tr
1098	**Chicken noodle soup**, dried, as served	2.7	0.3[a]	Tr	Tr	0.2	Tr	0	0.2	N	N	N	N	N	N
1099	**Chicken soup**, cream of, canned	3.4	1.1	Tr	0.1	0.6	0	0.4	Tr	Tr	0.6	2.0	1.0	0.1	N
1100	cream of, canned, condensed	4.6	1.4	Tr	0.2	0.4	0	0.8	Tr	Tr	0.8	3.0	1.4	N	4
1101	cream of, canned, condensed, as served	2.3	0.7	Tr	0.1	0.2	0	0.4	Tr	Tr	0.4	1.5	0.7	0.1	2
1102	**Instant soup**, dried, as served	2.8	1.7[a]	0.2	0.2	0.6	0.6	0.1	0.2	0.5	0.8	0.3	0.1	Tr	1
1103	**Lentil soup**, canned	7.3	1.2	0.5	0.7	Tr	0	0	1.2	N	N	N	N	Tr	0
1104	**Low calorie soup**, canned	3.8	2.4	1.2	1.2	Tr	0	0	N	0.7	0.2	N	N	Tr	0
1105	**Minestrone soup**, canned	4.8	1.8	N	N	N	N	0	0.7	0.9	0.1	Tr	Tr	Tr	Tr
1106	**Mushroom soup**, carton, chilled	3.3	1.4[a]	0.1	0.2	0.3	0	0.7	0.3	0.3	1.4	0.9	0.2	0.2	1
1107	cream of, canned	3.1	0.8	Tr	0.1	0.3	0	0.4	0.1	N	0.5	1.6	0.9	0.1	1
1108	**Oxtail soup**, canned	4.2	0.9	0.2	0.2	0.5	Tr	0	0.1	N	0.6	0.6	0.2	N	7
1109	**Tomato soup**, carton, chilled	1.0	3.3	1.0	1.1	1.1	Tr	0.2	0.8	1.4	0.9	0.8	0.1	0.1	4

[a] Not including oligosaccharides

Inorganic constituents per 100g edible portion

No.	Food	Na	K	Ca	Mg	P	Fe	Cu	Zn	Cl	Mn	Se	I
						mg						µg	
Soups													
1096	**Broccoli and stilton soup**, carton, chilled	200	125	53	8	47	0.2	0.03	0.3	340	0.11	1	6
1097	**Carrot and coriander soup**, carton, chilled	180	124	22	5	18	0.1	0.02	0.1	280	0.06	Tr	Tr
1098	**Chicken noodle soup**, dried, as served	220	14	4	3	15	0.2	0.01	0.1	320	0.04	N	N
1099	**Chicken soup**, cream of, canned	240	41	27	5	27	0.4	0.02	0.3	370	Tr	Tr	2
1100	cream of, canned, condensed	490	62	41	7	41	0.5	0.03	0.5	740	Tr	Tr	4
1101	cream of, canned, condensed, as served	250	31	20	4	20	0.3	0.02	0.3	380	Tr	Tr	2
1102	**Instant soup**, dried, as served	229	75	10	Tr	20	0.1	0.01	0.1	344	Tr	Tr	N
1103	**Lentil soup**, canned	200	97	11	9	40	0.8	0.08	0.3	300	0.11	N	N
1104	**Low calorie soup**, canned	170	130	13	7	17	0.3	0.01	0.1	270	0.05	N	N
1105	**Minestrone soup**, canned	200	101	18	9	24	0.3	0.04	0.2	310	0.10	0	1
1106	**Mushroom soup**, carton, chilled	280	131	24	6	38	0.4	0.07	0.3	444	0.08	6	5
1107	cream of, canned	230	55	30	4	30	0.3	0.04	0.3	370	Tr	1	3
1108	**Oxtail soup**, canned	220	93	40	6	37	1.0	0.04	0.4	330	Tr	Tr	1
1109	**Tomato soup**, carton, chilled	198	189	17	9	20	0.3	0.04	0.1	305	0.11	Tr	Tr

Soups, sauces and miscellaneous foods

Vitamins per 100g edible portion

No.	Food	Retinol µg	Carotene µg	Vitamin D µg	Vitamin E mg	Thiamin mg	Ribo-flavin mg	Niacin mg	Trypt 60 mg	Vitamin B6 mg	Vitamin B12 µg	Folate µg	Panto-thenate mg	Biotin µg	Vitamin C mg
	Soups														
1096	**Broccoli and stilton soup**, carton, chilled	48	129	Tr	0.34	0.01	0.06	0.4	0.4	0.04	Tr	25	0.29	2	3
1097	**Carrot and coriander soup**, carton, chilled	4	1979	Tr	0.29	0.02	0.02	0.4	0.1	0.03	Tr	4	0.11	Tr	Tr
1098	**Chicken noodle soup**, dried, as served	Tr	0	0	N	0.01	0.01	0.2	0.2	N	Tr	N	N	N	0
1099	**Chicken soup**, cream of, canned	39	16	Tr	0.55	0.01	0.03	0.2	0.3	0.01	Tr	1	0.04	0	0
1100	cream of, canned, condensed	96	39	0	0.93	0.02	0.04	0.6	0.5	0.01	Tr	1	0.06	0	0
1101	cream of, canned, condensed, as served	48	20	0	0.46	0.01	0.02	0.3	0.2	0.01	Tr	Tr	0.03	0	0
1102	**Instant soup**, dried, as served	0	68	0	0.17	Tr	Tr	Tr	0.1	0.01	0	1	0.03	Tr	0
1103	**Lentil soup**, canned	0	N	0	N	Tr	0.02	3.2	0.6	0.01	0	N	N	N	0
1104	**Low calorie soup**, canned	0	N	0	N	0.35	0.14	2.0	0.1	0.20	0	10	N	N	Tr
1105	**Minestrone soup**, canned	4	340	0	0.27	0.02	0.01	0.2	0.2	0.04	0	5	0.05	Tr	2
1106	**Mushroom soup**, carton, chilled	40	17	Tr	0.23	0.02	0.08	1.3	0.2	0.03	Tr	5	0.10	1	Tr
1107	cream of, canned	40	16	0	0.54	Tr	0.05	0.3	0.2	0.01	Tr	2	0.10	1	0
1108	**Oxtail soup**, canned	0	0	0	0.20	0.02	0.03	0.7	0.5	0.03	0	1	0.05	0	0
1109	**Tomato soup**, carton, chilled	18	324	Tr	1.10	0.02	0.02	0.6	0.1	0.06	Tr	4	0.19	3	Tr

Composition of food per 100g edible portion

No.	Food	Description and main data sources	Main data reference	Water g	Total nitrogen g	Protein g	Fat g	Carbo-hydrate g	Energy value kcal	Energy value kJ
Soups *continued*										
1110	**Tomato soup**, cream of, canned	Analytical data, 2011	72	89.0	0.14	0.9	2.0	7.8	51	215
1111	**Vegetable soup**, canned	Analytical data, 1992; and industry data, 2013	35	87.8	0.22	1.4	0.6	7.4	39	164
1112	homemade	Recipe		89.0	0.15	1.0	4.2	3.7[a]	55	230
Dairy sauces										
1113	**Bread sauce**, homemade with semi-skimmed milk	Recipe		76.6	0.65	4.0	2.5	15.6[a]	97	411
1114	**Cheese sauce**, homemade with semi-skimmed milk	Recipe		68.3	1.29	8.2	12.8	9.0	182	757
1115	packet mix, made up with semi-skimmed milk	Recipe		77.6	0.92	5.8	5.2	9.7	106	447
1116	**White sauce**, savoury, homemade with semi-skimmed milk	Recipe		75.8	0.71	4.4	8.0	11.1	131	548
Salad sauces, dressings and pickles										
1117	**Chutney**, mango, sweet	Analytical data, 1992	35	44.3	0.11	0.7	0.1	48.3	189[b]	806[b]
1118	tomato	Analytical data, 1992	35	63.8	0.19	1.2	0.2	31.0	128[c]	542[c]
1119	**Dips**, sour-cream based	Assorted flavours. Analytical data, 1993-1994	50	54.1	0.46	2.9	37.0	4.0[a]	360	1482
1120	sour-cream based, reduced fat	Industry data, 2013		74.0	0.61	3.9	15.2	7.3	180	746

[a] Includes oligosaccharides

[b] Includes 3kcal and 14kJ per 100g from acetic acid

[c] Includes 4kcal and 18kJ per 100g from acetic acid

Composition of food per 100g edible portion

No.	Food	Starch g	Total sugars g	Individual sugars					Dietary fibre		Fatty acids				Cholest- erol mg
				Gluc g	Fruct g	Sucr g	Malt g	Lact g	NSP g	AOAC g	Satd g	Mono- unsatd g	Poly- unsatd g	Trans g	
Soups continued															
1110	**Tomato soup**, cream of, canned	2.4	5.5	1.3	1.5	2.2	Tr	0.5	0.5	0.6	0.3	1.2	0.5	Tr	3
1111	**Vegetable soup**, canned	4.8	2.6	0.7	0.8	1.1	0	0	1.5	N	N	N	N	N	N
1112	homemade	1.5	1.8[a]	0.5	0.5	0.8	0	0	0.9	N	2.4	1.0	0.2	0.1	10
Dairy sauces															
1113	**Bread sauce**, homemade with semi-skimmed milk	9.8	5.4[a]	0.6	0.5	0.5	0.5	3.2	N	N	1.4	0.6	0.2	0.1	7
1114	**Cheese sauce**, homemade with semi-skimmed milk	4.8	4.2	Tr	Tr	0	0	4.1	0.2	0.7	8.0	3.3	0.4	0.5	36
1115	packet mix, made up with semi-skimmed milk	4.5	5.3	Tr	Tr	0	Tr	5.2	N	0.2	3.3	N	N	N	N
1116	**White sauce**, savoury, homemade with semi-skimmed milk	5.9	5.1	Tr	Tr	0	0	5.1	0.3	0.3	5.0	2.0	0.2	0.3	22
Salad sauces, dressings and pickles															
1117	**Chutney**, mango, sweet	2.6	45.7	20.6	19.5	5.6	0	0	N	N	Tr	Tr	Tr	N	0
1118	tomato	2.9	28.1	13.6	14.2	0.3	0	0	1.3	1.4	Tr	Tr	0.1	N	0
1119	**Dips**, sour-cream based	Tr	2.0[a]	0.9	0.7	0.4	Tr	Tr	N	N	N	N	N	N	60
1120	sour-cream based, reduced fat	4.0	3.4	N	N	Tr	Tr	N	0.1	0.1	4.4	N	N	N	N

[a] Not including oligosaccharides

Inorganic constituents per 100g edible portion

No.	Food	Na	K	Ca	Mg	P	Fe	Cu	Zn	Cl	Mn	Se	I
		mg										µg	
Soups continued													
1110	**Tomato soup**, cream of, canned	245	179	14	8	19	0.2	0.04	0.1	420	0.05	Tr	2
1111	**Vegetable soup**, canned	230	110	12	8	29	0.4	0.04	0.2	350	0.07	N	N
1112	homemade	315	120	14	6	20	0.3	0.02	0.1	241	0.07	Tr	N
Dairy sauces													
1113	**Bread sauce**, homemade with semi-skimmed milk	93	166	105	13	88	0.4	0.05	0.5	181	0.13	N	22
1114	**Cheese sauce**, homemade with semi-skimmed milk	213	163	247	16	183	0.2	0.02	1.2	342	0.05	2	34
1115	packet mix, made up with semi-skimmed milk	382	194	171	15	184	0.1	Tr	0.7	545	0.04	N	N
1116	**White sauce**, savoury, homemade with semi-skimmed milk	100	183	137	13	111	0.2	0.01	0.5	187	0.05	1	35
Salad sauces, dressings and pickles													
1117	**Chutney**, mango, sweet	1300	42	9	19	8	1.1	Tr	Tr	1530	0.07	N	N
1118	tomato	410	300	14	12	27	0.6	0.09	0.2	790	0.12	N	N
1119	**Dips**, sour-cream based	330	130	72	10	79	0.4	0.98	0.9	N	0.10	Tr	N
1120	sour-cream based, reduced fat	150	175	97	13	106	0.5	1.32	1.2	230	0.13	Tr	N

Soups, sauces and miscellaneous foods *continued*

Vitamins per 100g edible portion

No.	Food	Retinol µg	Carotene µg	Vitamin D µg	Vitamin E mg	Thiamin mg	Ribo-flavin mg	Niacin mg	Trypt 60 mg	Vitamin B$_6$ mg	Vitamin B$_{12}$ µg	Folate µg	Panto-thenate mg	Biotin µg	Vitamin C mg
Soups continued															
1110	**Tomato soup**, cream of, canned	Tr	147	0	1.42	Tr	0.11	0.6	0.1	0.06	Tr	14	0.04	1	1
1111	**Vegetable soup**, canned	0	18	0	N	0.09	0.02	2.5	0.2	0.01	0	10	N	N	Tr
1112	homemade	44	1206	0	0.24	0.07	0.01	0.2	0.1	0.07	Tr	6	0.08	Tr	2
Dairy sauces															
1113	**Bread sauce**, homemade with semi-skimmed milk	25	17	Tr	0.12	0.11	0.16	0.4	0.8	0.06	0.6	9	0.43	2	1
1114	**Cheese sauce**, homemade with semi-skimmed milk	140	70	0.1	0.25	0.04	0.26	0.2	1.9	0.07	1.1	7	0.57	3	1
1115	packet mix, made up with semi-skimmed milk	36	28	0.1	N	0.04	0.28	0.2	1.1	0.08	1.0	10	N	N	1
1116	**White sauce**, savoury, homemade with semi-skimmed milk	91	55	0.1	0.21	0.04	0.24	0.2	0.8	0.06	0.9	5	0.61	3	1
Salad sauces, dressings and pickles															
1117	**Chutney**, mango, sweet	0	N	0	N	0	0.01	0.2	0.8	N	0	N	N	N	Tr
1118	tomato	0	N	0	N	0.05	0.15	0.1	0.2	0.02	0	N	N	N	Tr
1119	**Dips**, sour-cream based	N	N	N	N	N	N	N	N	N	Tr	N	N	N	N
1120	sour-cream based, reduced fat	N	N	N	N	N	N	N	N	N	Tr	N	N	N	N

Soups, sauces and miscellaneous foods *continued*

Composition of food per 100g edible portion

No.	Food	Description and main data sources	Main data reference	Water g	Total nitrogen g	Protein g	Fat g	Carbo- hydrate g	Energy value kcal	kJ
Salad sauces, dressings and pickles continued										
1121	**Dressing**, blue cheese	Analytical data, 1992; and industry data, 2013	35	51.0	0.31	2.0	35.9	9.8	368	1519
1122	French	Analytical data, 1992; and industry data, 2013	35	55.3	0.05	0.3	32.2	11.7	335	1384
1123	French, fat free	Industry data (Kraft), 2013		N	0.02	0.1	Tr	8.7	33	141
1124	thousand island	Analytical data, 1992; and industry data, 2013	35	66.6	0.11	0.7	16.4	15.9	210	873
1125	**Mayonnaise**	Analytical data, 2011	72	19.3	0.17	1.1	74.8	2.4	686	2824
1126	reduced fat	Analytical data, 1995[a]	50	59.5	0.16	1.0	28.1	8.2	288	1188
1127	**Piccalilli**	Mild, saucy and sweet varieties. Analytical data, 1992; and industry data, 2013	35	79.1	0.16	1.0	0.5	17.6[b]	84[c]	360[c]
1128	**Pickle**, sweet	Analytical data, 1992; and industry data, 2013	35	67.8	0.10	0.6	0.1	28.0	111[d]	476[d]
1129	**Salad cream**	Analytical data, 1989; and industry data, 2013	30	50.1	0.23	1.5	26.7	21.2	326	1353
1130	reduced fat	Industry data, 2013		72.4	0.16	1.0	10.6	15.5	157	657
1131	**Tzatziki**, homemade	Recipe		85.6	0.54	3.4	5.5	3.4	76	314
Table sauces										
1132	**Barbecue sauce**	Literature sources, 1980; and industry data, 2013	145	61.6	0.16	1.0	0.1	36.1	140	598
1133	**Brown sauce**	Fruity. Analytical data, 1992; and industry data, 2013	35	68.2	0.19	1.2	0.1	22.2	98[e]	418[e]
1134	reduced salt/sugar	Estimated from brown sauce and industry data, 2013		79.2	0.11	0.7	0.1	20.0	88[e]	374[e]
1135	**Chilli sauce**	Assorted types, including garlic chilli sauce. Analytical data, 1992; and industry data, 2013	35	82.1	0.21	1.3	0.8	7.3[f]	40	169
1136	**Horseradish sauce**	Creamed and plain samples. Analytical data, 1992	35	64.0	0.40	2.5	8.4[g]	17.9[g]	153[g]	640[g]

[a] Extra light products contain 4.6g fat, 0.7g saturated fat, 90kcal and 370kJ per 100g

[b] Carbohydrate typically varies from 10.4g to 25.4g per 100g

[c] Includes 10kcal and 43kJ per 100g from acetic acid

[d] Includes 3kcal and 14kJ per 100g from acetic acid

[e] Includes 9kcal and 39kJ per 100g from acetic acid

[f] Values in sweet chilli varieties typically vary from 33g to 64g per 100g

[g] Products are very variable: range 6.0g to 29.3g fat, 8.0g to 28.9g carbohydrate, 110kcal to 341kcal and 450kJ to 1412kJ per 100g

Soups, sauces and miscellaneous foods *continued*

Composition of food per 100g edible portion

No.	Food	Starch g	Total sugars g	Gluc g	Fruct g	Sucr g	Malt g	Lact g	NSP g	AOAC g	Satd g	Mono-unsatd g	Poly-unsatd g	Trans g	Cholesterol mg
				Individual sugars					Dietary fibre		Fatty acids				
Salad sauces, dressings and pickles continued															
1121	**Dressing**, blue cheese	2.1	7.7	4.0	3.5	0.2	0	Tr	N	1.3	6.6	7.9	19.9	N	32
1122	**French**	5.0	6.7	N	N	N	0	0	N	0.5	N	N	N	N	0
1123	**French**, fat free	0.1	8.6	N	N	N	0	0	0.3	0.5	Tr	Tr	Tr	Tr	0
1124	thousand island	2.5	13.4	N	N	N	0	0	0.4	0.4	2.0	6.4	7.0	N	N
1125	**Mayonnaise**	Tr	2.4	0.3	0.4	1.7	Tr	Tr	0	0	5.7	45.6	19.9	Tr	57
1126	reduced fat	3.6	4.6	1.1	1.0	2.5	0	0	0	0	2.1	17.1	7.5	Tr	22
1127	**Piccalilli**	2.8	14.8	6.5	6.8	1.5	0	0	1.0	N	0.1	0.1	0.3	N	0
1128	**Pickle**, sweet	3.4	24.6	8.0	8.4	8.2	0	0	1.2	1.2	Tr	Tr	Tr	Tr	0
1129	**Salad cream**	4.5	16.7	1.9	1.9	12.9	0	0	N	0.5	N	N	N	N	43
1130	reduced fat	6.3	9.2	2.5	2.3	4.4	0	0	N	0.5	1.6	2.9	5.6	0	4
1131	**Tzatziki**, homemade	0.4	3.0[a]	0.4	0.3	0	Tr	1.9	0.3	0.3	3.6	1.3	0.2	0.1	9
Table sauces															
1132	**Barbecue sauce**	6.2	29.9	N	N	N	0	0	0.5	1.2	0	0	0.1	N	0
1133	**Brown sauce**	2.6	19.6	7.3	8.3	4.0	0	0	0.7	N	Tr	Tr	Tr	0	0
1134	reduced salt/sugar	5.8	14.1	5.2	5.9	3.0	0	0	0.7	N	Tr	Tr	Tr	0	0
1135	**Chilli sauce**	0.4	6.9[b]	3.1	3.8	Tr	0	0	1.1	2.2	Tr	Tr	Tr	0	0
1136	**Horseradish sauce**	3.0	15.0	4.0	3.6	7.4	0	0[c]	2.5	2.5	1.1	3.8	3.2	0.2	14

[a] Contains galactose

[b] Values in sweet chilli varieties typically vary from 31g to 61g per 100g

[c] Most creamed varieties contain lactose

No.	Food	Na	K	Ca	Mg	P	Fe	Cu	Zn	Cl	Mn	Se	I
						mg						μg	

Salad sauces, dressings and pickles continued

No.	Food	Na	K	Ca	Mg	P	Fe	Cu	Zn	Cl	Mn	Se	I
1121	**Dressing**, blue cheese	840	52	58	7	61	0.6	0.02	0.4	1060	0.10	1	6
1122	French	600	N	N	N	N	N	N	N	N	N	N	N
1123	French, fat free	1190	N	N	N	N	N	N	N	N	N	N	N
1124	thousand island	470	130	24	9	34	0.3	0.05	0.2	730	0.07	1	5
1125	**Mayonnaise**	131	4	2	Tr	5	0.2	Tr	0.1	330	Tr	Tr	7
1126	reduced fat	N	7	5	1	10	0.3	Tr	0.1	N	Tr	1	14
1127	**Piccalilli**	740	40	16	6	17	0.6	0.03	0.1	N	0.10	N	N
1128	**Pickle**, sweet	1130	94	15	6	12	0.6	Tr	0.1	1230	0.15	N	N
1129	**Salad cream**	700	40	18	9	48	0.5	0.02	0.3	1090	0.10	N	11
1130	reduced fat	530	N	N	N	N	N	N	N	N	N	N	N
1131	**Tzatziki**, homemade	369	168	75	11	97	0.2	0.01	0.3	600	0.05	1	22

Table sauces

No.	Food	Na	K	Ca	Mg	P	Fe	Cu	Zn	Cl	Mn	Se	I
1132	**Barbecue sauce**	630	240	17	23	27	0.6	0.11	0.2	970	0.10	Tr	1
1133	**Brown sauce**	510	330	35	53	21	1.2	0.10	0.2	N	0.34	N	N
1134	reduced salt/sugar	390	221	23	36	14	0.8	0.07	0.1	445	0.23	N	N
1135	**Chilli sauce**	1250	140	17	15	28	2.8	0.07	0.1	1770	0.17	Tr	2
1136	**Horseradish sauce**	910[a]	220	43	18	42	0.6	0.05	0.4	1710	0.18	N	N

[a] Na typically varies from 400mg to 1600mg per 100g

Vitamins per 100g edible portion

No.	Food	Retinol	Carotene	Vitamin D	Vitamin E	Thiamin	Ribo-flavin	Niacin	Trypt 60	Vitamin B6	Vitamin B12	Folate	Panto-thenate	Biotin	Vitamin C
		µg	µg	µg	mg	mg	mg	mg	mg	mg	µg	µg	mg	µg	mg
Salad sauces, dressings and pickles *continued*															
1121	**Dressing**, blue cheese	N	N	0.2	4.58	0.01	0.04	0	0.7	0.01	0	5	0.12	1	0
1122	French	0	0	0	N	0	0	0	0	0	0	0	0	0	0
1123	French, fat free	0	0	0	N	Tr	Tr	Tr	Tr	Tr	0	Tr	Tr	Tr	Tr
1124	thousand island	N	N	0.1	4.40	0.01	0.02	0.1	0.2	0.02	0	4	0.10	1	Tr
1125	**Mayonnaise**	78	Tr	Tr	22.10	Tr	0.10	Tr	0.1	0.09	0.3	9	0.15	1	Tr
1126	reduced fat	N	Tr	Tr	8.33	Tr	0.21	Tr	0.2	0.19	0.6	18	0.32	1	0
1127	**Piccalilli**	0	N	0	N	Tr	0.02	0.1	0.2	0.01	0	N	N	Tr	Tr
1128	**Pickle**, sweet	0	250	0	N	0.03	0.01	0.1	0.1	0.01	0	Tr	N	Tr	Tr
1129	**Salad cream**	9	17	0.2	13.58	N	N	N	0.3	0.03	0.5	3	N	N	0
1130	reduced fat	N	N	N	N	N	N	N	0.2	N	N	N	N	N	0
1131	**Tzatziki**, homemade	61	27	0	0.23	0.08	0.07	0.1	0.9	0.03	0.1	7	N	N	1
Table sauces															
1132	**Barbecue sauce**	0	505	0	0.91	0.03	0.02	0.4	0.1	0.04	0	5	0.10	1	3
1133	**Brown sauce**	0	40	0	N	0.13	0.09	0.1	0.2	0.10	0	8	N	N	Tr
1134	reduced salt/sugar	0	40	0	N	0.09	0.06	0.1	0.1	0.07	0	5	N	N	Tr
1135	**Chilli sauce**	0	570	0	1.97	0.01	0.09	0.6	0.3	0.10	0	10	0.22	1	8
1136	**Horseradish sauce**	Tr	Tr	Tr	N	N	N	N	N	N	Tr	N	N	N	Tr

Composition of food per 100g edible portion

No.	Food	Description and main data sources	Main data reference	Water g	Total nitrogen g	Protein g	Fat g	Carbo-hydrate g	Energy value kcal	Energy value kJ
Table sauces continued										
1137	**Mint sauce**	Analytical data, 1992; and industry data, 2013	35	68.7	0.26	1.6	Tr	21.5	101[a]	432[a]
1138	**Relish**, tomato based	Including chilli and burger relish. Analytical data, 1992	35	68.4	0.19	1.2	0.1	27.6	114[b]	485[b]
1139	corn/cucumber/onion	Analytical data, 1992; and industry data, 2013	35	60.6	0.16	1.0	0.3	36.6	144	614
1140	**Soy sauce**	Light and dark varieties. Analytical data, 1992; and industry data, 2013	35	65.4	0.48	3.0	Tr	17.9	79	337
1141	**Sweet and sour sauce**, take-away	Purchased from Chinese restaurants, sundry-style dipping sauce. Analytical data, 1992	35	65.3	0.03	0.2	3.4	32.8	157[c]	666[c]
1142	**Tartare sauce**	Analytical data, 1992; and industry data, 2013	35	53.5	0.21	1.3	24.6	17.9	299[d]	1241[d]
1143	**Tomato ketchup**	Analytical data, 1992; and industry data, 2013	35	68.0	0.26	1.6	0.1	28.6	115	489
1144	**Worcestershire sauce**	Analytical data, 1992; and industry data, 2013	35	65.3	0.22	1.4	0.1	28.3	113	480
Cooking sauces										
1145	**Curry paste**	Analytical data, 1992; and industry data, 2013	35	49.9	0.75	4.7	21.3	11.3	253	1049
1146	**Pesto**, green	Analytical data, 2002; and industry data, 2013	66	39.0	0.58	5.6	42.5	3.9	420	1730
1147	red	Analytical data, 2002; and industry data, 2013	66	47.6	0.78	5.0	30.6	5.9	317	1311
1148	**Sauce, Chinese cook in**, sweet & sour	Analytical data, 2002; and industry data, 2013	65	74.3	0.08	0.5	1.0	22.1	94	399
1149	**Sauce, Chinese**, stir fry	Including black bean and Szechuan. Analytical data, 2002; and industry data, 2013	65	72.8	0.23	1.4	1.3	19.9	92	390

[a] Includes 14kcal and 61kJ per 100g from acetic acid

[b] Includes 3kcal and 14kJ per 100g from acetic acid

[c] Includes 3kcal and 12kJ per 100g from acetic acid

[d] Includes 5kcal and 22kJ per 100g from acetic acid

| No. | Food | Starch g | Total sugars g | Individual sugars | | | | | Dietary fibre | | Fatty acids | | | | Cholest- erol mg |
				Gluc g	Fruct g	Sucr g	Malt g	Lact g	NSP g	AOAC g	Satd g	Mono- unsatd g	Poly- unsatd g	Trans g	
Table sauces *continued*															
1137	**Mint sauce**	0	21.5	4.9	4.8	11.8	0	0	N	N	Tr	Tr	Tr	Tr	0
1138	**Relish**, tomato based	2.5	25.1	6.5	6.8	11.8	0	0	1.3	N	Tr	Tr	Tr	Tr	0
1139	corn/cucumber/onion	7.7	28.9	9.0	9.4	10.5	0	0	1.2	1.5	Tr	0.1	0.2	N	0
1140	**Soy sauce**	1.5	16.4	4.8	2.0	9.6	0	0	0	Tr	0	0	0	0	0
1141	**Sweet and sour sauce**, take-away	5.3	27.5	9.5	9.7	8.3	0	0	N	N	N	N	N	N	0
1142	**Tartare sauce**	1.7	16.2	6.5	6.3	3.4	0	0	Tr	0.6	N	N	N	N	49
1143	**Tomato ketchup**	1.1	27.5	5.9	6.4	15.2	0	0	0.9	0.9	Tr	Tr	Tr	Tr	0
1144	**Worcestershire sauce**	N	21.5	N	N	N	0	0	Tr	Tr	Tr	Tr	Tr	Tr	0
Cooking sauces															
1145	**Curry paste**	4.3	7.0	N	N	N	0	0	N	6.8	N	N	N	N	0
1146	**Pesto**, green	1.6	2.3	1.1	0.4	Tr	0.4	0.4	1.1	N	6.5	16.6	17.6	0.3	8
1147	red	0.7	5.2	N	N	N	N	N	N	3.3	4.7	11.9	12.6	0.2	6
1148	**Sauce, Chinese cook in**, sweet & sour	2.7	19.4	4.8	4.8	9.7	0	0	0.9	0.8	Tr	N	N	0	0
1149	**Sauce, Chinese**, stir fry	3.2	16.7	3.7	3.6	9.3	Tr	0	0.8	0.9	0.1	0.6	0.5	Tr	0

461

Soups, sauces and miscellaneous foods continued

Inorganic constituents per 100g edible portion

No.	Food	mg										µg	
		Na	K	Ca	Mg	P	Fe	Cu	Zn	Cl	Mn	Se	I
Table sauces continued													
1137	**Mint sauce**	480ᵃ	210	120	46	27	7.4	0.30	0.2	780	0.86	Tr	Tr
1138	**Relish**, tomato based	480	290	13	12	26	0.3	0.07	0.1	980	0.10	N	N
1139	corn/cucumber/onion	420	110	13	9	24	0.3	0.07	0.2	820	0.07	N	N
1140	**Soy sauce**	5500ᵇ	180	17	37	47	2.4	0.01	0.2	8200	0.18	N	N
1141	**Sweet and sour sauce**, take-away	150	16	6	2	4	6.0	Tr	Tr	240	0.04	N	N
1142	**Tartare sauce**	1080	42	15	17	36	0.5	0.03	0.3	2080	0	1	8
1143	**Tomato ketchup**	800	350	13	19	31	0.3	0.05	0.1	880	0.10	N	N
1144	**Worcestershire sauce**	1500	600	190	73	31	10.1	0.21	0.4	2610	0.98	1	1
Cooking sauces													
1145	**Curry paste**	1520	520	150	75	110	12.8	0.29	0.8	3740	1.12	N	N
1146	**Pesto**, green	840	180	209	44	141	1.1	0.24	1.1	950	0.50	4	4
1147	red	770	N	N	N	N	N	N	N	N	N	N	N
1148	**Sauce, Chinese cook in**, sweet & sour	250	93	11	6	11	0.2	0.03	0.1	410	0.19	N	N
1149	**Sauce, Chinese**, stir fry	570	106	15	11	24	1.1	0.07	0.2	890	0.18	Tr	13

ᵃ Na typically varies from 120mg to 1300mg per 100g

ᵇ Na typically varies from 4400mg to 7200mg per 100g

Vitamins per 100g edible portion

No.	Food	Retinol	Carotene	Vitamin D	Vitamin E	Thiamin	Ribo-flavin	Niacin	Trypt 60	Vitamin B_6	Vitamin B_{12}	Folate	Panto-thenate	Biotin	Vitamin C
		µg	µg	µg	mg	mg	mg	mg	mg	mg	µg	µg	mg	µg	mg
Table sauces continued															
1137	**Mint sauce**	0	Tr	0	Tr	Tr	Tr	Tr	0.3	Tr	0	Tr	Tr	Tr	Tr
1138	**Relish**, tomato based	0	N	0	N	0.06	0.05	0.2	0.2	N	0	N	N	N	N
1139	corn/cucumber/onion	0	N	0	N	N	N	N	0.2	N	0	N	N	N	N
1140	**Soy sauce**	0	0	0	N	0.05	0.13	3.4	1.4	N	0	11	N	N	0
1141	**Sweet and sour sauce**, take-away	0	N	0	N	0.11	Tr	0	Tr	N	0	N	N	N	N
1142	**Tartare sauce**	24	150	0.2	10.10	0.02	0.02	Tr	0.3	0.02	0	4	0.12	1	2
1143	**Tomato ketchup**	0	473	0	N	1.00	0.09	2.1	0.2	0.03	0	1	N	N	2
1144	**Worcestershire sauce**	0	8	0	N	Tr	0.01	0.4	0.2	N	0	1	N	N	0
Cooking sauces															
1145	**Curry paste**	0	N	0	N	0.09	0.13	1.8	N	N	Tr	N	N	N	0
1146	**Pesto**, green	32	990	0.7	16.68	0.06	0.12	0.6	1.2	0.03	0	16	0.20	3	Tr
1147	red	13	1944	N	N	N	N	N	Tr	0	N	N	N	Tr	Tr
1148	**Sauce, Chinese cook in**, sweet & sour	0	584	0	0.50	0.02	Tr	0.3	Tr	0.03	0	3	0.14	2	1
1149	**Sauce, Chinese**, stir fry	0	121	0	0.27	0.02	0.03	0.3	0.1	0.04	0	6	0.20	1	2

Composition of food per 100g edible portion

No.	Food	Description and main data sources	Main data reference	Water g	Total nitrogen g	Protein g	Fat g	Carbohydrate g	Energy value kcal	kJ
Cooking sauces continued										
1150	**Sauce, dry**, casserole mix	Including liver and bacon, sausage, beef bourguignon mixes. Analytical data, 1992	35	7.3	1.55	9.7	3.9	68.2	330	1400
1151	**Sauce, Indian cook in**, korma/tikka masala	Analytical data, 2002; and industry data, 2013	65	75.8	0.28	1.7	9.5	10.9	133	555
1152	other	Including balti, rogan josh, jalfrezi. Analytical data, 2002; and industry data, 2013	65	82.6	0.23	1.4	3.2	8.7[a]	67	282
1153	**Sauce, pasta**, carbonara type	Chilled and ambient. Analytical data, 2002; and industry data, 2013	66	76.3	0.78	4.9	13.0	3.8	151	625
1154	four cheese	Chilled and ambient. Analytical data, 2002; and industry data, 2013	66	76.7	0.80	5.1	9.7	5.8	129	538
1155	tomato based, for bolognese	Ambient. Analytical data, 2002; and industry data, 2013	66	84.8	0.24	1.5	1.3	6.9	44	184
1156	tomato based, napoletana	Ambient, including tomato and basil sauce. Analytical data, 2002; and industry data, 2013	66	85.9	0.23	1.5	3.8	6.5	65	270
1157	tomato based, reduced fat	Ambient. Analytical data, 2002; and industry data, 2013	66	86.5	0.22	1.4	0.3	6.7	33	142
1158	tomato based, with added vegetables	Ambient. Analytical data, 2002; and industry data, 2013	66	84.9	0.23	1.4	2.1	5.7	46	193
1159	**Sauce, traditional cook in**, tomato based	Including chasseur and red wine sauce. Analytical data, 2002; and industry data, 2013	65	86.2	0.15	0.9	1.0	8.1[a]	43	182
1160	white sauce based	Including white wine sauces, cheese sauces and creamy sauces. Analytical data, 2002; and industry data, 2013	65	81.7	0.25	1.6	8.6	5.7[a]	105	437

[a] Includes oligosaccharides

Composition of food per 100g edible portion

No.	Food	Starch	Total sugars	Individual sugars					Dietary fibre		Fatty acids				Cholest-erol
				Gluc	Fruct	Sucr	Malt	Lact	NSP	AOAC	Satd	Mono-unsatd	Poly-unsatd	Trans	
		g	g	g	g	g	g	g	g	g	g	g	g	g	mg

Cooking sauces continued

No.	Food	Starch	Total sugars	Gluc	Fruct	Sucr	Malt	Lact	NSP	AOAC	Satd	Mono-unsatd	Poly-unsatd	Trans	Cholesterol
1150	**Sauce, dry**, casserole mix	56.0	12.2	3.8	2.3	4.8	0	1.3	N	N	N	N	N	N	0
1151	**Sauce, Indian cook in**, korma/tikka masala	3.5	7.4	1.6	2.0	3.2	0	0.5	1.5	2.5	4.4	2.4	2.2	0.1	8
1152	other	2.6	6.1[a]	1.9	2.3	1.9	0	Tr	1.5	2.5	0.5	1.2	1.3	Tr	N
1153	**Sauce, pasta**, carbonara type	3.0	0.8	Tr	Tr	Tr	0	0.8	0.9	1.3	7.7	3.8	0.8	0.4	31
1154	four cheese	3.9	1.9	Tr	Tr	N	Tr	N	0.9	1.3	5.7	2.8	0.6	0.3	23
1155	tomato based, for bolognese	0.8	6.1	2.2	2.6	1.3	0	0	1.3	2.0	0.2	0.7	0.4	Tr	Tr
1156	tomato based, napoletana	0.2	6.3	2.9	2.7	0.7	0	0	1.8	2.3	0.5	1.8	1.3	Tr	0
1157	tomato based, reduced fat	1.1	5.6	2.1	2.4	1.1	0	0	1.3	2.0	0.1	Tr	0.1	Tr	0
1158	tomato based, with added vegetables	0.6	5.1	1.8	2.1	1.2	0	0	2.4	2.4	0.3	1.1	0.6	Tr	0
1159	**Sauce, traditional cook in**, tomato based	3.1	4.9[a]	1.5	1.7	1.6	0	0	1.2	1.5	0.2	0.4	0.5	Tr	0
1160	white sauce based	2.8	2.8[a]	0.5	0.5	1.2	0.1	0.5	1.9	2.3	1.7	2.8	3.7	0.1	8

[a] Not including oligosaccharides

465

Inorganic constituents per 100g edible portion

No.	Food	Na	K	Ca	Mg	P	Fe	Cu	Zn	Cl	Mn	Se	I
		mg										µg	
Cooking sauces continued													
1150	**Sauce, dry**, casserole mix	5400	800	92	62	210	3.9	0.26	1.0	7470	0.54	N	N
1151	**Sauce, Indian cook in**, korma/tikka masala	270	193	34	17	40	0.8	0.06	0.3	460	0.35	1	3
1152	other	300	236	33	18	32	1.0	0.09	0.2	520	0.29	1	2
1153	**Sauce, pasta**, carbonara type	340	80	100	7	126	0.2	Tr	0.6	470	0.03	3	11
1154	four cheese	325	70	169	10	149	0.1	Tr	0.7	416	0.04	3	18
1155	tomato based, for bolognese	290	387	31	19	33	0.7	0.12	0.2	500	0.15	1	Tr
1156	tomato based, napoletana	290	356	33	18	32	0.6	0.12	0.2	500	0.15	1	Tr
1157	tomato based, reduced fat	230	387	31	19	33	0.7	0.12	0.2	400	0.15	1	Tr
1158	tomato based, with added vegetables	230	354	24	17	35	0.6	0.16	0.2	410	0.15	1	3
1159	**Sauce, traditional cook in**, tomato based	300	194	26	11	23	0.6	0.06	0.2	510	0.12	1	1
1160	white sauce based	370	67	28	5	56	0.1	0.02	0.2	610	0.05	1	4

Soups, sauces and miscellaneous foods *continued*

Vitamins per 100g edible portion

No.	Food	Retinol	Carotene	Vitamin D	Vitamin E	Thiamin	Ribo-flavin	Niacin	Trypt 60	Vitamin B$_6$	Vitamin B$_{12}$	Folate	Panto-thenate	Biotin	Vitamin C
		µg	µg	µg	mg	mg	mg	mg	mg	mg	µg	µg	mg	µg	mg

Cooking sauces continued

No.	Food	Retinol	Carotene	Vitamin D	Vitamin E	Thiamin	Ribo-flavin	Niacin	Trypt 60	Vitamin B$_6$	Vitamin B$_{12}$	Folate	Panto-thenate	Biotin	Vitamin C
1150	**Sauce, dry,** casserole mix	0	N	0	N	N	N	N	N	N	Tr	N	N	N	0
1151	**Sauce, Indian cook in,** korma/tikka masala	35	395	Tr	1.65	0.02	0.14	0.5	0.2	0.06	Tr	6	0.18	2	1
1152	other	0	384	0	2.34	0.03	0.03	0.8	0.1	0.08	Tr	11	0.31	3	3
1153	**Sauce, pasta,** carbonara type	87	49	Tr	0.55	N	0.09	0.6	0.9	0.12	Tr	5	0.20	1	Tr
1154	four cheese	87	49	Tr	0.55	Tr	0.11	0.1	1.1	0.15	Tr	6	0.20	1	Tr
1155	tomato based, for bolognese	0	577	0	1.99	0.06	0.02	1.0	0.2	0.27	0	2	0.40	3	Tr
1156	tomato based, napoletana	0	592	0	3.60	0.06	0.02	1.0	0.2	0.23	0	8	0.30	3	Tr
1157	tomato based, reduced fat	Tr	577	0	N	0.06	0.02	1.0	0.2	0.27	0	2	0.40	3	Tr
1158	tomato based, with added vegetables	0	472	0	1.05	Tr	0.07	1.2	0.2	0.23	0	15	0.20	2	4
1159	**Sauce, traditional cook in,** tomato based	0	315	0	1.38	0.12	0.03	0.7	0.1	0.06	0	5	0.27	3	3
1160	white sauce based	18	228	Tr	3.50	0.29	0.06	0.2	0.3	0.02	Tr	7	0.20	1	Tr

Soups, sauces and miscellaneous foods *continued*

1161 to 1177

Composition of food per 100g edible portion

No.	Food	Description and main data sources	Main data reference	Water g	Total nitrogen g	Protein g	Fat g	Carbo-hydrate g	Energy value kcal	Energy value kJ
Miscellaneous foods										
1161	**Baking powder**	MW4, 1978	4	6.3	0.91	5.2	0	37.8	163	693
1162	**Beef extract**	Including Bovril and own brands. Analytical data, 1992	35	39.0	6.64	40.4	0.6	3.2	179	760
1163	**Gelatine**	Literature sources, 1990	143	13.0	15.20	84.4	0	0	338	1435
1164	**Gravy instant granules**	Analytical data, 1992; and industry data, 2013	35	4.0	0.70	4.4	16.1[a]	65.2[b,c]	407	1714
1165	made up with water	Calculated from 23.5g granules to 300ml water		93.0	0.05	0.3	1.2	4.7[c]	30	125
1166	**Mustard**, smooth	Including English and French. Analytical data, 1992	35	63.7	1.14	7.1	8.2	9.7	139	579
1167	wholegrain	Analytical data, 1992	35	65.0	1.31	8.2	10.2	4.2	140	584
1168	**Salt**	Table salt. Analytical data, 1994	43	Tr	0	0	0	0	0	0
1169	**Stock**, chicken, ready made	Retail. Industry data, 2013		97.3	0.37	2.3	0.2	0.2	12	50
1170	**Stock cubes**, beef	Analytical data, 1993[d]	50	6.1	2.85[e]	16.8[f]	9.2	N	N	N
1171	chicken	Analytical data, 1992; and industry data, 2013[d]	35	5.8	2.50[g]	15.4[f]	15.4	N	N	N
1172	chicken, made up with water	Calculated from 7g stock cube to 190ml water		96.7	0.09	0.5	0.5	N	N	N
1173	vegetable	Analytical data, 1992; and industry data, 2013[d]	35	5.7	2.16	13.5	17.3	N	N	N
1174	**Stock gel**	Including stock pots, stock melts and squeezy tubes. Industry data, 2013	35	43.7	1.07	6.7	3.6	27.8	163	692
1175	**Tomato puree**	Double concentrate. Analytical data, 2012	74	72.5	0.71	4.4	0.2	12.9	67	287
1176	**Vinegar**	Including malt, cider and wine vinegar. Analytical data, 1994	43	N	0.07	0.4	0	0.6	22[h]	89[h]
1177	**Water**, distilled	For recipe calculations		100.0	0	0	0	0	0	0

[a] Fat typically varies from 5.5g to 30.0g per 100g

[b] Carbohydrate typically varies from 50.0g to 76.0g per 100g

[c] Oligosaccharides may be present, but levels are unknown

[d] Values for protein, fat, carbohydrate and energy can vary greatly between products

[e] Includes 0.17g purine nitrogen

[f] (Total N - purine N) x 6.25

[g] Purine nitrogen forms about 10% of total nitrogen

[h] Includes 18kcal and 73kJ per 100g from acetic acid

Soups, sauces and miscellaneous foods *continued*

No.	Food	Starch g	Total sugars g	Gluc g	Fruct g	Sucr g	Malt g	Lact g	NSP g	AOAC g	Satd g	Mono- unsatd g	Poly- unsatd g	Trans g	Cholest- erol mg
						Individual sugars			Dietary fibre		Fatty acids				

Miscellaneous foods

No.	Food	Starch	Total sugars	Gluc	Fruct	Sucr	Malt	Lact	NSP	AOAC	Satd	Mono-unsatd	Poly-unsatd	Trans	Cholesterol
1161	**Baking powder**	37.8	0	0	0	0	0	0	0	0	0	0	0	0	0
1162	**Beef extract**	2.8	0.4	0.2	0.2	Tr	0	0	0	0	N	N	N	N	N
1163	**Gelatine**	0	0	0	0	0	0	0	0	0	0	0	0	0	0
1164	**Gravy instant granules**	N	5.3	N	N	N	0	0	N	1.6	10.7	N	N	N	N
1165	made up with water	N	0.4	N	N	N	0	0	N	0.1	0.8	N	N	N	N
1166	**Mustard**, smooth	1.9	7.8	3.4	2.9	1.5	0	0	N	N	0.5	5.8	1.6	N	0
1167	wholegrain	0.3	3.9	2.0	1.9	Tr	0	0	4.9	N	0.6	7.2	1.9	N	0
1168	**Salt**	0	0	0	0	0	0	0	0	0	0	0	0	0	0
1169	**Stock**, chicken, ready made	0.1	0.1	N	N	N	0	0	N	0.3	0.1	N	N	N	N
1170	**Stock cubes**, beef	N	N	N	N	N	0	0	0	0	3.5	3.3	1.4	0.3	Tr
1171	chicken	N	N	N	N	N	0	0	N	0.6	N	N	N	N	Tr
1172	chicken, made up with water	N	N	N	N	N	0	0	N	0	N	N	N	N	Tr
1173	vegetable	N	N	N	N	N	0	N	N	1.8	N	N	N	N	0
1174	**Stock gel**	22.1	5.7	N	N	N	0	0	N	1.8	1.7	N	N	N	N
1175	**Tomato puree**	Tr	12.9	5.5	7.4	Tr	0	0	3.0	4.7	Tr	Tr	0.1	Tr	0
1176	**Vinegar**	0	0.6	0.3	0.3	0	0	0	0	0	0	0	0	0	0
1177	**Water**, distilled	0	0	0	0	0	0	0	0	0	0	0	0	0	0

Soups, sauces and miscellaneous foods *continued*

Inorganic constituents per 100g edible portion

No.	Food	Na	K	Ca	Mg	P	Fe	Cu	Zn	Cl	Mn	Se	I
		mg										µg	
	Miscellaneous foods												
1161	**Baking powder**	11800[a]	49	1130[a]	9	8430[a]	Tr	Tr	2.8	29	Tr	Tr	Tr
1162	**Beef extract**	4370	970	37	65	400	8.1	0.26	1.5	6550	0.08	N	N
1163	**Gelatine**	330	7	250	15	32	2.1	0.05	0.2	N	0.13	19	6
1164	**Gravy instant granules**	5300[b]	150	22	15	71	0.5	0.24	0.3	8370	0.40	N	N
1165	made up with water	385	11	2	1	5	Tr	0.02	Tr	608	Tr	N	N
1166	**Mustard**, smooth	2950	200	70	82	190	2.9	0.19	1.0	3550	0.70	N	N
1167	wholegrain	1620	220	120	93	200	2.8	0.21	1.2	2210	0.70	N	N
1168	**Salt**	39300	89	10	76	1	0.3	0.08	0.1	59900	Tr	N	44[c]
1169	**Stock**, chicken, ready made	225	N	N	N	N	N	N	N	N	N	N	N
1170	**Stock cubes**, beef	14560[d]	490	40	32	240	1.2	0.70	0.8	21010	0.20	N	N
1171	chicken	16300[d]	400	120	47	200	4.9	0.10	1.2	N	0.27	N	N
1172	chicken, made up with water	579	14	4	2	7	0.2	0	0	N	0.01	N	N
1173	vegetable	16800[d]	390	47	44	120	2.8	0.05	0.4	N	0.26	N	N
1174	**Stock gel**	6450	N	N	N	N	N	N	N	9930	N	N	N
1175	**Tomato puree**	49	1257	45	57	94	1.5	0.41	0.6	297	0.34	1	N
1176	**Vinegar**	5	34	3	4	10	0.1	0.01	0.1	47	0.01	1	N
1177	**Water**, distilled	0	0	0	0	0	0	0	0	0	0	0	0

[a] The sodium, calcium and phosphorus content will depend on the brand

[b] Na typically varies from 4830mg to 5910mg per 100g

[c] Iodised salt typically contains 1150µg iodine per 100g

[d] Reduced salt products contain 25-75% less salt than standard stock cubes

Miscellaneous foods

No.	Food	Retinol µg	Carotene µg	Vitamin D µg	Vitamin E mg	Thiamin mg	Ribo-flavin mg	Niacin mg	Trypt 60 mg	Vitamin B6 mg	Vitamin B12 µg	Folate µg	Panto-thenate mg	Biotin µg	Vitamin C mg
1161	**Baking powder**	0	0	0	Tr	Tr	Tr	Tr	1.0	Tr	0	Tr	Tr	Tr	0
1162	**Beef extract**	N	0	0	N	9.70	8.50	87.0	3.0	0.57	8	1300	N	N	0
1163	**Gelatine**	0	0	0	0	Tr	Tr	Tr	Tr	Tr	0	Tr	Tr	Tr	0
1164	**Gravy instant granules**	N	Tr	Tr	N	N	N	N	0.8	N	Tr	Tr	N	N	0
1165	made up with water	N	0	0	N	N	N	N	0.1	N	0	0	N	N	0
1166	**Mustard**, smooth	0	N	0	N	N	N	N	2.1	N	0	0	N	N	0
1167	wholegrain	0	N	0	N	N	N	N	2.4	N	0	0	N	N	0
1168	**Salt**	0	0	0	0	0	0	0	0	0	0	0	0	0	0
1169	**Stock**, chicken, ready made	N	N	0	N	N	N	N	N	N	N	N	N	N	0
1170	**Stock cubes**, beef	N	N	0	N	N	N	N	N	N	N	N	N	N	0
1171	chicken	N	N	0	N	N	N	N	N	N	N	N	N	N	0
1172	chicken, made up with water	N	N	0	N	N	N	N	N	N	N	N	N	N	0
1173	vegetable	0	N	0	N	N	N	N	N	N	Tr	N	N	N	0
1174	**Stock gel**	N	N	0	N	N	N	N	N	N	N	N	N	N	0
1175	**Tomato puree**	0	1750	0	5.22	0.98	0.12	3.6	0.4	0.28	0	39	0.11	6	43
1176	**Vinegar**	0	0	0	0	0	0	0	0	0	0	0	0	0	0
1177	**Water**, distilled	0	0	0	0	0	0	0	0	0	0	0	0	0	0

Composition of food per 100g edible portion

No.	Food	Description and main data sources	Main data reference	Water g	Total nitrogen g	Protein g	Fat g	Carbo-hydrate g	Energy value kcal	kJ
	Miscellaneous foods continued									
1178	**Yeast extract**	Including Marmite and own brands. Analytical data, 1992; and industry data, 2013	35	26.7	6.78[a]	40.7[b]	0.4	23.1	253	1076
1179	**Yeast,** bakers, compressed	MW4, 1978	4	70.0	2.02[c]	11.4[b]	0.4	1.1	53	226
1180	dried	MW4, 1978	4	5.0	6.32[c]	35.6[b]	1.5	3.5	169	717

[a] Includes 0.27g purine nitrogen

[b] (Total N - purine N) x 6.25

[c] Purine nitrogen forms about 10% of total nitrogen

No.	Food	Starch g	Total sugars g	Gluc g	Fruct g	Sucr g	Malt g	Lact g	NSP g	AOAC g	Satd g	Mono- unsatd g	Poly- unsatd g	Trans g	Cholest- erol mg

Individual sugars columns: Gluc, Fruct, Sucr, Malt, Lact. Dietary fibre columns: NSP, AOAC. Fatty acids columns: Satd, Mono-unsatd, Poly-unsatd, Trans.

Miscellaneous foods continued

No.	Food	Starch	Total sugars	Gluc	Fruct	Sucr	Malt	Lact	NSP	AOAC	Satd	Mono-unsatd	Poly-unsatd	Trans	Cholesterol
1178	**Yeast** extract	21.5	1.6	Tr	1.5	0.2	0	0	N	3.4	N	N	N	N	0
1179	**Yeast**, bakers, compressed	1.1	Tr	Tr	Tr	Tr	0	0	N	N	N	N	N	N	0
1180	dried	3.5	Tr	Tr	Tr	Tr	0	0	N	N	N	N	N	N	0

Inorganic constituents per 100g edible portion

No.	Food	Na	K	Ca	Mg	P	Fe	Cu	Zn	Cl	Mn	Se	I
						mg						µg	
Miscellaneous foods *continued*													
1178	**Yeast extract**	3780	2100	70	160	950	2.9	0.20	2.7	5830	0.19	N	49
1179	**Yeast**, bakers, compressed	16	610	25	59	390	5.0	1.60	3.2	20	N	N	N
1180	dried	50	2000	80	230	1290	20.0	5.00	8.0	N	N	N	N

Vitamins per 100g edible portion

No.	Food	Retinol	Carotene	Vitamin D	Vitamin E	Thiamin	Ribo-flavin	Niacin	$\frac{Trypt}{60}$	Vitamin B6	Vitamin B12	Folate	Panto-thenate	Biotin	Vitamin C
		µg	µg	µg	mg	mg	mg	mg	mg	mg	µg	mg	µg	mg

Miscellaneous foods continued

No.	Food	Retinol	Carotene	Vitamin D	Vitamin E	Thiamin	Ribo-flavin	Niacin	Trypt/60	Vitamin B6	Vitamin B12	Folate	Panto-thenate	Biotin	Vitamin C
1178	**Yeast extract**	0	0	0	N	4.10	11.90	64.0	9.0	1.60	15[a]	2620	N	N	0
1179	**Yeast**, bakers, compressed	0	Tr	0	Tr	0.71	1.70	11.0	2.0	0.60	Tr	1250	3.50	60	Tr
1180	dried	0	Tr	0	Tr	2.33[b]	4.00	8.5	7.0	2.00	Tr	4000	11.00	200	Tr

[a] Value relates to fortified products. Unfortified products contain 1µg per 100g

[b] Value for bakers yeast. Brewers yeast contains 15.6mg thiamin per 100g

Additional Tables

3.1 CAROTENOID FRACTIONS

The tables in this section detail the carotenoid fractions present in selected foods. β-carotene is the main or only source of vitamin A activity in most fruit and vegetables. Where *cis* and *trans* β-carotene were analysed separately, the sum of the two forms is presented in the table. Although there is some evidence to suggest a difference in activity for the two forms (Fernández-García *et al.,* 2012)[124], they have been treated as equal in these tables. The majority of naturally present β-carotene is in the *trans* form, and the conversion to retinol equivalents is based on the activity of this form.

Although β-carotene is the predominant source of vitamin A activity in foods, other carotenoids are present, most notably α-carotene and cryptoxanthins, though these forms only have half the vitamin A activity of β-carotene. Approximately 30% of carotenoids present in carrots are α-carotene. When there are known to be significant amounts of α-carotene and cryptoxanthins, these are given in the tables below. The values for cryptoxanthins were often analysed as total cryptoxanthins with the β and α forms unspecified; the β form is likely to predominate with smaller amounts of the α form present. Analysis of individual carotenoids is difficult because of several factors, including extraction from the food matrix and instability, and can lead to inconsistencies in data (Rodriguez-Amaya, 2001)[161]. Where β-cryptoxanthin values are reported as 0, it is possible that small quantities may be present.

β-Carotene and retinol equivalents are also given in the tables due to differences in the vitamin A activity of the carotenoids. The carotene equivalents reflect the carotene values given in the main tables. The β-carotene equivalent is the sum of the β-carotene and half of any α-carotene or cryptoxanthins present, and the retinol equivalent is one sixth of the β-carotene equivalent plus retinol. The retinol values given in the main tables reflect retinol content only and do not represent retinol equivalents. In the UK the requirement for vitamin A is expressed as retinol equivalents and relates to the lower biological efficiency of carotenoids compared with retinol (see Introduction, Section 1.4.12). Retinol equivalents are calculated as retinol + (β-carotene equivalents/6).

Lycopene and lutein do not have vitamin A activity as they cannot be converted to retinol, and are therefore not included in the tables, although footnotes have been included for foods with significant content.

It should be noted that absorption and utilisation of carotenes vary, for example with the amount of fat in the diet and β-carotene concentrations (Thurnham, 2007)[168], and there is still debate about the ratios used for calculating retinol equivalents (Fernández-García *et al.,* 2012)[124].

Further information on retinol equivalents can be found in the introduction (section 1.4.12).

No.	Food	Carotene fractions, µg per 100g edible portion				
		Carotene fractions				
		α-carotene	β-carotene	β-crypto-xanthin	Carotene equiv	Retinol equiv

Cereals and cereal products

No.	Food	α-carotene	β-carotene	β-crypto-xanthin	Carotene equiv	Retinol equiv
21	**Rice, savoury**, dried, cooked	33	133	18	159	26
34	**Noodles, egg**, dried, raw	13	36	0	43	11
91	**Cornflakes**, fortified	16	117	0	125	21
156	**Gateau**, chocolate based, frozen	19	70	0	80	115
157	fruit, frozen	14	48	0	55	118
158	**Jaffa cakes**	2	5	7	10	17
218	**Pizza**, vegetarian, retail and takeaway	24	103	0	114	61

Milk and milk products

303	**Ice cream bars/choc ices**, chocolate coated, luxury	30	174	0	189	502
326	**Rice pudding**, canned	2	9	0	10	19
329	**Torte**, fruit	20	67	0	77	112

Spreading fats

351	**Fat spread**, reduced fat (62-75%), not polyunsaturated	7	676	0	680	N
353	**Fat spread**, reduced fat (41-62%), not poly-unsaturated, with olive oil	14	488	0	495	817
354	**Fat spread**, reduced fat (41-62%), polyunsaturated	6	458	0	461	683
356	**Fat spread**, low fat (26-39%), not poly-unsaturated, with olive oil	19	620	0	630	892
357	**Fat spread**, low fat (26-39%), polyunsaturated	15	895	0	903	962

Cooking fats

| 358 | **Baking fat and margarine** (75-90% fat), hard block | 6 | 652 | 0 | 655 | 905 |

Meat products and meat dishes

508	**Beef pie, puff or shortcrust pastry**, family size	14	37	0	44	7
509	individual	3	30	0	32	N
553	**Chicken chow mein**, takeaway	12	104	0	110	18

No.	Food	Carotene fractions			Carotene equiv	Retinol equiv
		α-carotene	β-carotene	β-crypto-xanthin		

Meat products and meat dishes *continued*

No.	Food	α-carotene	β-carotene	β-crypto-xanthin	Carotene equiv	Retinol equiv
554	**Chicken curry**, average, takeaway	6	111	9	119	35
558	Thai green, takeaway and restaurant	61	343	25	386	66
559	**Chicken fajita**, meat only, takeaway and restaurant	0	0	43	22	31
560	**Chicken satay**, takeaway	0	18	9	23	9
588	**Spring rolls**, meat, takeaway	49	150	0	175	29
589	**Sweet and sour chicken**, takeaway	42	116	0	135	25
	Fish and fish products					
621	**Salmon**, farmed, raw	0	0	1	1	16
633	**Sardines**, canned in tomato sauce, whole contents	57	246	2	276	56
673	**Szechuan prawns with vegetables**, takeaway	100	510	17	569	95
	Potatoes					
695	**Potato wedges**, retail, cooked	0	8	4	10	2
	Beans and lentils					
698	**Beans**, green, raw	0	179	147	253	42
699	green, boiled	28	129	0	143	24
700	**Beansprouts**, mung, raw	20	20	20	40	7
701	mung, stir-fried in rapeseed oil	12	12	12	24	4
703	**Broad beans**, boiled	8	142	0	145	24
	Peas					
726	**Peas**, raw	19	290	0	300	50
727	boiled	7	245	0	250	42
728	**Peas**, canned, re-heated, drained	15	526	0	534	89
729	frozen, raw	0	266	0	266	44
	Vegetables, general					
732	**Asparagus**, raw	10	310	0	315	53
734	**Aubergine**, raw	60	40	0	70	12
735	fried in corn oil	110	70	0	125	21

No.	Food	Carotene fractions			Carotene equiv	Retinol equiv
		α-carotene	β-carotene	β-crypto-xanthin		
Vegetables, general *continued*						
736	**Beetroot**, boiled	27	14	0	27	5
747	**Carrots,** old, raw	5230	9150	0	11800	1960
748	old, boiled	2960	9620	0	11100	1850
749	old, microwaved	2870	9890	0	11300	1890
750	young, raw	3380	6120	0	7810	1300
751	young, boiled	3420	5990	0	7700	1280
752	canned, re-heated, drained	729	1710	0	2070	345
758	**Courgette**, raw	0	550	0[a]	610	100
760	fried in corn oil	0	450	0[a]	500	83
762	**Curly kale**, raw	0	3130	32	3150	525
763	boiled	0	3350	33	3380	560
771	**Mixed vegetables**, frozen, boiled	705	2155	26	2520	420
776	**Okra**, raw	30	500	0	515	85
777	boiled	29	450	0	465	77
778	stir-fried in corn oil	35	545	0	560	94
783	**Pak choi**, steamed	221	217	0	328	55
787	**Peppers, capsicum**, green, raw	9	260	0	265	44
788	green, boiled	8	235	0	240	40
789	red, raw	0	544	72	580	97
790	red, boiled	0	586	62	617	103
791	yellow, raw	0	115	37	134	22
795	**Pumpkin**, boiled	29	940	0	955	160
798	**Rocket**, raw	0	1130	17	1140	190
800	**Spinach**, mature, boiled	0	3820	39	3840	640
802	baby, raw	0	1560	0	1560	260
803	baby, boiled	0	2170	0	2170	362
805	**Squash**, butternut, baked	1810	2350	0	3260	545
810	**Sweetcorn**, kernels, canned in water, drained	13	23	22	41	7
811	kernels, boiled 'on the cob'	0	18	20	28	5
812	**Tomatoes**, standard, raw	0	333	31[b]	349	58
813	standard, grilled, flesh and seeds, only	0	343	23	355	59
814	cherry, raw	0	463	32	479	80
815	canned, whole contents	0	300	55	328	55

[a] Courgettes raw and fried in corn oil contain 120µg and 100µg α-cryptoxanthin per 100g, respectively

[b] Raw tomatoes also contain 507µg lycopene and 108µg lutein per 100g

No.	Food	Carotene fractions			Carotene equiv	Retinol equiv
		α-carotene	β-carotene	β-crypto-xanthin		
Vegetable dishes						
824	**Coleslaw**, not low calorie	184	602	0	694	153
827	**Curry**, Thai, stir-fry vegetable, takeaway and restaurant	93	456	22	514	89
828	vegetable, ready meal, cooked	136	502	20	580	112
839	**Quiche**, vegetable	13	190	10	202	155
847	**Sushi**, vegetable	13	147	18	163	27
853	**Vegetables, stir-fried**, takeaway	73	534	8	575	96
Fruit						
881	**Apricots**, raw, flesh and skin	2	405	0	405	67
882	ready-to-eat	8	540	0	545	91
883	**Avocado**, average	4	14	0	16	3
884	**Bananas**, flesh only	12	20	0	26	4
890	**Cherries**, raw, flesh and skin	4	23	0	25	4
892	**Citrus fruit**, soft/easy peelers, flesh only	0	67	76	105	18
899	**Gooseberries**, cooking, stewed with sugar	3	40	0	41	7
900	**Grapefruit**, raw, flesh only	9	12	0	17	3
908	**Mandarin oranges**, canned in juice	7	92	0	95	16
909	**Mangoes**, ripe, raw, flesh only	0	682	27	696	116
910	**Melon**, Canteloupe-type, flesh only	19	1760	0	1770	294
917	**Oranges**, flesh only	0	6	98	55	9
918	**Passion fruit**, flesh and pips	410	360	370	750	125
928	**Plums**, average, raw, flesh and skin	23	355	19	376	63
930	**Pomegranate**, flesh and pips	26	20	0	33	5
931	**Prunes**, canned in juice	15	135	0	140	23
932	ready-to-eat	27	125	0	140	23
Nuts and seeds						
962	**Trail mix**	3	45	0	47	8
Sugars, preserves and snacks						
996	**Chew sweets**	0	144	16	152	25
1007	**Corn snacks**	7	174	109	232	39
1016	**Tortilla chips**	30	141	103	208	35

No.	Food	Carotene fractions			Carotene equiv	Retinol equiv
		α-carotene	β-carotene	β-crypto-xanthin		

Beverages

No.	Food	α-carotene	β-carotene	β-crypto-xanthin	Carotene equiv	Retinol equiv
1061	**Orange juice**, chilled	0	16	48	40	7

Soups

1096	**Broccoli and stilton soup**, carton, chilled	1	128	1	129	70
1097	**Carrot and coriander soup**, carton, chilled	521	1712	12	1979	334
1102	**Instant soup**, dried, as served	18	57	4	68	11

Cooking sauces

1148	**Sauce, Chinese cook in**, sweet & sour	118	496	57	584	97
1149	**Sauce, Chinese**, stir fry	17	101	22	121	20
1151	**Sauce, Indian cook in**, korma/tikka masala	15	354	66	395	101
1152	other	16	327	98	384	64
1159	**Sauce, traditional cook in**, tomato based	41	274	41	315	53
1160	white sauce based	38	209	0	228	56

3.2 VITAMIN E FRACTIONS

The vitamin E activity of foods can be derived from a number of different tocopherols and tocotrienols. Where vitamin E is present, and the amount of each tocopherol is known, the values are shown below for selected foods which contain significant amounts of tocopherols other than α-tocopherol. The total vitamin E activity is also shown as α-tocopherol equivalents, which has been taken as the sum of the α-tocopherol, 40% of the β-tocopherol, 10% of the γ-tocopherol and 1% of the δ-tocopherol. For foods that also contain tocotrienols, their contribution to total vitamin E activity has been included, taken as 30% of α-tocotrienol, 5% of the β-tocotrienol, 1% of the γ-tocotrienol and 1% of δ-tocotrienol (McLaughlin and Weihrauch, 1979)[149]. The vitamin E equivalents reflect the vitamin E values given in the main tables.

No.	Food	Vitamin E fractions, mg per 100g edible portion				
		α-Toco-pherol	β-Toco-pherol	γ-Toco-pherol	δ-Toco-pherol	Vitamin E equiv
Cereals						
1	**Bran**, wheat	0.35	0.21	5.90	Tr	1.02
4	**Couscous**, plain, cooked	0.03	0.04	0.19	Tr	0.06
5	**Flour, chapati**, brown	0.61	0.36	4.14	Tr	1.17
7	**Flour, soya**	2.39	0.56	16.23	8.64	4.33
8	**Flour, wheat**, brown	0.61	0.38	1.44	0.06	0.90
9	white, bread/strong	0.25	0.15	1.15	Tr	0.43
12	wholemeal	0.37	0.19	2.41	Tr	0.69
15	**Wheatgerm**	13.42	6.66	1.30	Tr	16.20
16	**Rice, brown**, wholegrain, raw	0.34	0.03	0.14	Tr	0.37
18	**Rice, egg fried**, ready cooked, re-heated	1.88	0.04	1.81	0.09	2.08
30	**Rice, wild**, raw	0.22	0.04	0.05	Tr	0.24
35	**Noodles, egg**, medium, dried, boiled in unsalted water	0.18	0.26	0.72	0.02	0.35
37	**Pasta, egg**, fresh, raw	0.39	0.06	1.08	0.03	0.52
42	**Pasta, spaghetti**, canned in tomato sauce	0.28	Tr	0.04	Tr	0.29
50	**Bread, ciabatta**	0.35	0.10	0.78	Tr	0.47
58	**Bread, wheatgerm**	0.34	0.19	0.66	0.02	0.48
60	**Bread, white**, farmhouse or split tin	0.13	0.11	0.43	0.02	0.22
67	**Bread**, wholemeal, average	0.19	0.12	0.52	0.02	0.28
75	**Croissants**	0.88	0.08	0.82	0.31	0.99
107	**Porridge oats**, unfortified	0.41	0.39	0.20	0.04	0.59
156	**Gateau**, chocolate based, frozen	0.85	0.21	0.73	0.01	1.01
160	**Muffins**, American, chocolate	3.08	Tr	2.62	Tr	3.34
161	American, not chocolate	2.17	Tr	2.25	Tr	2.40

No.	Food	α-Toco-pherol	β-Toco-pherol	γ-Toco-pherol	δ-Toco-pherol	Vitamin E equiv
Cereals *continued*						
217	**Pizza**, meat topped, retail and takeaway	0.72	0.31	0.91	Tr	0.93
218	vegetarian, retail and takeaway	1.34	0.29	0.62	Tr	1.52
Milk and milk products						
227	**Whole milk,** pasteurised, average	0.06	Tr	Tr	Tr	0.06
242	**Soya, non-dairy alternative to milk**, unsweetened, fortified	0.15	0.03	1.56	0.68	0.32
243	**Cream,** fresh, single	0.46	0.01	0.02	Tr	0.47
244	fresh, whipping	1.29	0.06	0.04	Tr	1.32
245	fresh, double, including Jersey cream	1.62	0.04	0.03	Tr	1.64
247	**Creme fraiche**	0.72	Tr	0.03	Tr	0.72
248	half fat	0.42	Tr	0.01	Tr	0.42
253	**Cream substitute**, double	1.13	0.12	1.54	0.21	1.33
256	**Cheese, cheddar**, English	0.43	0.12	0.40	0.06	0.52
262	**Cheese, Danish blue**	0.71	Tr	0.04	0.13	0.71
266	**Cheese, goats milk**, soft, white rind	0.59	0.09	0.06	Tr	0.63
267	**Cheese, gouda**	0.56	0.02	0.02	Tr	0.57
269	**Cheese, mascarpone**	1.13	0.03	0.03	Tr	1.14
270	**Cheese, mozzarella**, fresh	0.30	0.02	0.03	Tr	0.31
272	**Cheese, parmesan**, fresh	0.73	0.07	0.03	Tr	0.76
279	**Cheese, stilton**, blue	0.60	Tr	0.02	0.01	0.60
293	**Yogurt, whole milk**, fruit	0.18	Tr	Tr	Tr	0.18
313	**Cheesecake**, fruit, individual	1.28	Tr	0.14	0.16	1.29
314	**Chocolate dairy desserts**	0.43	Tr	0.86	0.04	0.52
317	**Custard**, ready to eat	0.28	Tr	0.16	Tr	0.29
321	**Mousse**, chocolate, low fat	0.75	Tr	0.35	Tr	0.79
326	**Rice pudding**, canned	0.16	Tr	Tr	Tr	0.16
329	**Torte**, fruit	1.26	0.26	0.70	0.02	1.43
330	**Trifle**, fruit	0.64	Tr	0.16	0.16	0.66
Eggs						
332	**Eggs, chicken**, whole, raw	1.23	0.05	0.24	Tr	1.29[a]
334	yolk, raw	5.16	Tr	Tr	Tr	5.21[b]
335	whole, boiled	1.56	0.03	0.42	Tr	1.63[c]
337	yolk, boiled	4.73	Tr	Tr	Tr	4.78[b]

[a] Includes contribution from 0.04mg α-tocotrienol and 0.02mg γ-tocotrienol

[b] Includes contribution from 0.15mg α-tocotrienol

[c] Includes contribution from 0.05mg α-tocotrienol

No.	Food	α-Toco-pherol	β-Toco-pherol	γ-Toco-pherol	δ-Toco-pherol	Vitamin E equiv
Fats						
346	**Butter**, salted	1.82	0.07	0.03	0.01	1.85
Oils						
366	**Coconut oil**	0.50	0	0	0.60	0.66[d]
368	**Corn oil**	11.20	0	60.20	1.80	17.24
371	**Olive oil**	5.10	0	Tr	0	5.10
372	**Palm oil**	25.60	0	31.60	7.00	33.12[e]
373	**Peanut (groundnut) oil**	13.00	0	21.40	2.10	15.16
374	**Rapeseed oil**	18.40	0	38.00	1.20	22.21
376	**Soya oil**	10.10	0	59.30	26.40	16.06
377	**Sunflower oil**	48.70	0	5.10	0.80	49.22
Meat dishes						
481	**Duck**, crispy, Chinese style, meat and skin	2.07	Tr	0.97	Tr	2.17
525	**Meat samosas**, takeaway	0.44	Tr	1.09	0.14	0.55
553	**Chicken chow mein**, takeaway	0.83	Tr	1.29	Tr	0.96
554	**Chicken curry**, average, takeaway	1.88	Tr	2.40	0.16	2.12
558	Thai green, takeaway and restaurant	0.93	Tr	0.67	Tr	0.99
559	**Chicken fajita**, meat only, takeaway and restaurant	1.82	Tr	0.83	Tr	1.90
588	**Spring rolls**, meat, takeaway	1.23	Tr	2.35	0.15	1.47
589	**Sweet and sour chicken**, takeaway	1.88	Tr	2.54	0.15	2.14
Fish dishes						
656	**Curry**, prawn, takeaway	2.88	Tr	2.75	0.17	3.16
670	**Sesame prawn toasts**, takeaway	4.63	Tr	4.16	0.11	5.05
673	**Szechuan prawns with vegetables**, takeaway	1.86	Tr	1.27	0.08	1.99
Vegetables						
694	**Potato products**, shaped, baked	2.66	Tr	0.36	Tr	2.70
696	**Baked beans**, canned in tomato sauce	0.25	0.01	0.97	0.05	0.35
698	**Beans**, green, raw	0.37	Tr	0.67	0.10	0.44
707	**Gram flour**	1.76	Tr	7.74	0.43	2.54
739	**Broccoli**, green, boiled	1.62	0.01	0.48	Tr	1.67
744	**Cabbage**, green, boiled	0.27	Tr	0.02	Tr	0.27
779	**Onions**, raw	0.28	Tr	0.06	Tr	0.29

[d] Includes contribution from 0.50mg α-tocotrienol
[e] Includes contribution from 14.30mg α-tocotrienol

No.	Food	α-Toco-pherol	β-Toco-pherol	γ-Toco-pherol	δ-Toco-pherol	Vitamin E equiv
Vegetables *continued*						
789	**Peppers, capsicum**, red, raw	0.89	0.10	0.16	0.02	0.95
810	**Sweetcorn**, kernels, canned in water, drained	0.34	0.37	1.36	0.27	0.63
811	kernels, boiled 'on the cob'	0.42	Tr	Tr	0.03	0.42
812	**Tomatoes**, standard, raw	0.39	0.26	0.22	Tr	0.52
813	standard, grilled, flesh and seeds only	0.85	0.03	0.23	Tr	0.89
814	cherry, raw	0.81	0.02	0.69	0.03	0.89
Vegetable dishes						
827	**Curry**, Thai, stir-fry vegetable, takeaway and restaurant	1.39	Tr	0.94	Tr	1.48
828	vegetable, ready meal, cooked	1.88	Tr	0.94	Tr	1.97
847	**Sushi**, vegetable	0.50	Tr	0.51	Tr	0.55
849	**Vegetable and cheese grill/burger**, in crumbs, baked/grilled	0.94	0.12	1.30	0.39	1.12
853	**Vegetables, stir-fried**, takeaway	1.11	Tr	1.45	0.12	1.26
Fruit						
884	**Bananas**, flesh only	0.16	Tr	0.01	Tr	0.16
885	**Blackberries**, raw	2.05	0	2.90	2.75	2.37
889	**Blueberries**	0.88	0.02	0.54	0.02	0.94
902	**Grapes**, green	0.14	0.01	0.33	0.01	0.18
903	red	0.18	0.01	0.17	Tr	0.20
912	**Melon**, yellow flesh, flesh only	0.07	Tr	0.04	Tr	0.07
916	**Olives**, in brine	1.97	0.02	0.12	Tr	1.99
928	**Plums**, average, raw, flesh and skin	0.60	0	0.07	0	0.61
934	**Raspberries**, raw	0.30	0	1.50	2.70	0.48
936	**Strawberries**, raw	0.38	0	0.14	0.01	0.39
Nuts						
938	**Almonds**	23.77	0.26	0.81	0	23.96
939	**Brazil nuts**	5.72	0.15	13.87	0.17	7.18
940	**Cashew nuts**, roasted and salted	0.77	0.04	5.09	0.38	1.30
941	**Chestnuts**, raw	0.50	0	7.00	0	1.20
942	**Coconut**, creamed block	1.34	0	0.57	0	1.40
943	desiccated	1.21	0	0.52	0	1.26
946	**Hazelnuts**	24.20	0.80	4.33	0.22	24.98
948	**Marzipan**	6.13	0.07	0.21	0	6.18
950	**Peanut butter**, smooth	4.70	Tr	2.90	Tr	4.99
952	**Peanuts**, plain	9.21	0.23	7.91	0.37	10.09

No.	Food	α-Toco-pherol	β-Toco-pherol	γ-Toco-pherol	δ-Toco-pherol	Vitamin E equiv
Nuts *continued*						
953	dry roasted	0.70	0.18	3.30	0.53	1.11
954	roasted and salted	0.41	0.14	1.90	0.37	0.66
955	**Pecan nuts**	1.45	1.31	23.56	0.66	4.34
956	**Pine nuts**	12.47	0.02	11.77	0.03	13.66
957	**Pistachio nuts**, roasted and salted	1.43	0.03	27.15	0.58	4.16
959	**Sesame seeds**	0.25	0	22.81	0.29	2.53
960	**Sunflower seeds**	37.20	1.20	0.92	0.34	37.77
963	**Walnuts**	1.35	0.09	24.46	2.29	3.85
Confectionery						
984	**Chocolate**, fancy and filled	1.35	0.05	2.73	0.31	1.65
986	plain	0.86	0.18	5.11	0.28	1.44
987	white	0.61	Tr	5.26	0.21	1.14
993	**Smartie-type sweets**	0.46	Tr	3.20	0.18	0.80[†]
Beverages						
1027	**Drinking chocolate powder**	0.28	Tr	1.36	0.09	0.41
1031	**Instant drinks powder**, chocolate, low calorie	0.54	0.18	1.27	0.07	0.74
Sauces						
1146	**Pesto**, green	16.37	0.58	0.80	0.08	16.68
1149	**Sauce, Chinese**, stir fry	0.21	Tr	0.55	Tr	0.27
1151	**Sauce, Indian cook in**, korma/tikka masala	1.62	Tr	0.25	Tr	1.65
1155	**Sauce, pasta**, tomato based, for bolognese	1.87	0.21	0.35	0.25	1.99
1159	**Sauce, traditional cook in**, tomato based	1.38	Tr	Tr	Tr	1.38
1160	white sauce based	3.44	Tr	0.63	Tr	3.50

[†] Includes contribution from 0.07mg α-tocotrienol, 0.06mg γ-tocotrienol

3.3 VITAMIN K

Information on the phylloquinone (vitamin K_1) content of foods has been accumulating over a number of years and values for selected foods are reported in this table. Phylloquinone is lipid soluble and is found in the photosynthetic tissue of plants. As such, the darker green the plant leaves, the more phylloquinone is present (Shearer et al., 1996; Bolton-Smith et al., 2000)[164,84,85]. Certain vegetable oils, namely rapeseed, soybean and olive oils are also relatively high in phylloquinone compared to corn (maize) and sunflower seed oil. The phylloquinone content of individual retail products and mixed dishes will vary considerably depending on the oil type used. The phylloquinone content of plants also varies by climate and soil conditions (Ferland & Sadowski, 1992)[123].

A second family of naturally occurring, functional vitamin K compounds, the menaquinones (MK_n, where n represents the number of isoprene units in the side chain) are formed by bacteria. The menaquinone (vitamin K_2) content of eggs was determined in the 2012 survey of UK hens' eggs (Department of Health, 2012)[71] and results have been included here. Menaquinones are also likely to occur in variable quantities in fermented foods, and to a minor extent in some cheeses, as a result of the bacterial inoculation during their production. Menaquinones may also be found in some meats, such as chicken, as a result of feeding with the synthetic form of vitamin K, menadione, which is activated in vivo by conversion to MK_4.

Vitamin K_1 and K_2 are reported based on direct analysis using HPLC in redox mode with electro-chemical or UV detection (McCarthy et al., 1997; Shearer et al., 1996)[148,164]. These analyses have enabled recipe calculations and led to a report of vitamin K_1 food composition data (Bolton-Smith et al., 2000)[84,85]. Whilst the phylloquinone content of many of the foods included have been determined on UK-representative composite samples based on 4 to 7 individual samples, other results are based on analysis of a single sample or non-UK-representative composite samples made up of only 2 or 3 sub samples. The latter have been included when evidence supporting these values was available from work in other countries (e.g. Booth et al., 1996; Koivu et al., 1998)[86,141].

No.	Food	Vitamin K_1, µg per 100g edible portion Vitamin K_1
Cereals and cereal products		
1	**Bran**, wheat	10.4
7	**Flour, soya**	25.3
10	**Flour, wheat**, white, plain, soft	0.8
16	**Rice, brown, wholegrain**, raw	0.8
43	**Pasta, white**, dried, raw	0.2[a]
44	spaghetti, dried, boiled	0.1
54	**Bread**, naan	3.8
63	white, sliced	0.4
67	wholemeal, average	2.0

[a] Value for spaghetti, raw

No.	Food	Vitamin K$_1$

Cereals and cereal products *continued*

No.	Food	Vitamin K$_1$
91	**Cornflakes**, fortified	0.1
116	**Wheat biscuits**, Weetabix type, fortified	1.7
122	**Biscuits, digestive**, plain	1.5
124	**Biscuits, fully coated with chocolate**	3.5
127	**Biscuits, ginger nuts**	1.6
131	**Biscuits, sandwich**, cream	3.8
132	**Biscuits, semi-sweet**	1.7
133	**Biscuits, short, sweet**	4.0
154	**Fruit cake**	7.3

Milk and milk products

No.	Food	Vitamin K$_1$
219	**Channel Islands milk**, whole, pasteurised	0.9
225	**Skimmed milk**, pasteurised, average	Tr
227	**Whole milk**, pasteurised, average	0.6
231	**Condensed milk**, sweetened	0.4
233	**Evaporated milk**, whole	0.5
238	**Goats milk**, pasteurised	0.5
245	**Cream**, fresh, double, including Jersey cream	6.4
254	**Cheese, Brie**	2.4
256	**Cheese, cheddar**, English	4.7
262	**Cheese, Danish blue**	4.1
273	**Cheese, processed**, plain	1.6
278	**Cheese, spreadable**, soft white, full fat	4.7
288	**Yogurt, low fat,** fruit	Tr
290	plain	Tr
307	**Ice cream**, non-dairy, vanilla, soft scoop	0.8

Eggs

No.	Food	Vitamin K$_1$
332	**Eggs, chicken,** whole, raw[b]	Tr
334	yolk, raw[c]	Tr
335	whole, boiled[d]	Tr
337	yolk, boiled[e]	Tr
338	whole, fried in sunflower oil[b]	Tr
339	whole, poached[f]	Tr

[b] Contains 7.0μg vitamin K$_2$ per 100g

[c] Contains 15.0μg vitamin K$_2$ per 100g

[d] Contains 5.0μg vitamin K$_2$ per 100g

[e] Contains 18.0μg vitamin K$_2$ per 100g

[f] Contains 10.0μg vitamin K$_2$ per 100g

No.	Food	Vitamin K$_1$
Fats and oils		
346	**Butter**, salted	7.4
359	**Compound cooking fat,** not polyunsaturated	13.8
360	**Dripping**, beef	24.5
366	**Coconut oil**	1.0
367	**Cod liver oil**	0.3
368	**Corn oil**	3.0
371	**Olive oil**[g]	57.5
372	**Palm oil**	7.9
374	**Rapeseed oil**	112.5
376	**Soya oil**	131.0
377	**Sunflower oil**	6.3
Meat and meat products		
401	**Beef, mince**, stewed	7.2
403	**Beef, rump steak**, raw, lean and fat	0.8
427	**Lamb, loin chops**, grilled, lean only[h]	0.3
440	**Pork, fat,** average, raw	0.2
441	average, cooked	0.4
449	**Pork, loin chops**, raw, lean and fat	Tr
450	barbecued, lean and fat[i]	0.2
457	**Chicken, dark meat**, raw	0.1
460	**Chicken, light meat**, roasted	Tr
519	**Corned beef**, canned	2.0
526	**Paté**, liver	1.0
529	**Salami**	1.1
569	**Cottage/Shepherd's pie**, reheated	1.1
577	**Lasagne**, reheated	2.7
Fish and fish products		
591	**Cod**, raw	Tr
639	**Tuna**, canned in brine, drained	0.3
646	**Prawns**, standard, cooked	0.1
Potatoes		
677	**Old potatoes**, raw, flesh only	0.9
679	baked, flesh and skin	0.9
693	**Instant potato powder**, made up with water	0.9

[g] Mean of extra virgin and standard olive oils
[h] Fat only contains 1.42µg vitamin K$_1$ per 100g
[i] Value is for grilled, lean only. Fat only contains 0.35µg vitamin K$_1$ per 100g

No.	Food	Vitamin K_1
Beans and lentils		
696	**Baked beans**, canned in tomato sauce	2.7
698	**Beans**, green, raw	39.0
700	**Beansprouts**, mung, raw	Tr
703	**Broad beans**, boiled	11.4
705	**Chick peas**, whole, dried, boiled	2.2
715	**Runner beans**, raw	26.0
716	boiled	26.0
Peas		
722	**Mange-tout peas**, boiled	15.0
725	**Mushy peas**, canned, re-heated	22.5
726	**Peas**, raw	39.0
727	boiled	39.0
728	canned, re-heated, drained	30.4
Vegetables, general		
733	**Asparagus**, boiled	51.8
734	**Aubergine**, raw	6.1
738	**Broccoli**, green, raw	185.0
739	green, boiled	135.0
741	**Brussels sprouts**, raw	153.0
742	boiled	127.0
743	**Cabbage**, green, raw	242.0
744	green, boiled	201.0
746	white, raw[j]	60.0
747	**Carrots**, old, raw	5.5
748	old, boiled	5.5
750	**Carrots**, young, raw	9.2
751	young, boiled	9.2
753	**Cauliflower**, raw	31.0
754	boiled	28.5
755	**Celery**, raw	4.9
758	**Courgette**, raw	3.3
760	fried in corn oil	3.7
761	**Cucumber**, raw, flesh and skin	20.9

[j] Cabbage, white, outer leaves only contain 137 μg per 100g vitamin K1

No.	Food	Vitamin K$_1$

Vegetables, general *continued*

No.	Food	Vitamin K$_1$
762	**Curly kale**, raw	623.0
765	**Fennel**, Florence, boiled	4.9
768	**Leeks**, raw	10.1
769	boiled	9.5
770	**Lettuce**, average, raw	129.0
772	**Mushrooms**, white, raw	0.3
775	**Mustard and cress**, raw	88.0
784	**Parsnip**, raw[k]	0.1
787	**Peppers, capsicum,** green, raw	6.4
788	green, boiled	6.4
789	red, raw	1.6
790	red, boiled	1.6
793	**Plantain**, boiled, flesh only	0.1
795	**Pumpkin**, boiled	2.0
799	**Spinach**, mature, raw	394.0
800	mature, boiled	575.0
801	frozen, boiled	840.0
811	**Sweetcorn**, kernels, boiled 'on the cob'	0.4
812	**Tomatoes**, standard, raw	6.0
813	standard, grilled, flesh and seeds only	12.1
815	canned, whole contents	6.0
816	**Turnip**, boiled	0.2
817	**Watercress**, raw	315.0

Herbs and spices

No.	Food	Vitamin K$_1$
873	**Parsley**, fresh	548.0

Fruit

No.	Food	Vitamin K$_1$
880	**Apples**, eating, raw, flesh and skin[l]	5.6
884	**Bananas**, flesh only	0.1
900	**Grapefruit**, raw, flesh only	Tr
909	**Mangoes**, ripe, raw, flesh only	0.5
913	**Melon**, watermelon, flesh only	0.3
915	**Nectarines**, flesh and skin	2.5
917	**Oranges**, flesh only	0.1
920	**Peaches**, raw, flesh and skin	5.8
923	**Pears**, raw, flesh and skin	3.6
925	**Pineapple**, raw, flesh only	0.2
928	**Plums**, average, raw, flesh and skin[m]	7.5

[k] Parsnip, roasted in corn oil is estimated to contain 0.2µg vitamin K1 per 100g

[l] Value refers to Cox's apples

[m] Value refers to Victoria plum

No.	Food	Vitamin K_1
Fruit *continued*		
933	**Raisins**	3.7
936	**Strawberries**, raw	3.0
Nuts and seeds		
953	**Peanuts**, dry roasted	0.3
Sugars, preserves and snacks		
968	**Jam**, fruit with edible seeds	0.9
986	**Chocolate**, plain	2.3
991	**Mars bar** and own brand equivalents	4.8
1007	**Corn snacks**	15.5
Beverages		
1020	**Cocoa, powder**	1.5
1021	**Coffee**, infusion, average	0.1
1023	**Coffee**, powder, instant	4.3
1024	**Coffeemate**, whitener, powder	6.0
1035	**Tea**, black, infusion, average	0.3

The
Appendices

4.1 ANALYTICAL TECHNIQUES USED FOR THE TABLES

The methods which have been used for the analysis of foods in the Tables are shown below. Details of methods used for individual foods may be available in the main data references column in the Tables (see also Section 4.6 References).

The nutrient values quoted in the tables have been determined by a variety of methods and in many cases laboratories would have used modified versions of the methods referenced below. Although most give results of the same order of accuracy, with new methods merely improving the efficiency of analysis, some methods give different results and these have been documented in the Tables only where they appear to be substantial.

The following abbreviations are used in the text:

AOAC   Association of Official Analytical Chemists
EN   European Norm of the CEN (Comité Européen de Normalisation)
GLC   Gas liquid chromatography
HPLC   High performance liquid chromatography
ICPMS   Inductively coupled plasma mass spectrometry
ICPOES   Inductively coupled plasma optical emission spectrophotometry
IUPAC   International Union of Pure and Applied Chemistry

Nutrient	Method
Water	Freeze drying Vacuum drying at 70°C Air drying at 100°C
Nitrogen	Kjeldahl procedure Dumas combustion method
Fat	Weibull Stoldt (Egan et al., 1981)[100] Werner Schmidt (Egan et al., 1981)[100] Rose-Gottlieb (Egan et al., 1981)[100] Weibull-Berntrop (IDF 125A, 1988)[137]
Fatty acids Trans fatty acids	GLC of methyl esters (IUPAC, 1976)[138] (IUPAC, 1979)[139]
Cholesterol	GLC
Alcohol	Standard Inland Revenue distillation method

Nutrient	Method
Carbohydrates	
Total sugars (as monosaccharides)	Boehringer enzyme kit (Egan et al., 1981)[100] HPLC Colorimetry
Starch	Enzymatic hydrolysis and measurement of glucose Polarimetry
Fibre	
Non-starch polysaccharides	Englyst et al. (1994)[105] Englyst et al. (1992)[104] Englyst and Cummings (1988)[103] Englyst and Cummings (1984)[102] Englyst et al. (1982)[101]
AOAC	Official method 985.29 (AOAC, 2011)[78]
Inorganics	
Sodium	ICPMS ICPOES Emission spectrometry (Moxon, 1983)[152] Atomic absorption spectrophotometry Flame photometry
Potassium	ICPMS ICPOES Emission spectrometry Atomic absorption spectrophotometry Flame photometry
Calcium	ICPMS ICPOES Atomic absorption spectrophotometry Titrimetry
Magnesium Copper Iron Zinc	ICPMS ICPOES Atomic absorption spectrophotometry Colorimetry
Phosphorus	ICPMS ICPOES Colorimetry
Chloride	ICPMS Colorimetry Titrimetry
Manganese	ICPMS Atomic absorption spectrophotometry
Selenium	ICPMS Hydride generation atomic absorption spectroscopy Fluorimetry (Michie et al., 1978)[150]

Iodine	ICPMS
	Spectrophotometry (Moxon and Dixon, 1980)[151]
	GLC

Nutrient	Method
Vitamins	
Fat soluble vitamins	
Retinol Carotenoids	HPLC (EN 12823-1:2000)[110] HPLC (EN 12823-2:2000)[111] Chromatographic separation and absorption spectrophotometry
Vitamin D	HPLC (EN 12821:2000)[117] Biological assay and spectrophotometry GLC
Vitamin E	HPLC (EN 12822:2000)[118] Colorimetry combined with GLC (Christie *et al.*, 1973)[93]
Vitamin K	HPLC in redox mode with electrochemical or UV detection (Bolton-Smith *et al.*, 2000; Shearer *et al.*, 1996)[84,164]
Water soluble vitamins	
Thiamin	HPLC with fluorimetric detection (EN 14122:2003, Finglas and Faulks, 1984)[112,125] Fluorimetry (Society of Public Analysts and Other Analytical Chemists: Analytical Methods Committee, 1951)[166] Microbiological assay (Bell, 1974)[80]
Riboflavin	HPLC with fluorimetric detection (EN 14152:2003, Finglas and Faulks, 1984)[113,125] Microbiological assay (Bell, 1974)[80]
Niacin	HPLC (Kwiatkowska *et al.*, 1989)[142] Microbiological assay (Bell, 1974)[80]
Tryptophan	HPLC
Vitamin B$_6$	HPLC with fluorimetric detection (EN 14166:2001, Kwiatkowska *et al.*, 1989; Brubacher *et al.*, 1985)[115,142,90] Microbiological assay (EN 14164:2001, Bell, 1974)[114,80]
Vitamin B$_{12}$ Pantothenate Biotin	Microbiological assay (Bell, 1974)[80]
Folate	Microbiological assay (EN 14131:2003, Phillips and Wright, 1983; Bell, 1974)[109,157,80]
Vitamin C	
Ascorbic acid	HPLC with fluorimetric detection (EN 14130:2003, Finglas and Faulks, 1984)[116,125]
Ascorbic acid and dehydroascorbic acid	Titrimetry (AOAC, 1975)[77] Fluorimetry (AOAC, 1975)[77]

4.2 EDIBLE CONVERSION FACTORS AND CALCULATION OF NUTRIENT CONTENT FOR FOODS 'AS PURCHASED' OR 'AS SERVED'

Many foods are purchased or served with material that is clearly inedible or material that might be discarded as inedible by some consumers. For the purposes of this publication, 'waste' encompasses both types of material, which might include for example:

- outer leaves or stalks of vegetables
- stones, pips or peel of fruit
- nut shells
- fish skin and bones
- meat fat and bones
- liquid content of canned foods.

Earlier editions of the food tables included data for foods both with and without waste, and this information is still made available to users in the Composition of Foods Integrated Dataset. All the nutrient values in this edition apply to the edible part of the food only, as described, and are expressed per 100g of edible portion. The edible conversion factor allows calculation of the nutrient content of foods when the inedible waste is included in the weight and refers to the proportion of edible material remaining after the inedible waste has been removed. For example, an unpeeled banana on average consists of 63% edible flesh and 37% inedible skin; therefore the edible portion is expressed in the tables below as 0.63. The edible conversion factor will vary between different samples of the same food and these values should be treated as a guide to the typical proportion of inedible waste.

For canned foods, such as vegetables and fish, the proportion of the edible contents after the liquid has been drained off is given below, and the values in the tables are for the drained contents only unless otherwise stated in the description, e.g. tomatoes, canned, whole contents.

For canned fruits, where the juice or syrup component is often consumed as well as the fruit, the proportion of the edible contents after the liquid has been drained off is given below. The values in the tables for canned fruit are for the whole contents of the can, including both juice/syrup and fruit. It is not possible to calculate the nutrient values for only the fruit component.

Food	Edible conversion factors	
	Inedible part(s)[a]	Edible conversion factor
Milk and milk products		
Brie	Rind	0.69
Eggs		
Eggs, chicken, whole, medium/large, raw	Shell	0.87
boiled	Shell	0.89
Bacon and ham		
Bacon rashers, back, raw	Rind	0.97
Ham, gammon joint, raw	Rind	0.92
Beef		
Braising steak, braised, lean only	Fat	0.90
Rump steak, raw, lean and fat	Gristle	0.99
	Fat, gristle	0.88
Rump steak, barbecued, lean and fat	Fat	0.91
fried, lean and fat	Fat	0.87
Stewing steak, raw, lean and fat	Fat	0.90
stewed, lean and fat	Fat	0.84
Topside, roasted medium-rare, lean and fat	Fat	0.87
Lamb		
Leg, half knuckle, pot-roasted, lean and fat	Bone	0.74
	Bone, fat	0.65
Leg, whole, roasted, medium, lean and fat	Bone	0.77
	Bone, fat	0.67
Loin chops, raw, lean and fat	Bone, gristle	0.79
	Bone, gristle, fat	0.53
grilled, lean and fat	Bone	0.81
	Bone, fat	0.61
microwaved, lean and fat	Bone	0.82
	Bone, fat	0.58
roasted, lean and fat	Bone	0.78
	Bone, fat	0.56
Shoulder, whole, roasted, lean and fat	Bone	0.79
	Bone, fat	0.60
Stewing lamb, stewed, lean and fat	Bone, gristle	0.68
	Bone, gristle, fat	0.56
Pork		
Belly joint/slices, grilled, lean and fat	Bone, gristle	0.85
Leg joint, raw, lean and fat	Bone	0.87
	Bone, fat	0.68

Food	Inedible part(s)[a]	Edible conversion factor
Pork		
Leg joint, roasted, medium, lean and fat	Bone	0.85
	Bone, fat (soft and crackling)	0.69
Loin chops, raw, lean and fat	Bone	0.84
	Bone, fat	0.59
barbecued, lean and fat	Bone	0.84
	Bone, fat	0.68
grilled, lean and fat	Bone	0.77
	Bone, fat (soft and crackling)	0.60
microwaved, lean and fat	Bone	0.80
	Bone, fat	0.65
roasted, lean and fat	Bone	0.76
lean only	Bone, fat	0.59
Chicken, other poultry and game		
Chicken, drumsticks, casseroled with skin	Bone	0.65
	Bone, skin	0.55
roasted	Bone	0.63
	Bone, skin	0.57
Chicken, whole, roasted	Bone	0.65
	Bone, skin	0.54
Duck, dressed carcase, raw	Bone, skin, fat	0.28
dressed carcase, roasted	Bone, skin, fat	0.21
	Bone	0.42
crispy, Chinese style	Bone	0.74
Goose, dressed carcase, roasted	Bone	0.65
Pheasant, dressed carcase, roasted	Bone, skin, fat	0.53
Rabbit, whole carcase, fresh and frozen, raw	Bone, gristle, fat	0.63
stewed	Bone, gristle, fat	0.60
Meat products and dishes		
Chicken pieces, coated, takeaway, including skin and coating	Bone	0.70
Chicken wings, marinated, barbecued	Bone	0.65
Pork spare ribs, 'barbecue style', reheated	Bone	0.35
White fish		
Cod, fillet, raw	Skin	0.90
baked	Skin	0.89
microwaved	Skin, bone	0.88
Coley, fillet, raw	Skin	0.91
Haddock, fillet, raw	Skin	0.88
grilled	Skin	0.88
steamed	Skin	0.87

Food	Inedible part(s)[a]	Edible conversion factor
Haddock, smoked, poached	Skin	0.89
Lemon sole fillet, raw	Skin	0.72
grilled	Skin	0.77
Plaice, fillet, raw	Skin	0.74
Sea bass, raw, whole	Skin, bone, head, tail, fins, other	0.60
raw, fillets	Skin	0.86
baked, whole	Skin, bone, head, tail, fins, other	0.61
baked, fillets	Skin	0.89
Fatty fish		
Anchovies, canned in oil	Drained oil	0.74
Herring, grilled, average of whole fish and fillets	Skin, bones, fins, head, tail, other	0.78
Kippers (no butter), grilled, whole	Skin, bones, fins, head, tail	0.77
grilled, fillets	Skin	0.89
Kippers, boil in the bag, with butter	Skin, fins	0.88
Mackerel, raw, whole	Skin, bones, fins, head, tail, other	0.61
raw, fillets with skin	Skin (fin & bones where applicable)	0.82
grilled, whole	Skin, bones, fins, head, tail, other	0.77
grilled, fillets	Skin	0.98
smoked, purchased cooked	Skin	0.91
Salmon, farmed, raw	Skin	0.93
grilled	Skin	0.87
steamed	Skin	0.87
baked	Skin	0.88
Salmon, wild, raw	Skin, bone	0.77
Salmon, hot-smoked, cooked	Skin	0.89
Salmon, pink, canned	Liquid, main bones	0.77
Salmon, red, canned, with skin and bones	Liquid, main bones	0.70
canned, skinless and boneless	Liquid	0.78
Sardines, whole, raw	Skin, bones, head, tail, fins, other	0.47
whole, grilled	Skin, bones, head, tail, fins, other	0.63
canned in brine	Liquid	0.75
canned in oil	Liquid	0.70

Food	Inedible part(s)[a]	Edible conversion factor
Trout, rainbow, raw, whole	Skin, bones, head, tail, fins, other	0.71
raw, fillets	Skin, other	0.85
baked, whole	Skin, bones, head, tail, fins, other	0.71
baked, fillets	Skin, other	0.87
Tuna, steak, raw	Skin, bone	0.76
steak, baked	Skin, bone	0.81
canned in brine	Liquid	0.71
canned in sunflower oil	Liquid	0.71
Crustacea and molluscs		
Crab, canned in brine	Liquid	0.70
brown/white meat, cooked whole	Shell, claws, waste	0.44
Prawns, king, raw, whole	Head, tail, shell, legs	0.54
purchased cooked	Tail	0.91
Prawns, standard, purchased cooked with shell	Head, shell, legs	0.35
Mussels in white wine sauce, cooked, retail	Shell, inedible material, sauce, herbs	0.57
Potatoes		
Potatoes, old, raw	Peel	0.85
Beans and lentils		
Beans, green, raw, whole	Trimmed tops, ends	0.91
raw, with trimmed tops	Trimmed ends	0.94
Butter beans, canned	Liquid	0.57
Chick peas, canned	Liquid	0.60
Red kidney beans, canned	Liquid	0.64
Runner beans, raw	Trimmed ends, sides	0.86
Peas		
Mange-tout peas, raw	Trimmed ends	0.92
Marrowfat peas, canned	Liquid	0.62
Peas, raw	Pods	0.37
canned	Liquid	0.67
Vegetables, general		
Asparagus, raw, trimmed	Tough ends only	0.75

Food	Inedible part(s)[a]	Edible conversion factor
Asparagus, soft tips only, boiled	Tough ends and stalks	0.48
Aubergine, raw	Trimmed ends	0.96
raw, peeled	Trimmed ends, peel	0.77
Beetroot, boiled	Trimmed top and root, peel	0.80
Beetroot, pickled	Liquid	0.65
Broccoli, raw, whole 'head'	Tough stems, 'trunk'	0.66
Brussels sprouts, raw	Trimmed base, outer leaves	0.69
Cabbage, whole, green, raw	Core, outer leaves	0.87
white, raw	Core, outer leaves	0.90
red, raw	Core, outer leaves	0.91
Carrots, old peeled	Trimmed tops and ends, peel	0.71
unpeeled	Trimmed tops and ends	0.91
Carrots, young, raw	Scrubbed, trimmed ends	0.87
Carrots, canned	Liquid	0.61
Cauliflower, whole, raw	Leaves, lower stump, core	0.53
Celery, raw	Leaves, trimmed ends	0.91
Chicory, raw	Stem, inner leaves	0.80
Courgette, raw	Trimmed ends	0.88
Cucumber, raw, flesh and skin	Ends	0.92
Curly kale, raw	Main ribs, stalks	0.85
Fennel, Florence, raw	Green tops, end	0.80
Garlic, raw	Peel	0.79
Gherkins, pickled	Liquid	0.67
Leeks, raw	Trimmed ends, outer leaves	0.57
bulb only	Ends, leaves	0.36
Lettuce, average, purchased whole	Stalks, inedible leaves	0.82
Mushrooms, white, raw	Trimmed stalk ends	0.96
Mustard and cress, raw, purchased on soil block	Soil block	0.27
Okra, raw	Trimmed ends	0.74

Food	Inedible part(s)[a]	Edible conversion factor
Onions, raw	Skin, top, root	0.90
Onions, pickled	Liquid	0.59
Pak choi, steamed	Bottom, inedible leaves	0.94
Parsnip, raw	Peel, trimmed ends	0.72
Peppers, capsicum, chilli, green, raw	Seeds, core, stalk	0.90
Peppers, capsicum, average	Seeds, core, stalk	0.84
Pumpkin, raw	Peel, seeds	0.67
Radish, red, raw	Trimmed ends	0.81
Spinach, mature, raw	Ribs, stems	0.81
Spring onions, bulbs and tops, raw	Peel, leaves	0.69
Squash, butternut, raw	Peel, seeds	0.82
Swede, raw	Peel	0.73
Sweet potato, raw	Peel	0.84
Sweetcorn, canned in water	Liquid	0.87
Sweetcorn kernels, boiled on the cob	Leaves, core	0.59
Tomatoes, standard, raw	Stalks	0.99
grilled, flesh and seeds only	Stalks, hard core, skin	0.90
Tomatoes, cherry, on the vine	Stalks	0.99
Turnip, raw	Peel	0.75
Watercress, raw	Large stalks	0.62
Yams, raw	Peel	0.81

Vegetable dishes

Sauerkraut, bottled and canned	Liquid	0.71

Fruit

Apples, cooking, stewed, flesh only	Core, peel	0.69
Apples, eating, flesh and skin	Core	0.87
Apricots, raw	Stone	0.92
Avocado, average, raw	Stone, skin	0.71
Bananas, raw	Peel	0.63
Blackcurrants, raw	Stalks	0.98
Cherries, raw	Stalk, stone	0.83
Citrus fruit, soft/easy peelers	Peel, pips	0.78
Dates, dried	Stone	0.84
Fruit cocktail, canned in juice	Liquid	0.65
canned in syrup	Liquid	0.66
Gooseberries, raw	Tops, tails	0.91
Grapefruit, raw	Peel, pips	0.68
canned in juice	Liquid	0.52
Kiwi fruit, raw	Skin	0.86
Lemons, whole, without pips	Pips	0.99
Lychees, raw	Skin, stone	0.62

Food	Inedible part(s)[a]	Edible conversion factor
Mangoes, ripe, raw	Seeds, skin	0.68
Melon, Canteloupe-type	Seeds, skin	0.59
Galia	Seeds, skin	0.64
yellow flesh	Seeds, skin	0.58
watermelon	Seeds and skin	0.57
Nectarines, raw	Stone	0.89
Olives, in brine	Liquid, stones	0.80
Oranges, raw	Peel and pips	0.71
Passion fruit, raw	Skin	0.61
Papaya, raw	Skin and seeds	0.75
Peaches, raw	Stone	0.90
canned in juice	Liquid	0.68
canned in syrup	Liquid	0.62
Pears, raw	Core and stalk	0.85
canned in juice	Liquid	0.60
Pineapple, raw	Skin, core, top and bottom	0.53
canned in juice	Liquid	0.54
canned in syrup	Liquid	0.56
Plums, average, raw	Stones	0.94
stewed with sugar	Stones	0.95
Pomegranate	Skin	0.65
Prunes, canned in juice, no stones	Liquid	0.46
ready-to-eat	Stones	0.86
Strawberries	Stalks	0.94
Nuts and seeds		
Almonds	Shell	0.37
Brazil nuts	Shell	0.46
Chestnuts, raw	Shell	0.83
Hazelnuts	Shell	0.38
Peanuts, plain	Shell	0.69
Pecan nuts	Shell	0.49
Pistachio nuts, roasted	Shell	0.55
Walnuts	Shell	0.43

[a] For some foods 'inedible parts' may be consumed, depending on consumer preference, e.g. meat fat, fruit skin

If the quantity of food consumed (including waste) is known, this can be multiplied by the edible conversion factor enabling the nutrient values given in the tables (as per 100g edible portion) to be used in calculations of nutrient content. Values in the tables for canned fruit are for the whole contents of the can, including both juice/syrup and fruit, therefore it is not possible to calculate the nutrient values for the fruit only component. For the calculation of the composition of cooked foods from raw materials, users should refer to Section 4.3.

The nutrient content of a food 'as purchased' is calculated by multiplying the nutrient content 'as consumed' by the edible conversion factor.

Foods 'as purchased' and 'as served' include inedible portions while foods 'as consumed' refer to the edible portion only.

Worked examples showing the calculation of nutrients in foods when weighed with waste (such as foods 'as purchased' or 'as served') are given below.

Example 1: Carbohydrate content of Bananas weighed with skin ('as purchased')

Carbohydrate in Bananas ('as consumed', i.e. flesh only)	=	20.3 g per 100g
Edible proportion of Bananas weighed with skin ('as purchased')	=	0.63
Carbohydrate in Bananas weighed with skin ('as purchased')	=	20.3 x 0.63
	=	12.8 g per 100g bananas weighed with skin ('as purchased')

Example 2: Protein content of Lamb, loin chop, grilled, lean ('as consumed'), but weighed and served with fat and bone ('as served')

Protein in Lamb, loin chop, grilled, lean ('as consumed')	=	29.2 g per 100g
Edible proportion of Lamb, loin chop, grilled, lean, weighed with fat and bone ('as served')	=	0.61
Protein in Lamb, loin chop, grilled, lean, weighed with fat and bone ('as served')	=	29.2 x 0.61
	=	17.8 g per 100g lamb, loin chop, grilled ('as served')

Example 3: Carbohydrate content of Apples, eating, average, raw ('as consumed'), weighed with core ('as purchased')

Carbohydrate in Apples, eating, average, raw (flesh and skin only, 'as consumed')	=	11.6 g per 100g

Edible proportion of Apples, eating, average,　　=　　0.87
raw, weighed with core ('as purchased')

Carbohydrate in Apples, eating, average,　　=　　11.6　x　0.87
raw, weighed with core ('as purchased')

　　　　　　　　　　　　　　　　　　　　=　　10.1 g per 100g apples, eating,
　　　　　　　　　　　　　　　　　　　　　　raw, with core ('as purchased')

Example data
The table below includes the above three examples with calculations for water, protein,
fat and carbohydrate. In the first line for each entry, the food is given as it appears in the
Tables (the 'as consumed' description), along with the relevant edible conversion factor
from this section. The second line for each food describes the food 'as purchased' or 'as
served' and shows the data from the first line recalculated using the ECF. All values are
presented as g/100g.

No.	Food	Edible conversion factor	Water (g)	Protein (g)	Fat (g)	Carbo-hydrate (g)
427	**Lamb, loin chops**, grilled, lean	0.61	59.6	29.2	10.7	0
	weighed with fat and bone		*36.4*	*17.8*	*6.5*	*0*
880	**Apples**, eating, average, raw	0.87	86.2	0.6	0.5	11.6
	weighed with core		*75.0*	*0.5*	*0.4*	*10.1*
884	**Bananas**, flesh only	0.63	75.0	1.2	0.1	20.3
	weighed with skin		*47.3*	*0.8*	*0.1*	*12.8*

4.3 COOKED FOODS AND DISHES

4.3.1 Weight changes on preparation of foods

The figures below show the percentage changes in weight recorded during the cooking of foods included in this edition. Many new values have been added, based on data collected in recent analytical surveys. In addition, older values were obtained by Holland et al. (1991)[10], Wiles et al. (1980)[174], Paul and Southgate (1977)[156], McCance and Shipp (1933)[146] and from previously unpublished determinations where a measure of weight change was available. There is a lot of variation in the weight change on cooking for any given food, depending on factors including the cooking method, length of cooking time, temperature, amount of water used and surface area of the food. The values shown here should be treated as guidelines only; for more accurate figures users should make their own determinations. The weight changes during cooking of recipe dishes have been included with each recipe.

The majority of changes result from the loss or gain of water, but for many meats and fried foods there will also have been a loss or gain of fat. The values have been calculated as:

$$\frac{\text{Weight of cooked food or dish - Weight of raw food(s)}}{\text{Weight of raw food(s)}} \times 100$$

A value of +200 thus means not that the food doubled its weight, but that it gained twice its original weight on cooking (i.e. tripled in weight), because:

$$\frac{300 - 100}{100} \times 100 = +200$$

A plus sign (+) indicates that the food or dish gained weight on cooking, while a minus sign (-) shows that it lost weight. Individual sub-samples were weighed before and after cooking and the mean weight change for each composite sample is given. Where data is available for the range of weight changes, it is given in brackets.

CEREALS AND CEREAL PRODUCTS

	% weight change	
	Mean	Range
Rice and other grains		
Rice, brown, boiled	+151	(114-191)
of which, wholegrain, boiled	+154	(138-176)
easy cook, boiled	+131	(114-155)
basmati, boiled	+167	(158-191)
Rice, ready-cooked, microwaved	-1	(+1 to -9)
Rice, red, boiled	+199	(154-224)

CEREALS AND CEREAL PRODUCTS *continued*

	% weight change	
	Mean	**Range**
Rice, savoury, boiled	+144	(111-177)
Rice, Thai fragrant, boiled	+190	(170-214)
Rice, white, average, boiled	+172	(124-249)
of which, basmati, boiled	+184	(143-249)
basmati, easy cook, boiled	+178	(151-200)
long grain, boiled	+171	(134-210)
long grain, easy cook, boiled	+154	(124-206)
Rice, white, Italian Arborio risotto, boiled	+151	(101-200)
Rice, wild, boiled	+146	(101-179)
Couscous, plain, cooked	+102	(63-185)
Polenta, hydrated, reheated	-14	(13-16)
Pasta		
Noodles, egg, dried, medium, cooked	+115	(109-128)
fine, cooked	+176	(156-224)
thick, cooked	+148	(144-152)
Noodles, rice, dried, fine, cooked	+281	(208-382)
Pasta, white, dried, spaghetti, cooked	+148	(109-177)
tubes, shells, bows, macaroni, cooked	+103	(63-148)
twists, cooked	+122	(104-141)
Pasta, wholewheat, dried, spaghetti, cooked	+138	(121-154)
Pasta, white, egg, fresh, tagliatelle, cooked	+86	(65-102)
Pasta, egg, fresh, filled, average, cooked	+38	(12-66)
Bread		
White bread, fried	-29	
toasted	-18	
'with added fibre', toasted	-16	
Wholemeal bread, toasted	-15	
Bread, garlic and herb, retail, baked	-8	(5-11)
Buns and pastries		
Crumpets, toasted	-11	

	% weight change	
	Mean	**Range**
Muffins, English style, white, toasted	-13	
Other cereal products		
Pastry, filo, retail, baked	-24	(20-27)
flaky/puff, retail, baked	-21	(19-23)
shortcrust, retail, baked	-17	(13-21)
Pizza, cheese and tomato, retail, chilled/frozen, baked	-13	(8-19)
Quiche, retail, baked	-8	(5-17)
MEAT AND MEAT PRODUCTS		
Bacon and ham		
Bacon rashers, back, dry-fried	-33	(23-40)
back, grilled	-32	(22-44)
back, grilled crispy	-53	(28-68)
back, microwaved	-39	(26-48)
back, fat trimmed, grilled	-33	(25-44)
middle, grilled	-38	(27-49)
streaky, grilled	-35	(21-51)
Ham, gammon joint, boiled	-29	(15-40)
Gammon rashers, grilled	-34	(32-50)
Beef and veal		
Braising steak, braised	-40	(36-46)
Mince, microwaved	-28	(19-43)
Mince, stewed	-18	(4-25)
extra lean, stewed	-18	(9-29)
Rump steak, barbecued	-31	(18-47)
fried	-27	(20-36)
grilled	-28	(18-35)
strips, stir-fried	-29	(17-40)
Stewing steak, stewed	-36	(26-47)
Topside, roasted, medium-rare	-32	(19-42)
Veal, escalope, fried	-38	(18-46)

	% weight change	
	Mean	**Range**
Lamb		
Breast, roasted	-28	(20-41)
Leg, whole, roasted, medium	-31	(20-35)
Loin chops, grilled	-31	(15-52)
microwaved	-33	(24-41)
roasted	-37	(17-57)
Mince, stewed	-28	(22-33)
Shoulder, whole, roasted, medium	-32	(21-40)
Stewing lamb, stewed	-27	(21-41)
Pork		
Belly joint/slices, grilled	-36	(29-61)
Diced, casseroled	-37	(31-41)
Fillet strips, stir-fried	-33	(26-40)
Leg joint, roasted, medium	-35	(23-41)
Loin chops, barbecued	-28	(15-48)
grilled	-32	(21-40)
microwaved	-32	(20-40)
Loin chops, roasted	-38	(24-57)
Steaks, grilled	-38	(28-47)
Chicken		
Breast, casseroled, meat only	-25	
grilled, without skin, meat only	-25	
Breast, strips, stir-fried	-21	(17-29)
Breast in crumbs, fried	-5	
Drumsticks, roasted, meat and skin	-26	(14-50)
Turkey		
Breast fillet, grilled	-32	(23-46)
strips, stir-fried	-23	(18-27)

	% weight change	
	Mean	**Range**
Meat products		
Beefburgers, 98-99% beef, fried	-38	
grilled	-34	
Beefburgers, 62-85% beef, grilled	-17	(11-23)
Black pudding, dry-fried	-12	
Chicken pie, individual, baked	-5	(3-9)
Chicken/turkey breasts/steaks/burgers/pieces, coated, baked	-13	(6-26)
Chicken/turkey pasties/slices, puff pastry, retail, baked	-3	(2-6)
Cornish pasty, retail, baked	-2	(1-4)
Pie, beef, puff or shortcrust pastry, retail, baked	-4	(2-9)
Sausages, beef, chilled, grilled	-25	
Sausages, pork, chilled, fried	-20	
chilled, grilled	-24	
reduced fat, chilled, grilled	-24	
Sausages, premium, chilled, grilled	-24	
Meat dishes		
Beef curry, reheated, baked	-5	
microwaved	-16	
Chicken curry, reheated, baked	-1	
microwaved	-24	
Chicken tandoori, reheated, baked	-18	
microwaved	-13	
Chicken tikka masala, reheated, baked	-3	(0-4)
microwaved	-6	(2-9)
Chicken, stir-fried with rice and vegetables, reheated	-19	(15-23)
Cottage/Shepherds pie, reheated, baked	-13	(1-48)
microwaved	-21	(1-40)
Faggots in gravy, reheated	-6	(4-10)
microwaved	-2	(2-3)
Lamb/Beef hot pot with potatoes, reheated, baked	-13	(6-21)
microwaved	-8	(1-14)

	% weight change	
	Mean	**Range**
Lasagne, reheated, baked	-17	(7-47)
Moussaka, reheated, baked	-9	(4-13)
microwaved	-7	(5-11)
Spaghetti bolognese, reheated, baked	-7	(6-8)
microwaved	-15	(11-19)

FISH AND FISH PRODUCTS

White fish

	Mean	Range
Fish, white[a], baked	-31	(18-49)
of which, chilled, baked	-22	(18-25)
frozen, baked	-36	(26-49)
Fish, white[a], grilled	-29	(19-43)
of which, chilled, grilled	-24	(19-26)
frozen, grilled	-33	(22-43)
Fish, white[a], steamed	-25	(12-43)
of which, chilled, steamed	-18	(12-25)
frozen, steamed	-32	(25-43)
Fish, white[a], poached	-25	(14-44)
of which, chilled, poached	-21	(14-30)
frozen, poached	-29	(15-44)
Sea bass, baked	-23	(14-43)
of which, chilled, baked	-19	(14-25)
frozen, baked	-31	(23-43)
Fatty fish		
Herring, whole, chilled, grilled	-27	(25-29)
baked	-20	(14-24)
Kippers, grilled	-18	(10-30)
Mackerel, grilled	-20	(14-36)
Salmon, farmed, grilled	-15	(11-18)
steamed	-13	(8-21)
baked	-17	(13-19)
Sardines, whole, grilled	-22	(20-24)

[a] White fish includes cod, haddock, Alaskan pollock, pangasius, and coley

	% weight change	
	Mean	**Range**
Trout, rainbow, baked	-20	(16-29)
Tuna, baked	-19	(12-24)
Crustacea and molluscs		
Crab, boiled	-20	
Mussels, boiled	-33	
Prawns, king, grilled from raw	-33	(25-45)
Coated fish and fish products		
Calamari, coated in batter, baked	-34	(24-43)
Cod, coated in batter or breadcrumbs, retail, baked	-12	(3-22)
coated in batter, frozen, fried	-16	(6-27)
Fishcakes, average, coated in breadcrumbs, baked	-12	(6-21)
Fish fingers, cod, frozen, grilled/baked	-13	(8-21)
fried	-2	(0-8)
Plaice, coated in breadcrumbs, baked	-17	(10-23)
Scampi, coated in breadcrumbs, baked	-23	(16-30)
fried	-16	(9-23)
Fish pie, white fish, retail, baked	-19	(9-28)
VEGETABLES, VEGETABLE PRODUCTS AND FRUIT		
Potatoes and potato products		
Potatoes, old, flesh only, boiled	-10	(6-18)
with skin, baked	-25	(21-32)
roasted	-33	(27-38)
wedges, with skin, baked	-41	(33-50)
with skin, microwaved	-25	(20-29)
Potatoes, new, with skin, boiled	-4	(2-9)
Potato chips, oven ready, baked	-29	(16-38)
Potato products, shaped, frozen, baked	-20	(15-23)
Potato wedges, retail, baked	-18	(15-21)
Beans and lentils		
Aduki beans, soaked and boiled	+155	
Black gram, urad gram, soaked and boiled	+208	

VEGETABLES, VEGETABLE PRODUCTS AND FRUIT *continued*

	% weight change	
	Mean	**Range**
Blackeye beans, soaked and boiled	+164	
Chick peas, whole, soaked and boiled	+163	
Lentils, green and brown, boiled	+139	
Lentils, red split, boiled	+227	
Mung beans, whole, soaked and boiled	+199	
Red kidney beans, soaked and boiled	+161	
Soya beans, soaked and boiled	+156	
Other vegetables		
Beans, green, boiled	-6	(2-11)
Broccoli, green, boiled	+12	(3-18)
steamed	+4	(2-7)
Cabbage, green, boiled	+12	(1-30)
Carrots, old, boiled	-13	(10-16)
microwaved	-20	(14-37)
Cauliflower, boiled	-3	(-6 to +2)
Mushrooms, white, stewed	-29	(23-37)
Mushrooms, white, fried	-9	(5-17)
Onions, boiled	-6	(2-16)
fried	-21	(14-28)
Pak choi, steamed	-5	(1-11)
Peas, frozen, microwaved	-7	(-20 to +5)
Peppers, red, boiled	-13	(10-16)
Sweetcorn, kernels, boiled on the cob	-2	(1-6)
Tomatoes, grilled	-19	(12-23)
Vegetables, canned, reheated	-5	(2-9)
Vegetable products and dishes		
Curry, vegetable, retail, reheated	-3	(1-8)
Soup, vegetable, chilled, reheated	-3	(1-7)

| | % weight change | |
	Mean	Range
Vegeburgers, baked/grilled	-12	(3-26)
fried	-6	(0-17)
Vegetarian sausages, grilled	-14	(11-16)
fried	-8	(5-10)
Fruit		
Apples, cooking, stewed	-3	(-9 to +3)

4.3.2   Calculation of cooked edible matter from raw foods

Section 4.2 shows the edible conversion factors and calculation of the nutrient content of foods weighed with waste. It is sometimes necessary to estimate the amount of cooked edible material that would be obtained from a known weight of the raw food as purchased with waste, e.g. meat with bone. This is done by multiplying the percentage weight loss on cooking with the edible conversion factor as follows:

Cooked edible matter as a proportion of raw food purchased with waste $= \dfrac{(\text{Wt. raw} \times \text{Edible conversion factor} \times (100 - \% \text{ wt. loss on cooking}))}{100}$

For example, the weight loss on grilling lamb chops is 31% and the edible proportion of grilled lamb, loin chops, lean and fat, weighed with bone is 0.81. 200g of raw lamb chops with lean, fat and bone will therefore yield:

Cooked edible matter as calculated from raw food or 'as purchased' $= \dfrac{200 \times 0.81 \times (100-31)}{100}$

$= 112\text{g}$ cooked lamb (lean and fat) to eat

4.3.3   Calculation of the composition of dishes prepared from recipes

The composition of cooked dishes in this book has been calculated, as in previous editions, from the recipes listed in Section 4.4, based on the composition of the ingredients, the changes in weight on cooking and the vitamin losses on cooking.

The change in weight on cooking is usually due only to the evaporation of water or to its gain by absorption. The composition of dishes where the method of preparation also involves a change in fat content cannot be calculated directly in this way. In these cases the cooked dishes were either analysed for fat and water before the calculations were made or the weight change corrected for fat uptake measured after preparation.

The method of calculation was as follows. The weights of the raw ingredients were used to calculate the total amounts of nutrients in the raw dish. A correction to allow for any wastage due to ingredients left on utensils and in the vessels used in preparation was made at this stage. The weight of the raw dish was then measured, using a scale accurate to approximately 1g. The dish was then cooked as specified and re-weighed (a minor correction to allow for the difference between weighing the dish hot and at room temperature is not usually necessary). Where the difference in weight was accounted for by water alone, the nutrient composition and the water content of the cooked dish were calculated as follows:

$$\text{Nutrient content of cooked dish per 100 grams} = \frac{\text{Total nutrient content of raw ingredients}}{\text{Weight of cooked dish}} \times 100$$

$$\text{Water content of cooked dish per 100 grams} = \frac{\text{Water in raw ingredients} - \text{weight loss on cooking}}{\text{Weight of cooked dish}} \times 100$$

Weight loss on cooking is calculated as shown in section 4.3.1.

An example of this calculation is shown below.

Cheese sauce made with semi-skimmed milk

Ingredient		Amount in recipe g	Water g	Protein g	Fat g	Carbo-hydrate g
Milk, semi-skimmed (350ml)		362	323.6	12.7	6.2	17.0
Cheddar cheese		75	27.5	19.1	26.2	0.1
Flour		25	2.9	2.3	0.4	20.2
Butter		25	3.7	0.2	20.6	0.2
Total in recipe (a)		487	357.7	34.3	53.4	37.5
Weight of cooked dish (b)		413				
Weight loss on cooking (c)	= a-b	74				
% weight loss on cooking (d)	= c/a x 100	15.2				
Nutrient content of cooked dish (per 100g) (e)	= a/b x 100			8.3	12.9	9.1
Water content of cooked dish (per 100g) (f)	= $\frac{a-c}{b}$ x100		68.7			

If a recipe is to be calculated from the ingredients, but the weight of the cooked dish is not known, this may be estimated by using the % weight change from a similar recipe as follows (provided that all the weight change can be attributed to water):

$$\text{Weight of cooked dish} = \frac{\text{Weight of raw ingredients} \times (100 - \% \text{ weight loss of similar dish})}{100}$$

521

For recipes which gain weight on cooking, for example dumplings:

$$\text{Weight of cooked dish} = \frac{\text{Weight of raw ingredients} \times (100 + \% \text{ weight gain of similar dish})}{100}$$

4.3.4 Vitamin loss estimation in foods and recipe calculations

The losses of heat and water-labile vitamins in cooked recipe dishes were estimated by assigning a set of factors for percentage vitamin losses to each ingredient in the recipe, according to its food group and the method of cooking. Vitamin losses were not assigned to minor ingredients such as herbs, spices and salt. The percentage vitamin losses used for each food group and cooking method are shown in the tables below. Estimated losses for vitamins and other micronutrients have also been published elsewhere (Bergstöm, 1999, Bognár & Piekarski, 2000)[82,83]. The estimated losses applied are subject to considerable variation, depending on the ingredients and preparation methods used, and are applied to estimate typical losses that may occur. The values in the tables should be treated as guidelines only, and for more accurate information the foods or composite dish should be analysed.

Cereals: typical percentage losses of vitamins on cooking

	% vitamin losses	
	Boiling	Baking
Thiamin	40	25[a]
Riboflavin	40	15
Niacin	40	5
Vitamin B$_6$	40	25
Folate	50	50
Pantothenate	40	25
Biotin	40	0

[a] 15% in bread-making and toasting

Milk: typical percentage losses of vitamins on cooking

	% vitamin losses		
	Boiling[a]	Sauces[b]	Baked dishes
Vitamin E	20	(20)	ND
Thiamin	10	20	25
Riboflavin	10	(10)	15
Niacin	(0)	(0)	5
Vitamin B$_6$	10	20	25
Vitamin B$_{12}$	5	(5)	ND
Folate	20	50	50
Pantothenate	10	20	25
Vitamin C	50	50	ND

[a] In milk-based drinks, custards, etc.
ND = Not determined

[b] For example, for cheese sauce
Values in brackets are estimates

Eggs: typical percentage losses of vitamins on cooking

	% vitamin losses		
	Scrambled	Omelette	Baked dishes
Thiamin	5	5	15
Riboflavin	20	20	15
Niacin	5	5	5
Vitamin B$_6$	15	15	25
Folate	30	30	50
Pantothenate	15	15	25

Meats: typical percentage losses of vitamins on cooking

	% vitamin losses	
	Meat, grilled or fried	Meat dishes[a]
Vitamin A	0	0
Vitamin E	20	20
Thiamin	20	20
Riboflavin	20	20
Niacin	20	20
Vitamin B$_6$	20	20
Vitamin B$_{12}$	20	20
Folate	ND[b]	50
Pantothenate	20	20
Biotin	10	10
Vitamin C	ND[b]	50

[a] Some vitamins are lost on heating but the vitamins (and minerals and fat) that leach into the liquid during cooking will not be lost if the sauce or the gravy is eaten as part of the dish. On average therefore, the losses in meat dishes are no higher than from grilled or fried meat even though the cooking times are longer.
[b] The amounts of folate and vitamin C in meat are too low to make meaningful calculations of losses.
ND = Not determined

Fish: typical percentage losses of vitamins on cooking[a]

	% vitamin losses			
	Poaching	Baking	Grilling	Frying
Vitamin A	0	0	0	0
Vitamin D	0	0	0	0
Vitamin E	0	0	0	0
Thiamin	10	30	10	20
Riboflavin	0	20	10	20
Niacin	10	20	10	20
Vitamin B$_6$	0	10	10	20
Vitamin B$_{12}$	0	10	0	0
Folate	0	20	0	0
Pantothenate	20	20	5	20
Biotin	10	10	0	10

[a] Apart from grilling, the losses are mainly based on those found on cooking cod.

Vegetables: typical percentage losses of vitamins on cooking

	% vitamin losses		
	Boiling	Frying	Cooked dishes
Carotene	ND	ND	0
Vitamin E	0	0	0
Thiamin	35	20	20
Riboflavin	20	0	20
Niacin	30	0	20
Vitamin B_6	40	25	20
Folate	40	55	50
Pantothenate	ND	ND	20
Biotin	ND	ND	20
Vitamin C	45	30	50

ND = Not determined

Fruit: typical percentage losses of vitamins on stewing

	% vitamin losses
Carotene	(0)
Thiamin	25
Riboflavin	25
Niacin	25
Vitamin B_6	20
Folate	80
Pantothenate	25
Biotin	25
Vitamin C	25

Values in brackets are estimates

4.4 RECIPES

All recipes in these tables that were previously published in the sixth edition or in a supplement have been recalculated using updated ingredient composition and standard portion sizes. Previous publications have included added salt in recipes but most recipes in this edition do not include added salt, in line with government health policy recommendations and changing trends in consumer preparation.

Where a recipe source indicated a portion, but not the quantity of an ingredient, the portion size was taken from Food Portion Sizes (FSA, 2002)[127] or weighed during recipe testing.

Portion sizes

Baking powder	1 level tsp = 3.5g
Curry paste	1 tbsp = 15g
Egg	50g
Egg white	32g
Egg yolk	18g
Flour	1 level tbsp = 20g, heaped = 30g
	1 level tsp = 3g
Garlic	1 clove = 4g
Herbs, dried	1 tsp = 1g
Milk	1 tbsp = 15g
Mustard powder	1 level tsp = 3g
Ground black pepper	1 level tsp = 2g
Soy sauce	1 tbsp = 15g
Spices, dried	1 tsp = 3g
Tomato puree	1 tbsp = 15g
Sugar	1 level tsp = 4g
Vegetable oil	1 tbsp = 11g
	1 tsp = 3g
Yeast extract	1 level tsp = 9g

The amounts of lemon juice, milk, double cream, stock, vinegar, water, wine, sherry and brandy are given in millilitres but for milk and wine, the millilitre measures were converted to gram weights (using specific gravity) for the purposes of recipe calculation. Stock was made up using 6g stock cube to 190ml water.

Quantities have not been included for recipes obtained in confidence from manufacturers.

For a number of recipes obtained from dietary survey records only the major ingredients were recorded. These recipes do not contain a measure for salt, spices or other 'lesser' ingredients and these were not therefore, included in the recipe calculation.

Unless specified, all the recipe items used were raw. Semi-skimmed pasteurised milk, cheddar cheese, dairy vanilla ice cream, plain white flour and distilled water were used. The bacon was without rind, the carrots, onions, potatoes and root ginger were peeled, the chilli peppers were deseeded, and except where otherwise specified, the turkey and chicken were skinless and boneless, and the beef, lamb and pork included both lean and fat.

Where canned fruit were used as ingredients, the nutrient composition was an average of the fruit canned in syrup and juice. Where canned tomatoes were used, the nutrient composition included the juice as well.

The type of fat used in the recipes has been specified. The vegetable oil was retail sunflower oil. Fat spread was either 41-62% fat, polyunsaturated or 62-75% fat, not polyunsaturated, depending on the recipe type. Butter was salted. For fried dishes, the fat used during frying has been included at the end of the ingredients list with the quantity absorbed shown in brackets.

The baking powder used was a proprietary preparation whose composition is listed in these tables (No. 1161). Use of another brand could result in a different composition in the cooked dish with respect to sodium, calcium and phosphorus.

19   Rice, pilau, plain, homemade

200g raw white, basmati, easy cook rice
45ml water absorbed on soaking
25g vegetable oil
½ tsp ground turmeric

90g onion, sliced
500ml boiling water
1 tsp cumin seeds

Soak the rice. Heat the oil and add cumin seeds. Add the onion and fry for 5 minutes. Reduce heat, add the remaining ingredients, cover and cook until all the water has been absorbed and the rice is soft.

Weight loss: 17%

32   Risotto, plain, homemade

224g risotto (Italian Arborio) rice
550ml beef stock
½ tsp ground black pepper

2 tbsp vegetable oil
84g onion, chopped

Heat the oil, add the onion and fry until soft. Add the washed rice and stir over a low heat for 10 minutes. Pour in the stock, bring to the boil and simmer until all the stock is absorbed and add the seasoning.

Weight loss: 37%

33   Macaroni cheese, homemade

280g cooked macaroni
350ml semi-skimmed milk
25g fat spread (62-75%) not polyunsaturated

25g flour
100g cheese, grated

Boil the macaroni and drain well. Make a white sauce from the fat spread, flour and milk. Add 75g of the cheese, add the macaroni and put in a pie dish. Sprinkle with the remaining cheese and brown under grill or in a hot oven at 220°C/mark 7.

Weight loss: 9.4%

83   Sandwich, white bread, bacon, lettuce and tomato

86g white sliced bread
29g grilled back bacon
20g tomato, sliced

16g lettuce, chopped
11g mayonnaise
7g fat spread (41-62%) polyunsaturated

Average weights from University of North London survey of commercial sandwiches (1997)[58]

84   Sandwich, white bread, cheddar cheese and pickle

75g white sliced bread
43g cheese, sliced

16g sweet pickle
7g fat spread (41-62%) polyunsaturated

Average weights from University of North London survey of commercial sandwiches (1997)[58]

85   Sandwich, white bread, chicken salad

89g white sliced bread
46g roasted chicken, sliced
20g tomato, sliced

12g lettuce, chopped
12g cucumber, sliced
7g fat spread (41-62%) polyunsaturated

Average weights from University of North London survey of commercial sandwiches (1997)[58]

86 Sandwich, white bread, egg mayonnaise

94g white sliced bread
42g boiled egg, sliced

10g mayonnaise
7g fat spread (41-62%) polyunsaturated

Average weights from University of North London survey of commercial sandwiches (1997)[58]

87 Sandwich, white bread, ham salad

88g white sliced bread
35g ham
17g tomato, sliced

11g lettuce, chopped
9g cucumber, sliced
7g fat spread (41-62%) polyunsaturated

Average weights from University of North London survey of commercial sandwiches (1997)[58]

88 Sandwich, white bread, tuna mayonnaise

93g white sliced bread
56g tuna, canned in brine, drained

15g mayonnaise
7g fat spread (41-62%) polyunsaturated

Average weights from University of North London survey of commercial sandwiches (1997)[58]

152 Crispie cakes, homemade

112g plain chocolate
33g crisp rice cereal
33g corn flake type cereal

Melt the chocolate in a bowl over hot water. Stir in the cereals. Place in cases and allow to cool and set.

155 Fruit cake, rich, iced, homemade

750g mixed fruit
250g flour
200g butter
200g brown sugar
150g mixed glacé fruit, chopped

4 eggs
20g black treacle
20ml brandy
1 tsp mixed spice

Cream the butter and sugar. Beat the eggs, treacle and brandy. Fold in the sifted flour and spices and mix in the fruit. Turn into a 20cm cake tin. Bake for 4 hours at 150°C/mark 2.

Weight loss: 5%

Royal icing:

70g apricot jam
410g marzipan
300g icing sugar

1 egg white
5ml lemon juice

When the fruit cake is cold, spread with a thin layer of apricot jam and cover with marzipan. Make the icing by beating the egg whites and icing sugar; finally add the lemon juice.

163   Sponge cake, homemade

150g self raising flour
1 tsp baking powder
150g butter

150g caster sugar
3 eggs

Cream the butter and sugar until light and fluffy. Add the beaten egg a little at a time and beat well. Fold in the sifted flour and baking powder. Bake for about 20 minutes at 190°C/mark 5.

Weight loss: 12.9%

164   Sponge cake, fatless, homemade

4 eggs
100g caster sugar
100g flour

Whisk the eggs and sugar in a basin over hot water until stiff. Fold in the flour. Bake for 25 minutes at 190°C/mark 5.

Weight loss: 13.8%

175   Shortcrust pastry, cooked, homemade

200g flour
30ml water

100g butter

Rub the butter into the flour, mix to a stiff dough with the water. Combine the pastry and cheese, roll out and bake at 200°C/mark 6.

Weight loss: 13.8%

176 Wholemeal pastry, cooked, homemade

200g wholemeal flour
100g butter

30ml water

Rub the butter into the flour, mix to a stiff dough with the water, roll out and bake at 220°C/mark 7.

Weight loss: 13.6%

191 Scones, plain, homemade

200g flour
125ml semi-skimmed milk
50g fat spread (62-75%) not polyunsaturated

4 tsp baking powder
10g sugar

Sift the flour, sugar and baking powder and rub in the fat spread. Mix in the milk. Roll out and cut into rounds. Bake in a hot oven at 220°C/mark 7 for about 10 minutes.

Weight loss: 18.5%

196 Crumble, fruit, wholemeal, homemade

400g prepared fruit (equal proportions of apple, gooseberry, plum, rhubarb)
100g wholemeal flour
50g butter
100g sugar

Prepare the fruit. Arrange in a dish and sprinkle with sugar. Rub together the other ingredients and pile on top. Bake for 40 minutes at 190°C/mark 5.

Weight loss: 7.4%

198 Fruit pie, one crust, homemade

200g raw shortcrust pastry (retail)
450g prepared raw fruit (equal proportions of apple, gooseberry, plum, rhubarb)
80g sugar

Mix the fruit and sugar, place in a pie dish and cover with pastry. Bake for 10 - 15 minutes at 200°C/mark 6 to set the pastry, then bake for approximately 20 minutes at 180°C/mark 4 to cook the fruit.

Weight loss: 4.2%

199 Fruit pie, pastry top and bottom, homemade

450g raw shortcrust pastry (retail)
450g prepared raw fruit (equal proportions of apple, gooseberry, plum, rhubarb)
80g sugar

Line a pie dish with half the pastry. Fill with the prepared fruit and sugar and cover with the remaining pastry. Bake for 10 - 15 minutes at 220°C/mark 7 to set the pastry, then bake for approximately 20 - 30 minutes at 180°C/mark 4 to cook the fruit.

Weight loss: 4.2%

204 Dumplings, homemade

100g flour   1 tsp baking powder
45g suet   75g water

Mix the dry ingredients together with the cold water to form a dough. Divide into balls, flour them and place in boiling water. Boil for 30 minutes.

Weight gain: + 52.7%

205 Pancakes, savoury, made with semi-skimmed milk, homemade

112g flour   2 tbsp vegetable oil
1 egg
300ml semi-skimmed milk

Sieve the flour into a bowl, add the egg and about 100ml of the milk, stirring until smooth. Add the rest of the milk and beat to a smooth batter. Heat a little of the oil in a frying pan and pour in enough batter to cover the bottom. Cook both sides. Repeat until all the batter is used, to give about 10 pancakes.

Weight loss: 20%

210 Stuffing, sage and onion, homemade

224g onion
112g white breadcrumbs
4g fresh sage, chopped
56g fat spread (62-75%) not polyunsaturated

¼ tsp ground black pepper
1 egg

Parboil the onions, drain and chop, mix with the breadcrumbs and add the sage. Soften the fat spread and add to the stuffing. Mix thoroughly. Stir in the egg and seasoning.

Weight loss: 19.0%

211 Yorkshire pudding, made with semi-skimmed milk, homemade

100g flour
1 egg
250ml semi-skimmed milk

20g vegetable oil

Sieve the flour into a bowl. Break in the egg and add about 100ml milk, stirring until smooth. Add the rest of the milk and beat to a smooth batter. Pour into a tin containing the hot oil. Bake for about 40mins at 220°C/mark 7.

Weight loss: 16%

300 Chocolate nut sundae

115g ice cream
45ml double cream
70g chocolate ice cream topping, retail

6g chopped nuts
wafer

Cover the ice cream with the whipped cream and chocolate sauce. Sprinkle with nuts.

316 Custard, made up with semi-skimmed milk

500ml semi-skimmed milk
25g custard powder
25g sugar

Blend the custard powder with a little of the milk. Add the sugar to the remainder of the milk and bring to the boil. Pour immediately over the paste, stirring all the time. Return to the pan and bring back to boiling point while stirring until it begins to thicken.

Weight loss: 20.9%

320 **Meringue, homemade**

4 egg whites   200g caster sugar

Whisk the egg whites until stiff. Fold in the sugar. Pipe onto baking sheet
and bake at 130°C/mark ½ for 3 hours.

Weight loss: 33.3%

328 **Rice pudding, made with semi-skimmed milk, homemade**

500ml semi-skimmed milk   50g pudding rice
25g sugar   15g butter
1g nutmeg

Simmer until cooked or bake in a moderate oven at 180°C/mark 4.

Weight loss: 19.1%

340 **Eggs, chicken, scrambled, with semi-skimmed milk**

2 eggs   20g butter
15ml semi-skimmed milk   ½ tsp ground black
                                                    pepper

Melt the butter in pan, stir in the beaten egg, milk and seasoning. Cook over
a gentle heat until the mixture thickens.

Weight loss: 10.9%

341 **Omelette, plain**

2 eggs   10ml water
10g vegetable oil

Beat the eggs with the water. Heat the oil in an omelette pan. Pour in the
mixture and stir until it begins to thicken evenly. While still creamy, fold the
omelette and serve.

Weight loss: 5.7%

342   Omelette, cheese

115g omelette, cooked
60g cheese, grated

Proportions are derived from a recipe review.

343   Quiche, cheese and egg, homemade

200g raw plain shortcrust pastry (retail)   3 eggs
150g cheese, grated
150g semi-skimmed milk

Line a 20cm flan ring with the shortcrust pastry. Fill with the grated cheese. Beat the eggs in the warmed milk and pour into the pastry case. Bake for 10 minutes at 200°C/mark 6 and then 30 minutes at 180°C/mark 4.

Weight loss: 10%

344   Quiche, cheese and egg, wholemeal, homemade

Recipe as for 343, substituting plain shortcrust pastry for homemade wholemeal shortcrust pastry

539   Steak and kidney pie, single crust, homemade

400g stewing beef, diced   15g flour
200g lamb's kidneys, diced   100ml water
350g flaky/puff pastry (retail)

Place the meat and kidneys rolled in flour in a pie dish with the water. Cover with pastry. Bake for 20 minutes at 200°C/mark 6 then lower the heat to 150°C/mark 2 and cover with greaseproof paper. Cook for a further 2-2½ hours.

Weight loss: 21%

541   Beef bourguignon, homemade

1 tbsp vegetable oil   5g tomato purée
100g onions, chopped   1 tsp dried mixed
1 clove garlic, crushed   herbs
500g stewing beef, diced   250ml red wine
50g streaky bacon rashers, chopped   250ml beef stock
15g flour   150g mushrooms,
¼ tsp ground black pepper   sliced

Brown the onions, garlic, meat and bacon in oil. Stir in the flour, tomato purée, mixed herbs, wine, stock and seasoning. Bring to the boil, cover and simmer for 1 hour, stirring occasionally. Add the mushrooms and cook for a further 30 minutes.

Weight loss: 33%

542   Beef casserole, made with cook-in sauce

500g braising steak, diced   390g tomato-based
                                                 cook-in sauce

Cook the meat with sauce in a covered casserole dish for 1½ hours at 180°C/mark 4.

Weight loss: 20%

546   Beef curry, reduced fat, homemade

1 clove garlic, crushed   ½ tsp ground turmeric
60g onions, chopped   8g root ginger, ground
500g lean braising steak, diced   300ml water
1 tbsp vegetable oil   5ml lemon juice
1 tbsp ground coriander   1 tsp garam masala
1 tsp chilli powder   ½ tsp ground cumin

Brown the garlic, onions and meat in oil. Add the spices and ginger. Stir in the water and lemon juice, cover and bring to the boil. Cook for 1½ hours stirring occasionally. Add the garam masala.

Weight loss: 34%

547   Beef stew, homemade

500g stewing beef, diced   500ml beef stock
150g onions, chopped   150g carrots, chopped
1 tbsp vegetable oil   30g flour
¼ tsp ground black pepper

Brown the meat and onions in oil, add the flour and cook for 1 minute. Blend in the stock, add the carrots and seasoning, transfer to a dish, cover and cook in the oven for 2 hours at 180°C/mark 4.

Weight loss: 27%

548 Beef, stir-fried with green peppers, homemade

500g rump steak, thinly sliced
2 tbsp vegetable oil
400g green peppers, sliced
60g spring onions, sliced
20g root ginger, grated

Marinade:
4 tsp sugar
1 red chilli, finely chopped
2 tbsp soy sauce

30ml sherry
20g cornflour
¼ tsp ground black pepper

Marinade the steak for 30 minutes. Stir-fry the peppers, spring onions and ginger in oil for a few minutes, then add the meat and stir-fry for 6 minutes.

Weight loss: 16%

549 Bolognese sauce (with meat), homemade

1 clove garlic, crushed
60g onions, chopped
500g minced beef
40g carrots, chopped
10g tomato pureé
¼ tsp dried mixed herbs

397g canned tomatoes
250ml beef stock
2 tsp vegetable oil
30g celery, chopped
¼ tsp ground black pepper

Brown the garlic, onions and mince in oil, add the carrots and celery. Stir in the other ingredients and simmer for 40 minutes with the lid on.

Weight loss: 32%

550 Bolognese sauce (with meat), homemade, with extra lean minced beef

Recipe as for 549, substituting minced beef for extra lean minced beef.

557 Chicken curry, made with cook-in sauce

1 tbsp vegetable oil
500g chicken breast

385g cook-in curry sauce

Brown the chicken in the oil. Add the sauce, cover and simmer for 45 minutes.

Weight loss: 30%

565   Chilli con carne, homemade

500g minced beef
150g onions, chopped
100g green peppers, chopped
1 tbsp vegetable oil
150ml beef stock
¼ tsp ground black pepper
2 tsp chilli powder

15ml vinegar
1 tsp sugar
30g tomato purée
397g canned tomatoes
115g red kidney beans, canned, drained

Brown the mince, onions and peppers in oil. Blend the other ingredients and stir into the meat. Cover and simmer gently for 40 minutes. Add the kidney beans and continue cooking for a further 10 minutes.

Weight loss: 15%

567   Coq au vin, homemade

100g back bacon rashers, chopped
1000g chicken leg quarters (weighed with bone)
50g butter
50g flour
1 tsp dried mixed herbs
100g mushrooms, sliced

¼ tsp ground black pepper
100g shallots, chopped
600ml red wine

Brown the bacon and chicken coated in flour, in butter. Add the shallots, mixed herbs and red wine, cover and simmer for 35-45 minutes. Add the mushrooms and cook for another 20 minutes.

Weight loss: 16% (with bone), 19% (without bone).

568   Coronation chicken, homemade

500g cooked light and dark chicken meat, diced
300g mayonnaise
1 tbsp curry paste
2 tbsp apricot jam

Mix the ingredients together.

573 Irish stew, homemade

500g lamb neck fillet, diced
150g onions, sliced
200g carrots, sliced
300ml beef stock
¼ tsp ground black pepper

1 tsp dried mixed
herbs
15g flour
500g potatoes, sliced
3g fresh parsley,
chopped

Make layers of meat, vegetables, herbs, flour and seasoning in a casserole dish, ending with a top layer of potatoes. Pour in the stock and cover. Bake for 1 hour at 170°C/mark 3, remove lid and cook for a further 30 minutes.

Weight loss: 13%

574 Lamb curry, made with cook-in sauce

500g stewing lamb, diced
1 tbsp vegetable oil

385g cook-in curry
sauce

Brown the lamb in oil. Add the sauce, cover and simmer for 45 minutes.

Weight loss: 30%

575 Lamb kheema, homemade

6 tbsp vegetable oil
75g onions, finely chopped
2 garlic cloves, crushed
500g minced lamb
8g root ginger, grated
220g canned tomatoes
2 green chillies, deseeded, finely chopped
1 tsp ground cumin

1 tsp cayenne pepper
200ml water
200g peas, frozen
2 tbsp fresh coriander
leaves, chopped
2 tsp garam masala
1 tsp coriander seeds,
crushed

Brown the onions, garlic and mince in oil. Add the ginger and spices. Stir in 150ml of the water, cover and simmer for 30 minutes. Add the remaining ingredients and bring back to the boil. Cover and cook for a further 10 minutes.

Weight loss: 21%

578 Lasagne, homemade

Meat sauce:
1 tbsp vegetable oil
50g onions, chopped
50g carrots, chopped
30g celery, chopped
300g minced beef
220g canned tomatoes
375ml beef stock
1 clove garlic, crushed
¼ tsp ground black pepper
½ tsp dried marjoram
1 bay leaf
50g mushrooms, sliced

Cheese sauce:
30g fat spread (62-75%) not polyunsaturated
30g flour
400ml semi-skimmed milk
75g cheese, grated

200g lasagne, raw

To top:
25g cheese, grated

Brown the onions, carrots, celery and mince in the oil. Stir in the remaining ingredients for the meat sauce and simmer for 15 minutes. For the cheese sauce, melt the fat spread, add flour and cook for a few minutes, stir in the milk and cheese and cook gently until mixture thickens. In a dish, add alternative layers of lasagne, meat and cheese sauce ending with a layer of lasagne and cheese sauce. Sprinkle with cheese and bake for 1 hour at 190°C/mark 5.

Weight loss: 26%

579 Lasagne, homemade with extra lean minced beef

As for 578, substituting minced beef for extra lean minced beef.

581 Pasta with meat and tomato sauce, homemade

340g minced beef
900g boiled pasta

475g pasta sauce, tomato-based

Brown the mince in a pan. Add the pasta sauce and simmer for 20 minutes. Stir in the pasta.

Weight loss: 17%

582 Pork casserole, made with cook-in sauce

675g pork steaks

390g cook-in sauce, tomato based

Pour the sauce over the pork steaks and cook in a covered casserole dish for 1½ hours at 180°C/mark 4.

Weight loss: 20%

584 Sausage casserole, homemade

400g diced pork
150g onions, chopped
200g streaky bacon rashers, chopped
1 tbsp vegetable oil
227g baked beans, in tomato sauce, canned
200g pork sausage, chopped

1 bay leaf
1 tsp dried mixed herbs
300ml beef stock
¼ tsp ground black pepper

Brown the pork, sausage, onions and bacon in the oil, add the remaining ingredients and bake, uncovered, for 1½ hours at 170°C/mark 3.

Weight loss: 15%

590 Sweet and sour pork, homemade

400g diced pork

Marinade:
1 tbsp soy sauce
30ml sherry
½ tsp sugar

Batter:
20g cornflour
1 tbsp water
½ egg
vegetable oil (16g)

Sauce:
1 tbsp vegetable oil
1 clove garlic, crushed
7g root ginger, grated
100g onions, chopped
75g green peppers, sliced
75g red peppers, sliced
30g sugar
30ml vinegar
5g cornflour
1 tbsp soy sauce
15ml sherry
1 tbsp tomato purée
5 tbsp water

Marinade the pork for 1 hour. Coat the pork with the batter ingredients and deep-fry for 4 minutes. For the sauce, stir-fry the garlic, ginger and onions in oil, add the remaining ingredients and cook until thickened. Add the pork, stir and heat through.

Weight loss: 28%

654 Curry, fish, Bangladeshi, homemade

450g boal (white fish), raw
450g rohu (white fish), raw
225g onions, chopped
75g vegetable oil
300g water

2 tsp chilli powder
2 tsp ground coriander
½ tsp ground cumin
1½ tsp ground
turmeric

Cut the fish into 1 inch slices and sprinkle with some of the chilli, turmeric and coriander. Add 2 tbsp of water and mix. Heat half the oil and fry the fish for 6 to 8 minutes then remove from the pan and set aside. Fry the onions in the remaining oil until brown, add the remaining spices and the remaining water and cook for 6 minutes. Add the fish and cook for 4 to 5 minutes. Cover and cook for 10 minutes.

Weight loss: 21%

666 Kedgeree, homemade

200g smoked haddock, cooked
25g fat spread (62-75%) not polyunsaturated

100g boiled white rice
2 eggs

Hard boil the eggs. Melt the fat spread and stir in the haddock and rice. Stir in the chopped hard boiled eggs and heat thoroughly.

Weight loss: 10%

820 Casserole, vegetable, homemade

240g potato, diced
120g carrot, sliced
120g onion, diced
120g swede, diced
120g parsnip, diced
90g sweetcorn, canned, drained

90g frozen peas
90g tomatoes,
chopped
450g canned
tomatoes
1 tsp yeast extract

Place all the ingredients in a casserole dish and stir. Cover and cook for approximately 1 hour at 190°C/mark 5.

Weight loss: 15%

822 Cauliflower cheese, homemade with semi-skimmed milk

100g cheese, grated
1 small cauliflower (700g)
100ml cauliflower water

25g fat spread (62-75%) not polyunsaturated
250ml semi-skimmed milk
25g flour

Boil the cauliflower until just tender, break into florets. Drain, saving 100ml water, place in a dish and keep warm. Make a white sauce from the fat spread, flour, milk and cauliflower water. Add 75g of the cheese and season. Pour over the cauliflower and sprinkle with the remaining cheese. Brown under a grill or in a hot oven at 220°C/mark 7.

Weight loss: 15%

823 Chilli, vegetable, homemade

120g onion, chopped
440g red kidney beans, canned, drained
330g sweetcorn, canned, drained
240g parsnips, diced
180g courgette, diced
400g canned tomatoes

240g carrots, diced
120g pepper, diced
10g chilli powder
14g vegetable stock cube
568ml water

Quantities are derived from dietary survey records.

Weight loss: 15%

826 Curry, chick pea dhal, homemade

225g dry chick pea dhal
200ml water absorbed on soaking
28g vegetable oil
60g onion, chopped
2g garlic, crushed

1 tsp chilli powder
½ tsp garam masala
7g green chilli, chopped
100g tomato, chopped
415ml water

Soak the chick pea dhal overnight. Fry the onion and garlic until brown. Add a little water together with the spices and tomatoes. Stir and cook until dry. Add the dhal and water, simmer until cooked.

Weight loss: 35%

829 Garlic mushrooms, not coated, homemade

250g mushrooms
2g garlic
40g butter

Clean the mushrooms and remove the stems. Crush the garlic and sauté in butter. Fill the mushroom caps with the garlic butter mixture and grill for 5-7 minutes.

Weight loss: 19%

834 Nut roast, homemade

90g onion, chopped
1 tbsp vegetable oil
20g flour
140ml water
225g chopped mixed nuts

115g wholemeal breadcrumbs
1 tsp yeast extract
1 tsp dried mixed herbs

Fry the onion in the oil. Add the flour and water and thicken. Mix in the nuts, breadcrumbs, yeast extract and herbs. Pack into a loaf tin and cover with foil. Bake at 190°C/mark 5 for 35-45 minutes.

Weight loss: 13%

836 Pancakes, stuffed with vegetables, homemade

320g prepared pancakes

Filling:
50g mushrooms, chopped
200g canned tomatoes

90g onion, chopped
1 tsp dried mixed herbs

Prepare the filling by cooking all the ingredients for approximately 15 minutes. Fill and roll up the pancakes. Place under a grill to reheat if necessary.

Weight loss: 20% for filling

837 Pasty, vegetable, homemade

50% cooked shortcrust pastry
15% potato, boiled, diced
7.5% water
6.3% carrot, boiled, diced
6.3% parsnip, boiled, diced

6.3% onion, boiled, diced
6.3% cabbage, boiled, chopped
2.5% flour

Proportions are derived from dietary survey records.

840 Ratatouille, homemade

150g onion, chopped
5g garlic, crushed
65g vegetable oil
420g aubergine, sliced
230g courgettes, sliced

135g green pepper, sliced
255g tomatoes, skinned, chopped

Fry the onion and garlic in the oil until soft. Add the remaining vegetables, stir and cover. Simmer gently for 50 minutes until tender.

Weight loss: 22%

841 Salad, green

150g lettuce, shredded
230g cucumber, sliced
30g celery, sliced

160g green pepper, sliced

Toss all the ingredients together.

843 Salad, rice, homemade

720g boiled white rice
240g spring onion, chopped
90g sweetcorn, canned, drained
60g cashew nuts

60g raisins
40g soy sauce
60g vegetable oil
80g green pepper, diced

Quantities are derived from dietary survey records.

850   Vegetable bake, homemade

210g carrots, chopped
120g courgettes, chopped
120g onions, chopped
210g potatoes, diced
45g fat spread (62-75%) not polyunsaturated
60g Leicester cheese, grated

30g flour
426ml semi-skimmed milk
½ tsp mustard powder
45g white breadcrumbs

Quantities are derived from dietary survey records.

Weight loss: 15%

851   Vegetable pie, homemade

100g onion, chopped
100g carrot, sliced
100g courgettes, sliced
60g celery, chopped
50g mushrooms, sliced
80g red pepper, diced
100g potatoes, diced
200g canned tomatoes

100ml water
2 tsp cornflour
1 tsp dried mixed herbs
1 tsp yeast extract
300g raw shortcrust pastry

Place the vegetables in a pan, together with the herbs and yeast extract. Bring to the boil and simmer for 20-25 minutes. Make the cornflour into a paste, add to the pan, boil and stir until the mixture thickens. Pour into a pie dish and leave to cool. Roll the pastry to fit dish size. Cut an additional 1 inch strip from the remaining pastry, wet and place around the edge of the dish. Cover with the pastry top and seal the edges. Bake at 200°C/mark 6 for 30-40 minutes.

Weight loss: 15%

898   Fruit salad, homemade

400g eating apples, sliced
120g kiwi fruit, sliced
320g oranges, sliced

110g grapes, halved
200g banana, sliced
110g strawberries, sliced

Syrup:
57g caster sugar
40ml lemon juice

114ml water

Dissolve the sugar in the water over a low heat. Bring to the boil and simmer for a minute, then remove from the heat and allow to cool. Prepare the fruit and sprinkle with the lemon juice. Mix the fruit with the cool syrup and refrigerate.

999   Fudge, homemade

450g granulated sugar
175ml evaporated milk
150ml semi-skimmed milk

75g butter
few drops of vanilla essence

Dissolve the sugar in the milks over a low heat and add the butter. Bring to the boil and boil gently to 125°C. Remove from the heat, add the vanilla essence. Beat the mixture until thick and grainy. Pour into a tin and cut into squares when almost set.

Weight loss: 28%

1112   Vegetable soup, homemade

100g carrots, chopped
100g onion, chopped
60g leeks, chopped
60g potatoes, chopped
50g celery, chopped

50g butter
700ml vegetable stock
50g peas
60g turnip, chopped
½ tsp ground black pepper

Fry the chopped vegetables in butter until soft. Add the stock, peas and seasoning and simmer for 30 minutes.

Weight loss: 12%

1113   Bread sauce, homemade with semi-skimmed milk

250ml semi-skimmed milk
50g fresh breadcrumbs

90g onion
5g butter

Put the milk and onion in a saucepan and bring to the boil. Add the breadcrumbs, and simmer for about 20 minutes over gentle heat. Remove the onion and stir in the butter.

Weight loss: 6.8%

1114 Cheese sauce, homemade with semi-skimmed milk

350ml semi-skimmed milk
75g cheese, grated

25g flour
25g butter

Melt the butter in a pan, add the flour and cook gently for a few minutes stirring all the time. Add the milk and cook until the mixture thickens, stirring continually. Add the grated cheese. Reheat to soften the cheese, serve immediately.

Weight loss: 15.2%

1115 Cheese sauce, packet mix, made up with semi-skimmed milk

1 packet cheese sauce mix (40g)
309ml semi-skimmed milk

Prepared as packet directions.

Weight loss: 9.1%

1116 White sauce, savoury, homemade with semi-skimmed milk

350ml semi-skimmed milk
25g flour

25g butter

Melt the butter in a pan. Add the flour and cook for a few minutes stirring constantly. Add milk, and cook gently until the mixture thickens.

Weight loss: 18.1%

1131 Tzatziki, homemade

250g Greek style yogurt
5g fresh garlic, crushed

213g cucumber, chopped
fresh mint, chopped

Recipe from yogurt manufacturers.

4.5 ALTERNATIVE AND TAXONOMIC NAMES

- Foods are listed below by food group.
- The alternative names listed in the left-hand column below are those that were most frequently encountered during data collection and are included to help in identifying foods. It is important to recognise that in some cases such names may be used for more than one food and that all such usages may not appear in this list.
- To see if a name is listed, the food index should be consulted first. If the term is included as an alternative name, a cross reference entry indicates the food name to which it refers. This allows all alternatives to be listed together.
- Taxonomic names listed in the right-hand column refer as specifically as possible to the varieties and species likely to be consumed in the UK. These are included to help users identify foods. However, the list is not comprehensive and users are advised to refer to the scientific literature for authoritative information on classification.
- The abbreviation 'var' is used to indicate the specific variety or unspecified variety(ies); 'sp' and 'spp' are used to indicate that one or more than one species of the specified Genus is included.

	Alternative names	Food names	Taxonomic names
Cereals			
		Oats	*Avena sativa*
		Rye	*Secale cereale*
		Wheat	*Triticum aestivum*
		Rice	*Oryza sativa*
	Durum wheat	Pasta wheat	*Triticum durum*
Meat			
		Beef	*Bos taurus*
		Lamb	*Ovis aries*
		Pork	*Sus scrofa*
		Veal	*Bos taurus*
Poultry			
		Chicken	*Gallus domesticus*
		Turkey	*Meleagris gallopavo*
		Duck	*Anas platyrhynchos*
		Goose	*Anser anser*
		Pheasant	*Phasianus colchicus*
Game			
		Rabbit	*Oryctolagus cuniculus*
		Venison	*Cervus spp*
Fish			
	White fish		
		Cod	*Gadus morhua*
	Coalfish Saithe	Coley	*Pollachius virens*
		Haddock	*Melanogrammus aeglefinus*

Alternative names	Food names	Taxonomic names
	Lemon sole	*Microstomus kitt*
Basa River cobbler Panga	**Pangasius**	*Pangasius hypophthalmus*
	Plaice	*Pleuronectes platessa*
Alaska pollack Pacific pollack Pacific pollock	**Pollock, Alaska**	*Theragra chalcogramma*
Bass	**Sea bass**	*Dicentrarchus labrax*
Fatty fish		
	Anchovies	All species of the family *Engraulidae*
Kipper	**Herring**	*Clupea harengus*
	Mackerel	All species of *Scomber*
	Salmon, Atlantic red	*Salmo salar* *Oncorhynchus nerka*
	Sardines	*Sardina pilchardus*
	Trout, rainbow	*Oncorhynchus mykiss*
	Tuna	All species of *Thunnus*
Crustacea		
	Crab	All species of the order *Brachyura* All species of the family *Lithodidae*
	Lobster	All species of *Homarus*
Prawns, cold-water	**Prawns***	All species of the families *Aristaeidae, Palaemonidae, Pandalidae, Penaeidae* Includes *Pandalus borealis*
Prawns, warm-water	**Prawns, king***	All species of the families *Aristaeidae, Palaemonidae, Penaeidae* Includes *Litopenaeus vannamei*
Langoustine Dublin Bay prawns Norway lobster	**Scampi**	*Nephrops norvegicus*
Molluscs		
	Cockles	All species of *Cerastoderma*
	Mussels	All species of the family *Mytilidae*

* The terms prawn and king prawn refer to the size of the prawn rather than specific species

Alternative names	Food names	Taxonomic names
	Squid	All species of *Illex* All species of *Loligo* *Ommastrephes sagittatus*

Vegetables

Potatoes

Aloo Batata	**Potatoes**	*Solanum tuberosum*

Beans and lentils

	Baked beans	*Phaseolus vulgaris* (navy beans)
	Beansprouts, mung	*Vigna radiata*
Alad Urad	**Black gram,** urad gram	*Vigna mungo*
Blackeye peas Cowpeas Chori Lobia	**Blackeye beans**	*Vigna unguiculata*
Fava bean	**Broad beans**	*Vicia faba*
Lima beans	**Butter beans**	*Phaseolus Lunatus*
Channa Common gram Garbanzo Yellow gram	**Chick peas**	*Cicer arietinum*
Fansi	**Green beans/French beans**	*Phaseolus vulgaris*
Masoor dhal Masur dhal	**Lentils,** red	*Lens culinaris*
Green gram Golden gram Moong beans	**Mung beans**	*Vigna radiata*
	Red kidney beans	*Phaseolus vulgaris*
	Runner beans	*Phaseolus coccineus*
	Soya beans	*Glycine max*

Peas

Snowpeas	**Mange-tout peas**	*Pisum sativum var macrocarpon*
Badla Mattar Vatana	**Peas**	*Pisum sativum*

Other vegetables

	Asparagus	*Asparagus officinalis*

Alternative names	Food names	Taxonomic names
Baingan Brinjal Eggplant Jew's apple Ringana	**Aubergine**	*Solanum melongena*
	Beetroot	*Beta vulgaris*
Calabrese	**Broccoli,** green	*Brassica oleracea var italica*
Chote bund gobhi Nhanu kobi	**Brussels sprouts**	*Brassica oleracea var gemmifera*
Bund gobhi Kobi	**Cabbage**	*Brassica oleracea var capitata*
	Cabbage, white	*Brassica oleracea var capitata*
Gajjar	**Carrots**	*Daucus carota*
Pangoli Phool gobhi Gobi	**Cauliflower**	*Brassica oleracea var botrytis*
	Celery	*Apium graveolens var dulce*
Belgian chicory Witloof	**Chicory**	*Cichorium intybus*
Zucchini	**Courgette**	*Cucurbita pepo*
Kakdi Khira	**Cucumber**	*Cucumis sativus*
Borecole Kale	**Curly kale**	*Brassica oleracea var acephala*
	Fennel, Florence	*Foeniculum vulgare var dulce*
Lassan Lehsan	**Garlic**	*Allium sativum*
	Gherkins	*Cucumis sativus*
	Leeks	*Allium ampeloprasum var porrum*
	Lettuce	*Lactuca sativa*
	Mushrooms, common	*Agaricus bisporus*
	Mustard and cress	*Brassica and Lepidium spp*
Bhendi Bhinda Bhindi Gumbo Lady's fingers	**Okra**	*Hibiscus esculentus Abelmoschus esculentus*

Alternative names	Food names	Taxonomic names
Dungli Kanda Piyaz	**Onions**	*Allium cepa*
Bok choi	**Pak choi**	*Brassica rapa chinensis*
	Parsnip	*Pastinaca sativa*
Pimento	**Peppers,** capsicum, chilli, green	*Capsicum annuum*
Bell peppers Motamircha Simila mirch Sweet peppers	**Peppers,** capsicum (green/red)	*Capsicum annuum*
	Plantain	*Musa paradisiaca*
Kumra Lal kaddu Lal phupala	**Pumpkin**	*Cucurbita sp*
	Quorn, myco-protein	*Fusarium venenatum*
	Radish, red	*Raphanus sativus*
Roquette Rucola Arugula	**Rocket**	*Eruca sativa*
Palak Saag	**Spinach**	*Spinacia oleracea*
Scallion	**Spring onions**	*Allium cepa*
Neeps (England) Rutabaga Yellow turnip	**Swede**	*Brassica napus var napobrassica*
Shakaria Yam (USA)	**Sweet potato**	*Ipomoea batatas*
	Sweetcorn	*Zea mays*
	Tomatoes	*Lycopersicon esculentum* *Solanum lycopersicum*
Neeps (Scotland) Shalgam	**Turnip**	*Brassica rapa var rapifera*
	Watercress	*Nasturtium officinale*
	Yam	*Dioscorea sp*

Herbs and spices

Sweet basil Tea bush	**Basil**	*Ocimum basilicum*
	Chives	*Allium schoenoprasum*
	Cinnamon	*Cinnamomum verum* *Cinnamomum aromaticum*

	Alternative names	Food names	Taxonomic names
	Chinese parsley Cilantro Dhana	**Coriander leaves**	*Coriandrum sativum*
		Coriander seeds	*Coriandrum sativum*
	Jeera	**Cumin seeds**	*Cuminum cyminum*
		Ginger	*Zingiber officinale*
		Mint	*Mentha spicata*
		Mustard	*Sinapis alba* *Brassica hirta*
		Nutmeg	*Myristica fragrans*
		Oregano	*Origanum vulgare*
		Paprika	*Capsicum annuum*
		Parsley	*Petroselinum crispum*
		Pepper, black	*Piper nigrum*
		Pepper, white	*Piper nigrum*
		Rosemary	*Rosmarinus officinalis*
		Thyme	*Thymus vulgaris*
Fruit	Tarel	**Apples**	*Malus pumila* *Malus domestica*
		Apricots	*Prunus armeniaca*
		Avocado	*Persea americana*
	Kula	**Bananas**	*Musa spp*
		Blackberries	*Rubus fruticosus*
		Blackcurrants	*Ribes nigrum*
		Blueberries	*Vaccinium spp or* *Vaccinium corymbosum* *Vaccinium darrowii*
		Cherries	*Prunus avium*
		Clementines	*Citrus reticulata var* *Clementine*
		Dates	*Phoenix dactylifera*
	Gullar	**Figs**	*Ficus carica*
		Gooseberries	*Ribes grossularia*
		Grapefruit	*Citrus paradisi*
		Grapes	*Vitis vinifera*
	Chinese gooseberry	**Kiwi fruit**	*Actinidia deliciosa*
		Lemons	*Citrus limon*
	Chinese cherry Lichee Lichi Litchee Litchi	**Lychees**	*Litchi chinensis*

Alternative names	Food names	Taxonomic names
	Mandarin oranges	*Citrus reticulata*
	Mangoes	*Mangifera indica*
	Melon, Canteloupe-type	*Cucumis melo var cantalupensis*
	Melon, Galia	*Cucumis melo var reticulata*
	Melon, Honeydew	*Cucumis melo var inodorus*
	Nectarines	*Prunus persica var nectarina*
	Olives	*Olea europaea*
	Oranges	*Citrus sinensis*
Purple grenadillo	**Passion fruit**	*Passiflora edulis f edulis*
Papai Paw-paw	**Papaya**	*Carica papaya*
	Peaches	*Prunus persica*
	Pears	*Pyrus communis*
	Pineapple	*Ananas comosus*
	Plums	*Prunus domestica subsp domestica*
Anar Granada	**Pomegranate**	*Punica granatum*
	Prunes	*Prunus domestica*
	Raisins	*Vitis vinifera*
	Raspberries	*Rubus idaeus*
	Rhubarb	*Rheum rhaponticum*
	Satsumas	*Citrus reticulata*
	Strawberries	*Fragaria sp*
	Sultanas	*Vitis vinifera*
	Tangerines	*Citrus reticulata*

Nuts and seeds

Alternative names	Food names	Taxonomic names
Badam	**Almonds**	*Prunus amygdalus* *Prunus dulcis*
	Brazil nuts	*Bertholletia excelsa*
Kaju	**Cashew nuts**	*Anacardium occidentale*
	Chestnuts	*Castanea vulgaris* *Castanea sativa* (European/sweet chestnut)
	Coconut	*Cocos nucifera*
	Hazelnuts	*Corylus avellana* *Corylus maxima*
Queensland nuts	**Macadamia nuts**	*Macadamia integrifolia* *Macadamia tetraphylla*
Groundnuts Monkey nuts	**Peanuts**	*Arachis hypogaea*
Hickory nuts	**Pecan nuts**	*Carya illinoensis*

Alternative names	Food names	Taxonomic names
Indian nuts Pignolias Pine kernels	**Pine nuts**	*Pinus pinea* *Pinus edulis*
Pista	**Pistachio nuts**	*Pistacia vera*
	Pumpkin seeds	*Cucurbita* spp
Beniseed Gingelly Til	**Sesame seeds**	*Sesamum indicum*
	Sunflower seeds	*Helianthus annuus*
Akhrot Madeira nuts	**Walnuts**	*Juglans regia*

4.6 REFERENCES

Reference number	Publications in 'The Composition of Foods' series
1	McCance, R.A. and Widdowson, E.M. (1940) *The Chemical Composition of Foods*. His Majesty's Stationery Office, London
2	McCance, R.A. and Widdowson, E.M. (1946) *The Chemical Composition of Foods*, 2nd edition. His Majesty's Stationery Office, London
3	McCance, R.A. and Widdowson, E.M. (1960) *The Composition of Foods*, 3rd edition. Her Majesty's Stationery Office, London
4	Paul, A.A. and Southgate, D.A.T. (1978) *McCance and Widdowson's The Composition of Foods*, 4th edition. Her Majesty's Stationery Office, London
5	Paul, A.A., Southgate, D.A.T. and Russell, J. (1980) *Amino acid composition (mg per 100g food) and fatty acid composition (g per 100g food)*. First supplement to 4th edition of *McCance and Widdowson's The Composition of Foods*. HMSO, London
6	Tan, S.P., Wenlock, R.W. and Buss, D.H. (1985) *Immigrant Foods*. Second supplement to 4th edition of *McCance and Widdowson's The Composition of Foods*. HMSO, London
7	Holland, B., Unwin, I.D. and Buss, D.H. (1988) *Cereals and Cereal Products*. Third supplement to 4th edition of *McCance and Widdowson's The Composition of Foods*. The Royal Society of Chemistry, Nottingham
8	Holland, B., Unwin, I.D. and Buss, D.H. (1989) *Milk Products and Eggs*. Fourth supplement to 4th edition of *McCance and Widdowson's The Composition of Foods*. The Royal Society of Chemistry, Cambridge
9	Holland, B., Unwin, I.D. and Buss, D.H. (1991) *Vegetables, Herbs and Spices*. Fifth supplement to 4th edition of *McCance and Widdowson's The Composition of Foods*. The Royal Society of Chemistry, Cambridge
10	Holland, B., Welch, A.A., Unwin, I.D., Buss, D.H., Paul, A.A. and Southgate, D.A.T. (1991) *McCance and Widdowson's The Composition of Foods*, 5th edition. The Royal Society of Chemistry, Cambridge

11   Holland, B., Unwin, I.D. and Buss, D.H. (1992) *Fruit and Nuts*. First supplement to 5th edition of *McCance and Widdowson's The Composition of Foods*. The Royal Society of Chemistry, Cambridge

12   Holland, B., Welch, A.A. and Buss, D.H. (1992) *Vegetable Dishes*. Second supplement to 5th edition of *McCance and Widdowson's The Composition of Foods*. The Royal Society of Chemistry, Cambridge

13   Holland, B., Brown, J. and Buss, D.H. (1993) *Fish and Fish Products*. Third supplement to 5th edition of *McCance and Widdowson's The Composition of Foods*. The Royal Society of Chemistry, Cambridge

14   Chan, W., Brown, J. and Buss, D.H. (1994) *Miscellaneous Foods*. Fourth supplement to 5th edition of *McCance and Widdowson's The Composition of Foods*. The Royal Society of Chemistry, Cambridge

15   Chan, W., Brown, J., Lee, S.M. and Buss, D.H. (1995) *Meat, Poultry and Game*. Fifth supplement to 5th edition of *McCance and Widdowson's The Composition of Foods*. The Royal Society of Chemistry, Cambridge

16   Chan, W., Brown, J., Church, S.M. and Buss, D.H. (1996) *Meat Products and Dishes*. Sixth supplement to 5th edition of *McCance and Widdowson's The Composition of Foods*. The Royal Society of Chemistry, Cambridge

17   Ministry of Agriculture, Fisheries and Food. (1998) *Fatty Acids*. Seventh supplement to 5th edition of *McCance and Widdowson's The Composition of Foods*. The Royal Society of Chemistry, Cambridge.

18   Food Standards Agency (2002) *McCance and Widdowson's The Composition of Foods*, 6th summary edition. The Royal Society of Chemistry, Cambridge

19   Composition of Foods Integrated Dataset (2008) http://tna.europarchive.org/20110116113217/http://www.food.gov.uk/science/dietarysurveys/dietsurveys/

Analytical Reports

20   Laboratory of the Government Chemist (1982-1983) Carcase meat and offal survey

21   Laboratory of the Government Chemist (1983-1984) Alcoholic beverages, soft drinks and tea and coffee survey

22   Laboratory of the Government Chemist (1983-1984) Poultry and game surveys

23   Laboratory of the Government Chemist (1984) The nutritional composition of fruit juice

24   Institute of Food Research (1984-1987) The nutritional composition of retail vegetables in the UK

25   Laboratory of the Government Chemist (1985) Canned and other processed vegetable products survey

26   Laboratory of the Government Chemist (1985) Frozen vegetable survey

27   Laboratory of the Government Chemist (1985-1986) Nutritional composition of fruit products

28   Laboratory of the Government Chemist (1985-1986) Nutritional composition of fresh fruit

29   Laboratory of the Government Chemist (1986-1987) Fish and fish products

30   Laboratory of the Government Chemist (1989) Dairy products and eggs

31   Laboratory of the Government Chemist (1989-1990) Fruit and vegetables

32   Laboratory of the Government Chemist (1990-1991) Analytical survey of meat products

33   Laboratory of the Government Chemist (1992) Analytical survey of confectionery items

34   Laboratory of the Government Chemist (1992) Nutritional analysis of foods for pre-school children

35   Leatherhead Food R.A. (1992) Nutrient analysis of miscellaneous foods

36   Laboratory of the Government Chemist (1992-1993) Nutrient analysis of carcase beef

37   Laboratory of the Government Chemist (1992-1993) Nutrient analysis of retail cuts of pork

38   Leatherhead Food R.A. (1993) Nutritional analysis of soft drinks

39   Laboratory of the Government Chemist (1993) Survey of the Nutritional Composition of savoury snacks and nuts

40   RHM Research and Engineering Ltd (1993) Fatty acids in foods

41   Laboratory of the Government Chemist (1993-1994) Nutrient analysis of retail cuts of bacon

42   Laboratory of the Government Chemist (1993-1994) Nutrient analysis of retail cuts of lamb

43   Laboratory of the Government Chemist (1994) Analysis of assorted foods

44   Laboratory of the Government Chemist (1994) Nutrient analysis of foods important in elderly people

45   Laboratory of the Government Chemist (1994-1995) Nutrient analysis of chicken and turkey

46   Laboratory of the Government Chemist (1994-1995) Nutritional analysis of meat and poultry products

47   Laboratory of the Government Chemist (1995) Added folic acid in supplements and fortified foods

48   Laboratory of the Government Chemist (1995) Nutrient analysis of foods commonly consumed by schoolchildren

49   RHM Technology (1995) Nutrient analysis of pizzas

50   RHM Technology (1995) Nutrient analysis of selected foods

51   ADAS Laboratory Services (1995-1996) Nutrient analysis of pasteurised liquid milk

52   Laboratory of the Government Chemist (1996) Individual folates in foodstuffs

53   Aspland and James Ltd (1997) Nutrient analysis of ethnic takeaway foods

54   Laboratory of the Government Chemist (1997) Determination of 25-OH vitamin D in selected foodstuffs

55   Laboratory of the Government Chemist (1997) Determination of cis carotenoids in foodstuffs

56   Laboratory of the Government Chemist (1997) The determination of different forms of iron in foodstuffs

57 RHM Technology (1997) Nutrient analysis of manufactured foods for vegetarians

58 University of London School of Life Sciences (1997) Analysis of composition of commercial sandwiches

59 Laboratory of Government Chemist (1998) Nutrient analysis of 'other' milk and cream

60 Campden and Chorleywood Food Research Association (1998) Nutrient analysis of yoghurts, fromage frais and chilled desserts

61 Laboratory of the Government Chemist (1999) Nutrient analysis of bread and morning goods

62 Laboratory of the Government Chemist (1999) Nutrient analysis of cheese

63 ADAS Laboratories (1999) Nutrient analysis of ice creams and desserts

64 Campden and Chorleywood Food Research Association (2003) Programme of mini-surveys: survey of sausages

65 Direct Laboratories (2003) Nutrient analysis catch up project

66 Laboratory of the Government Chemist (2004) Nutrient analysis of pasta and pasta sauces

67 Laboratory of the Government Chemist (2004) Nutrient survey of breakfast cereals

68 Laboratory of the Government Chemist (2005) Nutrient survey of flours and grains

69 University of Leeds (2007) Nutritional analysis of commonly consumed South Asian foods in the UK

70 Department of Health (2011) Nutrient analysis survey of biscuits, buns, cakes and pastries

71 Department of Health (2012) Nutrient analysis of eggs

72 Department of Health (2013) Nutrient analysis of a range of processed foods with particular reference to trans fatty acids, revised version

73	Department of Health (2013) Nutrient analysis of fish and fish products

74	Department of Health (2013) Nutrient analysis of fruit and vegetables

Additional references

75	Anderson, B.A., Kinsella, J.A. and Watt, B.K. (1975) Comprehensive evaluation of fatty acids in foods. II. Beef products. *J. Am. Diet. Assoc.* 67, 35-41

76	Anderson, B.A. (1976) Comprehensive evaluation of fatty acids in foods. VII. Pork products. *J. Am. Diet. Assoc.* 69, 44-49

77	AOAC (1975) *Official methods of analysis, 12th edition.* Association of Official Analytical Chemists, Washington DC

78	AOAC. (2011) In W. Horwitz, G. Latimer (Eds.), *Official methods of analysis (18th ed., Revision 4).* ISBN: 0-935584-82-X

79	Bath, S.C., Button, S. and Rayman, M.P. (2011) Iodine concentration of organic and conventional milk: implications for iodine intake. *Br. J. Nutr.*, 5, 1–6

80	Bell, J.G. (1974) Microbiological assay of vitamins of the B group in foodstuffs. *Lab. Pract.* 23, 235-242, 252

81	Benelam, B., Roe, M., Pinchen, H., Church, S., Buttriss, J., Gray, J., Farron-Wilson, M. and Finglas, P. (2012) New data on the nutritional composition of UK hens' eggs. *Nutrition Bulletin*, 37, 344–349

82	Bergstom, L. (1999) Nutrient losses and gains in the preparation of foods. NLG - Project Rapport 32/94, revised. National Food Administration, Uppsala/Sweden.

83	Bognar, A. and Piekarski, J. (2000) Guidelines for recipe information and calculation of nutrient composition of prepared foods (dishes). *J. Food Compos. Anal.* 13, 391-410

84	Bolton-Smith, C., Price, R.J.G., Fenton, S.T., Harrington, D.J. and Shearer, M.J. (2000) Compilation of a provisional UK database for the phylloquinone (vitamin K_1) content of foods. *Br. J. Nutr.* 83, 389-399

85	Bolton-Smith, C. and Shearer, M.J. (2000) The extension and verification of the provisional UK phylloquinone (vitamin K_1) food composition database. Report to the Food Standards Agency

86   Booth, S.L., Pennington, J.A.T. and Sadowski, J.A. (1996) Dihydro-vitamin K_1: primary food sources and estimated dietary intakes in the American diet. *Lipids* 31, 715-720

87   Bouckaert, K.P., Slimani, N., Nicolas, G., Vignat, J., Wright, A.J.A, Roe, M., Witthoft, C.M. and Finglas, P.M. (2011) Critical evaluation of folate data in European and international databases: Recommendations for standardization in international nutritional studies. *Mol. Nutr. Food Res.* 55, 166–180

88   The Bread and Flour Regulations (1998) *Statutory Instrument No. 141.* The Stationery Office, London

89   Breese Jones, D., (1941) Factors for Converting Percentages of Nitrogen in Foods and Feeds into Percentages of Proteins. *United States Department of Agriculture, Circular* 183, 1931 (slightly revised August, 1941)

90   Brubacher, G., Müller-Mulot, W. and Southgate, D.A.T. (1985) *Methods for the determination of vitamins in food.* Elsevier Applied Science Publishers Ltd, London

91   Cashel, K., English, R. and Lewis, J. (1989) *Composition of Foods, Australia. Volume 1.* Department of Community Services and Health, Canberra

92   Castenmiller, J.J.M. and West, C.E. (1998) Bioavailability and bioconversion of carotenoids. *Annu. Rev. Nutr.* 18, 19-38

93   Christie, A.A., Dean, A.C. and Millburn, B.A. (1973) The determination of vitamin E in food by colorimetry and gas- liquid chromatography. *Analyst* 98, 161-167

94   Church, S. M. (2009) EuroFIR synthesis report no. 7: Food composition explained. *Nutrition Bulletin*, 34, 250-272

95   Cummings, J.H. and Stephen, A.M. (2007) Carbohydrate terminology and classification. In supplement: "Joint FAO/WHO Scientific update on carbohydrates in human nutrition". *Eur. J. Clin. Nutr.*, 61 (Suppl 1), S5-S18

96   Cutrufelli, R. and Matthews, R.H. (1986) *Composition of foods: beverages, raw, processed and prepared*. Agriculture Handbook No. 8-14, US Department of Agriculture, Washington DC

97   Department of Health and Social Security (1977) *The composition of mature human milk*. Report on Health and Social Subjects No 12, HMSO, London

98   Department of Health (1991) *Dietary reference values for food energy and nutrients for the United Kingdom.* Report on Health and Social Subjects No. 41, HMSO, London

99   Diet and physical activity measurement toolkit. Medical Research Council. http://dapa-toolkit.mrc.ac.uk/ (accessed March 2014)

100   Egan, H., Kirk, R.S. and Sawyer, R. (1981) *Pearson's Chemical Analysis of Foods,* 8th edition. Churchill Livingstone, Edinburgh

101   Englyst, H.N., Wiggins, H.S. and Cummings, J.H. (1982) Determination of the non-starch polysaccharides in plant foods by gas-liquid chromatography of constituent sugars as alditol acetates. *Analyst* 107, 307-318

102   Englyst, H.N. and Cummings, J.H. (1984) Simplified method for the measurement of total non-starch polysaccharides by gas-liquid chromatography of constituent sugars as alditol acetates. *Analyst* 109, 937-942

103   Englyst, H.N. and Cummings, J.H. (1988) An improved method for the measurement of dietary fibre as the non-starch polysaccharides in plant foods. *J. Assoc. Off. Anal. Chem.* 71, 808-814

104   Englyst, H.N., Quigley, M.E., Hudson, J.G. and Cummings, J.H. (1992) Determination of dietary fibre as non-starch polysaccharides by gas-liquid-chromatography. *Analyst* 117, 1707-1714

105   Englyst, H. N., Quigley, M. E. and Hudson, G. J. (1994). Determination of dietary fibre as non-starch polysaccharides with gas–liquid chromatographic, high performance liquid chromatographic or spectrophotometric measurement of constituent sugars. Analyst, 119, 1497–1509

106   European Commission Directive 90/496/EEC (1990) Nutrition Labelling For Foodstuffs

107   European Commission Directive 2003/120/EC (2003) Amendment of Nutrition Labelling For Foodstuffs

108   European Commission Directive 2008/100/EC (2008) Amendment of Nutrition Labelling For Foodstuffs as regards recommended daily allowances, energy conversion factors and definitions

109   European Committee for Standardization, Technical Committee CEN/TC 275 (2003) Foodstuffs – determination of folate by microbiological assay, EN 14131

110   European Committee for Standardization, Technical Committee CEN/TC 275 (2000) Foodstuffs – determination of Vitamin A by high performance liquid chromatography – Part 1: measurement of all-*trans*-Retinol and 13-*cis*-Retinol, EN 12823-1

111   European Committee for Standardization, Technical Committee CEN/TC 275 (2000) Foodstuffs – determination of Vitamin A by high performance liquid chromatography – Part 2: measurement of β-Carotene, EN 12823-2

112   European Committee for Standardization, Technical Committee CEN/TC 275 (2003) Foodstuffs – determination of Vitamin B_1 by HPLC, EN 14122

113   European Committee for Standardization, Technical Committee CEN/TC 275 (2003) Foodstuffs – determination of Vitamin B_2 by HPLC, EN 14152

114   European Committee for Standardization, Technical Committee CEN/TC 275 (2001) Foodstuffs – determination of Vitamin B_6 by HPLC, EN 14164

115   European Committee for Standardization, Technical Committee CEN/TC 275 (2001) Foodstuffs – determination of Vitamin B_6 by microbiological assay, EN 14166

116   European Committee for Standardization, Technical Committee CEN/TC 275 (2003) Foodstuffs – determination of Vitamin C by HPLC, EN 14130

117   European Committee for Standardization, Technical Committee CEN/TC 275 (2000) Foodstuffs – determination of Vitamin D by high performance liquid chromatography – measurement of cholecalciferol (D_3) and ergocalciferol (D_2), EN 12821

118   European Committee for Standardization, Technical Committee CEN/TC 275 (2000) Foodstuffs – determination of Vitamin E by high performance liquid chromatography – measurement of α-, β-, γ- and δ-Tocopherols, EN 12822

119   European Union Regulation 1169/2011 (2011) The Provision of Food Information to Consumers

120   Exler, J., Kinsella, J.E. and Watt, B.K. (1975) Lipids and fatty acids of important finfish. New data for nutrient tables. *J. Am. Oil Chem.* Soc. 52, 154-159

121   Fairweather-Tait, S.J. (1998) Trace element bioavailability. In: *Role of trace elements for health promotion and disease prevention. Edited by Sandstrom, B. and Walter, P. Bibliotheca Nutritio et Dieta* 54, 29-39

122   FAO (2003) Food Energy—Methods of Analysis and Conversion Factors. Report of a Technical Workshop. FAO Food and Nutrition Paper no. 77. Food and Agriculture Organization of the United Nations, Rome

123   Ferland, G. and Sadowski, J.A. (1992) The vitamin k_1 (phylloquinone) content of green vegetables: effects of plant maturation and geographical growth location. *J. Ag. Food Chem.* 40, 1874-1877

124   Fernández-García, E., Carvajal-Lérida, I., Jarén-Galán, M., Garrido-Fernández, J., Pérez-Gálvez, A. and Hornero-Méndez, D. (2012) Carotenoids bioavailability from foods: From plant pigments to efficient biological activities. *Food Res. Int.* 46, 438-450

125   Finglas, P.M. and Faulks, R.M. (1984) The HPLC analysis of thiamin and riboflavin in potatoes. *Food Chem.* 15, 37-44

126   Food Standards Agency (2000) Guidance Note dated 22 September 2000. http://www.food.gov.uk/multimedia/pdfs/nutlabel2.pdf

127   Food Standards Agency (2002) Food portion sizes. Third edition. TSO, London

128   Foster E., Hawkins, A. and Adamson, A. (2011) Young person's food atlas: Pre-school. Food Standards Agency. http://multimedia.food.gov.uk/multimedia/pdfs/publication/foodatlaspreschool0310.pdf

129   Gebhardt, S.E., Cutrufelli, R. and Matthews, R.H. (1982) *Composition of foods: fruits and fruit juices, raw, processed and prepared*, Agriculture Handbook No 8-9, US Department of Agriculture, Washington DC

130   Gibson, R.S. (2005) *Principles of nutrition assessment (2nd edition).* Oxford University Press

131   Gopalan, C., Rama Sastri, B.V. and Balasubramanian, S.C. (1980) *Nutritive value of Indian foods*, National Institute of Nutrition, Indian Council of Medical Research, Hyderabad

132   Gregory, J. F. (1988) Methods for determination of vitamin B_6 in foods and other biological materials: A critical review. J. Food Compos. Anal. 1: 105-123

133   Gregory, J.F., Trumbo, P.R., Bailey, L.B., Toth, J P.,Baumgartner, T.G. and Cerda, J.J. (1991) Bioavailability of pyridoxine-5'-B-D-glucoside determined in humans by stable-isotopic methods. *J. Nutr.* 121:177-186

134   Greenfield, H. and Southgate, D.A.T. (2003) *Food composition data: Production, management and use* (2nd edition). Elsevier: London and New York

135   Haytowitz, D.B. and Matthews, R.H. (1986) *Composition of foods: legumes and legume products, raw, processed and prepared.* Agriculture Handbook No. 8-11, US Department of Agriculture, Washington DC

136   Institute of Medicine (2001) Dietary Reference Intakes for Vitamin A, Vitamin K, Arsenic, Boron, Chromium, Copper, Iodine, Iron, Manganese, Molybdenum, Nickel, Silicon, Vanadium, and Zinc, Food and Nutrition Board. Washington, DC, National Academy Press

137   International Dairy Federation (1988) *Edible ices and ice mixes: Determination of fat content: Weibull-Berntrop gravimetric method (Reference method).* Joint IDF/ISO/AOAC Publication. Brussels

138   IUPAC (1976) *Standard methods for the analysis of oils, fats and soaps. 4th supplement to the 5th edition.* Method II D.19 Preparation of fatty acid methyl esters. Method II D.25 Gas liquid chromatography of fatty acid methyl esters

139   IUPAC (1979) *Standard methods for the analysis of oils, fats and derivatives. 6th Edition.* Oxford: Pergamon Press

140   Jakobsen, J. (2007) Bioavailability and bioactivity of vitamin D_3 active compounds – Which potency should be used for 25-hydroxyvitamin D_3? *International Congress Series* 1297, 133–142

141   Koivu, T.J., Piironen, V.I. and Mattila, P.H. (1998) Phylloquinone (vitamin K_1) in cereal products. *Cereal Chem.* 75, 113-116

142   Kwiatkowska, C.A., Finglas, P.M. and Faulks, R.M. (1989) The vitamin content of retail vegetables in the UK. J. Hum. Nut. Diet. 2, 159-172

143   Lewis, J. and English, R. (1990) *Composition of foods, Australia. Volume 5, nuts and legumes, beverages, miscellaneous foods.* Department of Community Services and Health, Canberra

144   Marsh, A.C., Moss, M.K. and Murphy, E.W. (1977) *Composition of foods: spices and herbs, raw, processed and prepared.* Agriculture Handbook No. 8-2, US Department of Agriculture, Washington, Washington DC

145   Marsh, A.C. (1980) *Composition of foods: soups, sauces and gravies, raw, processed and prepared.* Agriculture Handbook No 8-6, US Department of Agriculture, Washington DC

146   McCance, R.A. and Shipp, H.L. (1933) *The chemistry of flesh foods and their losses on cooking*. Medical Research Council Special Report Series, No. 187. HMSO, London

147   McCarthy, M.A. and Matthews, R.H. (1984) *Composition of foods: nut and seed products, raw, processed and prepared*. Agriculture Handbook No. 8-12, US Department of Agriculture, Washington DC

148   McCarthy, P.T., Harrington, D. and Shearer, M.J. (1997) Assay of phylloquinone in plasma. *Methods in Enzymology* 282, 421-433

149   McLaughlin, P.J. and Weihrauch, J.L. (1979) Vitamin E content of foods. *J. Am. Diet. Assoc.* 75, 647-665

150   Michie, N.D., Dixon E.J. and Bunton, N.G. (1978) Critical review of AOAC fluorimetric method for determining selenium in foods. *J. Assoc. Off. Analyt. Chem.* 61, 48-51

151   Moxon, R.E.D. and Dixon, E.J. (1980) Semi-automated method for the determination of total iodine in food. *Analyst* 105, 344-352

152   Moxon, R.E.D. (1983) A rapid method for the determination of sodium in butter. *J. Assoc. Publ. Analysts* 21, 83-87

153   Nelson, M., Atkinson, M. and Meyer, J. (2002) *Food portion sizes. A photographic atlas*. Food Standards Agency, London

154   Ollilainen, V., Van den Berg, H., Finglas, P.M. and de Froidmont-Goertz, I. (2001) Certification of B-group vitamins (B_1, B_2, B_6 and B_{12}) in four food reference materials. *J. Agric. Food Chem.* 48 (12), 6325-6331

155   Olson, J.A. (1989) Pro vitamin A function of carotenoids: The conversion of b-carotene into vitamin A. *J. Nutr.* 119, 105-108

156   Paul, A.A. and Southgate, D.A.T. (1977) A study on the composition of retail meat: dissection into lean, separable fat and inedible portion. *J. Hum. Nutr.* 31, 259-272

157   Phillips, D.R. and Wright A.J.A. (1983) Studies on the response of *Labtobacillus casei* to folate vitamin in foods. *Br. J. Nutr.* 49, 181-186

158   Phillips, D.I.W., Nelson, M., Baker, D.J.P., Morris, J.A. and Wood, T.J. (1988) Iodine in milk and the incidence of thyrotoxicosis in England. *Clin. Endocrinol.* 28, 61-66

159   Polacchi, W., McHargue, J.S. and Perloff, B.P. (1982) *Food composition tables for the near east*, Food and Agriculture Organization of the United Nations, Rome

160   Posati, L.P., Kinsella, J.E. and Watt, B.K. (1975) Comprehensive evaluation of fatty acids in foods. III. Eggs and egg products. *J. Am. Diet. Assoc.* 67, 111-115

161   Rodriguez-Amaya D.B. (2001) *A Guide to Carotenoid Analysis in Foods.* ILSI Press, Washington DC.

162   Royal Society (1972) *Metric units, conversion factors and nomenclature in nutritional and food sciences.* Report of the subcommittee on metrication of the British National Committee for Nutritional Sciences

163   Scott, K.J. and Rodriguez-Amaya, D. (2000) Pro-vitamin A carotenoid conversion factors: retinol equivalents – fact or fiction? *Food Chemistry* 69, 125-127

164   Shearer, M.J., Bach, A. and Kohlmeier, M. (1996) Chemistry, nutritional sources, tissue distribution and metabolism of vitamin K with special reference to bone health. *J. Nutr.* 126, S1181-S1186

165   Sivell, L.M., Bull, N.L., Buss, D.H., Wiggins, R.A., Scuffam, D., and Jackson, P.A. (1984) Vitamin A activity in foods of animal origin. *J. Sci. Food Agric.* 35, 931-939

166   Society of Public Analysts and Other Analytical Chemists: Analytical Methods Committee (1951) The chemical assay of aneurine in foodstuffs. *Analyst* 76, 127-133

167   Southgate, D.A.T. and Durnin, J.V.G.A. (1970) Calorie conversion factors: an experimental reassessment of the factors used in the calculations of the energy value of human diets. *Brit. J. Nutr.* 24, 517-535

168   Thurnham, D. I. (2007) Bioequivalence of β-carotene and retinol. *J. Sci. Food. Agric.* 87, 13-39

169   U.S. Department of Agriculture, Agricultural Research Service (2013) USDA National Nutrient Database for Standard Reference, Release 26. Nutrient Data Laboratory Home Page, http://www.ars.usda.gov/ba/bhnrc/ndl

170   Weihrauch, J.L., Kinsella, J.E. and Watt, B.K. (1976) Comprehensive evaluation of fatty acids in foods. VI. Cereal products. *J. Am. Diet. Assoc.* 68, 335-340

171   Westenbrink, S., Brunt, K. and van der Kamp, J-W. (2013) Dietary fibre: Challenges in production and use of food composition data. *Food Chem.* 140, 162-167

172   Wharton, P.A., Eaton, P.M. and Day, K.C. (1983) Sorrento Asian food tables: food tables, recipes and customs of mothers attending Sorrento Maternity Hospital, Birmingham, England. *Hum. Nutr. Appli. Nutr.,* 37A, 378-402

173   Widdowson, E.M. and McCance, R.A. (1943) Food tables. Their scope and limitations. *Lancet* i: 230-2

174   Wiles, S.J., Nettleton, P.A., Black A.E. and Paul, A.A. (1980) The nutrition composition of some cooked dishes eaten in Britain: A supplementary food composition table. *J. Hum. Nutr.* 34, 189-223

175   Wrieden, W.L. and Barton, K.L. (2006) Calculation and collation of typical food portion sizes for adults aged 19-64 and older people aged 65 and over. Food Standards   Agency. http://www.foodbase.org.uk//admintools/reportdocuments/82-1-441_82-1-188_Adult_Food_Portion_Project_Draft_Final_Report_28th_February_2006_amended_dec_2007.pdf

176   Wu Leung, W.T., Butrum, R.R., Chang, F.H., Narayama Rao, M. and Polacchi, W. (1972) *Food composition table for use in East Asia*, Food and Agriculture Organization and US Department of Health, Education and Welfare, Bethesda

4.7 FOOD INDEX

Foods are indexed by their publication number and, for ease of reference, each food has been assigned a consecutive publication number for the purposes of this edition only. In addition, each food has a unique food code number which will allow read-across to the fifth edition, sixth edition or the Composition of Foods Integrated Dataset (CoFID), where appropriate.

For foods that have already been included in the CoFID and for which there are no new data, their food code number (including the unique 2 digit prefix) has been repeated. These prefixes are 11- *Cereals and Cereal Products*, 12 – *Milk Products and Eggs*, 13 – *Vegetables, Herbs and Spices*, 14 – *Fruit and Nuts*, 15 – *Vegetable Dishes*, 16 – *Fish and Fish Products*, 17 – *Miscellaneous Foods*, 18 – *Meat, Poultry and Game*, 19 – *Meat Products and Dishes*, and 50 – *Fifth Edition*. Foods that have not previously been included have been given a new food code number using the most appropriate prefix (e.g. peshwari naan (11-910)). Where new data have been incorporated for an existing food, a new food code has been allocated but with the same prefix code (e.g. homemade sausage casserole was 19-351, now 19-484). For ease of use the original food code number is given alongside the new food code. These are the numbers that will be used in the CoFID and nutrient databank applications.

The index includes two kinds of cross-reference. The first is the normal coverage of alternative names (e.g. Stewing steak see **Beef, stewing steak**). The second is to other commonly used and scientific names (e.g. Akhrot see **Walnuts**).

	Publication number	Current code	Previous code
Abelmoschus esculentus	See **Okra**		
Actinidia deliciosa	See **Kiwi fruit**		
Agaricus bisporus	See **Mushrooms, white**		
Akhrot	See **Walnuts**		
Alaskan pollack	See **Pollock, Alaskan**		
Alaskan pollock, baked	612	16-436	
Alaskan pollock, raw	611	16-378	16-123
Allium ampeloprasum var porrum	See **Leeks**		
Allium cepa	See **Onions** and **Spring onions**		
Allium sativum	See **Garlic**		
Allium schoenoprasum	See **Chives**		
Almonds	938	14-870	
Aloo	See **Potatoes**		
American muffins, chocolate	160	11-737	
American muffins, not chocolate	161	11-738	
American style chocolate chip cookies	119	11-816	

	Publication number	Current code	Previous code
Anacardium occidentale	See **Cashew nuts**		
Ananas comosus	See **Pineapple**		
Anar	See **Pomegranate**		
Anas platyrhynchos	See **Duck**		
Anchovies, canned in oil, drained	614	16-448	16-323
Anser anser	See **Goose**		
Apium graveolens var dulce	See **Celery**		
Apple juice, clear, ambient and chilled	1055	14-331	14-271
Apple pie, pastry, double crust	193	11-921	
Apples, cooking, stewed with sugar, flesh only	878	14-332	14-004
Apples, cooking, stewed without sugar, flesh only	879	14-320	14-005
Apples, eating, raw, flesh and skin	880	14-319	14-012
Apricots, raw, flesh and skin	881	14-025	
Apricots, ready-to-eat	882	14-036	
Arachis hypogaea	See **Peanuts**		
Aristaeidae	See **Prawns** and **Prawns, king**		
Arugula	See **Rocket**		
Asparagus officinalis	See **Asparagus**		
Asparagus, boiled in unsalted water	733	13-538	
Asparagus, raw	732	13-157	50-737
Aubergine, fried in corn oil	735	13-162	50-740
Aubergine, raw	734	13-161	50-739
Avena sativa	See **Porridge oats**		
Avocado, average	883	14-037	50-685
Baby spinach, boiled in unsalted water	803	13-550	
Baby spinach, raw	802	13-521	
Baby sweetcorn, fresh and frozen, boiled in unsalted water	809	13-552	
Bacon rashers, back, dry-fried	381	19-498	19-002
Bacon rashers, back, fat trimmed, grilled	385	19-499	19-008
Bacon rashers, back, grilled	382	19-500	19-003
Bacon rashers, back, grilled crispy	383	19-501	19-004
Bacon rashers, back, microwaved	384	19-502	19-005
Bacon rashers, back, raw	380	19-497	19-001
Bacon rashers, middle, grilled	386	19-503	19-015
Bacon rashers, streaky, fried in corn oil	387	19-504	19-017
Bacon rashers, streaky, grilled	388	19-018	50-359
Bacon, fat only, average, cooked	389	19-537	50-339

	Publication number	Current code	Previous code
Bacon, lettuce and tomato sandwich, white bread	83	11-955	11-563
Badam	See **Almonds**		
Badla	See **Peas**		
Bagels, plain	48	11-970	11-534
Baingan	See **Aubergine**		
Baked beans, canned in tomato sauce	696	13-532	13-044
Baked beans, canned in tomato sauce, reduced sugar, reduced salt	697	13-535	13-046
Bakers yeast, compressed	1179	17-378	50-1187
Bakewell tarts, iced	177	11-845	11-426
Baking and margarine fats (75-90% fat), hard block	358	12-500	17-539
Baking powder	1161	17-355	50-1174
Baklava	185	11-842	11-248
Balti, chicken	552	19-449	
Banana/strawberry flavoured milk, pasteurised	235	12-326	12-034
Bananas, flesh only	884	14-318	14-045
Banoffee pie	311	12-394	
Barbecue sauce	1132	17-705	17-289
Barley water, undiluted	1046	17-743	17-185
Basa	See **Pangasius**		
Basil, fresh	855	13-804	
Basmati rice, white, boiled in unsalted water	23	11-858	
Basmati rice, white, easy cook, boiled in unsalted water	24	11-860	
Basmati rice, white, raw	22	11-857	11-041
Bass	See **Sea bass**		
Batata	See **Potatoes**		
Battenberg cake	146	11-835	11-574
Beans, blackeye, dried, boiled in unsalted water	702	13-063	50-701
Beans, broad, boiled in unsalted water	703	13-066	
Beans, butter, canned, re-heated, drained	704	13-559	13-429
Beans, green, boiled in unsalted water	699	13-515	13-432
Beans, green, raw	698	13-514	13-431
Beans, mung, whole, dried, boiled in unsalted water	711	13-097	50-715
Beans, red kidney beans, boiled in unsalted water	713	13-110	50-717

	Publication number	Current code	Previous code
Beans, red kidney, canned, re-heated, drained	714	13-561	13-435
Beans, red kidney, dried, raw	712	13-109	50-716
Beans, runner, boiled in unsalted water	716	13-114	50-720
Beans, runner, raw	715	13-112	50-719
Beans, soya, dried, boiled in unsalted water	718	13-116	50-722
Beans, soya, dried, raw	717	13-115	50-721
Beansprouts, mung, raw	700	13-426	13-052
Beansprouts, mung, stir-fried in rapeseed oil	701	13-567	13-427
Beef bourguignon, homemade	541	19-471	19-330
Beef casserole, made with cook-in sauce	542	19-470	19-332
Beef chow mein, reheated	543	19-519	19-165
Beef curry, reduced fat, homemade	546	19-472	19-333
Beef curry, reheated	544	19-488	19-169
Beef curry, reheated, with rice	545	19-529	19-170
Beef dripping	360	17-487	17-006
Beef extract	1162	17-514	17-361
Beef pie, puff or shortcrust pastry, family size	508	18-505	
Beef pie, puff or shortcrust pastry, individual	509	18-506	
Beef sausages, grilled	531	19-489	19-077
Beef stew, homemade	547	19-473	19-334
Beef stock cubes	1170	17-515	17-368
Beef, braising steak, braised, lean and fat	398	18-009	
Beef, braising steak, braised, lean only	397	18-008	
Beef, fat, average, cooked	395	18-005	50-362
Beef, fat, average, raw	394	18-003	50-361
Beef, lean, average, raw	396	18-468	18-001
Beef, mince, extra lean, stewed	402	18-507	18-041
Beef, mince, microwaved	400	18-037	
Beef, mince, raw	399	18-469	
Beef, mince, stewed	401	18-470	18-038
Beef, rump steak, barbecued, lean	404	18-045	
Beef, rump steak, fried in corn oil, lean and fat	406	18-472	18-048
Beef, rump steak, fried in corn oil, lean only	405	18-473	18-047
Beef, rump steak, from steakhouse, lean only	408	18-050	

	Publication number	Current code	Previous code
Beef, rump steak, grilled, lean only	407	18-474	18-049
Beef, rump steak, raw, lean and fat	403	18-471	18-044
Beef, rump steak, strips, stir-fried in corn oil, lean	409	18-052	
Beef, stewing steak, raw, lean	410	18-076	
Beef, stewing steak, raw, lean and fat	411	18-077	50-383
Beef, stewing steak, stewed, lean and fat	413	18-081	50-384
Beef, stewing steak, stewed, lean only	412	18-080	
Beef, stir-fried with green peppers, homemade	548	19-530	19-335
Beef, topside, roasted medium-rare, lean and fat	415	18-089	50-386
Beef, topside, roasted medium-rare, lean only	414	18-088	50-387
Beefburgers, 62-85% beef, grilled	500	19-546	19-043
Beefburgers, 98-99% beef, fried in vegetable oil	498	19-490	19-029
Beefburgers, 98-99% beef, grilled	499	19-491	19-030
Beefburgers, 98-99% beef, raw	497	19-492	19-309
Beer, bitter, average	1067	17-506	17-207
Beer, bitter, best, premium	1068	17-208	
Beer, bitter, strong	1069	17-748	
Beetroot, boiled in unsalted water	736	13-539	
Beetroot, pickled, drained	737	13-166	50-743
Belgian chicory	See **Chicory**		
Bell peppers	See **Peppers, capsicum (green/red)**		
Belly joint/slices, pork, grilled, lean and fat	443	18-209	50-418
Benniseed	See **Sesame seeds**		
Bertholletia excelsa	See **Brazil nuts**		
Beta vulgaris	See **Beetroot**		
Bhendi	See **Okra**		
Bhinda	See **Okra**		
Bhindi	See **Okra**		
Bhindi subji, homemade	819	15-627	
Big Mac, takeaway	501	19-493	19-310
Biscuits, cheese flavoured	118	11-821	
Biscuits, cookies, chocolate chip, American style	119	11-816	
Biscuits, cookies, chocolate chip, standard	120	11-815	11-508
Biscuits, digestive, half coated in chocolate	121	11-807	11-512
Biscuits, digestive, plain	122	11-799	11-513

	Publication number	Current code	Previous code
Biscuits, digestive, with oats, plain	123	11-803	11-517
Biscuits, fully coated with chocolate	124	11-809	11-506
Biscuits, fully coated with chocolate, with cream	125	11-810	11-507
Biscuits, fully coated with chocolate, with marshmallow	126	11-811	11-419
Biscuits, ginger nuts	127	11-798	11-514
Biscuits, iced	128	11-808	
Biscuits, jam filled	129	11-804	11-516
Biscuits, plain, reduced fat	130	11-801	
Biscuits, sandwich, cream	131	11-813	11-519
Biscuits, semi-sweet	132	11-797	11-521
Biscuits, short or sweet, half coated in chocolate	134	11-806	11-415
Biscuits, short, sweet	133	11-796	11-522
Bitter, beer, average	1067	17-506	17-207
Bitter, beer, best, premium	1068	17-208	
Bitter, beer, strong	1069	17-748	
Black pepper	874	13-880	13-846
Black pudding, dry-fried	510	19-114	50-505
Black treacle	978	17-826	17-068
Blackberries, raw	885	14-048	50-869
Blackberries, stewed without sugar	886	14-050	50-871
Blackcurrant juice drink/squash, undiluted	1047	17-737	17-187
Blackcurrants, raw	887	14-053	50-872
Blackcurrants, stewed without sugar	888	14-055	
Blackeye beans, dried, boiled in unsalted water	702	13-063	50-701
Blackeye peas	See **Blackeye beans**		
Blue cheese dressing	1121	17-715	17-300
Blueberries	889	14-325	
Boiled eggs, chicken, white	336	12-941	
Boiled eggs, chicken, whole	335	12-940	12-806
Boiled eggs, chicken, yolk	337	12-942	
Boiled sweets	995	17-101	50-1025
Bok choi	See **Pak choi**		
Bolognese pasta sauce, tomato based	1155	17-618	17-323
Bolognese sauce (with meat), homemade	549	19-476	19-352
Bolognese sauce (with meat), homemade, with extra lean minced beef	550	19-475	
Bolognese sauce (with meat), reheated	551	19-542	19-328

	Publication number	Current code	Previous code
Bombay mix	1006	17-764	14-807
Borecole	See **Curly kale**		
Bos taurus	See **Beef** and **Veal**		
Bounty bar and own brand equivalents	979	17-766	17-546
Brachyura	See **Crab**		
Braising steak	See **Beef, braising steak**		
Bran flakes, fortified	90	11-763	11-486
Bran type cereal, fortified	89	11-767	11-485
Bran, wheat	1	11-906	11-005
Brassica	See **Mustard and cress**		
Brassica hirta	See **Mustard**		
Brassica napus var napobrassica	See **Swede**		
Brassica oleracea var acephala	See **Curly kale**		
Brassica oleracea var botrytis	See **Cauliflower**		
Brassica oleracea var capitata	See **Cabbage** and **Cabbage, white**		
Brassica oleracea var gemmifera	See **Brussels sprouts**		
Brassica oleracea var italica	See **Broccoli, green**		
Brassica rapa chinensis	See **Pak choi**		
Brassica rapa var rapifera	See **Turnip**		
Brazil nuts	939	14-871	14-808
Bread rolls, brown, soft	69	11-983	11-478
Bread rolls, malted wheat	70	11-984	11-479
Bread rolls, white, crusty	71	11-985	11-482
Bread rolls, white, soft	72	11-1006	11-483
Bread rolls, wholemeal	73	11-986	11-484
Bread sauce, homemade with semi-skimmed milk	1113	17-664	17-520
Bread, brown, average	49	11-971	11-456
Bread, ciabatta	50	11-969	11-609
Bread, garlic and herb	51	11-937	11-460
Bread, malt, fruited	52	11-462	11-084
Bread, malted wheat	53	11-972	11-461
Bread, naan	54	11-973	11-463
Bread, naan, peshwari	55	11-910	
Bread, pitta, white	56	11-974	11-465
Bread, seeded	57	11-947	
Bread, wheatgerm	58	11-975	11-467
Bread, white, Danish style	59	11-976	11-466
Bread, white, farmhouse or split tin	60	11-977	11-470
Bread, white, French stick	61	11-978	11-471

	Publication number	Current code	Previous code
Bread, white, premium	62	11-979	11-474
Bread, white, sliced	63	11-980	11-468
Bread, white, sliced, toasted	64	11-1001	11-475
Bread, white, 'with added fibre'	65	11-1003	11-472
Bread, white, 'with added fibre', toasted	66	11-1004	11-473
Bread, wholemeal, average	67	11-981	11-476
Bread, wholemeal, toasted	68	11-982	11-611
Breadsticks	135	11-826	17-123
Breakfast cereal, bran flakes, fortified	90	11-763	11-486
Breakfast cereal, bran type, fortified	89	11-767	11-485
Breakfast cereal, cornflakes, crunchy/honey nut coated, fortified	93	11-746	11-491
Breakfast cereal, cornflakes, fortified	91	11-742	11-490
Breakfast cereal, cornflakes, frosted, fortified	94	11-749	11-492
Breakfast cereal, cornflakes, unfortified	92	11-745	
Breakfast cereal, crunchy clusters type cereal, without nuts, unfortified	95	11-938	11-783
Breakfast cereal, crunchy/crispy muesli type cereal, with nuts, unfortified	96	11-939	11-783
Breakfast cereal, fruit and fibre type cereal, fortified	97	11-779	11-493
Breakfast cereal, honey loops and hoops, fortified	98	11-755	
Breakfast cereal, malted flake, fortified	99	11-760	11-501
Breakfast cereal, malted wheat, fortified	100	11-761	11-500
Breakfast cereal, multigrain hoops, fortified	103	11-1019	11-623
Breakfast cereal, oat cereal, instant, plain, fortified, cooked, made up with semi-skimmed milk	105	11-793	
Breakfast cereal, oat, instant, flavoured, unfortified, cooked, made up with semi-skimmed milk	106	11-795	
Breakfast cereal, oat, instant, plain, fortified, raw	104	11-792	11-496
Breakfast cereal, puffed wheat, honey coated, fortified	110	11-757	11-503
Breakfast cereal, puffed wheat, unfortified	109	11-756	11-144
Breakfast cereal, rice, chocolate flavoured, fortified	112	11-753	11-488
Breakfast cereal, rice, toasted/crisp, fortified	111	11-750	11-497

	Publication number	Current code	Previous code
Breakfast cereal, shredded wheat type with fruit, unfortified	114	11-777	50-079
Breakfast cereal, shredded wheat type, unfortified	113	11-775	11-499
Breakfast cereal, wheat and multigrain, chocolate flavoured, fortified	115	11-762	50-092
Breakfast cereal, wheat biscuits, Weetabix type, fortifed	116	11-773	11-505
Breakfast cereal, wheat biscuits, Weetabix type, unfortified	117	11-774	
Breast, chicken	See **Chicken, breast**		
Breast, lamb	See **Lamb, breast**		
Breast, turkey	See **Turkey, breast**		
Brie	254	12-344	50-226
Brinjal	See **Aubergine**		
Broad beans, boiled in unsalted water	703	13-066	
Broccoli and stilton soup, carton, chilled	1096	17-637	
Broccoli, green, boiled in unsalted water	739	13-503	13-172
Broccoli, green, raw	738	13-502	13-170
Broccoli, green, steamed	740	13-504	
Brown bread rolls, soft	69	11-983	11-478
Brown bread, average	49	11-971	11-456
Brown rice, wholegrain, boiled in unsalted water	17	11-869	11-443
Brown rice, wholegrain, raw	16	11-868	11-442
Brown sauce	1133	17-706	17-293
Brown sauce, reduced salt/sugar	1134	17-678	
Brown sugar	974	17-060	
Brown wheat flour	8	11-892	11-437
Brussels sprouts, boiled in unsalted water	742	13-179	50-747
Brussels sprouts, raw	741	13-177	50-746
Build-up, powder, shake	1018	17-823	17-534
Build-up, powder, soup	1019	17-728	17-535
Bund gobhi	See **Cabbage**		
Buns, currant	77	11-1009	11-536
Buns, currant, toasted	78	11-948	
Buns, iced	186	11-828	
Burger relish, tomato based	1138	17-354	
Burger, chicken, takeaway	503	19-315	19-041
Burger, chicken/turkey, coated, baked	504	18-502	
Burger/grill, vegetable and cheese, in crumbs, baked/grilled	849	15-657	15-363

	Publication number	Current code	Previous code
Burgers, beef	See **Beefburgers, Big Mac, Cheese burger, Hamburger, Quarterpounder with cheese** and **Whopper burger**		
Butter beans, canned, re-heated, drained	704	13-559	13-429
Butter, salted	346	17-685	17-485
Butter, spreadable (75-80% fat)	348	17-655	17-486
Butter, spreadable, light (60% fat)	349	17-656	
Butter, unsalted	347	17-661	
Cabbage, green, boiled in unsalted water	744	13-511	13-444
Cabbage, green, raw	743	13-510	13-468
Cabbage, red, boiled in unsalted water	745	13-540	
Cabbage, white, raw	746	13-509	13-445
Cake bars, chocolate	147	11-740	
Cake, battenberg	146	11-835	11-574
Cake, carrot, iced	149	11-836	
Cake, chocolate fudge	151	11-527	
Cake, chocolate, with filling and icing	150	11-830	
Cake, fruit	154	11-829	11-529
Cake, fruit, rich, iced, homemade	155	11-991	11-578
Cake, loaf	159	11-833	
Cake, sponge, fatless, homemade	164	11-957	11-581
Cake, sponge, homemade	163	11-956	11-580
Cake, sponge, soft iced	167	11-832	
Cake, sponge, with dairy cream and jam	165	11-532	11-215
Cake, sponge, with jam and butter cream	166	11-831	
Cakes from 'healthy eating' ranges	148	11-840	11-617
Cakes, crispie, homemade	152	11-990	11-576
Cakes, eccles	183	11-838	11-589
Cakes, fancy iced	153	11-839	11-528
Calabrese	See **Broccoli, green**		
Calamari, coated in batter, baked	650	16-404	16-266
Calf, liver, fried in corn oil	492	18-410	50-484
Camembert	255	12-345	12-133
Canteloupe-type melon, flesh only	910	14-339	14-295
Cappuccino, latte	1022	17-632	
Capsicum annuum	See **Peppers, capsicum, chilli, green, Peppers, capsicum (green/red)** and **Paprika**		
Caramel bars and sweets, chocolate covered	980	17-649	17-492
Carbonara type pasta sauce	1153	17-625	

	Publication number	Current code	Previous code
Carica papaya	See **Papaya**		
Carrot and coriander soup, carton, chilled	1097	17-634	
Carrot cake, iced	149	11-836	
Carrots, canned in water, re-heated, drained	752	13-565	13-450
Carrots, old, boiled in unsalted water	748	13-497	13-447
Carrots, old, microwaved	749	13-498	
Carrots, old, raw	747	13-496	13-446
Carrots, young, boiled in unsalted water	751	13-449	50-757
Carrots, young, raw	750	13-448	50-756
Carya illinoensis	See **Pecan nuts**		
Cashew nuts, roasted and salted	940	14-812	50-976
Casserole mix sauce, dry	1150	17-329	
Casserole, beef, made with cook-in sauce	542	19-470	19-332
Casserole, pork, made with cook-in sauce	582	19-536	19-348
Casserole, sausage, homemade	584	19-484	19-351
Casserole, vegetable, homemade	820	15-638	15-368
Castanea sativa	See **Chestnuts**		
Castanea vulgaris	See **Chestnuts**		
Cauliflower cheese	821	15-637	
Cauliflower cheese, homemade with semi-skimmed milk	822	15-639	15-369
Cauliflower, boiled in unsalted water	754	13-513	13-217
Cauliflower, raw	753	13-512	13-215
Celery, boiled in unsalted water	756	13-544	
Celery, raw	755	13-451	13-221
Cerastoderma	See **Cockles**		
Cereal bars, with fruit and/or nuts, no chocolate, unfortified	137	11-819	17-494
Cereal bars, with fruit and/or nuts, with chocolate, unfortified	136	11-818	17-494
Cervus spp	See **Venison**		
Channa	See **Chick peas**		
Channel Islands milk, whole, pasteurised	219	12-321	50-194
Chapati flour, brown	5	11-895	11-433
Chapatis, made with fat	74	11-987	11-458
Cheddar cheese and pickle sandwhich, white bread	84	11-963	11-564
Cheddar type, '30% less fat'	257	12-548	12-348
Cheddar, English	256	12-346	50-228
Cheese and onion rolls, pastry	203	11-997	11-550

	Publication number	Current code	Previous code
Cheese and tomato pizza, retail	213	11-936	11-553
Cheese flavoured biscuits	118	11-821	
Cheese omelette	342	12-947	12-922
Cheese sauce, homemade with semi-skimmed milk	1114	17-665	17-522
Cheese sauce, packet mix, made up with semi-skimmed milk	1115	17-666	17-524
Cheese spread, plain	258	12-540	12-349
Cheese spread, reduced fat	259	12-537	12-350
Cheese straws/twists	139	11-824	
Cheese, Brie	254	12-344	50-226
Cheese, Camembert	255	12-345	50-227
Cheese, Cheddar type, '30% less fat'	257	12-548	12-348
Cheese, Cheddar, English	256	12-346	50-228
Cheese, cottage, plain	260	12-539	12-351
Cheese, cottage, plain, reduced fat	261	12-550	12-352
Cheese, Danish blue	262	12-354	50-236
Cheese, Double Gloucester	263	12-487	12-153
Cheese, Edam	264	12-355	50-237
Cheese, Feta	265	12-525	12-356
Cheese, goats milk, soft, white rind	266	12-357	12-162
Cheese, Gouda	267	12-358	50-243
Cheese, Halloumi	268	12-496	
Cheese, Mascarpone	269	12-490	
Cheese, Mozzarella, fresh	270	12-360	12-170
Cheese, Paneer	271	12-495	
Cheese, Parmesan, fresh	272	12-526	12-361
Cheese, processed, plain	273	12-527	12-362
Cheese, processed, slices, reduced fat	274	12-549	12-363
Cheese, Red Leicester	275	12-485	12-167
Cheese, spreadable, soft white, full fat	278	12-551	12-364
Cheese, spreadable, soft white, low fat	276	12-541	12-366
Cheese, spreadable, soft white, medium fat	277	12-538	12-365
Cheese, Stilton, blue	279	12-367	50-249
Cheese, Wensleydale	280	12-489	12-182
Cheeseburger, takeaway	502	19-545	19-314
Cheesecake, fruit, frozen	312	12-395	50-274
Cheesecake, fruit, individual	313	12-542	12-396
Cherries, glace	891	14-335	14-068

	Publication number	Current code	Previous code
Cherries, raw, flesh and skin	890	14-061	50-876
Cherry tomatoes, raw	814	13-519	13-388
Chestnuts, raw	941	14-813	50-977
Chew sweets	996	17-647	17-104
Chick pea dhal curry, homemade	826	15-641	15-371
Chick peas, canned, re-heated, drained	706	13-560	13-078
Chick peas, whole, dried, boiled in unsalted water	705	13-430	50-705
Chicken balti	552	19-449	
Chicken breast/steak, coated, baked	511	18-504	
Chicken burger, takeaway	503	19-315	19-041
Chicken chow mein, takeaway	553	19-321	
Chicken curry, average, takeaway	554	19-322	19-300
Chicken curry, made with cook-in sauce	557	19-534	19-336
Chicken curry, reheated	555	19-520	19-188
Chicken curry, reheated, with rice	556	19-528	19-189
Chicken curry, Thai green, takeaway and restaurant	558	19-465	
Chicken fajita, meat only, takeaway and restaurant	559	19-464	
Chicken noodle soup, dried, as served	1098	17-714	17-254
Chicken pie, individual, baked	512	19-515	19-055
Chicken pieces, coated, takeaway	513	18-501	
Chicken pizza, retail	214	11-1012	11-559
Chicken portions, battered, deep fried, takeaway	515	18-500	
Chicken salad sandwich, white bread	85	11-964	11-565
Chicken satay, takeaway	560	19-323	
Chicken slices	516	19-538	19-126
Chicken soup, cream of, canned	1099	17-695	17-250
Chicken soup, cream of, canned, condensed	1100	17-696	17-251
Chicken soup, cream of, canned, condensed, as served	1101	17-697	17-252
Chicken stock cubes	1171	17-726	17-369
Chicken stock cubes, made up with water	1172	17-774	
Chicken stock, ready made	1169	17-681	
Chicken tandoori, reheated	561	19-540	19-127
Chicken tikka masala, reheated	562	19-296	19-325
Chicken wings, marinated, barbecued	563	19-541	19-204
Chicken, breast, casseroled, meat only	463	18-307	

	Publication number	Current code	Previous code
Chicken, breast, grilled without skin, meat only	464	18-323	
Chicken, breast, strips, stir-fried in corn oil	465	18-326	
Chicken, dark meat, raw	457	18-289	50-434
Chicken, dark meat, roasted	458	18-329	50-441
Chicken, drumsticks, casseroled, meat and skin	466	18-311	
Chicken, drumsticks, roasted, meat and skin	467	18-335	
Chicken, light meat, raw	459	18-290	50-433
Chicken, light meat, roasted	460	18-330	50-440
Chicken, liver, fried in corn oil	493	18-412	50-486
Chicken, meat, average, raw	461	18-488	50-431
Chicken, meat, average, roasted	462	18-331	50-438
Chicken, skin, dry roasted/grilled	468	18-332	18-448
Chicken, stir-fried with rice and vegetables, reheated	564	19-521	19-201
Chicken, sweet and sour, takeaway	589	19-324	
Chicken, whole, roasted, meat and skin	469	18-341	
Chicken/turkey burger, coated, baked	504	18-502	
Chicken/turkey pasties/slices, puff pastry	517	19-469	
Chicken/turkey pieces, coated, baked	514	18-503	19-121
Chicory, raw	757	13-225	50-763
Chilli con carne, homemade	565	19-478	19-337
Chilli con carne, reheated, with rice	566	19-527	19-209
Chilli peppers, capsicum, green, raw	786	13-316	50-801
Chilli powder	856	13-873	13-812
Chilli sauce	1135	17-719	17-294
Chilli, vegetable, homemade	823	15-640	15-370
Chinese 5 spice	857	13-813	
Chinese cherry	See **Lychees**		
Chinese cook in, sweet & sour sauce	1148	17-628	17-335
Chinese gooseberry	See **Kiwi fruit**		
Chinese parsley	See **Coriander leaves**		
Chinese style duck, crispy, meat and skin	481	18-490	
Chinese, stir fry sauce	1149	17-629	
Chips, fine cut, from fast food outlets	687	13-486	13-423
Chips, fried in commercial oil, from takeaway fish and chip shops	688	13-485	
Chips, homemade, fried in rapeseed oil	689	13-555	13-407
Chips, microwave, cooked	690	13-557	13-028

	Publication number	Current code	Previous code
Chips, oven ready, no batter, baked	691	13-487	13-029
Chips, oven ready, with batter, baked	692	13-488	
Chives, fresh	858	13-887	13-814
Choc ices/ice cream bars, chocolate coated, luxury	303	12-510	12-391
Choc ices/ice cream bars, non-dairy, with chocolate flavoured coating	304	12-384	50-263
Chocolate based gateau, frozen	156	11-526	11-421
Chocolate biscuits, fully coated	124	11-809	11-506
Chocolate biscuits, with cream, fully coated	125	11-810	11-507
Chocolate cake bars	147	11-740	
Chocolate cake, with filling and icing	150	11-830	
Chocolate chip cookies, American style	119	11-816	
Chocolate chip cookies, standard	120	11-815	11-508
Chocolate coated biscuits, with marshmallow	126	11-811	11-419
Chocolate covered and filled swiss rolls	168	11-834	11-533
Chocolate covered bar with caramel and cereal	981	17-658	17-550
Chocolate covered caramel and biscuit fingers	983	17-657	17-550
Chocolate covered caramel bars and sweets	980	17-649	17-492
Chocolate covered wafer biscuit	982	11-812	11-509
Chocolate dairy desserts	314	12-398	12-912
Chocolate eclairs, cream filled	184	11-844	11-247
Chocolate flavoured milk, pasteurised	236	12-535	12-325
Chocolate fudge cake	151	11-527	
Chocolate mousse, low fat	321	12-401	12-914
Chocolate muffins, American	160	11-737	
Chocolate nut spread	965	17-687	17-070
Chocolate nut sundae	300	12-518	12-411
Chocolate spread	964	17-659	17-069
Chocolate, dark, with crème or mint fondant centres	989	17-650	
Chocolate, fancy and filled	984	17-690	17-088
Chocolate, milk	985	17-648	17-089
Chocolate, plain	986	17-491	50-1016
Chocolate, white	987	17-091	50-1017
Chori	See **Blackeye beans**		
Chorizo	518	19-516	19-099

	Publication number	Current code	Previous code
Chote bund gobhi	See **Brussels sprouts**		
Chow mein, beef, reheated	543	19-519	19-165
Chow mein, chicken, takeaway	553	19-321	
Christmas pudding	194	11-1022	11-291
Chutney, mango, sweet	1117	17-343	
Chutney, tomato	1118	17-345	
Ciabatta	50	11-969	11-609
Cicer arietinum	See **Chick peas**		
Cichorium intybus	See **Chicory**		
Cider, dry	1078	17-222	50-1104
Cider, low alcohol	1079	17-223	
Cider, sweet	1080	17-224	50-1105
Cider, strong	1081	17-225	17-822
Cilantro	See **Coriander leaves**		
Cinnamomum aromaticum	See **Cinnamon**		
Cinnamomum verum	See **Cinnamon**		
Cinnamon, ground	859	13-874	13-815
Citrus fruit, soft/easy peelers, flesh only	892	14-326	
Citrus limon	See **Lemons**		
Citrus paradisi	See **Grapefruit**		
Citrus sinensis	See **Oranges**		
Citrus reticulata	See **Citrus fruit**		
Clementines	See **Citrus fruit**		
Clotted cream, fresh	246	12-592	12-117
Clupea harengus	See **Herring** and **Kippers**		
Coalfish	See **Coley**		
Cockles, boiled	651	16-252	50-644
Cocoa, powder	1020	12-545	12-082
Coconut milk	944	14-889	14-820
Coconut milk, reduced fat	945	14-890	
Coconut oil	366	17-031	50-320
Coconut, creamed block	942	14-872	50-978
Coconut, desiccated	943	14-873	50-979
Cocos nucifera	See **Coconut**		
Cod in batter, baked	594	16-369	16-025
Cod in batter, fried in rapeseed oil	595	16-426	16-021
Cod in batter, fried, takeaway	596	16-368	16-023
Cod in breadcrumbs, baked	597	16-370	
Cod liver oil	367	17-488	50-321

	Publication number	Current code	Previous code
Cod, baked	592	16-373	16-013
Cod, microwaved	593	16-374	
Cod, raw	591	16-372	16-012
Coffee, cappuccino, latte	1022	17-632	
Coffee, infusion, average	1021	17-833	17-152
Coffee, powder, instant	1023	17-158	50-1054
Coffeemate, whitener powder	1024	12-546	12-027
Cola	1038	17-175	50-1080
Cola, diet	1039	17-505	
Coleslaw, not low calorie	824	15-635	15-077
Coleslaw, with reduced calorie dressing	825	15-636	15-078
Coley, baked	599	16-429	
Coley, raw	598	16-383	16-031
Common gram	See **Chick peas**		
Complan, powder, original and sweet	1025	17-729	17-540
Complan, powder, savoury	1026	17-730	17-541
Compound cooking fat, not polyunsaturated	359	12-501	17-004
Condensed milk, sweetened	231	12-520	12-029
Cook in sauce, traditional, tomato based	1159	17-630	17-295
Cook in sauce, traditional, white sauce based	1160	17-631	17-295
Cookies, chocolate chip, American style	119	11-816	
Cookies, chocolate chip, standard	120	11-815	11-508
Cooking apples, stewed with sugar, flesh only	878	14-332	14-004
Cooking apples, stewed without sugar, flesh only	879	14-320	14-005
Coq au vin, homemade	567	19-486	19-338
Coriander leaves, fresh	860	13-888	13-817
Coriander seeds	861	13-875	13-819
Coriandrum sativum	See **Coriander leaves** and **Coriander seeds**		
Corn oil	368	17-033	50-322
Corn snacks	1007	17-645	17-125
Corned beef, canned	519	19-128	50-507
Cornetto type ice cream cone	301	12-507	12-386
Cornflakes, crunchy/honey nut coated, fortified	93	11-746	11-491
Cornflakes, fortified	91	11-742	11-490
Cornflakes, frosted, fortified	94	11-749	11-492

	Publication number	Current code	Previous code
Cornflakes, unfortified	92	11-745	
Cornflour	2	11-1045	11-435
Cornish pasty	520	19-466	
Coronation chicken, homemade	568	19-477	19-339
Corylus avellana	See **Hazelnuts**		
Corylus maxima	See **Hazelnuts**		
Cottage cheese, plain	260	12-539	12-351
Cottage cheese, plain, reduced fat	261	12-550	12-352
Cottage/Shepherd's pie, reheated	569	19-494	19-216
Courgette, boiled in unsalted water	759	13-231	50-765
Courgette, fried in corn oil	760	13-232	50-766
Courgette, raw	758	13-230	50-764
Couscous, plain, cooked	4	11-902	
Couscous, plain, raw	3	11-901	
Cowpeas	See **Blackeye beans**		
Crab, canned in brine, drained	641	16-452	16-234
Crab, cooked	642	16-441	16-331
Cranberry fruit juice drink	1056	17-744	17-537
Cream crackers	138	11-820	11-510
Cream filled pastries	178	11-843	11-654
Cream liqueurs	1091	17-768	17-242
Cream substitute, double	253	12-342	50-224
Cream substitute, single	252	12-544	12-340
Cream, dairy, extra thick (24% fat)	249	12-337	
Cream, dairy, UHT, canned spray, 85% cream	250	12-338	50-218
Cream, dairy, UHT, half fat, canned spray	251	12-339	
Cream, fresh, clotted	246	12-592	12-117
Cream, fresh, double, including Jersey cream	245	12-334	50-215
Cream, fresh, single	243	12-332	50-212
Cream, fresh, whipping	244	12-333	50-214
Creme caramel	315	12-397	50-275
Creme egg	988	17-763	17-544
Creme fraiche	247	12-335	12-896
Creme fraiche, half fat	248	12-336	
Cress and mustard, raw	775	13-297	50-788
Crispbread, rye	140	11-822	11-511
Crispie cakes, homemade	152	11-990	11-576
Crisps, potato, fried in sunflower oil	1011	17-671	

	Publication number	Current code	Previous code
Croissants	75	11-988	11-480
Crumble, fruit	195	11-1020	11-546
Crumble, fruit, wholemeal, homemade	196	11-994	11-595
Crumpets, toasted	76	11-989	11-535
Crunchy clusters type cereal, without nuts, unfortified	95	11-938	11-783
Crunchy/crispy muesli type cereal, with nuts, unfortified	96	11-939	11-783
Crunchy/honey nut coated cornflakes, fortified	93	11-746	11-491
Cucumber, raw, flesh and skin	761	13-523	13-233
Cucumis melo var cantalupensis	See **Melon, Canteloupe-type**		
Cucumis melo var inodorus	See **Melon, yellow flesh**		
Cucumis melo var reticulata	See **Melon, Galia**		
Cucumis sativus	See **Cucumber** and **Gherkins**		
Cucurbita pepo	See **Courgette**		
Cucurbita sp	See **Pumpkin**		
Cucurbita spp	See **Pumpkin seeds**		
Cumin seeds	862	13-889	13-820
Cuminum cyminum	See **Cumin seeds**		
Curly kale, boiled in unsalted water	763	13-541	
Curly kale, raw	762	13-234	50-768
Currant buns	77	11-1009	11-536
Currant buns, toasted	78	11-948	
Curry paste	1145	17-720	17-297
Curry powder	863	13-876	13-822
Curry, beef, reduced fat, homemade	546	19-472	19-333
Curry, beef, reheated	544	19-488	19-169
Curry, beef, reheated, with rice	545	19-529	19-170
Curry, chick pea dhal, homemade	826	15-641	15-371
Curry, chicken, average, takeaway	554	19-322	19-300
Curry, chicken, made with cook-in sauce	557	19-534	19-336
Curry, chicken, reheated	555	19-520	19-188
Curry, chicken, reheated, with rice	556	19-528	19-189
Curry, chicken, Thai green, takeaway and restaurant	558	19-465	
Curry, fish, Bangladeshi, homemade	654	16-446	16-336
Curry, fish, homemade	655	16-364	
Curry, lamb, made with cook-in sauce	574	19-535	19-344
Curry, prawn, takeaway	656	16-333	16-278

	Publication number	Current code	Previous code
Curry, Thai, stir-fry vegetable, takeaway and restaurant	827	15-634	
Curry, vegetable, ready meal, cooked	828	15-619	
Custard tarts, individual	179	12-461	11-537
Custard, made up with semi-skimmed milk	316	12-519	12-413
Custard, ready to eat	317	12-543	12-399
Dhal, mixed, homemade	831	13-484	
Danish blue	262	12-354	50-236
Danish pastries	180	11-841	11-538
Dark chocolate with crème or mint fondant centres	989	17-650	
Dates, dried, flesh and skin	893	14-085	
Daucus carota	See **Carrots**		
Demerara sugar	975	17-061	50-1010
Dhana	See **Coriander leaves**		
Dicentrarchus labrax	See **Sea bass**		
Digestive biscuits, half coated in chocolate	121	11-807	11-512
Digestive biscuits, plain	122	11-799	11-513
Digestive biscuits, with oats, plain	123	11-803	11-517
Dioscorea sp	See **Yam**		
Dips, sour-cream based	1119	17-299	
Dips, sour-cream based, reduced fat	1120	17-677	
Doner kebab in pitta bread with salad	571	19-526	19-130
Doner kebabs, meat only	570	19-539	19-129
Double cream, fresh, including Jersey cream	245	12-334	50-215
Double Gloucester	263	12-487	12-153
Doughnuts ring, iced	182	11-850	11-244
Doughnuts, with jam	181	11-849	11-242
Dressing, blue cheese	1121	17-715	17-300
Dressing, French	1122	17-701	17-509
Dressing, French, fat free	1123	17-716	17-538
Dressing, thousand island	1124	17-717	17-306
Dried mixed fruit	894	14-087	50-888
Dried skimmed milk	232	12-521	12-030
Dried yeast	1180	17-379	50-1188
Drinking chocolate, powder	1027	17-498	50-1064
Drinking chocolate, powder, made up with semi-skimmed milk	1028	17-532	50-1066
Drinking chocolate, powder, reduced fat	1029	17-499	
Dripping, beef	360	17-487	50-317

	Publication number	Current code	Previous code
Drumsticks, chicken	See **Chicken, drumsticks**		
Dry roasted peanuts	953	14-878	50-989
Dublin Bay prawns	See **Scampi**		
Duck, crispy, Chinese style, meat and skin	481	18-490	
Duck, raw, meat only	480	18-489	50-445
Duck, roasted, meat only	482	18-372	50-447
Duck, roasted, meat, fat and skin	483	18-374	50-448
Dumplings, homemade	204	11-962	11-603
Dungli	See **Onions**		
Eating apples, raw, flesh and skin	880	14-319	14-012
Eccles cakes	183	11-838	11-589
Eclairs, chocolate, cream filled	184	11-844	11-247
Edam	264	12-355	50-237
Egg fried rice, ready cooked, re-heated	18	11-885	
Egg mayonnaise sandwich, white bread	86	11-966	11-567
Egg noodles, dried, raw	34	11-719	11-055
Egg noodles, medium, dried, boiled in unsalted water	35	11-724	11-056
Egg pasta, fresh, filled with cheese only, boiled in unsalted water	39	11-728	11-451
Egg pasta, fresh, filled with meat, boiled in unsalted water	40	11-732	
Egg pasta, fresh, raw	37	11-726	11-449
Egg pasta, tagliatelle, white, fresh, boiled in unsalted water	38	11-727	
Eggplant	See **Aubergine**		
Eggs, chicken, scrambled, with semi-skimmed milk	340	12-945	12-926
Eggs, chicken, white, boiled	336	12-941	
Eggs, chicken, white, raw	333	12-938	12-804
Eggs, chicken, whole, boiled	335	12-940	12-806
Eggs, chicken, whole, fried in sunflower oil	338	12-944	12-919
Eggs, chicken, whole, poached	339	12-943	12-810
Eggs, chicken, whole, raw	332	12-937	12-918
Eggs, chicken, yolk, boiled	337	12-942	
Eggs, chicken, yolk, raw	334	12-939	12-805
Energy drink, carbonated	1040	17-672	
English style muffins, white	79	11-541	11-260
English style muffins, white, toasted	80	11-542	11-260
Engraulidae	See **Anchovies**		
Eruca sativa	See **Rocket**		

	Publication number	Current code	Previous code
Evaporated milk, light	234	12-324	12-890
Evaporated milk, whole	233	12-522	12-033
Evening primrose oil	369	17-035	17-420
Faggots in gravy, reheated	572	19-131	50-509
Fajita, chicken, meat only, takeaway and restaurant	559	19-464	
Fancy iced cakes	153	11-839	11-528
Fansi	See **Green beans**		
Fat spread, low fat (26-39%), not polyunsaturated, including dairy type	355	12-497	17-552
Fat spread, low fat (26-39%), not polyunsaturated, with olive oil	356	12-498	
Fat spread, low fat (26-39%), polyunsaturated	357	12-499	17-027
Fat spread, reduced fat (41-62%), not polyunsaturated	352	12-504	
Fat spread, reduced fat (41-62%), not polyunsaturated, with olive	353	12-505	17-025
Fat spread, reduced fat (41-62%), polyunsaturated	354	12-503	17-024
Fat spread, reduced fat (62-75%), not polyunsaturated	351	12-506	17-022
Fat spread, reduced fat (62-75%), polyunsaturated	350	17-710	17-551
Fat, beef, average, cooked	395	18-005	50-362
Fat, beef, average, raw	394	18-003	50-361
Fat, lamb, average, cooked	418	18-100	50-389
Fat, lamb, average, raw	417	18-098	50-388
Fat, pork	See **Pork, fat**		
Fava bean	See **Broad beans**		
Fennel, Florence, boiled in unsalted water	765	13-542	
Fennel, Florence, raw	764	13-241	50-770
Fermented milk drink with probiotics	281	12-513	
Feta	265	12-525	12-356
Ficus carica	See **Figs**		
Figs, ready-to-eat	895	14-095	50-890
Filo pastry, cooked	170	11-856	
Filo pastry, uncooked	169	11-855	
Fish curry, Bangladeshi, homemade	654	16-446	16-336
Fish curry, homemade	655	16-364	
Fish fingers, cod, fried in rapeseed oil	660	16-444	16-289
Fish fingers, cod, fried in sunflower oil	661	16-445	16-291

	Publication number	Current code	Previous code
Fish fingers, cod, grilled/baked	659	16-405	16-288
Fish fingers, pollock, grilled	662	16-371	
Fish fingers, salmon, grilled/baked	663	16-406	
Fish paste	664	16-450	16-334
Fish pie, white fish	665	16-410	16-295
Fish pizza, takeaway	215	11-1011	11-560
Fishcakes, salmon, coated in breadcrumbs, baked	658	16-408	
Fishcakes, white fish, coated in breadcrumbs, baked	657	16-407	16-281
Flaky/puff pastry, cooked	172	11-854	
Flaky/puff pastry, uncooked	171	11-852	11-224
Flapjacks	141	11-814	
Flavoured milk, pasteurised, chocolate	236	12-535	12-325
Flavoured milk, pasteurised, strawberry, banana	235	12-326	50-203
Flour, chapati, brown	5	11-895	11-433
Flour, gram	707	11-896	13-073
Flour, rye	6	11-897	11-436
Flour, soya	7	11-898	11-025
Flour, wheat, bread/strong, white	9	11-887	11-438
Flour, wheat, brown	8	11-892	11-437
Flour, wheat, white, plain, soft	10	11-886	11-439
Flour, wheat, white, self raising	11	11-888	11-440
Flour, wheat, wholemeal	12	11-889	11-441
Foeniculum vulgare var dulce	See **Fennel, Florence**		
Four cheese pasta sauce	1154	17-624	
Fragaria sp	See **Strawberries**		
Frankfurter	521	19-495	19-100
French dressing	1122	17-701	17-509
French dressing, fat free	1123	17-716	17-538
Fried eggs, chicken, whole, fried in sunflower oil	338	12-944	12-919
Fromage frais, fruit, children's, fortified	282	12-534	12-908
Fromage frais, virtually fat free, fruit	283	12-372	50-241
Fromage frais, virtually fat free, natural	284	12-528	12-371
Frosted cornflakes, fortified	94	11-749	11-492
Frozen ice cream desserts	302	12-385	50-266
Fruit and fibre type cereal, fortified	97	11-779	11-493
Fruit cake	154	11-829	11-529
Fruit cake, rich, iced, homemade	155	11-991	11-578

	Publication number	Current code	Previous code
Fruit cheesecake, frozen	312	12-395	50-274
Fruit cheesecake, individual	313	12-542	12-396
Fruit cocktail, canned in juice	896	14-336	14-096
Fruit cocktail, canned in syrup	897	14-097	50-892
Fruit crumble, wholemeal, homemade	196	11-994	11-595
Fruit gateau, frozen	157	11-530	11-420
Fruit gums/jellies	997	17-107	
Fruit juice drink, carbonated, no added sugar, ready to drink	1042	17-673	
Fruit juice drink, carbonated, ready to drink	1041	17-735	17-177
Fruit juice drink, no added sugar, ready to drink	1051	17-742	17-196
Fruit juice drink, no added sugar, undiluted	1050	17-739	17-191
Fruit juice drink/squash, ready to drink	1049	17-741	17-195
Fruit juice drink/squash, undiluted	1048	17-738	17-189
Fruit juice, mixed	1060	17-746	
Fruit mousse	322	12-402	
Fruit pastilles	998	17-824	17-108
Fruit pie, individual	197	11-847	11-547
Fruit pie, one crust, homemade	198	11-1007	11-596
Fruit pie, pastry top and bottom, homemade	199	11-1008	11-597
Fruit salad, homemade	898	14-333	14-303
Fruit scones	189	11-993	11-543
Fruit sorbet	310	12-393	
Fruit torte	329	12-408	
Fruit trifle	330	12-409	
Fruit, crumble	195	11-1020	11-546
Fudge, homemade	999	17-683	17-518
Fusarium venenatum	See **Quorn**		
Gadus morhua	See **Cod**		
Gajjar	See **Carrots**		
Galia melon, flesh only	911	14-159	50-921
Gallus domesticus	See **Chicken**		
Gammon joint, boiled	392	19-021	
Gammon joint, raw	391	19-020	
Gammon rashers, grilled	393	19-505	19-022
Garam masala	864	13-829	50-841
Garbanzo	See **Chick peas**		

	Publication number	Current code	Previous code
Garlic and herb bread	51	11-937	11-460
Garlic mushrooms, not coated, homemade	829	15-642	15-373
Garlic, raw	766	13-244	50-772
Gateau, chocolate based, frozen	156	11-526	11-421
Gateau, fruit, frozen	157	11-530	
Gelatine	1163	17-360	
Ghee made from vegetable oil	362	12-502	17-009
Ghee, butter	361	17-640	17-007
Gherkins, pickled, drained	767	13-246	50-773
Gingelly	See **Sesame seeds**		
Ginger nut biscuits	127	11-798	11-514
Ginger, fresh	866	13-831	
Ginger, ground	865	13-832	
Glace cherries	891	14-335	14-068
Glycine max	See **Soya beans**		
Goats milk cheese, soft, white rind	266	12-357	12-162
Goats milk, pasteurised	238	12-328	
Gobi	See **Cauliflower**		
Golden gram	See **Mung beans**		
Golden syrup	977	17-065	
Goose, roasted, meat, fat and skin	484	18-376	
Gooseberries, cooking, stewed with sugar	899	14-101	50-896
Gouda	267	12-358	50-243
Gram flour	707	11-896	13-073
Granada	See **Pomegranate**		
Grape juice, unsweetened	1057	17-745	14-273
Grapefruit juice, unsweetened	1058	14-275	
Grapefruit, canned in juice	901	14-107	50-901
Grapefruit, raw, flesh only	900	14-292	
Grapes, green	902	14-322	
Grapes, red	903	14-323	
Grapeseed oil	370	17-036	
Gravy instant granules	1164	17-724	17-310
Gravy instant granules, made up with water	1165	17-725	17-311
Greek pastries, Baklava	185	11-842	11-248
Greek style yogurt, fruit	286	12-377	
Greek style yogurt, plain	287	12-555	12-376
Green beans, boiled in unsalted water	699	13-515	13-432

	Publication number	Current code	Previous code
Green beans, raw	698	13-514	13-431
Green cabbage, boiled in unsalted water	744	13-511	13-444
Green cabbage, raw	743	13-510	13-468
Green gram	See **Mung beans**		
Green peppers, capsicum, boiled in unsalted water	788	13-548	
Green peppers, capsicum, raw	787	13-318	50-802
Green salad	841	15-648	15-380
Green tea, infusion	1036	17-171	
Groundnut oil	373	17-040	
Groundnuts	See **Peanuts**		
Guinness	1077	17-767	17-219
Gullar	See **Figs**		
Gumbo	See **Okra**		
Haddock, grilled	601	16-376	16-045
Haddock, raw	600	16-375	16-044
Haddock, smoked, poached	603	16-402	16-066
Haddock, steamed	602	16-377	16-049
Haggis, boiled	522	19-132	
Halloumi	268	12-496	
Ham	390	19-496	19-308
Ham and pineapple pizza, retail	216	11-1013	11-558
Ham salad sandwich, white bread	87	11-965	11-566
Ham, gammon joint, boiled	392	19-021	
Ham, gammon joint, raw	391	19-020	
Ham, gammon rashers, grilled	393	19-505	19-022
Hamburger, takeaway	505	19-544	19-311
Hard block margarine and baking fats (75-90% fat)	358	12-500	17-539
Hazelnuts	946	14-874	
Heart, lamb, roasted	489	18-492	
Helianthus annuus	See **Sunflower seeds**		
Herbal tea, infusion	1037	17-172	
Herring, grilled	615	16-176	
Hibiscus esculentus	See **Okra**		
Hickory nuts	See **Pecan nuts**		
High juice drink, no added sugar, undiluted	1053	17-674	
High juice drink, undiluted	1052	17-740	17-197
Honey	966	17-050	

	Publication number	Current code	Previous code
Honey loops and hoops, fortified	98	11-755	
Horlicks, powder	1030	17-731	17-503
Horseradish sauce	1136	17-314	
Hot pot, lamb/beef, with potatoes, reheated	576	19-522	19-231
Houmous	708	13-556	13-433
Human milk, mature	239	12-536	12-040
Ice cream bars/choc ices, chocolate coated, luxury	303	12-510	12-391
Ice cream bars/choc ices, non-dairy, with chocolate flavoured coating	304	12-384	50-263
Ice cream cone, Cornetto type	301	12-507	12-386
Ice cream desserts, frozen	302	12-385	
Ice cream sauce, topping	967	17-689	17-053
Ice cream wafers, plain, not filled	145	11-800	12-212
Ice cream, dairy, luxury, with chocolate/caramel	306	12-511	
Ice cream, dairy, vanilla, soft scoop	305	12-508	12-387
Ice cream, non dairy, vanilla, soft scoop	307	12-509	12-388
Iced biscuits	128	11-808	
Iced buns	186	11-828	
Iced ring doughnuts	182	11-850	11-244
Illex	See **Calamari**		
Indian cook in sauce, korma/tikka masala	1151	17-626	17-298
Indian cook in sauce, other	1152	17-627	17-298
Indian nuts	See **Pine nuts**		
Instant drinks powder, chocolate, low calorie	1031	17-732	17-500
Instant drinks powder, malted, unfortified	1032	17-825	17-501
Instant potato powder, made up with water	693	13-558	13-032
Instant soup, dried, as served	1102	17-660	17-508
Ipomoea batatas	See **Sweet potato**		
Irish stew, homemade	573	19-479	19-341
Jaffa cakes	158	11-739	11-515
Jam doughnuts	181	11-849	11-242
Jam filled biscuits	129	11-804	11-516
Jam tarts	187	11-846	11-540
Jam, fruit with edible seeds	968	17-073	
Jam, reduced sugar	969	17-075	
Jam, stone fruit	970	17-688	17-074

	Publication number	Current code	Previous code
Jeera	See **Cumin seeds**		
Jellies/fruit gums	997	17-107	
Jelly, made with water	318	12-237	50-282
Jelly, sugar free, made with water	319	12-516	
Jew's apple	See **Aubergine**		
Juglans regia	See **Walnuts**		
Kaju	See **Cashew nuts**		
Kakdi	See **Cucumber**		
Kale	See **Curly kale**		
Kanda	See **Onions**		
Kebab, doner, in pitta bread with salad	571	19-526	19-130
Kebab, doner, meat only	570	19-539	19-129
Kebab, shish, in pitta bread with salad	586	19-525	19-151
Kebab, shish, meat only	585	19-150	
Kedgeree, homemade	666	16-447	16-337
Kheema, lamb, homemade	575	19-480	19-343
Khira	See **Cucumber**		
Kidney, lamb, fried in corn oil	490	18-493	
Kidney, ox, stewed	491	18-405	
King prawns	See **Prawns, king**		
Kippers, boil in the bag, with butter, cooked	617	16-398	16-190
Kippers, grilled	616	16-397	16-188
Kiwi fruit, flesh and seeds	904	14-293	
Kobi	See **Cabbage**		
Kula	See **Bananas**		
Kumra	See **Pumpkin**		
Lactuca sativa	See **Lettuce**		
Lady's fingers	See **Okra**		
Lager, alcohol-free	1071	17-212	
Lager, extra strong	1074	17-676	17-214
Lager, low alcohol	1072	17-750	17-213
Lager, premium	1073	17-751	17-211
Lager, standard	1070	17-749	
Lal kaddu	See **Pumpkin**		
Lal phupala	See **Pumpkin**		
Lamb curry, made with cook-in sauce	574	19-535	19-344
Lamb kheema, homemade	575	19-480	19-343
Lamb, breast, roasted, lean and fat	421	18-114	
Lamb, breast, roasted, lean only	420	18-113	

	Publication number	Current code	Previous code
Lamb, fat, average, cooked	418	18-100	50-389
Lamb, fat, average, raw	417	18-098	50-388
Lamb, heart, roasted	489	18-492	
Lamb, kidney, fried in corn oil	490	18-493	
Lamb, lean only, average, raw	419	18-475	
Lamb, leg, average, raw, lean and fat	422	18-478	
Lamb, leg, half knuckle, pot-roasted, lean and fat	423	18-129	
Lamb, leg, whole, roasted, lean and fat	425	18-480	
Lamb, leg, whole, roasted, lean only	424	18-479	
Lamb, liver, fried in corn oil	494	18-494	
Lamb, loin chops, grilled, lean and fat	428	18-477	
Lamb, loin chops, grilled, lean only	427	18-141	
Lamb, loin chops, microwaved, lean and fat	429	18-147	
Lamb, loin chops, raw, lean and fat	426	18-476	
Lamb, loin chops, roasted, lean and fat	431	18-151	
Lamb, loin chops, roasted, lean only	430	18-149	
Lamb, mince, raw	432	18-481	
Lamb, mince, stewed	433	18-159	
Lamb, neck fillet, strips, stir-fried in corn oil, lean only	434	18-164	
Lamb, shoulder, diced, kebabs, grilled, lean and fat	435	18-172	
Lamb, shoulder, whole, roasted, lean and fat	437	18-180	
Lamb, shoulder, whole, roasted, lean only	436	18-179	
Lamb, stewing lamb, stewed, lean and fat	439	18-187	
Lamb, stewing lamb, stewed, lean only	438	18-186	
Lamb/beef hot pot with potatoes, reheated	576	19-522	19-231
Langoustine	See **Scampi**		
Lard	363	17-010	
Lasagne, homemade	578	19-481	19-346
Lasagne, homemade, with extra lean minced beef	579	19-482	
Lasagne, reheated	577	19-523	19-238
Lasagne, vegetable	830	15-651	15-189
Lassan	See **Garlic**		
Lassi, sweetened	285	12-373	
Latte, cappuccino	1022	17-632	
Leeks, boiled in unsalted water	769	13-452	

	Publication number	Current code	Previous code
Leeks, raw	768	13-466	
Leg joint, pork	See **Pork, leg joint**		
Leg, lamb	See **Lamb, leg**		
Lehsan	See **Garlic**		
Lemon curd	971	17-762	17-490
Lemon juice, fresh	1059	14-277	
Lemon meringue pie	200	11-548	
Lemon peel	905	14-337	14-127
Lemon sole, grilled	605	16-380	16-083
Lemon sole, raw	604	16-379	16-082
Lemonade	1043	17-179	
Lemons, whole, without pips	906	14-128	50-910
Lens culinaris	See **Lentils, red**		
Lentil soup, canned	1103	17-698	17-263
Lentils, red, split, dried, boiled in unsalted water	710	13-434	
Lentils, red, split, dried, raw	709	13-091	50-712
Lepidium spp	See **Mustard and cress**		
Lettuce, average, raw	770	13-520	13-453
Lichee	See **Lychees**		
Lichi	See **Lychees**		
Lima beans	See **Butter beans**		
Lime juice cordial, undiluted	1054	17-200	
Liqueurs, high strength	1092	17-244	
Liqueurs, low-medium strength	1093	17-245	
Liquorice allsorts	1000	17-777	17-112
Litchee	See **Lychees**		
Litchi	See **Lychees**		
Litchi chinensis	See **Lychees**		
Lithodidae	See **Crab**		
Litopenaeus vannamei	See **Prawns, king**		
Liver pate	526	19-317	
Liver sausage	523	19-106	
Liver, calf, fried in corn oil	492	18-410	
Liver, chicken, fried in corn oil	493	18-412	50-486
Liver, lamb, fried in corn oil	494	18-494	
Liver, ox, stewed	495	18-416	
Liver, pig, stewed	496	18-418	
Loaf cake	159	11-833	
Lobia	See **Blackeye beans**		

	Publication number	Current code	Previous code
Loin chops, lamb	See **Lamb, loin chops**		
Loin chops, pork	See **Pork, loin chops**		
Loligo	See **Calamari**		
Lollies, containing ice-cream	308	12-390	
Lollies, with real fruit juice	309	12-389	
Long grain rice, white, boiled in unsalted water	28	11-862	11-050
Long grain rice, white, easy cook, boiled in unsalted water	29	11-864	11-446
Long grain rice, white, raw	27	11-861	11-049
Low calorie soup, canned	1104	17-699	17-265
Low fat yogurt, fruit	288	12-380	
Low fat yogurt, hazelnut	289	12-904	
Low fat yogurt, plain	290	12-379	
Low fat yogurt, toffee	291	12-905	
Lucozade	1044	17-761	17-543
Lychees, raw, flesh only	907	14-142	50-911
Lycopersicon esculentum	See **Tomatoes**		
Macadamia integrifolia	See **Macadamia nuts**		
Macadamia nuts, salted	947	14-891	14-823
Macadamia tetraphylla	See **Macadamia nuts**		
Macaroni cheese, homemade	33	11-954	11-562
Mackerel, grilled	619	16-394	16-325
Mackerel, raw	618	16-393	16-324
Mackerel, smoked	620	16-414	16-196
Madeira nuts	See **Walnuts**		
Malt bread, fruited	52	11-462	
Malted flake cereal, fortified	99	11-760	11-501
Malted wheat bread	53	11-972	11-461
Malted wheat bread rolls	70	11-984	11-479
Malted wheat cereal, fortified	100	11-761	11-500
Maltesers and similar products	990	17-651	
Malus domestica	See **Apples**		
Malus pumila	See **Apples**		
Mandarin oranges, canned in juice	908	14-146	50-914
Mandarins	See **Citrus fruit**		
Mange-tout peas, boiled in unsalted water	722	13-547	
Mange-tout peas, raw	721	13-122	50-725
Mange-tout peas, stir-fried in rapeseed oil	723	13-568	13-124
Mangifera indica	See **Mangoes**		

	Publication number	Current code	Previous code
Mango chutney, sweet	1117	17-343	
Mangoes, ripe, raw, flesh only	909	14-294	
Margarine and baking fats (75-90% fat), hard block	358	12-500	17-539
Marmalade	972	17-078	
Marrowfat peas, canned, re-heated, drained	724	13-562	13-125
Mars bar and own brand equivalents	991	17-668	17-547
Marshmallows	1001	17-114	
Marzipan	948	14-875	
Mascarpone	269	12-490	
Masoor dhal	See **Lentils, red**		
Masur dhal	See **Lentils, red**		
Mattar	See **Peas**		
Mayonnaise	1125	17-654	17-510
Mayonnaise, reduced fat	1126	17-679	17-511
Meat pate, reduced fat	527	19-145	
Meat samosas, takeaway	525	19-326	
Meat spread	524	19-506	19-139
Meat topped pizza, retail and takeaway	217	11-1015	11-556
Melanogrammus aeglefinus	See **Haddock**		
Meleagris gallopavo	See **Turkey**		
Melon, Canteloupe-type, flesh only	910	14-339	14-295
Melon, Galia, flesh only	911	14-159	50-921
Melon, watermelon, flesh only	913	14-296	
Melon, yellow flesh, flesh only	912	14-328	14-162
Mentha spicata	See **Mint**		
Meringue, homemade	320	12-517	12-414
Microstomus kitt	See **Lemon sole**		
Microwave chips, cooked	690	13-557	13-028
Milk alternative, non-dairy, soya, sweetened, fortified	241	12-523	12-330
Milk alternative, non-dairy, soya, unsweetened, fortified	242	12-524	12-331
Milk chocolate	985	17-648	17-089
Milk drink, fermented, with probiotics	281	12-513	
Milk shake, powder	1033	17-733	12-104
Milk, 1% fat, pasteurised	220	12-512	
Milk, coconut	944	14-889	
Milk, coconut, reduced fat	945	14-890	
Milk, condensed, sweetened	231	12-520	12-029

	Publication number	Current code	Previous code
Milk, dried, skimmed	232	12-521	12-030
Milk, evaporated, light	234	12-324	12-890
Milk, evaporated, whole	233	12-522	12-033
Milk, flavoured, pasteurised, chocolate	236	12-535	12-325
Milk, flavoured, pasteurised, strawberry, banana	235	12-326	
Milk, goats, pasteurised	238	12-328	
Milk, human, mature	239	12-536	12-040
Milk, semi-skimmed, pasteurised, summer and autumn	222	12-418	
Milk, semi-skimmed, pasteurised, winter and spring	223	12-419	
Milk, semi-skimmed, UHT	224	12-314	
Milk, semi-skimmed, pasteurised, average	221	12-313	
Milk, sheeps, raw	240	12-329	
Milk, skimmed, pasteurised, average	225	12-307	
Milk, skimmed, UHT	226	12-310	
Milk, whole, Channel Islands, pasteurised	219	12-321	
Milk, whole, pasteurised, average	227	12-596	12-316
Milk, whole, pasteurised, summer and autumn	228	12-598	12-317
Milk, whole, pasteurised, winter and spring	229	12-597	12-318
Milk, whole, UHT	230	12-599	12-320
Milkshake, thick, takeaway	237	12-327	
Milky Way and own brand equivalents	992	17-669	17-548
Mince pies	188	11-848	
Mince, beef, extra lean, stewed	402	18-507	18-041
Mince, beef, microwaved	400	18-037	
Mince, beef, raw	399	18-469	
Mince, beef, stewed	401	18-470	
Mincemeat	973	17-765	17-080
Minestrone soup, canned	1105	17-711	17-542
Minibreads, toasted	142	11-825	
Mint sauce	1137	17-707	17-319
Mint, fresh	867	13-836	50-842
Mixed dhal, homemade	831	13-484	
Mixed fruit juice	1060	17-746	
Mixed fruit, dried	894	14-087	50-888
Mixed herbs, dried	868	13-884	13-871
Mixed nuts	949	14-880	50-985

	Publication number	Current code	Previous code
Mixed peel	914	14-338	14-167
Mixed vegetables cooked with onion, spice and tomatoes, homemade	832	15-621	
Mixed vegetables, frozen, boiled in unsalted water	771	13-543	13-281
Monkey nuts	See **Peanuts**		
Moong beans	See **Mung beans**		
Motamircha	See **Peppers, capsicum (green/red)**		
Moussaka, reheated	580	19-507	19-248
Moussaka, vegetable	833	15-652	15-206
Mousse, chocolate, low fat	321	12-401	12-914
Mousse, fruit	322	12-402	
Mozzarella, fresh	270	12-360	12-170
Muesli type cereal, crunchy/crispy, with nuts, unfortified	96	11-939	
Muesli, Swiss style, no added sugar or salt, unfortified	102	11-781	11-495
Muesli, Swiss style, unfortified	101	11-780	11-494
Muffins, American, chocolate	160	11-737	
Muffins, American, not chocolate	161	11-738	
Muffins, English style, white	79	11-541	11-260
Muffins, English style, white, toasted	80	11-542	11-260
Multigrain hoops, fortified	103	11-1019	11-623
Mung beans, whole, dried, boiled in unsalted water	711	13-097	50-715
Musa paradisiaca	See **Plantain**		
Musa spp	See **Bananas**		
Mushroom soup, carton, chilled	1106	17-635	
Mushroom soup, cream of, canned	1107	17-713	17-270
Mushrooms, white, fried in rapeseed oil	774	13-507	50-785
Mushrooms, white, raw	772	13-505	13-284
Mushrooms, white, stewed	773	13-506	13-285
Mushy peas, canned, re-heated	725	13-563	13-437
Mussels in white wine sauce, cooked	653	16-411	
Mussels, cooked	652	16-390	16-256
Mustard and cress, raw	775	13-297	50-788
Mustard powder	869	17-362	50-843
Mustard, smooth	1166	17-364	
Mustard, wholegrain	1167	17-365	
Myristica fragrans	See **Nutmeg**		
Mytilidae	See **Mussels**		

	Publication number	Current code	Previous code
Naan bread	54	11-973	11-463
Naan, peshwari	55	11-910	
Napoletana pasta sauce, tomato based	1156	17-619	
Nasturtium officinale	See **Watercress**		
Navy beans	See **Baked beans**		
Nectarines, flesh and skin	915	14-297	
Neeps (England)	See **Swede**		
Neeps (Scotland)	See **Turnip**		
Nephrops norvegicus	See **Scampi**		
New and salad potatoes, boiled in unsalted water, flesh and skin	676	13-495	13-420
Nhanu kobi	See **Brussels sprouts**		
Noodles, egg, dried, raw	34	11-719	11-055
Noodles, egg, medium, dried, boiled in unsalted water	35	11-724	11-056
Noodles, rice, fine, dried, boiled in unsalted water	36	11-725	
Norway lobster	See **Scampi**		
Nut roast, homemade	834	15-643	15-374
Nutmeg, ground	870	13-877	13-840
Nuts, almonds	938	14-870	
Nuts, Brazil	939	14-871	
Nuts, cashew, roasted and salted	940	14-812	50-976
Nuts, chestnuts, raw	941	14-813	50-977
Nuts, coconut milk	944	14-889	
Nuts, coconut milk, reduced fat	945	14-890	
Nuts, coconut, creamed block	942	14-872	
Nuts, coconut, desiccated	943	14-873	
Nuts, hazelnuts	946	14-874	
Nuts, macadamia, salted	947	14-891	14-823
Nuts, mixed	949	14-880	50-985
Nuts, peanuts, dry roasted	953	14-878	
Nuts, peanuts, plain	952	14-877	
Nuts, peanuts, roasted and salted	954	14-834	50-990
Nuts, pecan	955	14-837	50-991
Nuts, pine	956	14-839	50-992
Nuts, pistachio, roasted and salted	957	14-840	
Nuts, walnuts	963	14-879	
Oat cereal, instant, flavoured, unfortified, cooked, made up with semi-skimmed milk	106	11-795	

	Publication number	Current code	Previous code
Oat cereal, instant, plain, fortified, cooked, made up with semi-skimmed milk	105	11-793	
Oat cereal, instant, plain, fortified, raw	104	11-792	11-496
Oatcakes, plain	143	11-823	11-518
Oats, porridge, unfortified	107	11-788	11-017
Oats, porridge, unfortified, cooked, made up with semi-skimmed milk	108	11-789	
Ocimum basilicum	See **Basil**		
Oil, coconut	366	17-031	50-320
Oil, cod liver	367	17-488	50-321
Oil, corn	368	17-033	50-322
Oil, evening primrose	369	17-035	17-420
Oil, grapeseed	370	17-036	
Oil, groundnut	373	17-040	
Oil, olive	371	17-038	
Oil, palm	372	17-039	
Oil, peanut (groundnut)	373	17-040	
Oil, rapeseed	374	17-041	
Oil, sesame	375	17-043	
Oil, soya	376	17-044	
Oil, sunflower	377	17-045	
Oil, vegetable, average	378	17-686	17-489
Oil, walnut	379	17-047	
Okra, boiled in unsalted water	777	13-301	50-790
Okra, raw	776	13-300	50-789
Okra, stir-fried in corn oil	778	13-302	50-791
Old potatoes	See **Potatoes, old**		
Olea europaea	See **Olives**		
Olive oil	371	17-038	
Olives, in brine	916	14-340	14-173
Omelette, cheese	342	12-947	12-922
Omelette, plain	341	12-946	12-921
Ommastrephes sagittatus	See **Calamari**		
Oncorhynchus mykiss	See **Trout, rainbow**		
Oncorhynchus nerka	See **Salmon, red**		
Onions, boiled in unsalted water	780	13-500	13-306
Onions, fried in sunflower oil	781	13-501	
Onions, pickled, drained	782	13-309	50-797
Onions, raw	779	13-499	13-304
Onions, spring, bulbs and tops, raw	804	13-352	50-818

	Publication number	Current code	Previous code
Orange juice, ambient, UHT	1062	14-330	14-301
Orange juice, chilled	1061	14-329	14-301
Oranges, flesh only	917	14-327	14-298
Oregano, dried, ground	871	13-878	13-842
Origanum vulgare	See **Oregano**		
Oryctolagus cuniculus	See **Rabbit**		
Oryza sativa	See **Rice**		
Ovaltine, powder	1034	17-734	17-504
Ovis aries	See **Lamb**		
Ox, kidney, stewed	491	18-405	
Ox, liver, stewed	495	18-416	
Oxtail soup, canned	1108	17-700	17-272
Pacific pollack	See **Pollock, Alaskan**		
Pacific pollock	See **Pollock, Alaskan**		
Pak choi, steamed	783	13-516	
Pakora/bhajia, vegetable	835	15-653	15-232
Palaemonidae	See **Prawns** and **Prawns, king**		
Palak	See **Spinach**		
Palm oil	372	17-039	
Pancakes, savoury, made with semi-skimmed milk, homemade	205	11-959	
Pancakes, Scotch	192	11-544	
Pancakes, stuffed with vegetables, homemade	836	15-645	15-376
Pandalidae	See **Prawns**		
Pandalus borealis	See **Prawns**		
Paneer	271	12-495	
Panga	See **Pangasius**		
Pangasius hypophthalmus	See **Pangasius**		
Pangasius, baked	607	16-432	
Pangasius, raw	606	16-382	
Pangoli	See **Cauliflower**		
Papadums, takeaway	206	11-998	11-464
Papai	See **Papaya**		
Papaya, raw, flesh only	919	14-180	50-935
Paprika	872	13-879	13-843
Parmesan, fresh	272	12-526	12-361
Parsley, fresh	873	13-844	50-846
Parsnip, boiled in unsalted water	785	13-454	
Parsnip, raw	784	13-312	50-799

	Publication number	Current code	Previous code
Passiflora edulis f edulis	See **Passion fruit**		
Passion fruit, flesh and pips	918	14-178	50-933
Pasta sauce, carbonara type	1153	17-625	
Pasta sauce, four cheese	1154	17-624	
Pasta sauce, tomato based, for bolognese	1155	17-618	17-323
Pasta sauce, tomato based, napoletana	1156	17-619	
Pasta sauce, tomato based, reduced fat	1157	17-620	
Pasta sauce, tomato based, with added vegetables	1158	17-621	
Pasta with meat and tomato sauce, homemade	581	19-483	19-347
Pasta, egg, fresh, filled with cheese only, boiled in unsalted water	39	11-728	11-451
Pasta, egg, fresh, filled with meat, boiled in unsalted water	40	11-732	
Pasta, egg, fresh, raw	37	11-726	11-449
Pasta, ravioli, meat filling, canned in tomato sauce	41	11-736	11-621
Pasta, spaghetti, canned, in tomato sauce	42	11-735	11-357
Pasta, white, dried, raw	43	11-716	11-452
Pasta, white, spaghetti, dried, boiled in unsalted water	44	11-722	11-453
Pasta, white, tagliatelle, egg, fresh, boiled in unsalted water	38	11-727	
Pasta, white, twists/fusilli, dried, boiled in unsalted water	45	11-720	
Pasta, wholewheat, spaghetti, dried, boiled in unsalted water	47	11-723	11-455
Pasta, wholewheat, spaghetti, dried, raw	46	11-718	11-454
Pasties/slices, chicken/turkey, puff pastry	517	19-469	
Pastinaca sativa	See **Parsnip**		
Pastries, cream filled	178	11-843	11-654
Pastries, Danish	180	11-841	11-538
Pastries, Greek, Baklava	185	11-842	11-248
Pastry, filo, cooked	170	11-856	
Pastry, filo, uncooked	169	11-855	
Pastry, flaky/puff, cooked	172	11-854	
Pastry, flaky/puff, uncooked	171	11-852	11-224
Pastry, shortcrust, cooked, homemade	175	11-1052	11-585
Pastry, shortcrust, uncooked	173	11-851	11-227
Pastry, shortcrust, cooked	174	11-853	
Pastry, wholemeal, cooked, homemade	176	11-961	11-587

	Publication number	Current code	Previous code
Pasty, Cornish	520	19-466	
Pasty, vegetable, homemade	837	15-646	15-377
Pate, liver	526	19-317	
Pate, meat, reduced fat	527	19-145	
Pate, tuna	675	16-451	16-308
Pavlova, toffee/chocolate, no fruit	324	12-475	12-403
Pavlova, with fruit and cream	323	12-552	12-404
Paw-paw	See **Papaya**		
Peaches, canned in juice	921	14-188	50-940
Peaches, canned in syrup	922	14-189	50-941
Peaches, raw, flesh and skin	920	14-299	
Peanut (groundnut) oil	373	17-040	
Peanut butter, smooth	950	14-892	14-876
Peanuts and raisins	951	14-882	
Peanuts, dry roasted	953	14-878	50-989
Peanuts, plain	952	14-877	
Peanuts, roasted and salted	954	14-834	50-990
Pears, canned in juice	924	14-197	50-945
Pears, raw, flesh and skin	923	14-321	14-190
Peas, boiled in unsalted water	727	13-439	
Peas, canned, re-heated, drained	728	13-564	13-441
Peas, chick peas, canned, re-heated, drained	706	13-560	13-078
Peas, chick peas, whole, dried, boiled in unsalted water	705	13-430	
Peas, frozen, boiled in unsalted water	730	13-536	13-440
Peas, frozen, microwaved	731	13-528	
Peas, frozen, raw	729	13-527	
Peas, mange-tout, boiled in unsalted water	722	13-547	
Peas, mange-tout, raw	721	13-122	50-725
Peas, mange-tout, stir-fried in rapeseed oil	723	13-568	13-124
Peas, marrowfat, canned, re-heated, drained	724	13-562	13-125
Peas, mushy, canned, re-heated	725	13-563	13-437
Peas, raw	726	13-438	
Pecan nuts	955	14-837	
Peel, mixed	914	14-338	14-167
Penaeidae	See **Prawns** and **Prawns, king**		
Pepper, black	874	13-880	13-846

	Publication number	Current code	Previous code
Pepper, capsicum, red, boiled in unsalted water	790	13-525	13-321
Pepper, capsicum, red, raw	789	13-524	13-320
Pepper, capsicum, yellow, boiled in unsalted water	792	13-537	
Pepper, capsicum, yellow, raw	791	13-526	13-322
Pepper, white	875	13-881	13-848
Peppermints	1002	17-117	
Peppers, capsicum, chilli, green, raw	786	13-316	50-801
Peppers, capsicum, green, boiled in unsalted water	788	13-548	
Peppers, capsicum, green, raw	787	13-318	50-802
Persea americana	See **Avocado**		
Peshwari naan	55	11-910	
Pesto, green	1146	17-622	
Pesto, red	1147	17-623	
Petroselinum crispum	See **Parsley**		
Phaseolus coccineus	See **Runner beans**		
Phaseolus Lunatus	See **Butter beans**		
Phaseolus vulgaris	See **Baked beans** (navy beans), **Green beans** and **Red kidney beans**		
Phasianus colchicus	See **Pheasant**		
Pheasant, roasted, meat only	485	18-383	
Phoenix dactylifera	See **Dates**		
Phool gobhi	See **Cauliflower**		
Piccalilli	1127	17-702	17-347
Pickle, sweet	1128	17-718	17-352
Pickled onions, drained	782	13-309	50-797
Pie, apple, pastry, double crust	193	11-921	
Pie, beef, puff or shortcrust pastry, family size	508	18-505	
Pie, beef, puff or shortcrust pastry, individual	509	18-506	
Pie, chicken, individual, baked	512	19-515	19-055
Pie, Cottage/Shepherd's, reheated	569	19-494	19-216
Pie, fish, white fish	665	16-410	16-295
Pie, fruit, individual	197	11-847	11-547
Pie, fruit, one crust, homemade	198	11-1007	11-596
Pie, fruit, pastry top and bottom, homemade	199	11-1008	11-597
Pie, lemon meringue	200	11-548	
Pie, pork, individual	528	19-467	

	Publication number	Current code	Previous code
Pie, Shepherd's, vegetable	846	15-655	15-313
Pie, steak and kidney, single crust, homemade	539	19-557	19-329
Pie, vegetable, homemade	851	15-647	15-379
Pies, mince	188	11-848	
Pig, liver, stewed	496	18-418	
Pignolias	See **Pine nuts**		
Pilau rice, plain, homemade	19	11-968	11-561
Pilau, vegetable, homemade	838	12-472	
Pimento	See **Peppers, capsicum, chilli, green**		
Pine kernels	See **Pine nuts**		
Pine nuts	956	14-839	50-992
Pineapple juice, unsweetened	1063	14-286	
Pineapple, canned in juice	926	14-211	50-948
Pineapple, canned in syrup	927	14-212	50-949
Pineapple, raw, flesh only	925	14-208	50-947
Pinus edulis	See **Pine nuts**		
Pinus pinea	See **Pine nuts**		
Piper nigrum	See **Pepper, black** and **Pepper, white**		
Pista	See **Pistachio nuts**		
Pistachio nuts, roasted and salted	957	14-840	
Pistacia vera	See **Pistachio nuts**		
Pisum sativum	See **Peas**		
Pisum sativum var macrocarpon	See **Mange-tout peas**		
Pitta bread, white	56	11-974	11-465
Piyaz	See **Onions**		
Pizza base, raw	212	11-1016	11-552
Pizza, cheese and tomato, retail	213	11-936	11-553
Pizza, chicken topped, retail	214	11-1012	11-559
Pizza, fish topped, takeaway	215	11-1011	11-560
Pizza, ham and pineapple, retail	216	11-1013	11-558
Pizza, meat topped, retail and takeaway	217	11-1015	11-556
Pizza, vegetarian, retail and takeaway	218	11-1014	11-557
Plaice, baked	609	16-434	
Plaice, in breadcrumbs, baked	610	16-403	
Plaice, raw	608	16-381	16-102
Plain biscuits, reduced fat	130	11-801	
Plain chocolate	986	17-491	50-1016
Plain peanuts	952	14-877	
Plain scones	190	11-827	

	Publication number	Current code	Previous code
Plain scones, homemade	191	11-958	11-592
Plantain, boiled in unsalted water, flesh only	793	13-324	50-807
Plantain, ripe, fried in rapeseed oil	794	13-569	13-325
Pleuronectes platessa	See **Plaice**		
Plums, average, raw, flesh and skin	928	14-300	
Plums, average, stewed with sugar	929	14-314	14-215
Poached eggs, chicken, whole	339	12-943	12-810
Polenta, hydrated, raw	13	11-905	
Pollachius virens	See **Coley**		
Pollock, Alaskan, baked	612	16-436	
Pollock, Alaskan, raw	611	16-378	16-123
Pomegranate juice, drink	1064	14-341	14-288
Pomegranate, flesh and pips	930	14-226	
Popcorn, candied	1008	17-691	17-130
Popcorn, salted	1009	17-692	17-131
Pork casserole, made with cook-in sauce	582	19-536	19-348
Pork pie, individual	528	19-467	
Pork sausages, fried in vegetable oil	533	19-512	19-079
Pork sausages, grilled	534	19-509	19-080
Pork sausages, raw	532	19-510	19-318
Pork sausages, reduced fat, grilled	535	19-511	19-086
Pork scratchings	1010	17-132	
Pork spare ribs, 'barbecue style', reheated	583	19-262	
Pork, belly joint/slices, grilled, lean and fat	443	18-209	
Pork, diced, casseroled, lean only	444	18-482	
Pork, fat, average, cooked	441	18-205	
Pork, fat, average, raw	440	18-203	
Pork, fillet strips, stir-fried in corn oil, lean	445	18-228	
Pork, lean, average, raw	442	18-201	
Pork, leg joint, raw, lean and fat	446	18-483	
Pork, leg joint, roast, lean and fat	448	18-485	
Pork, leg joint, roast, lean only	447	18-484	
Pork, loin chops, barbecued, lean and fat	450	18-249	
Pork, loin chops, grilled, lean and fat	452	18-252	
Pork, loin chops, grilled, lean only	451	18-251	
Pork, loin chops, microwaved, lean and fat	453	18-254	
Pork, loin chops, raw, lean and fat	449	18-246	
Pork, loin chops, roasted, lean and fat	454	18-256	
Pork, steaks, grilled, lean and fat	456	18-286	

	Publication number	Current code	Previous code
Pork, steaks, grilled, lean only	455	18-285	
Pork, sweet and sour, homemade	590	19-485	19-349
Porridge oats, unfortified	107	11-788	11-017
Porridge oats, unfortified, cooked, made up with semi-skimmed milk	108	11-789	
Port	1088	17-234	
Pot savouries, made up	208	17-682	17-144
Potato crisps, fried in sunflower oil	1011	17-671	
Potato crisps, low fat	1012	17-693	17-496
Potato powder, instant, made up with water	693	13-558	13-032
Potato products, shaped, baked	694	13-533	13-425
Potato rings	1013	17-643	17-142
Potato salad, with mayonnaise	842	15-654	15-297
Potato snacks, pringle type, fried in vegetable oil	1014	17-642	
Potato wedges, retail, cooked	695	13-483	
Potatoes, new and salad, boiled in unsalted water, flesh and skin	676	13-495	13-420
Potatoes, old, baked, flesh and skin	679	13-491	13-010
Potatoes, old, boiled in unsalted water, flesh only	678	13-490	13-421
Potatoes, old, mashed with butter	681	13-553	13-481
Potatoes, old, mashed with reduced fat spread	682	13-554	
Potatoes, old, microwaved, flesh and skin	680	13-494	
Potatoes, old, raw, flesh only	677	13-489	13-009
Potatoes, old, roasted in rapeseed oil	683	13-534	
Potatoes, old, roasted in sunflower oil	684	13-492	
Potatoes, old, wedges with skin, homemade, cooked in rapeseed oil	685	13-493	
Potatoes, old, wedges with skin, homemade, cooked in sunflower oil	686	13-566	
Potatoes, sweet, boiled in unsalted water, flesh only	808	13-551	
Potatoes, sweet, raw, flesh only	807	13-463	
Prawn crackers, takeaway	207	11-1023	11-551
Prawn curry, takeaway	656	16-333	16-278
Prawns, cold-water	See **Prawns**		
Prawns, king, cooked	645	16-389	
Prawns, king, grilled from raw	644	16-388	
Prawns, king, raw	643	16-387	

	Publication number	Current code	Previous code
Prawns, standard, cooked	646	16-384	16-239
Prawns, warm-water	See **Prawns, king**		
Premium sausages, grilled	536	19-513	19-095
Pre-mixed spirit based drinks	1095	17-758	
Pringle type potato snack types, fried in vegetable oil	1014	17-642	
Processed cheese, plain	273	12-527	12-362
Processed cheese, slices, reduced fat	274	12-549	12-363
Profiteroles with sauce	325	12-405	
Prunes, canned in juice	931	14-237	50-955
Prunes, ready-to-eat	932	14-239	50-957
Prunus amygdalus	See **Almonds**		
Prunus armeniaca	See **Apricots**		
Prunus avium	See **Cherries**		
Prunus domestica	See **Prunes**		
Prunus domestica subsp domestica	See **Plums**		
Prunus dulcis	See **Almonds**		
Prunus persica	See **Peaches**		
Prunus persica var nectarina	See **Nectarines**		
Pudding, Christmas	194	11-1022	11-291
Pudding, sponge, canned	202	11-1021	11-549
Puffed wheat cereal, honey coated, fortified	110	11-757	11-503
Puffed wheat cereal, unfortified	109	11-756	11-144
Pumpkin seeds	958	14-842	
Pumpkin, boiled in unsalted water	795	13-549	
Punica granatum	See **Pomegranate**		
Puri	81	11-911	
Purple grenadillo	See **Passion fruit**		
Pyrus communis	See **Pears**		
Quarter pounder with cheese, takeaway	506	19-487	19-312
Queensland nuts	See **Macadamia nuts**		
Quiche Lorraine with shortcrust pastry	345	12-936	
Quiche, cheese and egg, homemade	343	12-948	12-923
Quiche, cheese and egg, wholemeal, homemade	344	11-995	12-924
Quiche, vegetable	839	12-949	
Quinoa, raw	14	14-843	
Quorn, pieces, as purchased	796	13-574	13-455
Rabbit, raw, meat only	486	18-387	

	Publication number	Current code	Previous code
Rabbit, stewed, meat only	487	18-388	
Radish, red, raw, flesh and skin	797	13-330	50-812
Rainbow trout, baked	637	16-396	
Rainbow trout, raw	636	16-395	16-225
Raisins	933	14-242	50-958
Rapeseed oil	374	17-041	
Raphanus sativus	See **Radish, red**		
Raspberries, raw	934	14-244	50-959
Ratatouille, homemade	840	15-659	15-571
Ravioli pasta, meat filling, canned in tomato sauce	41	11-736	11-621
Ready cooked rice, plain, re-heated	20	11-884	
Red cabbage, boiled in unsalted water	745	13-540	
Red kidney beans, canned, re-heated, drained	714	13-561	13-435
Red kidney beans, dried, boiled in unsalted water	713	13-110	50-717
Red kidney beans, dried, raw	712	13-109	50-716
Red Leicester	275	12-485	12-167
Red pepper, capsicum, boiled in unsalted water	790	13-525	13-321
Red pepper, capsicum, raw	789	13-524	13-320
Red wine	1082	17-752	17-228
Reduced fat biscuits, plain	130	11-801	
Reduced fat pasta sauce, tomato based	1157	17-620	
Relish, corn/cucumber/onion	1139	17-708	17-353
Relish, tomato based	1138	17-354	
Rheum rhaponticum	See **Rhubarb**		
Rhubarb, stewed with sugar	935	14-253	50-962
Ribes grossularia	See **Gooseberries**		
Ribes nigrum	See **Blackcurrants**		
Rice cakes	1015	17-633	11-618
Rice cereal, chocolate flavoured, fortified	112	11-753	11-488
Rice cereal, toasted/crisp, fortified	111	11-750	11-497
Rice noodles, fine, dried, boiled in unsalted water	36	11-725	
Rice pudding, canned	326	12-580	12-406
Rice pudding, canned, low fat	327	12-553	12-407
Rice pudding, made with semi-skimmed milk, homemade	328	12-514	
Rice salad, homemade	843	15-649	15-381

	Publication number	Current code	Previous code
Rice, brown, wholegrain, boiled in unsalted water	17	11-869	11-443
Rice, brown, wholegrain, raw	16	11-868	11-442
Rice, egg fried, ready cooked, re-heated	18	11-885	
Rice, pilau, plain, homemade	19	11-968	11-561
Rice, ready cooked, plain, re-heated	20	11-884	
Rice, savoury, dried, cooked	21	11-881	11-620
Rice, white, basmati, boiled in unsalted water	23	11-858	
Rice, white, basmati, easy cook, boiled in unsalted water	24	11-860	
Rice, white, basmati, raw	22	11-857	11-041
Rice, white, Italian Arborio risotto, boiled in unsalted water	26	11-879	
Rice, white, Italian Arborio risotto, raw	25	11-878	
Rice, white, long grain, boiled in unsalted water	28	11-862	11-050
Rice, white, long grain, easy cook, boiled in unsalted water	29	11-864	11-446
Rice, white, long grain, raw	27	11-861	11-049
Rice, wild, boiled in unsalted water	31	11-873	
Rice, wild, raw	30	11-872	
Ringana	See **Aubergine**		
Risotto rice, Italian Arborio, white, boiled in unsalted water	26	11-879	
Risotto rice, Italian Arborio, white, raw	25	11-878	
Risotto, plain, homemade	32	11-999	11-605
River cobbler	See **Pangasius**		
Roasted and salted peanuts	954	14-834	50-990
Rocket, raw	798	13-522	
Roquette	See **Rocket**		
Rose wine, medium	1083	17-754	17-229
Rosemary, dried	876	13-882	13-851
Rosmarinus officinalis	See **Rosemary**		
Rubus fruticosus	See **Blackberries**		
Rubus idaeus	See **Raspberries**		
Rucola	See **Rocket**		
Runner beans, boiled in unsalted water	716	13-114	50-720
Runner beans, raw	715	13-112	50-719
Rutabaga	See **Swede**		
Rye flour	6	11-897	11-436
Rye, crispbread	140	11-822	11-511

	Publication number	Current code	Previous code
Saag	See **Spinach**		
Sage and onion stuffing, homemade	210	11-1000	11-606
Saithe	See **Coley**		
Salad and new potatoes, boiled in unsalted water, flesh and skin	676	13-495	13-420
Salad cream	1129	17-703	17-512
Salad cream, reduced fat	1130	17-704	17-327
Salad, green	841	15-648	15-380
Salad, potato, with mayonnaise	842	15-654	15-297
Salad, rice, homemade	843	15-649	15-381
Salami	529	19-517	19-110
Salami snack	530	19-508	19-108
Salmon en croute	667	16-453	16-304
Salmon, farmed, baked	624	16-359	
Salmon, farmed, grilled	622	16-357	16-327
Salmon, farmed, raw	621	16-356	16-326
Salmon, farmed, steamed	623	16-358	16-205
Salmon, pink, canned in brine, drained	628	16-420	16-346
Salmon, red, canned in brine, drained	629	16-418	16-211
Salmon, red, skinless and boneless, canned in brine, drained	630	16-419	16-210
Salmon, smoked (cold-smoked)	626	16-412	16-207
Salmon, smoked (hot-smoked)	627	16-413	
Salmon, wild, raw	625	16-360	16-326
Salt	1168	17-367	
Samosas, meat, takeaway	525	19-326	
Samosas, vegetable	844	15-305	
Sandwich biscuits, cream	131	11-813	11-519
Sandwich, white bread, bacon, lettuce and tomato	83	11-955	11-563
Sandwich, white bread, cheddar cheese and pickle	84	11-963	11-564
Sandwich, white bread, chicken salad	85	11-964	11-565
Sandwich, white bread, egg mayonnaise	86	11-966	11-567
Sandwich, white bread, ham salad	87	11-965	11-566
Sandwich, white bread, tuna mayonnaise	88	11-967	11-568
Sardina pilchardus	See **Sardines**		
Sardines, canned in brine, drained	632	16-424	16-328
Sardines, canned in olive oil, drained	635	16-440	16-329
Sardines, canned in sunflower oil, drained	634	16-439	16-329

	Publication number	Current code	Previous code
Sardines, canned in tomato sauce, whole contents	633	16-422	16-217
Sardines, grilled	631	16-438	
Satay, chicken, takeaway	560	19-323	
Satsumas	See **Citrus fruit**		
Sauce, barbecue	1132	17-705	17-289
Sauce, bolognese (with meat), homemade	549	19-476	19-352
Sauce, bolognese (with meat), homemade, with extra lean minced beef	550	19-475	
Sauce, bolognese (with meat), reheated	551	19-542	19-328
Sauce, bread, homemade with semi-skimmed milk	1113	17-664	17-520
Sauce, brown	1133	17-706	17-293
Sauce, brown, reduced salt/sugar	1134	17-678	
Sauce, cheese, homemade with semi-skimmed milk	1114	17-665	17-522
Sauce, cheese, packet mix, made up with semi-skimmed milk	1115	17-666	17-524
Sauce, chilli	1135	17-719	17-294
Sauce, Chinese cook in, sweet & sour	1148	17-628	17-335
Sauce, Chinese, stir fry	1149	17-629	
Sauce, dry, casserole mix	1150	17-329	
Sauce, horseradish	1136	17-314	
Sauce, Indian cook in, korma/tikka masala	1151	17-626	17-298
Sauce, Indian cook in, other	1152	17-627	17-298
Sauce, mint	1137	17-707	17-319
Sauce, pasta, carbonara type	1153	17-625	
Sauce, pasta, four cheese	1154	17-624	
Sauce, pasta, tomato based, for bolognese	1155	17-618	17-323
Sauce, pasta, tomato based, napoletana	1156	17-619	
Sauce, pasta, tomato based, reduced fat	1157	17-620	
Sauce, pasta, tomato based, with added vegetables	1158	17-621	
Sauce, soy	1140	17-721	17-334
Sauce, sweet and sour, take-away	1141	17-336	
Sauce, tartare	1142	17-722	17-337
Sauce, traditional cook in, tomato based	1159	17-630	17-295
Sauce, traditional cook in, white sauce based	1160	17-631	17-295
Sauce, white, savoury, homemade with semi-skimmed milk	1116	17-667	17-528

	Publication number	Current code	Previous code
Sauce, Worcestershire	1144	17-723	17-340
Sauerkraut	845	13-336	
Sausage casserole, homemade	584	19-484	19-351
Sausage roll, flaky pastry, ready-to-eat	537	19-468	
Sausages, beef, grilled	531	19-489	19-077
Sausages, pork, fried in vegetable oil	533	19-512	19-079
Sausages, pork, grilled	534	19-509	19-080
Sausages, pork, raw	532	19-510	19-318
Sausages, pork, reduced fat, grilled	535	19-511	19-086
Sausages, premium, grilled	536	19-513	19-095
Sausages, vegetarian, baked/grilled	854	15-658	15-365
Savoury rice, dried, cooked	21	11-881	11-620
Scallion	See **Spring onions**		
Scampi, coated in breadcrumbs, baked	647	16-409	
Scampi, coated in breadcrumbs, fried in rapeseed oil	648	16-442	16-243
Scampi, coated in breadcrumbs, fried in sunflower oil	649	16-443	16-244
Scomber	See **Mackerel**		
Scones, fruit	189	11-993	11-543
Scones, plain	190	11-827	
Scones, plain, homemade	191	11-958	11-592
Scotch eggs	538	19-518	19-320
Scotch pancakes	192	11-544	
Scrambled eggs, chicken, with semi-skimmed milk	340	12-945	12-926
Sea bass, baked	613	16-386	
Seafood selection	668	16-454	16-306
Seafood sticks	669	16-415	16-273
Secale cereale	See **Rye**		
Seeded bread	57	11-947	
Seeds, coriander	861	13-875	13-819
Seeds, cumin	862	13-889	13-820
Seeds, pumpkin	958	14-842	
Seeds, sesame	959	14-844	50-944
Seeds, sunflower	960	14-845	50-955
Semi-skimmed milk, pasteurised, average	221	12-313	
Semi-skimmed milk, pasteurised, summer and autumn	222	12-418	
Semi-skimmed milk, pasteurised, winter and spring	223	12-419	

	Publication number	Current code	Previous code
Semi-skimmed milk, UHT	224	12-314	
Semi-sweet biscuits	132	11-797	11-521
Sesame oil	375	17-043	
Sesame prawn toast, takeaway	670	16-367	16-321
Sesame seeds	959	14-844	50-944
Sesamum indicum	See **Sesame seeds**		
Sevyian, homemade	201	11-915	11-676
Shakaria	See **Sweet potato**		
Shalgam	See **Turnip**		
Shandy, 50% lager	1076	17-760	17-218
Shandy, bottled or canned	1075	17-821	17-217
Sheeps milk, raw	240	12-329	
Shepherd's pie, vegetable	846	15-655	15-313
Sherbert sweets	1003	17-828	17-119
Sherry, medium	1089	17-236	
Shish kebab in pitta bread with salad	586	19-525	19-151
Shish kebab, meat only	585	19-150	
Short or sweet biscuits, half coated in chocolate	134	11-806	11-415
Short, sweet biscuits	133	11-796	11-522
Shortbread	144	11-802	11-523
Shortcake, caramel, chocolate covered	162	11-837	
Shortcrust pastry, cooked, homemade	175	11-1052	11-585
Shortcrust pastry, uncooked	173	11-851	11-227
Shortcrust pastry, cooked	174	11-853	
Shoulder, lamb	See **Lamb, shoulder**		
Shredded wheat type cereal with fruit, unfortified	114	11-777	50-079
Shredded wheat type cereal, unfortified	113	11-775	11-499
Simila mirch	See **Peppers, capsicum (green/red)**		
Sinapis alba	See **Mustard**		
Single cream, fresh	243	12-332	50-212
Skimmed milk, dried	232	12-521	12-030
Skimmed milk, pasteurised, average	225	12-307	
Skimmed milk, UHT	226	12-554	12-310
Smartie-type sweets	993	17-096	
Smoked haddock, poached	603	16-402	16-066
Smoked salmon (cold-smoked)	626	16-412	16-207
Smoked salmon (hot-smoked)	627	16-413	
Smoothies	1065	17-747	

	Publication number	Current code	Previous code
Snickers/Topic and own brand equivalents	994	17-670	17-549
Snowpeas	See **Mange-tout peas**		
Solanum lycopersicum	See **Tomatoes**		
Solanum tuberosum	See **Potatoes**		
Solanum melongena	See **Aubergine**		
Sorbet, fruit	310	12-393	
Soup, broccoli and stilton, carton, chilled	1096	17-637	
Soup, carrot and coriander, carton, chilled	1097	17-634	
Soup, chicken noodle, dried, as served	1098	17-714	17-254
Soup, chicken, cream of, canned	1099	17-695	17-250
Soup, chicken, cream of, canned, condensed	1100	17-696	17-251
Soup, chicken, cream of, canned, condensed, as served	1101	17-697	17-252
Soup, instant, dried, as served	1102	17-660	17-508
Soup, lentil, canned	1103	17-698	17-263
Soup, low calorie, canned	1104	17-699	17-265
Soup, minestrone, canned	1105	17-711	17-542
Soup, mushroom, carton, chilled	1106	17-635	
Soup, mushroom, cream of, canned	1107	17-713	17-270
Soup, oxtail, canned	1108	17-700	17-272
Soup, tomato, carton, chilled	1109	17-636	
Soup, tomato, cream of, canned	1110	17-652	17-278
Soup, vegetable, canned	1111	17-712	17-284
Soup, vegetable, homemade	1112	17-684	17-607
Sour-cream based dips	1119	17-299	
Sour-cream based dips, reduced fat	1120	17-677	
Soy sauce	1140	17-721	17-334
Soya beans, dried, boiled in unsalted water	718	13-116	50-722
Soya beans, dried, raw	717	13-115	50-721
Soya flour	7	11-898	11-025
Soya oil	376	17-044	
Soya yogurt, non-dairy alternative to yogurt, fruit, fortified	292	12-529	12-381
Soya, non-dairy alternative to milk, sweetened, fortified	241	12-523	12-330
Soya, non-dairy alternative to milk, unsweetened, fortified	242	12-524	12-331
Spaghetti bolognese, reheated, with spaghetti	587	19-524	19-353
Spaghetti, canned, in tomato sauce	42	11-735	11-357

	Publication number	Current code	Previous code
Spaghetti, white, dried, boiled in unsalted water	44	11-722	11-453
Spaghetti, wholewheat, dried, boiled in unsalted water	47	11-723	11-455
Spaghetti, wholewheat, dried, raw	46	11-718	11-454
Spare ribs, pork, 'barbecue style', reheated	583	19-262	
Spinach, baby, boiled in unsalted water	803	13-550	
Spinach, baby, raw	802	13-521	
Spinach, frozen, boiled in unsalted water	801	13-458	
Spinach, mature, boiled in unsalted water	800	13-573	13-457
Spinach, mature, raw	799	13-572	13-456
Spinacia oleracea	See **Spinach**		
Spirit based drinks, pre-mixed	1095	17-758	
Spirits, 40% volume	1094	17-247	
Sponge cake, fatless, homemade	164	11-957	11-581
Sponge cake, homemade	163	11-956	11-580
Sponge cake, soft iced	167	11-832	
Sponge cake, with dairy cream and jam	165	11-532	
Sponge cake, with jam and butter cream	166	11-831	
Sponge pudding, canned	202	11-1021	11-549
Spread, cheese, plain	258	12-540	12-349
Spread. cheese, reduced fat	259	12-537	12-350
Spreadable cheese, soft white, full fat	278	12-551	12-364
Spreadable cheese, soft white, low fat	276	12-541	12-366
Spreadable cheese, soft white, medium fat	277	12-538	12-365
Spring onions, bulbs and tops, raw	804	13-352	50-818
Spring rolls, meat, takeaway	588	19-327	
Squash, butternut, baked	805	13-356	
Steak and kidney pie, single crust, homemade	539	19-557	19-329
Steak, beef, rump	See **Beef, rump steak**		
Steak, beef, stewing	See **Beef, stewing steak**		
Steak, braising, braised, lean and fat	398	18-009	
Steak, braising, braised, lean only	397	18-008	
Steak, pork	See **Pork, steaks**		
Stew, beef, homemade	547	19-473	19-334
Stew, Irish, homemade	573	19-479	19-341
Stewed apples, cooking, stewed with sugar, flesh only	878	14-332	14-004

	Publication number	Current code	Previous code
Stewed apples, cooking, stewed without sugar, flesh only	879	14-320	14-005
Stewed blackberries, stewed without sugar	886	14-050	
Stewed blackcurrants, stewed without sugar	888	14-055	
Stewed gooseberries, cooking, stewed with sugar	899	14-101	50-896
Stewed plums, average, stewed with sugar	929	14-314	
Stewed rhubarb, stewed with sugar	935	14-253	50-962
Stewing lamb	See **Lamb, stewing**		
Stewing steak	See **Beef, stewing steak**		
Stilton, blue	279	12-367	50-249
Stir-fried beef, rump steak, strips, stir-fried in corn oil, lean	409	18-052	
Stir-fried lamb, neck fillet, strips, stir-fried in corn oil, lean only	434	18-164	
Stir-fried vegetables, takeaway	853	15-364	
Stir-fry mix, vegetable, fried in rapeseed oil	852	15-661	15-346
Stir-fry sauce, Chinese	1149	17-629	
Stir-fry vegetable curry, Thai, takeaway and restaurant	827	15-634	
Stock cubes, beef	1170	17-515	
Stock cubes, chicken	1171	17-726	17-369
Stock cubes, chicken, made up with water	1172	17-774	
Stock cubes, vegetable	1173	17-727	17-370
Stock gel	1174	17-680	
Stock, chicken, ready made	1169	17-681	
Stout, Guinness	1077	17-767	17-219
Strawberries, raw	936	14-324	14-260
Strawberry/banana flavoured milk, pasteurised	235	12-326	
Stuffing mix, dried, assorted flavours, made up	209	17-372	
Stuffing, sage and onion, homemade	210	11-1000	11-606
Suet, shredded	364	17-011	
Suet, vegetable, reduced fat	365	17-759	17-012
Sugar, brown	974	17-060	
Sugar, Demerara	975	17-061	50-1010
Sugar, white	976	17-063	
Sultanas	937	14-263	50-969

	Publication number	Current code	Previous code
Sunflower oil	377	17-045	
Sunflower seeds	960	14-845	50-995
Sus scrofa	See **Pork**		
Sushi, salmon nigiri	671	16-361	
Sushi, tuna nigiri	672	16-362	
Sushi, vegetable	847	15-617	
Swede, boiled in unsalted water, flesh only	806	13-361	50-820
Sweet and sour chicken, takeaway	589	19-324	
Sweet and sour pork, homemade	590	19-485	19-349
Sweet and sour sauce, Chinese cook in	1148	17-628	17-335
Sweet and sour sauce, take-away	1141	17-336	
Sweet basil	See **Basil**		
Sweet peppers	See **Peppers, capsicum (green/red)**		
Sweet pickle	1128	17-718	17-352
Sweet potato, boiled in unsalted water, flesh only	808	13-551	
Sweet potato, raw, flesh only	807	13-463	
Sweetcorn, baby, fresh and frozen, boiled in unsalted water	809	13-552	
Sweetcorn, kernels, boiled 'on the cob' in unsalted water	811	13-508	13-370
Sweetcorn, kernels, canned in water, drained	810	13-529	13-459
Sweets, boiled	995	17-101	
Sweets, chew	996	17-647	17-104
Sweets, sherbert	1003	17-828	17-119
Sweets, Smartie-type	993	17-096	
Swiss rolls, chocolate covered and filled	168	11-834	11-533
Syrup, golden	977	17-065	
Szechuan prawns with vegetables, takeaway	673	16-335	
Tagliatelle pasta, white, egg, fresh, boiled in unsalted water	38	11-727	
Tahini paste	961	14-847	50-996
Tandoori, chicken, reheated	561	19-540	19-127
Tangerines	See **Citrus fruit**		
Taramasalata	674	16-449	16-307
Tarel	See **Apples**		
Tartare sauce	1142	17-722	17-337
Tarts, bakewell, iced	177	11-845	11-426
Tarts, custard, individual	179	12-461	11-537

	Publication number	Current code	Previous code
Tarts, jam	187	11-846	11-540
Tea bush	See **Basil**		
Tea, black, infusion, average	1035	17-165	
Tea, green, infusion	1036	17-171	
Tea, herbal, infusion	1037	17-172	
Theragra chalcogramma	See **Pollock, Alaskan**		
Thousand island dressing	1124	17-717	17-306
Thunnus	See **Tuna**		
Thyme, dried, ground	877	13-883	13-860
Thymus vulgaris	See **Thyme**		
Tikka masala, chicken, reheated	562	19-296	19-325
Til	See **Sesame seeds**		
Tiramisu	331	12-476	
Toffees, mixed	1004	17-646	17-120
Tofu, soya bean, steamed	719	13-570	13-119
Tofu, soya bean, steamed, fried	720	13-571	13-120
Tomato based cook in sauce, traditional	1159	17-630	17-295
Tomato based pasta sauce, for bolognese	1155	17-618	17-323
Tomato based pasta sauce, napoletana	1156	17-619	
Tomato based pasta sauce, reduced fat	1157	17-620	
Tomato based pasta sauce, with added vegetables	1158	17-621	
Tomato chutney	1118	17-345	
Tomato juice	1066	13-382	50-1093
Tomato ketchup	1143	17-709	17-513
Tomato puree	1175	13-531	17-516
Tomato soup, carton, chilled	1109	17-636	
Tomato soup, cream of, canned	1110	17-652	17-278
Tomatoes, canned, whole contents	815	13-530	13-461
Tomatoes, cherry, raw	814	13-519	13-388
Tomatoes, standard, grilled, flesh and seeds only	813	13-518	13-467
Tomatoes, standard, raw	812	13-517	13-460
Tonic water	1045	17-736	17-184
Topic/Snickers and own brand equivalents	994	17-670	17-549
Topside, beef, roasted medium-rare, lean and fat	415	18-089	
Topside, beef, roasted medium-rare, lean only	414	18-088	
Torte, fruit	329	12-408	
Tortilla chips fried in sunflower oil	1016	17-644	17-497

	Publication number	Current code	Previous code
Tortilla, wheat, soft	82	11-925	11-632
Trail mix	962	14-849	50-1041
Treacle, black	978	17-826	17-068
Trifle, fruit	330	12-409	
Triticum aestivum	See **Wheat**		
Trout, rainbow, baked	637	16-396	
Trout, rainbow, raw	636	16-395	16-225
Tuna mayonnaise sandwich, white bread	88	11-967	11-568
Tuna pate	675	16-451	16-308
Tuna, baked	638	16-400	
Tuna, canned in brine, drained	639	16-416	16-339
Tuna, canned in sunflower oil, drained	640	16-417	16-230
Turkey slices	540	19-543	19-157
Turkey, breast, fillet, grilled, meat only	476	18-356	
Turkey, breast, strips, stir-fried in corn oil	477	18-357	
Turkey, dark meat, raw	470	18-348	
Turkey, dark meat, roasted	471	18-358	
Turkey, light meat, raw	472	18-349	
Turkey, light meat, roasted	473	18-359	
Turkey, meat, average, raw	474	18-350	
Turkey, meat, average, roasted	475	18-361	
Turkey, skin, dry, roasted	478	18-362	
Turkey, thighs, diced, casseroled, meat only	479	18-355	
Turkish delight, without nuts	1005	17-122	
Turnip, boiled in unsalted water	816	13-391	50-834
Twiglets	1017	17-694	17-150
Tzatziki, homemade	1131	12-547	12-410
UHT cream, dairy, canned spray, 85% cream	250	12-338	
UHT cream, dairy, half fat, canned spray	251	12-339	
UHT milk, semi-skimmed	224	12-314	
UHT milk, skimmed	226	12-554	12-310
UHT milk, whole	230	12-599	12-320
Vaccinium corymbosum	See **Blueberries**		
Vaccinium darrowii	See **Blueberries**		
Vaccinium spp	See **Blueberries**		
Vatana	See **Peas**		
Veal, escalope, fried in corn oil	416	18-487	
Vegeburger, grilled	848	15-656	15-331

	Publication number	Current code	Previous code
Vegetable and cheese grill/burger, in crumbs, baked/grilled	849	15-657	15-363
Vegetable bake, homemade	850	15-650	15-382
Vegetable casserole, homemade	820	15-638	15-368
Vegetable chilli, homemade	823	15-640	15-370
Vegetable curry, ready meal, cooked	828	15-619	
Vegetable lasagne	830	15-651	15-189
Vegetable moussaka	833	15-652	15-206
Vegetable oil, average	378	17-686	17-489
Vegetable pakora/bhajia	835	15-653	15-232
Vegetable pasty, homemade	837	15-646	15-377
Vegetable pie, homemade	851	15-647	15-379
Vegetable pilau, homemade	838	12-472	
Vegetable quiche	839	12-949	
Vegetable samosas	844	15-305	
Vegetable Shepherd's pie	846	15-655	15-313
Vegetable soup, canned	1111	17-712	17-284
Vegetable soup, homemade	1112	17-684	17-607
Vegetable stir-fry mix, fried in rapeseed oil	852	15-661	15-346
Vegetable stock cubes	1173	17-727	17-370
Vegetable sushi	847	15-617	
Vegetables, mixed, cooked with onion, spice and tomatoes, homemade	832	15-621	
Vegetables, mixed, frozen, boiled in unsalted water	771	13-543	13-281
Vegetables, stir-fried, takeaway	853	15-364	
Vegetarian pizza, retail and takeaway	218	11-1014	11-557
Vegetarian sausages, baked/grilled	854	15-658	15-365
Venison, roasted	488	18-491	
Vermouth, dry	1090	17-239	
Vicia faba	See **Broad beans**		
Vigna radiata	See **Beansprouts, mung** and **Mung beans**		
Vigna unguiculata	See **Blackeye beans**		
Vinegar	1176	17-339	
Vitis vinifera	See **Grapes, Raisins** and **Sultanas**		
Wafers, plain ice cream wafers, not filled	145	11-800	12-212
Walnut oil	379	17-047	
Walnuts	963	14-879	
Water, distilled	1177	17-377	
Watercress, raw	817	13-462	

	Publication number	Current code	Previous code
Watermelon, flesh only	913	14-296	
Weetabix type cereal, wheat biscuits, fortifed	116	11-773	11-505
Weetabix type cereal, wheat biscuits, unfortified	117	11-774	
Wensleydale	280	12-489	12-182
Wheat and multigrain cereal, chocolate flavoured, fortified	115	11-762	50-092
Wheat biscuits, Weetabix type, fortifed	116	11-773	11-505
Wheat biscuits, Weetabix type, unfortified	117	11-774	
Wheat flour, bread/strong, white	9	11-887	11-438
Wheat flour, brown	8	11-892	11-437
Wheat flour, white, plain, soft	10	11-886	11-439
Wheat flour, white, self raising	11	11-888	11-440
Wheat flour, wholemeal	12	11-889	11-441
Wheat tortilla, soft	82	11-925	11-632
Wheat, bran	1	11-906	11-005
Wheatgerm	15	11-907	11-622
Wheatgerm bread	58	11-975	11-467
Whipping cream, fresh	244	12-333	50-214
White bread rolls, crusty	71	11-985	11-482
White bread rolls, soft	72	11-1006	11-483
White bread, Danish style	59	11-976	11-466
White bread, farmhouse or split tin	60	11-977	11-470
White bread, French stick	61	11-978	11-471
White bread, premium	62	11-979	11-474
White bread, sliced	63	11-980	11-468
White bread, sliced, toasted	64	11-1001	11-475
White bread, 'with added fibre'	65	11-1003	11-472
White bread, 'with added fibre', toasted	66	11-1004	11-473
White cabbage, raw	746	13-509	13-445
White chocolate	987	17-091	50-1017
White pasta, dried, raw	43	11-716	11-452
White pasta, spaghetti, dried, boiled in unsalted water	44	11-722	11-453
White pasta, tagliatelle, egg, fresh, boiled in unsalted water	38	11-727	
White pasta, twists/fusilli, dried, boiled in unsalted water	45	11-720	
White pepper	875	13-881	13-848
White pitta bread	56	11-974	11-465

	Publication number	Current code	Previous code
White rice, basmati, boiled in unsalted water	23	11-858	
White rice, basmati, easy cook, boiled in unsalted water	24	11-860	
White rice, basmati, raw	22	11-857	11-041
White rice, Italian Arborio risotto, boiled in unsalted water	26	11-879	
White rice, Italian Arborio risotto, raw	25	11-878	
White rice, long grain, boiled in unsalted water	28	11-862	11-050
White rice, long grain, easy cook, boiled in unsalted water	29	11-864	11-446
White rice, long grain, raw	27	11-861	11-049
White sauce based cook in sauce, traditional	1160	17-631	17-295
White sauce, savoury, homemade with semi-skimmed milk	1116	17-667	17-528
White sugar	976	17-063	
White wine, dry	1084	17-755	17-230
White wine, medium	1085	17-756	17-231
White wine, sparkling	1086	17-757	17-232
White wine, sweet	1087	17-233	
Whitener powder, Coffeemate	1024	12-546	12-027
Whole milk yogurt, fruit	293	12-375	
Whole milk yogurt, infant, fruit flavour	294	12-530	12-378
Whole milk yogurt, plain	295	12-184	
Whole milk yogurt, twin pot, not fruit	296	12-515	
Whole milk yogurt, twin pot, thick and creamy with fruit	297	12-531	12-374
Whole milk, Channel Islands, pasteurised	219	12-321	
Whole milk, evaporated	233	12-522	12-033
Whole milk, pasteurised, average	227	12-596	12-316
Whole milk, pasteurised, summer and autumn	228	12-598	12-317
Whole milk, pasteurised, winter and spring	229	12-597	12-318
Whole milk, UHT	230	12-599	12-320
Wholegrain mustard	1167	17-365	
Wholemeal bread rolls	73	11-986	11-484
Wholemeal bread, average	67	11-981	11-476
Wholemeal bread, toasted	68	11-982	11-611
Wholemeal pastry, cooked, homemade	176	11-961	11-587
Wholewheat pasta, spaghetti, dried, boiled in unsalted water	47	11-723	11-455

	Publication number	Current code	Previous code
Wholewheat pasta, spaghetti, dried, raw	46	11-718	11-454
Whopper burger, takeaway	507	19-514	19-313
Wild rice, boiled in unsalted water	31	11-873	
Wild rice, raw	30	11-872	
Wine, red	1082	17-752	17-228
Wine, rose, medium	1083	17-754	17-229
Wine, white, dry	1084	17-755	17-230
Wine, white, medium	1085	17-756	17-231
Wine, white, sparkling	1086	17-757	17-232
Wine, white, sweet	1087	17-233	
Witloof	See **Chicory**		
Worcestershire sauce	1144	17-723	17-340
Yam (USA)	See **Sweet potato**		
Yam, boiled in unsalted water, flesh only	818	13-400	50-837
Yeast extract	1178	17-753	17-517
Yeast, bakers, compressed	1179	17-378	
Yeast, dried	1180	17-379	50-1188
Yellow gram	See **Chick peas**		
Yellow pepper, capsicum, boiled in unsalted water	792	13-537	
Yellow pepper, capsicum, raw	791	13-526	13-322
Yellow turnip	See **Swede**		
Yogurt, Greek style, fruit	286	12-377	
Yogurt, Greek style, plain	287	12-555	12-376
Yogurt, low fat, fruit	288	12-380	
Yogurt, low fat, hazelnut	289	12-904	
Yogurt, low fat, plain	290	12-379	
Yogurt, low fat, toffee	291	12-905	
Yogurt, soya, non-dairy alternative to yogurt, fruit, fortified	292	12-529	12-381
Yogurt, virtually fat free/diet, fruit	298	12-532	12-382
Yogurt, virtually fat free/diet, plain	299	12-533	12-383
Yogurt, whole milk, fruit	293	12-375	
Yogurt, whole milk, infant, fruit flavour	294	12-530	12-378
Yogurt, whole milk, plain	295	12-184	
Yogurt, whole milk, twin pot, not fruit	296	12-515	
Yogurt, whole milk, twin pot, thick and creamy with fruit	297	12-531	12-374
Yorkshire pudding, made with semi-skimmed milk, homemade	211	11-960	
Zea mays	See **Sweetcorn**		

	Publication number	Current code	Previous code
Zingiber officinale	See **Ginger**		
Zucchini	See **Courgette**